Handbook of Perception and Action

Volume 1: Perception

Handbook of Perception and Action

Volume 1: Perception

Edited by

Wolfgang Prinz[1] and Bruce Bridgeman[2]

[1]*Department of Psychology, University of Munich, Germany*
Max Planck Institute for Psychological Research, Munich, Germany

[2]*Program in Experimental Psychology, University of California, Santa Cruz, USA*

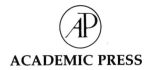

ACADEMIC PRESS

Harcourt Brace & Company, Publishers

London, San Diego, New York, Boston, Sydney, Tokyo, Toronto

ACADEMIC PRESS LIMITED
24–28 Oval Road
LONDON NW1 7DX

U.S. Edition Published by
ACADEMIC PRESS INC.
San Diego, CA 92101

This book is printed on acid-free paper

The German original is published under the title "Wahrnehmung"
as volume 1 of the "Enzyklopädie der Psychologie".
Copyright © 1994 by Hogrefe-Verlag
Rohnsweg 25, 37085 Göttingen, Germany

A catalogue record for this book is available from the British Library

ISBN 0 12 516161 1

Typeset by Doyle Graphics, Tullamore, Co. Offaly, Republic of Ireland
Printed and bound in Great Britain by Hartnolls Ltd, Bodmin, Cornwall

Contents

I Basic Processes and Mechanisms

II Perception of Objects, Events and Actions

List of Contributors

Bruce Bridgeman
Program in Experimental Psychology
University of California
Santa Cruz, CA 95064
USA

Heiner Deubel
Max Planck Institute
for Psychological Research
Leopoldstr. 24
D-80802 Munich
Germany

Diana Deutsch
Department of Psychology
University of California
San Diego, La Jolla, CA 92093
USA

Martin Eimer
Department of Psychology
University of Munich
Leopoldstr. 13
D-80802 Munich
Germany

Oded M. Flascher
Department of Psychology
Center for the Ecological Study
of Perception and Action
University of Connecticut
Storrs, CT 06269-1020
USA

Joachim Hoffmann
Lehrstuhl für Psychologie III
Universität Würzburg
Röntgemring 11
D-97070 Würzburg
Germany

Bernhard Hommel
Max Planck Institute
for Psychological Research
Leopoldstr. 24
D-80802 Munich
Germany

Lothar Kehrer
Department of Psychology
University of Bielefeld
Postfach 100131
D-33501 Bielefeld
Germany

William M. Mace
Department of Psychology
Trinity College
Hartford, CT 06106
USA

Cristina Meinecke
Department of Psychology
University of Munich
Leopoldstr. 13
D-80802 Munich
Germany

Aaron L. Peters
Department of Psychology
Texas A & M University
College Station, TX 77843
USA

Wolfgang Prinz
[1]Department of Psychology
University of Munich
Leopoldstr. 13
D-80802 Munich
Germany

[2]Max Planck Institute
for Psychological Research
Leopoldstr. 24
D-80802 Munich
Germany

Adam Reeves
Department of Psychology
Northeastern University
360 Huntington Avenue
Boston, MA 02115
USA

Robert E. Shaw
Department of Psychology
Center for the Ecological Study
of Perception and Action
University of Connecticut
Storrs, CT 06269-1020
USA

Wayne L. Shebilske
Department of Psychology
Texas A & M University
College Station, TX 77843
USA

Werner X. Schneider
Department of Experimental Psychology
Ludwig-Maximilians-University
Leopoldstr. 13
D-80802 Munich
Germany

Jürgen Stränger
Faculty of Psychology
Ruhr University, Bochum
Universitätsstr. 150
D-44801 Bochum
Germany

Preface

The idea of editing a *Handbook of Perception and Action* as a three-volume set evolved at the end of a study year on *Perception and Action* at the Center for Interdisciplinary Studies (ZiF) in Bielefeld, Germany, which was held in 1984/85. During the course of the year, scholars from various disciplines met at the Center in order to explore how the mechanisms and processes involved in generating representations of the world are related to the mechanisms and processes involved in generating action. At the end of the project some of us felt that it might be worthwhile pursuing the issue further, in a systematic way, and we decided to embark on assembling a *Handbook of Perception and Action* that, in addition to giving overviews of the state of the art in these two areas of study, also stresses the functional relationships between them. From the outset we distinctly felt that this goal was impossible to achieve without including the field of attention as a third area of study.

Now, as they have been published, the volumes look back on a long and complex history. Two categories of people are involved in this history: the visible and the nonvisible ones. Authors and editors are the visible ones.

As to the invisible persons, this volume has received substantial support from a number of individuals and it would certainly never have reached its final shape without their help. In fact, some of our colleagues in Munich virtually served as associate editors in processing the manuscripts. This applies first and foremost to Martin Eimer, but also to Heiner Deubel, Bernhard Hommel, Cristina Meinecke, Werner X. Schneider and Stefan Vogt. They were involved, in one way or another, in various stages of the editorial procedure, starting from reviewing first drafts through checking final versions of chapter translations and producing the index. Thanks are due to Jonathan Harrow who translated the German manuscripts most proficiently. Finally, we are very much obliged to Heidi John, the most important invisible person in the enterprise, for doing all the secretarial work.

Wolfgang Prinz and Bruce Bridgeman
Munich, Germany and Santa Cruz, USA
December 1992

Introduction

Wolfgang Prinz* and Bruce Bridgeman[†]

*University of Munich and †University of California, Santa Cruz

1 DIVERSITY AND UNITY

'Perception is a rich, diverse and difficult field.' This assertion, which opens the Preface to the first volume of Carterette's and Friedman's enormous *Handbook of Perception* (Carterette and Friedman, 1974, p. xv) is even more true today than when it was made 20 years ago. Yet, at the same time, this statement was simply true in the early 1970s; in the 1990s it certainly understates the issue. Over the last 20 years the field has become even richer, more diverse and, hence, more difficult.

In some ways, though, theoretical advances have helped to simplify and organize the flood of data. For example, differentiation of cognitive (symbolic) and sensorimotor-oriented visual systems has resolved apparent contradictions among studies of spatial orientation by vision (Bridgeman, 1991; Paillard, 1987). From a more physiological point of view, the separation of visual information into magnocellular and parvocellular pathways has helped to organize the understanding of the psychophysical interactions of color, form and motion.

The field's diversity can be traced back to its creation in the nineteenth century when scientists like Helmholtz, Hering and Fechner started to discuss, in the light of new scientific observations, the old epistemological problem of the way in which our knowledge about the world relates to the world itself. These observations came from studies in sensory physiology which, at that time, mainly relied on 'subjective methods', i.e. on an analysis of sensory experience under controlled conditions. As the field was thus created in a liaison between philosophy and physiology the diversity entailed with this parenthood is hardly surprising. One of the philosophical burdens of the field has always been to understand the implications of our growing knowledge of perceptual functioning for basic epistemological issues (like the realism versus constructivism debate). Another, perhaps more serious burden is that the area of perception has become one of the main battlefields for metaphysical controversies about the relationship between physical and mental events (such as the monism versus dualism debate).

This issue is closely related to the main burden that the field has inherited from physiology. From the neurophysiological perspective it is obvious that

Handbook of Perception and Action: Volume 1
ISBN 0-12-516161-1

the psychological analysis of perceptual awareness cannot be isolated from the physiological analysis of the functions of the sense organs and the brain systems involved. The attempt to understand this relationship forms the empirical counterpart of the metaphysical mind–body problem.

Over the last 20 years the field's richness and diversity has increased still more. First, as far as richness is concerned, there has been an enormous growth of knowledge about the coding of sensory information in the brain. Two important results (among many others) stand out: first, the brain operates on the principle of multiple coding of sensory information, and that it is the activity of large cell assemblies (rather than of single units) that forms the functional basis of this coding. Second, as far as diversity is concerned, the last two decades have seen the emergence of new theoretical tools for the analysis of perceptual functioning. These tools refer to the algorithmic analysis of basic perceptual achievements and to the implementation of such algorithms in connectionist networks, i.e. in artificial systems that mirror some functional characteristics of human and animal brains. At first glance this development adds another subdiscipline to the already existing diversity of the field. It might turn out, however, that these algorithmic models could, at the same time, provide a theoretical language which is neutral in the sense that it could bridge the gap between the physical language for the description of brain events and the mental language for the description of mind events – and thereby contribute to reducing diversity.

How could the scope of the field of perception be delineated? As has already been pointed out by Attneave (1962), it is not easy to give a satisfactory and theoretically neutral definition of perception. Instead of defining perception proper Attneave offers a crude operational definition of what counts as a study of perception: 'Perception has to do with the input side of the organism, with certain short-term consequences... of variations in stimulating conditions' (1962, p. 620). The wisdom of this definition lies in the fact that it leaves entirely open the nature of these short-term consequences, thereby allowing such diverse measures as psychophysical judgements, phenomenal reports, single-unit recordings, brain images or even movements and actions. The only thing that it does specify is the scientist's manipulative control over the stimulating conditions and his/her concern about their short-term effects. This is perhaps the sole viable way of creating at least some unity in the diversity of the field: by specifying the proper manner of its study.

2   THEORETICAL ATTITUDES

Within the framework provided by Attneave's formula one can still distinguish a few theoretical approaches that differ in various respects. One way to describe them is to give a historical account of which approaches were developed and how they emerged (see, for example, Hochberg, 1992; Prinz, 1990a, b). Another way is to give a more systematic account in terms of some basic theoretical attitudes. For the present purpose four such attitudes may help to structure the theoretical landscape. They differ in the way they define the field and the proper way of studying it.

2.1 Experience/Performance

This distinction refers to the nature of short-term consequences of stimulation. More traditional approaches to perception, such as Gestalt psychology, have always stressed perceptual experience as the critical output of perceptual functioning. This is particularly obvious in Koffka's famous question: 'Why do things look as they do?' (Koffka, 1935). According to this question the field's main goal is to explain the nature of perceptual experiences arising under various conditions of stimulation. The same applies to Metzger who, in the very first sentence of his editorial introduction to the Perception volume of the *Handbuch der Psychologie,* simply stated that the study of perception (*Wahrnehmungslehre*) forms part of the study of conscious awareness (*Bewußtseinslehre*) (Metzger, 1966, p. 3). Again, the same applies to all brands of psychophysics where perceptual experience is explored and measured as a function of controlled stimulation.

Yet analysis of experience is not the only game in town. The organism's performance in terms of its coordinated movements and goal-directed actions forms another type of short-term consequence of stimulation that can be explored as a source for understanding perceptual functioning. This approach is not only characteristic of the motor control domain (where it is prevalent by definition), rather, it is also broadly used in perceptual studies, sometimes explicitly as part of a research program (such as the ecological approach to perception; see, for example, Gibson, 1950, 1966, 1979; Turvey and Kugler, 1984), sometimes more implicitly as part of the standard research routines in experimental studies (those that use time- and error-dependent performance measures such as reaction times, search times, percent-correct, etc. as dependent variables in a variety of perceptual tasks). All of these studies are concerned with the perceptual control of performance and not with perceptual experience.

It is, of course, also widespread use to take performance as an indicator of experience. We believe, for example, that the subject presses her response key (performance) at the very moment when she has attained a certain state of perceptual knowledge (experience), or that she reaches for an object at a certain location (performance) because she has seen it there (experience). Yet we cannot be sure how valid this folk-psychology type of reasoning is. There are also clear dissociations between experience and performance that should warn us to take the distinction more seriously and not simply reduce one to the other (see Chapter 6).

2.2 Transformation/Interaction

This distinction refers to the types of input information that are taken into consideration and are included in the theoretical approach. The transformational approach concentrates on stimulus information as the critical input for perception whereas the interactional approach considers both stimulus information and information stored in memory.

In the transformational framework, perceptual processes are regarded as a chain of more or less complex transformations of the input information delivered by the stimulus. What is to be explained are the properties of the output (experience or performance) as far as they can be derived from and related to corresponding properties of the stimulation. The leading question is: What is the nature of these transformations, how can they be described and which models are needed to account for them? Within the general transformational framework a variety of approaches has been developed. Some of them stress single, isolated stimulus dimensions and corresponding dimensions of experience (like traditional psycho-physics), whereas others stress more complex patterns of stimulation and their percepts (like the Gestalt approach and more recent algorithmic models). The common defining feature of transformational approaches is that the information delivered by the stimulation is considered the sole source of information that enters into the generation of the output.

In contrast, interactional approaches consider two such sources of information. Interactional approaches study how information derived from the stimulation interacts with information stored in memory and how the output depends on this interaction. When one adopts this view one can account not only for those aspects of the output that 'mirror', as it were, corresponding properties of the stimulation, but also for aspects that go beyond the information given and refer to the meaning of perceived objects and events. Though it may be trivial to posit this in such general terms, the explicit introduction of this view was initially felt to represent a 'New Look' at perception by the majority of researchers in the field who, at that time (i.e. in the early 1950s), were still strong believers in the transformational approach. If one broadens the scope of the study of perception to encompass the attainment of meaning and knowledge, one also has to broaden the theoretical framework of explanation. One of the core theoretical problems of the interactional approach is how information derived from stimulation can interact with informa-tion stored in memory. Again, this question can be attacked from either side: How does a given stimulus find access to appropriate memory structures (perceptual recognition, identification, etc.) and how does a given state of the memory system affect the analysis of stimulus information (selective attention, attentional tuning of perception, etc.)?

2.3   Processing/Discovery

This distinction refers to the goal of scientific inquiry in the field. Characteristic of mainstream research in perception is the processing type of theoretical attitude. The basic idea is that, in order to yield the desired output, the input information inherent in the stimulus always has to be processed according to certain rules or principles – either in the transformational or in the interactional sense. The history of perception has seen a variety of concepts that stand for a variety of different views of the nature of such processing, such as unconscious inference, organiza-tional laws, algorithmic computation and production rules.

Although these conceptual metaphors differ deeply in the nature of the assumed operations and mechanisms, they share the assumption that more or less complex operations are needed in order to compute the desired output variables on the basis of the given input variables. With this type of approach the output cannot be directly picked up from the input. This is exactly what the discovery type of attitude claims. According to this approach, the problem that perceptual systems have to solve is not to process the stimulus in a way suitable for the output but rather to discover in the stimulus the information that leads to the desired output in a direct way, i.e. without any further processing. The pickup perspective sees the stimulus as a potentially rich source of information and believes that the ecologically relevant information does not reside in its basic physical dimensions but in higher-order invariants of stimulation instead. From this viewpoint processing-oriented approaches are criticized for starting from a misconceived notion of the stimulus. The true functional stimulus is not an impoverished bundle of elementary physical properties that then becomes enriched through processing. Rather, stimulation is regarded as inherently rich and is believed to contain a vast amount of potentially relevant information. Hence, there is no need for complex processing of simple information. Instead, perception relies on simple discovery of complex information.

There is another way to interpret the direct pickup approach to perception, as championed by Gibson. In his conception, the directness of perception refers neither to internal processing nor the lack of it—that is not his concern. Rather, direct perception means that it is the surfaces and objects of the world along with their transformations that are perceived, not any intermediate physiological stages. These intermediates, whatever they may be, simply do not enter into the Gibsonian analysis because they are not perceived. The starting point for human experience is the surfaces and objects that make up the perceptual world, and it is here according to Gibson that the study of perception must start also.

Independent of these two interpretations of the notion of directness, some researchers tend to relate the distinction between discovery and processing to the epistemological distinction between realism and idealism (or constructivism). However, it seems to us that equating these two distinctions is far from compelling. While the epistemological distinction refers to the relationship between properties of the world and properties of our knowledge about the world, the psychological distinction refers to the nature and the complexity of the operations that relate these two classes of properties to each other. Although these two distinctions may be correlated, one does not follow from the other by necessity.

2.4   In–out/out–in

This distinction refers to the preferred direction of inquiry (cf. Prinz, 1990a). In in–out approaches the basic question is which output (e.g. which experience and/or which performance) is produced under given stimulus conditions. In out–in approaches the direction of inquiry is reversed, the basic research question being which input variables contribute to a given output. The in–out mode represents the traditional type of approach, such as in psychophysics. It starts with a description of the stimulus input (usually in terms of its basic physical dimensions) and ends up with an analysis of those aspects of the output that can be accounted for in terms of the input dimensions. Conversely, in the out–in mode output variables are considered first, and only then does one start to look for pertinent aspects of the input—pertinent in the sense that they account for some aspects of the output.

The history of the field has so far seen two major shifts in emphasis from the in–out to the out–in direction which has now become the standard approach to the study of perception. The first of them was Gestalt psychology which claimed that in order to achieve a functionally adequate description of stimulation one has to start from a thorough analysis of perceptual experience. This analysis can then guide the search for both a suitable description of the stimulation and the laws that mediate between stimulation and experience. The second of them was Gibson who, in the core of his theoretical program, claimed that the main task of perceptual research is to detect functionally adequate ways of describing the stimulation. According to this approach an adequate description must capture those abstract properties (or invariants) of the stimulation that specify a given output (experience and/or performance) in a direct way, such that, in order to achieve that output, it need only be picked up (cf. Gibson, 1966, 1979).

The common conviction in these two claims seems to be that the out–in mode is more suitable than the in–out mode to guide us in the search for a functionally adequate description of the stimulation. This conviction has since been shared by the majority of researchers in the field.

3   ORGANIZATION OF THIS VOLUME

This brief outline of the theoretical landscape can serve as a background against which the chapters of this volume can be viewed. In the planning for the volume we made no explicit attempt to give equal weight to all of these attitudes. Rather, we assembled a representative collection of views – representative in the sense that all major attitudes are represented, roughly according to their relative weight in the field. In trying this, however, we found that, given the limitations of a single volume, we could not at the same time strive for representativeness with regard to the major domains and subdomains of the whole field. Instead, we decided to focus on vision (though not exclusively) and to represent this broad and richly developed domain by a collection of chapters that samples the current landscape of theoretical and methodological attitudes in a fairly representative way.

Given this general guideline it does not come as a surprise that the majority of contributions (1) emphasize experience over performance; (2) put more weight on bottom-up transformations than on interactions between bottom-up and top-down information; (3) seek to model the processing mechanisms that underlie these transformations; and (4) stress the out–in over the in–out direction of inquiry. This combination of theoretical attitudes represents, in our view, the mainstream line of research which is prevalent throughout the field.

The organization of the volume goes from basic to more complex functions. Although our emphasis on the out–in mode of inquiry might suggest reversing that order and starting from functionally relevant output of perceptual processes, we have decided to follow the more conventional organization that has always been used in handbooks and textbooks on perception (see, for example, Boff, Kaufman and Thomas 1986; Carterette and Friedman, 1974; von Fieandt and Moustgaard, 1977; Kling and Riggs, 1971; Metzger, 1966; Schiffman, 1976): from 'low' to 'high', from 'simple' to 'complex', from 'early' to 'late' (presumably, at least).

In the first section, which considers basic processes and mechanisms, we go from very early vision (Reeves) via early vision (Kehrer and Meinecke; Eimer; Schneider) to not-so-early, but still basic vision (Deubel; Bridgeman). In the second section, which focuses on more complex perceptual achievements, we start with an account of perceptual constancies (Shebilske and Peters), then proceed to pattern and object perception (Deutsch; Hoffmann) and finally conclude with the perception of events and actions (Shaw, Flascher and Mace; Stränger and Hommel).

Although the aforementioned group of theoretical attitudes appears to be the dominant type of approach, other theoretical attitudes are represented as well. Performance-related consequences of stimulation play an important role in the chapters by Bridgeman, Deubel and Shebilske and Peters. Bridgeman shows that experience and performance can become dissociated within the same task. Conversely, Shebilske and Peters stress the relevance of experience to performance by demonstrating that constancy mechanisms serve to furnish perceivers with experiences tailored to guide their actions. Deubel considers oculomotor performance as an indicator of what the involved perceptual modules are computing.

Reeves' chapter, which deals with a very basic constraint on vision, is perhaps the sole pure example of the classic in–out direction of inquiry. It starts from some basic facts about the nature of light and proceeds to drawing conclusions about the limits of temporal resolution of a photon detector like the eye. If one accepts his argument, the output of such a detector is unequivocally determined by certain properties of the stimulus. However, when the stimulus input is regarded as a source of information that can be used, or processed, in one or the other way the inquiry has to proceed in the out–in direction, using the output as a guideline for finding out which way of processing is actually used. This can be seen in Deutsch's chapter on the perception of auditory patterns and it can even be seen in the chapters on early vision by Kehrer and Meinecke, Eimer and Schneider. Although these chapters start the discussion of their respective areas from descriptions of basic properties of the stimulus input (such as luminance changes, edges, contours and line orientations) they make clear, at the same time, that the logic of inquiry in these fields is guided by known properties of the output: What kind of computation must be invoked and/or what kind of invariant must be picked up in order to produce a given segmentation, a given depth value or a given illusory contour? Hence, even early vision research, although it is still very close to the stimulus, has to follow the out–in direction of inquiry.

Hoffmann's chapter makes explicit reference to the issue of how information from the stimulus and information from memory interact in the perceptual recognition of objects. It represents an interactional approach to the study of perception. Another aspect of the interactional attitude is brought out in Deubel's analysis of how top-down factors such as attention and expectancy interact with stimulus-dependent factors in the control of saccadic eye movements. Stränger and Hommel make their way from a transformationalist view of the perception of abstract motion to a more interactionalist view of the perception of complex human action.

Shaw, Flascher and Mace's chapter on event perception forms again the sole pure example of an attitude that stresses discovery over processing. This chapter proposes searching for those higher-order input variables that form the direct counterpart of given output (seen motion) rather than dwelling on complex computation from simple stimulus characteristics. Some related ideas can also be found in Shebilske and Peters' chapter.

REFERENCES

Attneave, F. (1962). Perception and related areas. In S. Koch (Ed.), *Psychology: A study of a Science*, vol. 4: *Biologically Oriented Fields: Their Place in Psychology and in Biological Science* (pp. 619-659). New York, San Francisco, Toronto: McGraw-Hill.

Boff, K. R., Kaufman, L. and Thomas, J. P. (1986). *Handbook of Perception and Human Performance*, vols. 1 and 2. New York, Brisbane: John Wiley,

Bridgeman, B. (1991). Complementary cognitive and motor image processing. In G. Obrecht and L. Stark (Eds), *Presbyopia Research: From Molecular Biology to Visual Adaptation*. New York: Plenum Press.

Carterette, E. C. and Friedman, M. P. (Eds) (1974). *Handbook of Perception*, vol 1: *Historical and Philosophical Roots of Perception*. New York, San Francisco, London: Academic Press.

Fieandt, K. von and Moustgaard, I. K. (1977). *The Perceptual World*. New York, San Francisco, London: Academic Press.

Gibson, J. J. (1950). *The Perception of the Visual World*. Boston, MA: Houghton-Mifflin.

Gibson, J. J. (1966). *The Senses Considered as Perceptual Systems*. Boston, MA: Houghton-Mifflin.

Gibson, J. J. (1979). *The Ecological Approach to Visual Perception*. Boston, MA: Houghton-Mifflin.

Hochberg, J. (1992). Perceptual theory toward the end of the twentieth century. *International Journal of Psychology*, **27**, *(3 and 4)*, 14–15 (Abstract from the XXV International Congress of Psychology, Brussels 1992).

Kling, J. W. and Riggs, L. A. (1971). *Woodworth and Schlosberg's Experimental Psychology*. New York, Chicago: Holt, Rinehart and Winston.

Koffka, K. (1935). *Principles of Gestalt Psychology*. London: Routledge and Kegan Paul.

Metzger, W. (1966). Der Ort der Wahrnehmungslehre im Aufbau der Psychologie. In W. Metzger (Ed.), *Wahrnehmung und Bewußtsein. Handbuch der Psychologie*, vol. I/1 (pp. 3–20). Göttingen: Hogrefe.

Paillard, J. (1987). Cognitive versus sensorimotor encoding of spatial information. In P. Ellen and C. Thinus-Blanc (Eds), *Cognitive Processes and Spatial Orientation in Animal and Man*. Dordrecht: Nijhoff.

Prinz, W. (1990a). Epilogue: Beyond Fechner. In H. G. Geissler, M. H. Müller and W. Prinz (Eds), *Psychophysical Explorations of Mental Structures* (pp. 491–498). Toronto, Göttingen: Hogrefe.

Prinz, W. (1990b). Wahrnehmung. In H. Spada (Ed.), *Lehrbuch der Allgemeinen Psychologie* (pp. 26–115). Bern, Stuttgart, Toronto: Huber.

Schiffman, H. R. (1976). *Sensation and Perception: An Integrated Approach*. New York, Chichester, Brisbane: John Wiley.

Turvey, M. T. and Kugler, P. N. (1984). An ecological approach to perception and action. In H. T. A. Whiting (Ed.), *Human Motor Actions – Bernstein Reassessed* (pp. 373–412). Amsterdam: North-Holland.

Part I
Basic Processes and Mechanisms

Chapter 1

Temporal Resolution in Visual Perception

Adam Reeves

Northeastern University, Boston

1 INTRODUCTION

Research on the temporal aspects of visual perception has developed somewhat slowly over the past century. While the fundamentals of color, space and motion perception are well known, this is not so in the case of time. Perhaps this is because the perception of time is to some extent subservient to the perception of spatial structure, for which the visual system is specialized. Indeed, the very act of spatial perception takes time to accomplish and to that extent temporal resolution must be lost. This chapter will explore a few ramifications of this point. Physical constraints on processing require that if spatial and chromatic information is to be recovered by the eye, a fundamental limit is imposed on temporal resolution. Although temporal resolution is not the only factor in time perception (James, 1890), it is an important one and does lend itself to analysis.

The approach taken here is to analyze the eye from the point of view of an ideal detector of photons. It will be argued that the temporal resolution obtained in various experiments is near the theoretical limit of what is physically possible, given the requirements of an ideal detector. In principle, this theoretical limit is not fixed but depends on the informational requirements imposed by the task of processing the sensory signal. However, this chapter will concentrate mainly on simple threshold tasks in which the informational requirements vary rather little.

The limit of temporal resolution can be defined operationally by the 'critical duration' measured at threshold. This is the duration of a visual stimulus below which time and intensity trade off for each other. For example, if the stimulus is both doubled in intensity and halved in duration, threshold does not change. This illustrates Bloch's law (Boynton, 1961; Brindley, 1954), which states that the product of time and intensity – which is energy – defines the outcome. Bloch's law generalizes to above-threshold stimuli as follows: two stimuli of different durations but the same energy must have the same visual effect, as long as both durations are within the critical duration.

To understand why the critical duration can be used to define temporal resolution, imagine two different visual stimuli of different durations. The two stimuli can be made perceptually indistinguishable by varying the intensity of one of them (to equate their energies), just so long as both stimuli are briefer than the

Handbook of Perception and Action: Volume 1
ISBN 0-12-516161-1

critical duration. In a word, two stimuli below the critical duration can be made *metamers*. On the other hand, if the two stimuli are discriminable in duration and either or both are longer than the critical duration, no reasonable variation in relative intensity can make them indiscriminable. Analogously, imagine two fine rods applied to the skin; if they are close to each other, that is, within a critical distance, the sensation is the same as that of a single rod applied with twice the force. If separated by more than the critical distance, if both are felt they will be felt as two, no matter what their relative intensity.

The argument of this chapter is relatively straightforward. The idea is to build an ideal detector of spatial and chromatic information, and then deduce what must be light intensity requirements of such a detector. Knowing this, it is then possible to deduce the ideal detector's temporal resolution. Each aspect of the ideal detector can be compared with optimal human performance. As far as possible, the argument will be made using only well-established facts. The data discussed will concern only foveal vision, on which the bulk of visual studies have concentrated.

2   IDEAL DETECTOR: AREA

2.1   Spatial Information

It is a commonplace that we can see fine details and delicate shadows, yet, when taking photographs, require light meters to establish the overall level of light. Indeed, in order to obtain spatially acute vision it is essential to enhance sensitivity to local contrasts, and reduce sensitivity to uniform areas of light. This principle was first argued by Mach, and demonstrated by the 'Mach band' illusion (Cornsweet, 1970). Gestalt psychology also emphasized that we perceive patterns of contrasts, not merely overall light intensity. Grossberg's neural network theory also assumes this principle for functional reasons, but in addition requires lowered sensitivity to uniform areas for a 'hardware' reason: to reduce the risk of saturating all neural signals at a single high level when the eye is exposed to a bright visual field (Grossberg, 1982). Assuming that the perception of spatial contrast is critical, how then might it be signalled?

A complete spatial model which can account for contrast perception is necessarily complex (e.g. Grossberg, 1982). However, it is simple to specify the minimal retinal anatomy needed to suppress uniform areas of light and enhance contrast: it is to subtract from the output of a receptor the mean outputs of its nearest neighbors (a so-called 'center-surround' anatomy). In the fovea, the photoreceptors (all cones) are arranged on an exact hexagonal matrix (Hirsch and Hylton, 1984; Williams, 1985). Such a matrix represents an 'ideal' packing geometry, in that it results when circular elements (here, cones) are packed as tightly as possible in a finite plane area. Thus, each foveal cone has six nearest neighbors, and so the width of the resulting circular receptive field is 3.2 times the cone diameter. This factor of 3.2 cone diameters provides an estimate for the area of spatial integration or spatial summation. It is the foveal cones that contribute to the tiniest receptive fields and provide the highest spatial acuity, so it is to these that the ideal detector should be compared. The area of spatial integration at the fovea can be estimated psycho-physically from Riccò's area, as will be explained below.

One might dispute this simple spatial contrast model on the grounds that it would be better to use information from each receptor independently, rather than pooling over seven of them (1 center and 6 surround). However, were independence to be maintained throughout the visual system, changes of contrast across borders could not be distinguished from variations in lighting that were nothing to do with the stimulus pattern (which might arise, for example, from variations in the brightness of the sky or passing clouds). This is not to say that one is insensitive to all variations in illumination. However, it is reasonable to suppose that the vast majority of visual cells (90% in primates) are specialized for the perception of patterns, borders and the like, and respond feebly or not at all to uniform illumination (see, for example, Livingstone and Hubel, 1988, for a recent summary). For these cells, isolation of contrast is essential and the geometry just described, involving seven receptors, is the bare minimum. (However, this does not imply that there are seven times more cones than receptive fields, because each cone contributes to more than one receptive field: Schein, 1988.)

2.2 Chromatic Vision

I turn next to the existence of color vision. How can an ideal detector, or photoreceptor, provide information concerning light? To be sensitive to light and to provide the enormous magnification needed to convert light energy to an electrical signal, photoreceptors must contain very many photo-sensitive molecules. To do this, given that the retinal mosaic is dense, photoreceptors must be long, narrow cylinders, each end-on to the retinal surface. Indeed, this is an adequate description of the outer segments (the light-sensitive part) of human foveal cones. Given that foveal cones are in fact cylinders, how large should their diameters be? This will determine the spatial integration area (3.2 cone diameters) already derived. The cone diameter should be as small as possible, to provide optimal spatial acuity, but cannot be indefinitely small, if the cone is to be selective for wavelength. Indeed, photoreceptors must be wider than the range of wavelengths of light to which they are selective, for optical reasons. Specifically, the propagation of light energy by a cone is a problem of wave-mode propagation. Such propagation in long circular cylinders, like foveal cones, is soluble theoretically, so that the relationship between cylinder diameter and the degree of selectivity can be calculated (Snyder and Hamer, 1972). Although cones are not perfect cylinders and so approximations are involved, it is clear that cones much narrower than the wavelength of light would be useless for color vision. Thus, the range of wavelengths to which the eye is sensitive provides a lower bound on cone diameters, and indeed on the diameter of the ideal detector. In fact, long-wave cones, whose diameter is $1.1\,\mu m$, are about 1.5 times wider than the longest wavelength they respond to: $0.7\,\mu m$ (or 700 nm). This is in line with the optical approximations, given the actual wavelength selectivity of the cones (Snyder and

Hamer, 1972). Therefore, combining these spatial and chromatic considerations for the ideal detector, the diameter of the smallest receptive field should be 3.2 times 1.1 μm, that is, 3.5 μm. Note that these numbers are derived from physical considerations alone, plus the functional consideration that contrast should be signalled.

A digression here on short-wave sensitive (SW) cones: according to these optical considerations, SW cones could have been half the diameter (say, 0.5 μm) and still have been selective for wavelength. Thus, one might have expected to see even smaller foveal receptive fields, receiving inputs from even smaller SW cones. However, SW cones are actually absent from the foveola and are very rare in the fovea. Thus, spatial acuity for stimuli detected only by SW cones is low. SW cones do not contribute to the highest acuity, smallest receptive fields, primarily because of another optical consideration: chromatic aberrations in the eye mean that short-wave light is badly out of focus. For example, light at 400 nm is out of focus by 1 to 2 diopters relative to middle and long-wave light (Bennett and Francis, 1962). The eye cannot focus adequately over the entire spectrum, given the nature of the lens and aqueous humor. When a full range of wavelengths is present, the eye focuses the middle wavelengths best, where both sun and moon provide the strongest illumination. Given good focus at these wavelengths, chromatic aberrations at short wavelengths are severe enough that signals from SW cones, which primarily reflect short-wave light, cannot be used to provide sharp acuity. (Outside the foveola, SW cones do contribute to pattern perception, but only very minimally: Boynton, Eskew and Olson, 1985.)

2.3   Riccò's Area

Using the standard schematic human eye (Le Grand, 1968), the predicted 3.5 μm diameter of the smallest ideal receptive field subtends about one minute of arc. Support for this prediction comes from the standard result that 1 min arc is the limit of acuity in the fovea, which is also the estimate of Riccò's area normally accepted in visual psychophysics (Le Grand, 1968). This area could not be smaller with insignificant loss of visual information, given the optical design of the eye. To see the significance of Riccò's area, note that it operates for space in the same way as the critical duration does for time. Thresholds for stimuli which fall within Riccò's area (e.g. a tiny spot) and within the critical duration (e.g. a pulse of light) are determined by stimulus energy, that is, by the product of area, intensity and duration. If any one of these is halved and another is doubled, thresholds do not change (Le Grand, 1968).

There are many examples of the so-called 'hyperacuities' (Westheimer, 1975), such as stereoscopic disparities which are around 10 sec arc or less (Fahle and Westheimer, 1988), whose existence might seem to shed doubt on this derivation of Riccò's area. However, hyperacuities can only be obtained with extended stimuli, and presumably involve pooling across many receptors in order to increase precision. In principle, the error in locating a line stimulus can be made vanishingly small, even given receptors of nonzero area, if the system is allowed to compute an appropriate statistic by averaging (pooling) all along its length. The statistic could be the center of gravity, or some shape descriptor (Watt, Ward and Casco, 1987). This assumption of pooling has been made many times and is necessary, given the relatively large size of foveal cones (about 20 sec arc). Given pooling, no direct estimate of Riccò's area can be made from hyperacuity measurements.

In summary, spatial and chromatic constraints of an essentially physical nature ensure that foveal cones are about 1.1 μm (equivalent to 20 sec arc) across. Thus, given the need to process contrast, the smallest receptive fields should be about 3.5 μm (1 min arc) across.

3   IDEAL DETECTOR: QUANTA

3.1   Light Intensity and Critical Duration

So far the size of the area of spatial summation has been deduced from physical principles. The next step along the route to obtaining the critical duration is to consider the threshold light intensity. To be just visible, a light which stimulates only foveal cones should produce about one troland (1 td) of retinal illumination, as shown by Hecht, Haig and Chase (1937) who used red light to avoid detection by rods. One may ask to what extent this figure agrees with ideal detector considerations. At this low light level (1 td) each foveal photoreceptor receives on average one photon of light in 240 ms (Baylor, Nunn and Schnapf, 1984). This follows directly from knowing the physical conversion from trolands to photons per second. In addition, some photons incident on the eye are reflected back by the pupil, and some are scattered by the optic media, but these factors were accounted for by Baylor, Nunn and Schnapf (1984). Assuming that cone outer segments abut each other with no gaps in the fovea, which is almost true, 1 td of illumination provides an average of one photon to each 7-cone receptive field every 240/ 7 = 34 ms. For readers unused to thinking about vision at this level, this figure should give pause for reflection. One photon is a very small amount of light! As one cannot have part of a photon, this calculation implies that the critical duration for the detection of a brief, weak flash of light cannot be less than 34 ms.

The theoretical critical duration of 34 ms compares well with a measured critical duration of 40 ms in Krauskopf and Mollon's (1971) extended study of the temporal properties of the long- and middle-wave cone pathways in the fovea. (One refers to 'cone pathways' rather than cones because the temporal summation involved is primarily neural. Cones themselves do summate information in time, but for less than 1 ms: Boynton, 1961.) Thus, the 34 ms critical duration and the 1 min arc spatial extent (which defines Riccò's area) specify a single spatiotemporal integration unit, which is justified both by experiment and by basic physical considerations. It should be emphasized here that the experimental determinations of the exact numbers are probably firmer, as some of the numbers in the theoretical calculations – particularly the effects of cone diameter (Snyder and Hamer, 1972) and the determination of the fraction of light scattered by the optic media (Baylor, Nunn and Schnapf, 1984) – involve approximations. However, the agreement between theory and experiment is not at all bad.

Large and long test flashes will fill many spatiotemporal integration units, and permit multiple observations by an ideal detector. By making many (say, N) observations of the same event, an ideal detector should be able to reduce noise in proportion to the square root of N, and so lower threshold to the same degree. This improvement in threshold is analogous to that found in spatial vision when conditions favor spatial averaging or pooling, as discussed in the section on Riccò's area. However, a brief, tiny test flash (34 ms, 1 min arc) will just fill one such integration unit, and in this case the measured threshold should provide a precise estimate of the sensitivity of one unit.

3.2   Photon Noise and the Absolute Threshold

The next part of the argument considers the statistics of light at the photon level in greater detail. It will be argued that visual thresholds are determined by the randomness of light itself, rather than by independently varying random factors in the nervous system. The argument will generally proceed by assuming an ideal detector with no internal sources of 'noise' (randomness), either at the information-sensing level or at the decision-making level. The assumption that the visual system is comparable to an ideal detector with virtually no internal noise is equivalent to arguing that the visual system has evolved to have the highest possible theoretical precision.

The assumption that visual thresholds are strongly influenced by random, Poisson-distributed 'photon noise' has long been accepted for brief, dim test lights seen near absolute threshold. This is so whether the test light is presented in total darkness or superimposed on very dim fields of uniform light (e.g. Barlow, 1956, 1977; Bouman, 1961; Hecht, Shlaer and Pirenne, 1942; Vimal, *et al.*, 1989). When dark-adapted, individual cones can respond to very few photons (Vimal *et al.*, 1989), so the statistical nature of light inevitably has an effect on the probability of detection. Thus, photon noise certainly contributes to absolute thresholds; this is not in debate. To obtain an exact account of performance at and near the absolute threshold, however, one must invoke a much smaller amount of internal noise, termed 'dark light' (Barlow, 1977). Some of the dark light occurs because of heat, which produces a very low level of activity indistinguishable from that produced by light. Therefore, it is not quite correct to say that the eye has completely achieved the ideal, although the effects of dark light are small at absolute threshold and negligible above it.

3.3   Photon Noise and the Increment Threshold

Does photon noise also contribute to increment thresholds? By 'increment threshold' is meant the threshold of visibility for a small test light flashed briefly on a large, steadily illuminated background field of light to which the observer is well adapted. This situation is somewhat analogous to noticing a small, low-contrast object, such as a bird or a 'plane, against a bright sky after having looked at the sky for long enough to be adapted to it.

The Poisson statistics of photon emissions ensure that light is variable in proportion to its mean intensity (i.e. mean rate of arrival of photons). More precisely, the 'photon noise' or standard deviation (SD) of the momentary rate of arrival of photons, $SD(I)$, is the square root of the mean rate, I, because the mean and variance of a Poisson distribution are equal. In the increment threshold situation, I refers to the intensity of the steady background, which contributes nearly all of the variability and so determines SD(I). Although the test light adds to the variability, it is so weak at threshold that its contribution – typically less than 2% of the total light – may be neglected.

The fact that light becomes more variable as it becomes more intense is well known. One might therefore expect that thresholds would be increasingly influenced by photon noise, or at least that such an influence would not abate, when the background field was made more intense. However, it is often assumed that the effect of photon noise is negligible above absolute threshold (e.g. Massof, 1987). In deed, one has no subjective experience of the variability of light; if one looks at a smoothly painted wall, for example, one's perceptual field does not seem to sparkle at random. Perhaps this is why photon noise is assumed to be irrelevant. However, the point here is that the visual system must integrate over space and time to average out the effects of photon noise. When stimuli are brief and weak, it is argued, the effects of photon noise can be revealed through threshold measurements.

Arguments more sophisticated than these have been made (e.g. Massof, 1987) to suggest that increment thresholds are determined by stimulus-independent neural noise, not by photon noise. As this position is contrary to the one adopted here, the reader should be aware that the issues are less clear-cut than so far in this chapter. The next few paragraphs argue that the visual system is comparable to the ideal detector at all intensities. It will be concluded that photon noise determines not just absolute thresholds in the dark, but also increment thresholds in the light, in agreement with Bouman (1961). To follow the argument, the reader must keep in mind both the intensity of the background light (I) and the intensity of the test flash needed to just make the test flash visible (the increment threshold). The question at issue is how the increment threshold varies with I, and in particular whether that variation can be accounted for by thinking about SD(I). In the relevant research, the test flash is considerably smaller than the background field, and the two can be thought of as acting independently. More exactly, the test flash can be thought of as a probe, used to discover the sensitivity of the visual system, given the presence of the background light. It was Stiles (1949) who demonstrated that small test lights and large adapting backgrounds have independent effects in this sense. (If the test and background have similar sizes, their contours can interact and independence of action is lost.)

The classic argument is that is the detection threshold for a test spot on field of intensity I is determined by the standard deviation of the photon noise, then thresholds should be proportional to SD(I) (De Vries, 1943). This prediction is called the square root law, or Rose–De Vries law, for thresholds. The square root law is obeyed with dim fields (low I) and all varieties of test flash, and with brighter fields and very brief and tiny test flashes (Bouman, 1961, p. 385). Thus, Bouman concluded that photon noise does control increment thresholds at all levels of light. However, in other experiments employing larger test flashes on bright fields, Weber's law (proportionality with I) holds very closely (e.g. Stiles, 1949). This fact has been taken to argue strongly against the classic argument for control of thresholds by photon noise (Massof, 1987), because if the square root law is true, it is predicted to be true for all stimuli, not just some.

Very recent theoretical work by Rudd, however, has shown that the transition to Weber's law for larger stimuli can be explained by an elaboration of the classic view. He analyzed an 'integrate-and-fire' model which assumes photon noise but no internal noise (Rudd, 1992). Rudd showed that to obtain square root behavior with large stimuli and no false alarms, as classically assumed, temporal integration would have to continue for ever. On the other hand, his model with finite temporal integration generates Weber-like behavior, appropriately short critical durations, and a limited (but not zero) number of false alarms for large stimuli. The model also correctly predicts the transition from square root to Weber behavior as stimulus diameter increases. Rudd's sole assumptions, of photon noise and an integrate-and-fire detector, are highly reasonable. (The proofs are mathematically complicated, which partly explains why these assumptions have not been used before.) Thus, Rudd has removed the main argument against the classic view that photon noise does control thresholds.

An additional point to consider is that any neural noise which is correlated with photon noise will be compound Poisson, and in this distribution, for which the mean and variance are proportional rather than identical, square root behavior is also predicted (Teich *et al.*, 1982). Only if the neural noise is generated independently will the square root prediction fail. Therefore, square root behavior is compatible with the occurrence of some neural or receptoral noise, as long as that noise is driven by the photon noise. In sumary, increment thresholds may well be controlled, directly or indirectly, by signal-induced (photon) noise.

3.3.1   Signal Detection Predictions

To illustrate the prediction of increment thresholds from photon noise considerations, assume an intensity $I = 10\,000$ td (that of a very bright sky). This produces an SD of 100. For a tiny, 'unit-sized' test, $N = 1$, and so the standard error (SE) is also 100. Let sensitivity be indexed by d', from signal-detection theory. Suppose $d' = 1.8$ at the threshold of visibility for this test; then the mean increment in light due to a just-visible test flash is predicted to be $1.8 \times 100 = 180$ quanta. How realistic is this number? In fact, on a $10\,000$ td field a just-visible 'unit-sized' test flash will deliver 180 quanta on average, given the empirical Weber fraction for foveal long- and middle-wave cones of 0.018 (Stiles, 1949). Thus, the amount of signal-induced noise predicts exactly the threshold intensity measured in increment threshold experiments.

For purposes of illustration, this argument was made unrealistically precise. Assuming $d' = 1.8$ is reasonable enough, given the methods used to set just-visible flashes in these experiments, but the exact value might be somewhat different. Moreover, the SD was assumed to be equal to the square root of I (Poisson), not proportional to it as would be the case for a compound Poisson. However, the point is still that ideal detector considerations do predict this increment threshold quite closely. Moreover, this calculation is not specific to the example given, but scales with I over most of the photopic range (the Weber part). Thus, increment thresholds for small, brief test flashes (i.e. within the critical area and critical duration) can be predicted entirely from ideal detector considerations.

3.4   Dark Adaptation and Photon Noise

A rather different line of attack on the role of photon noise stems from an analysis of vision at the start of dark adaptation. In these experiments, threshold is measured for a small spot flashed either on a large background field (the increment threshold), or just after the field has been turned off. In the Weber region, the elimination of photon noise consequent on turning the background field off predicts, for an ideal detector, a drop in threshold proportional to SD(I). This prediction implies that the log threshold obtained just after turning off the field should be exactly half the log threshold obtained before the field was turned off. That log thresholds behaved in just this way was confirmed using moderately bright chromatic fields in Krauskopf and Reeves (1980), who give the mathematical derivation of the prediction. The experiment was recently repeated in my laboratory with very intense background fields, sufficient to raise threshold 5 log units above absolute threshold. Within 100 ms after turning off the field, test threshold had dropped 2.5 log units (unpublished observation), again just as predicted.

The drop in threshold at the start of dark adaptation is usually attributed to a remarkably fast recovery of sensitivity by the eye. Indeed, this is such a commonplace idea that sensitivity is often defined as the inverse of threshold! However, such a large and rapid change in sensitivity (2.5 log units in 100 ms) strains the imagination, as no physiological recordings show such fast recovery at the cell level. In contrast, the photon noise account generates exactly the correct, predictions, while assuming that sensitivity does not change at all over the 100 ms interval. As the photon noise predictions are compatible with physical principles and known physiology, their agreement with the dark adaptation results offer additional support for the line of argument developed here.

3.5   Other Detection Studies

Further reasons for assuming that signal-dependent noise affects vision in the light comes from signal-detection experiments in which field intensity is fixed. The aim here is to study the precise details of visual performance at one light level, rather than the variation of performance over a large range of light levels as in the increment threshold studies. In one of these experiments, the slopes of Yes–No receiver–operator characteristics (ROC) curves on normal–normal probability axes were found to have slopes greater than one for light increments and less than one for light decrements. The precise slopes were explained on the assumption that the signal itself contributes Poisson-distributed variability (Cohn, 1976), which it should if the photon noise hypothesis is correct. In another study, Rudd (1988) showed that photon noise effects predict that processing times (indexed by reaction times) should be linearly related to the square of sinusoidal grating frequency, as was reported by Breitmeyer (1975). Finally, Geissler (1989) has shown that several different types of visual discrimination, including the hyperacuity case, can be understood as limited by photon noise. Geissler (1989) has even shown that thresholds for variations in luminance are lower than those for variations in chromaticity, not because the eye is less sensitive to color, but almost entirely because of photon noise effects. All of these results were explained by assuming that variability arises in the light, rather than in the nervous system, just as for an ideal detector.

In summary, if the visual system is to capture light (and have some sensitivity to color), and is to signal contrast, it can only have limited temporal resolution. The quantal and spectral nature of light firmly constrain the 'minimum visible' in both space and time.

4   TEMPORAL ORDER

4.1   Two-flash Experiments

If the critical duration of 34 ms defines a temporal integration unit, pairs of flashes presented to the same retinal location but less than 34 ms apart should tend to 'run into' each other and be seen as one flash; flashes more than 34 ms apart should be seen as two. The exact prediction depends on whether the 34 ms integration period is exogenous, being triggered by stimulus onset, or endogenous, triggered by some biological clock that runs independently of the stimulus (e.g. Kristofferson, 1967). An endogenous trigger could in principle have any period, depending on the putative biological clock. However, if the photon noise considerations are valid, it would be pointless to trigger much faster than 34 ms because many intervals would collect nothing (in the case of a dim test light in darkness) or noise (in the case of an incremental flash). Also, it would be wasteful to trigger much more slowly than every 34 ms, because potentially discriminative stimulus information would be smeared together. In either the endogenous or the exogenous cases, if energy is summed linearly during the integration period, the psychophysical function for discriminating pairs of flashes separated in time should be linear over most of its range, as is typically obtained (cf. Baron, 1969).

Numerous experiments have measured the temporal separation needed to resolve two stimuli. Hirsch and Sherrick (1961) reported an 18 ms separation at threshold (75% correct) for two momentary flashes presented to separate locations. Exner (1875) found that two visual stimuli needed to be separated by 44 ms, if they were flashed to the same retinal location. Allan, Kristofferson and Wiens (1971) found that a separation of 35 ms between two flashes to the same location produced a d' of 1.2. (When the separation was 50 ms, performance was perfect.)

If temporal integration is exogenous, one would predict a mean separation at a threshold of 17 ms for flashes to different locations, and of 51 ms for flashes to the same location. It is assumed here that the integration process is spatially local, so that stimuli only fall into the same epoch of temporal integration if they are delivered to the same location. Thus, there is an uncertainty region of 34 ms around each stimulus. Consider two stimuli delivered to different spatial locations: if they are 34 ms apart or more in time, their temporal order will always be judged correctly; if $0.5 \times 34 = 17$ ms apart, their order will be correctly seen on 50% of the trials and correctly guessed on half of the remaining trials, for a total of 75% correctly judged (threshold); if 0 ms apart (simultaneous), then order will be guessed correctly on half the trials. Similarly, two stimuli delivered to the same location would have to be $2 \times 34 = 68$ ms apart to ensure 100% order judgements, and $1.5 \times 34 = 51$ ms for 75% correct order judgements.

If the integration trigger was endogenous, one would predict the same temporal separations at threshold, no matter what the stimulus location, as the location would have no effect on the trigger process by hypothesis. Thus, the measured separations are satisfactorily predicted by the exogenous model. This is itself consistent with a sensory stage of integration, in which the stimulus itself controls the epoch of summation, and thus with photon noise considerations.

4.1.1 Some Caveats

First, the temporal separation needed for threshold performance may be quite large in certain situations; for example, 75 ms for foveal–temporal flash pairs (Rutschman, 1966), or up to 98 ms for subjects judging pairs of light onsets rather than light pulses (Oatley, Robertson and Scanlan, 1969). Photon noise considerations place a lower bound on temporal resolution, but the effect of noise on the rate of extraction of information from the stimulus must also be considered, and this has been left out of account here. In the case of Rutschman's experiment, the temporal flash excited peripheral retina for which all the parameters discussed here (chromatic, spatial and intensity) may differ; in addition, neural noise may be non-negligible in the periphery. Second, the Poisson distribution of photon noise predicts ROC curves for temporal discriminations which deviate upwards from those predicted by the normal distribution. Baron (1969) reported this tendency but his ROCs are very variable across subjects, and better data do not seem to exist elsewhere. Third, other evidence supports a central timing mechanism independent of sensory modality (e.g. Hirsch and Sherrick, 1961; Stroud, 1956), but perhaps influenced by attention (Stone, 1926). This raises issues which photon noise explanations obviously do not address. Nonetheless, to the extent that evolutionary pressures drive the visual system to minimize temporal, spatial and wavelength uncertainty, photon noise considerations must be primal.

4.2 Rapid Serial Visual Presentation (RSVP)

Finally, one might consider the effects of temporal integration on multiple stimuli experiments such as RSVP, in which a stream of displays is presented to the same retinal area. Sperling *et al.* (1971) showed that scanning RSVP displays for letters or numbers was maximally efficient when the displays were changed every 40 or 50 ms; that is, just over the integration period of 34 ms suggested here for the fovea. When the separation time was reduced below 34 ms, performance dropped off very fast. These results are in close agreement with the single-flash and threshold studies reviewed above. However, the signal detection aspects of identifying one symbol from a small alphabet of symbols in the presence of spatially random (photon) noise are not simple. To specify the precise time needed, given these additional spatial complexities, would require an entire model of the character recognition process. If the photon noise considerations discussed above are correct, then these RSVP data show that the additional complexity is handled with very little additional loss in temporal resolution.

5   CONCLUSIONS

This chapter has emphasized ways in which physical considerations can place limits on temporal processing in the visual system. In doing this, theory and data have been taken from different lines of research which are not usually considered together in one place. In places the argument has become rather technical, and in one place (the increment threshold analysis) controversial. However, the results for foveal stimulation appear to support the general line of argument that the eye is closely analogous to an ideal detector – an old idea (De Vries, 1943) but one which has recently become popular again (Geissler, 1989).

The argument has been put forward that for a variety of conditions, temporal resolution in foveal vision should be about 34 ms. To what extent should one canonize this as a 'time atom', an indestructible unit of temporal processing? At one level, it should be noted that chromatic, contrast, spatial and intensity considerations were all invoked before the 34 ms period was calculated. In each case, some trade-offs may exist. Thus, for example, temporal processing could be speeded at the loss of spatial acuity and sensitivity to contrast, and this indeed occurs in a relatively small number of transient ('Y' type) retinal ganglion cells. Signalling motion may well rely on such transient signals; the issues raised by motion perception have been bypassed here. Again, at very high intensities of light sufficient photons may be available to permit some improvement in temporal resolution, as in the integrate-and-fire model of Rudd (1992). Nonetheless, the available trade-offs may be so limited that temporal resolution is in practice rather stable, particularly for the range of conditions (foveal stimulation, moderate light levels) typically used in visual and cognitive studies. At a somewhat deeper level, however, it may not be justifiable to give such a time atom psychological significance. To do this means that the system in some sense 'knows' that its resolution is 34 ms, and so does not attempt to break temporal intervals down into subjective units smaller than this, at least when representing visual information. (Shorter temporal intervals between two flashes may be coded, if the two flashes are separated spatially, in nontemporal terms; that is, by variations in apparent intensity, or by apparent motion. Such encoding does not affect the point at issue.) The time atom refers to only one aspect of the perception of temporal events. Whether such an atom affects the subjective experience of time is quite another matter. To make a somewhat far-fetched analogy, it appears that objective spatial acuity influences the grain of visual imagery (Kosslyn, 1980). Perhaps the time atom has some influence on the subjective grain of time – but perhaps not.

REFERENCES

Allan, L. G., Kristofferson, A. B. and Wiens, E. W. (1971). Duration discrimination of brief light flashes. *Perception and Psychophysics* **9**, 327–334.
Barlow, H. B. (1956). Retinal noise and absolute threshold. *Journal of the Optical Society of America*, **46**, 634–639.

Barlow, H. B. (1977). Retinal and central factors in human vision limited by noise. In H. B. Barlow and P. Fatt (Eds), *Photoreception in Vertebrates* (pp. 337–358). New York: Academic Press.

Baron, J. (1969) Temporal ROC curves and the psychological moment. *Psychonomic Science,* **15,** 299–300.

Baylor, D. A., Nunn, B. J. and Schnapf, J. L. (1984). The photocurrent noise and spectral sensitivity of rods of the monkey *Macaca fascicularis. Journal of Physiology,* **357,** 575–607.

Bennett, A. G. and Francis, J. L. (1962). The eye as an optical system. In H. Davson (Ed.), *The Eye.* New York: Academic Press.

Bouman, M. A. (1961). History and present status of quantum theory in vision. In W. A. Rosenblith (Ed.), *Sensory Communication* (pp. 377–402). New York: John Wiley.

Boynton, R. M. (1961). Some temporal factors in vision. In W. A. Rosenblith (Ed.), *Sensory Communication.* Cambridge, MA: MIT Press.

Boynton, R. M., Eskew, R. T. and Olson, C. X. (1985). Blue cones contribute to border distinctness. *Vision Research,* **25,** 1349–1352.

Breitmeyer, B. G. (1975). Simple reaction time as a measure of the temporal response properties of transient and sustained channels. *Vision Research,* **15,** 1411–1412.

Brindley, G. S. (1954). The order of coincidence required for visual threshold. *Proceedings of the Royal Society London, B,* **LXVII,** 673–676.

Cohn, T. E. (1976). Quantum fluctuation limit in foveal vision. *Vision Research,* **16,** 573–579.

Cornsweet, T. (1970). *Visual Perception.* New York: Academic Press.

De Vries, H. (1943). The quantum character of light and its bearing on the threshold of vision, the differential sensitivity, and the visual acuity of the eye. *Physica,* **10,** 553–564.

Exner, S. (1875). *Pflueger's Archiv 11.* Quoted in W. James, *op. cit.*

Fahle, M. and Westheimer, G. (1988). Local and global factors in disparity detection of rows of points. *Vision Research,* **28,** 171–178.

Geissler, W. S. (1989). Sequential ideal-observer analysis of visual discriminations. *Psychological Review,* **96,** 267–314.

Grossberg, S. (1982). *Studies of Mind and Brain.* Boston, MA: Reidel Press.

Hecht, S., Haig, C. and Chase, A. M. (1937). The influence of light adaptation on subsequent dark-adaptation of the eye. *Journal of General Physiology,* **20,** 831–843.

Hecht, S., Shlaer, S. and Pirenne, M. H. (1942). Energy, quanta, and vision. *Journal of General Physiology,* **25,** 819–840.

Hirsch, J. and Hylton, R. (1984). Quality of the primate photoreceptor lattice and limits of spatial vision. *Vision Research,* **24,** 347–356.

Hirsch, I. J. and Sherrick, C. E. (1961). Perceived order in different sense modalities. *Journal of Experimental Psychology,* **62,** 423–432.

James, W. (1890). *The Principles of Psychology* vol. 1. New York: Holt.

Kosslyn, S. M. (1980). *Image and Mind.* Cambridge, MA: Harvard University Press.

Krauskopf, J. and Mollon, J. D. (1971). The independence of the temporal integration properties of individual chromatic mechanisms in the human eye. *Journal of Physiology,* **219,** 611–623.

Krauskopf, J. and Reeves, A. (1980). Measurement of the effect of photon noise on detection. *Vision Research,* **20,** 193–196.

Kristofferson, A. B. (1967). Successiveness discrimination as a two-state quantal process. *Science,* **158,** 1337–1339.

Le Grand, Y. (1968). *Light, Colour, and Vision,* 2nd edn. (R. W. G. Hunt, J. W. T. Walsh and F. R. W. Hunt, Transl.) Somerset, NJ: Halsted Press.

Livingstone, M. and Hubel, D. H. (1988). Segregation of form, color, movement, and depth: Anatomy, physiology, and perception. *Science,* **240,** 740–749.

Massof, R. W. (1987). Relation of the normal–deviate vision ROC curve slope to *d'. Journal of the Optical Society of America,* **4,** 548–550.

Oatley, K., Robertson, A. and Scanlan, P. M. (1969). Judging the order of visual stimuli. *Quarterly Journal of Experimental Psychology,* **21,** 172–179.

Riccò, A. (1877). Relazione fra il minimo angolo visuale e l'intensità luminosa. *Annali d'Ottalmologia*, **6**, 373–479.

Rudd, M. E. (1988). Quantal fluctuation limitations on reaction time to sinusoidal gratings. *Vision Research*, **28**, 179–186.

Rudd, M. E. (1992). Photon fluctuations and visual adaptation. *Investigative Ophthalmology and Visual Science*, **33**, 1259.

Rutschman, R. (1966). Perception of temporal order and relative visual latency. *Science*, **152**, 1099–1101.

Schein, S. J. (1988). Anatomy of macaque fovea and spatial densities of neurons in foveal representation. *Journal of Comparative Neurology*, **269**, 479–505.

Snyder, A. W. and Hamer, M. (1972). The light-capture area of a photoreceptor. *Vision Research* **12**, 1749–1753

Sperling, G., Budiansky, J., Spivak, J. G. and Johnson, M. (1971). Extremely rapid visual search: The maximum rate of scanning letters for the presence of a numeral. *Science*, **174**, 307–311.

Stiles, W. S. (1949). Increment thresholds and the mechanisms of colour vision. *Documenta Opthalmologica*, **3**, 138–165.

Stone, S. A. (1926). Prior entry in the auditory-tactual complication. *American Journal of Psychology*, **37**, 284–287.

Stroud, J. M. (1956). The fine structure of psychological time. In H. Quastler (Ed.), *Information Theory in Psychology*. Glencoe, IL: Free Press.

Teich, M. C., Prucnal, P. R., Vannucci, G., Breton, M. E., McGill, W. J. and Kelly, D. H. (1982). Multiplication noise in the human visual system at threshold: 1. Quantum fluctuations and minimum detectable energy. *Journal of the Optical Society of America*, **72**, 419–431.

Vimal, R. L. P., Pokorny, J., Smith, V. C. and Shevell, S. K. (1989). Foveal cone thresholds. *Vision Research*, **29**, 61–78.

Watt, R. J., Ware, R. M. and Casco, C. (1987). The detection of deviation from straightness in lines. *Vision Research*, **27**, 1659–1675.

Westheimer, G. (1975). Visual acuity and hyperacuity. *Investigative Ophthalmology and Visual Science*, **14**, 570–572.

Williams, D. (1985). Aliasing in human foveal vision. *Vision Research*, **25**, 195–205.

Chapter 2

Perceptual Organization of Visual Patterns: The Segmentation of Textures

Lothar Kehrer* and Cristina Meinecke[†]

*University of Bielefeld and [†]University of Munich

1 INTRODUCTION

Research that is concerned with how the human visual system operates has often discriminated between two subfunctions. Neisser (1967), in particular, has been a major promoter of this division, and it has been widely accepted since this time. Neisser's central assumption is that visual input information, that is, that which is projected onto the retinas of our eyes when we look at the environment, is processed in two successive stages, and different levels of information processing are assigned to each of these two stages. According to this concept, the first so-called 'preattentive' stage uses characteristic image features to perform an initially coarse segmentation of the total input image. This segmentation is relatively rapid. The second so-called 'attentive' stage can then concentrate on single areas previously isolated by the first stage in subsequent, finer analyses of the image. Compared with the preattentive stage, the processing in the attentive stage is relatively slow.[1]

This chapter deals exclusively with the 'earlier' preattentive stages of visual information processing and investigates which specific stimulus properties facilitate image segmentation. However, we will only consider some of the theoretically conceivable stimulus properties, or, more succinctly, stimulus dimensions. At least five stimulus dimensions could be involved in image segmentation: (1) relative movement between parts of the image; (2) binocular disparity (i.e. a relative shift of parts of the image on the two retinas); (3) color differences; (4) differences in luminance; and (5) differences in the texturing of areas of the image. This chapter concentrates on the last stimulus dimension (texture differences) and considers which specific properties of textures could underlie image segmentation.

The chapter is divided into four main sections. The first contains older, but in no way obsolete, ideas and findings on the mechanisms and processes thought to be involved in the segmentation of visual input information. The second section views image segmentation as a problem of information processing and focuses on general

---

[1]For the sake of completeness, it should be noted here that Neisser (1967) has assigned other characteristic properties to his postulated stages of information processing than those named here. However, these are not dealt with here as they are unrelated to the issues discussed in this chapter.

Handbook of Perception and Action: Volume 1
ISBN 0-12-516161-1

principles that apply to any image processing system, regardless of which kind. This particularly concerns an effective system-internal representation of images, that is, one that has been cleared of redundancies. It is pointed out that segmentation processes and the 'database' (i.e. image representation) on which these processes draw should not be viewed in isolation. The third section presents a more recent model of image segmentation based on the general principles presented in the second section, while the fourth section reflects back on the concepts presented in the first section.

2   THEORIES OF PERCEPTUAL SEGMENTATION

2.1   The Gestalt Movement

We can hardly provide a more vivid introduction to perceptual segmentation performance from the perspective of Gestalt psychology than the introductory comments to Max Wertheimer's (1923) widely acclaimed article 'Untersuchungen zur Lehre von der Gestalt II' (Studies on Gestalt theory II), published in *Psychologische Forschung*:

> 'I stand at the window and I see a house, trees, and the sky.
>   And, theoretically speaking, I could now try to count up and say: There are…327 levels of light (and color).
>   (Do I have "327?" No: I have sky, house, trees; and nobody can be aware of the "327" as such.)
>   And if, in this curious calculation, house, for example, has 120, and trees 90, and sky 117, then, at any rate, I have *this* combination, this separation, and not, for example, 127 and 100 and 100; or 150 and 177.
>   I *see* it in this specific combination, this specific separation; and the type of combination, of separation in which I see it is not simply a matter of my will: I am completely unable simply to put them together in any other way that I desire.
>   …*Are there principles* underlying the type of "togetherness" and "separatedness" that result? *Which ones*? (p. 301, translated)

The search for Wertheimer's principles led to the Gestalt laws that are cited frequently even (or particularly) today (see, for example, Beck, Prazdny and Rosenfeld, 1983; Beck, Rosenfeld and Ivry, 1989; Boldt, Weiss and Riseman, 1989; Calis and Leeuwenberg, 1981; Conners and Ng, 1989; Driver and Baylis, 1989; Fox and Mayhew, 1979; Graham, 1989; Grossberg and Mingolla, 1985; Gurnsey and Browse, 1987; Jáñez, 1984; Klymenko and Weisstein, 1986; Marr, 1982; Olson and Attneave, 1970; Oyama, 1986; Smits, Voss and van Oeffelen, 1985; Wong and Weisstein, 1983; Zucker and Davis, 1988). Some of the elementary Gestalt laws will be sketched in the following, focusing on those that are particularly relevant to perceptual segmentation performance. Particular reference will be made to Wertheimer (1923; see also Katz, 1969; Koffka, 1935; Köhler, 1924, 1933; Metzger, 1975; Rubin, 1921).

In his characteristic style, Wertheimer (1923) has described very vividly the phenomenal impression that can arise when observing nonhomogeneous fields:

> 'In a homogeneous field, specific stimulus differences (nonhomogeneities) are required if the field is to separate in a special way so that any specific form can appear in it (stand

out from it) . A homogeneous field appears as a unified ganzfeld; it opposes a "separation", "tearing apart", or "interruption"; this requires relatively strong non-homogeneities, and particular kinds of nonhomogeneity are preferred for this.' (p. 348, translated)

The Gestalt laws demonstrate an attempt to provide a more precise description of the factors that bring about the separation of nonhomogeneous fields. With a glance toward the problem of perceptual segmentation, the stimulus displays to which the Gestalt laws refer can be divided roughly into two typical classes. In class 1, several, frequently identical, individual elements (e.g. points) are arranged on the stimulus display. In class 2, line configurations are found in the stimulus. We will first deal with class 1 and its particular laws. In principle, the individual elements arranged on the stimulus surface in a particular way can also be perceived as individual elements. However, under particular conditions, an impression of groups of elements arises for the observer of these stimuli. Figures 2.1 and 2.2 present examples of this kind of stimulus display and the phenomenal impression of grouping described here. The law of proximity and the law of similarity make statements on the groupings that occur.

The *law of proximity* deals with the effect of the spatial arrangement of the individual elements. It states that if individual elements are very close together, there is an increased probability that these elements will be perceived as a group. This law is illustrated in Figure 2.1: the observer sees a row of small, slanted groups sloping from left up to right (and none that slope, for example, from right up to left). Wertheimer performed a closer analysis of what can be understood by 'high proximity' in this stimulus display (conceivable meanings are, for example, absolute size of the interval, difference between intervals, relationship between intervals). We will, however, not discuss this in any more detail here.

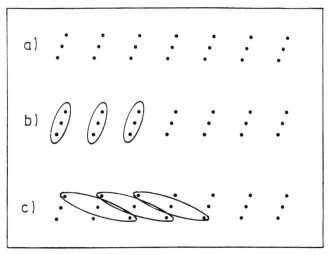

Figure 2.1. *Gestalt law of proximity. (a) Stimulus display: pattern of points. Slanted groups are perceived as in (b) but not as in (c). [(a) from Wertheimer, 1923, p. 305. © 1923 Springer; reprinted with kind permission.]*

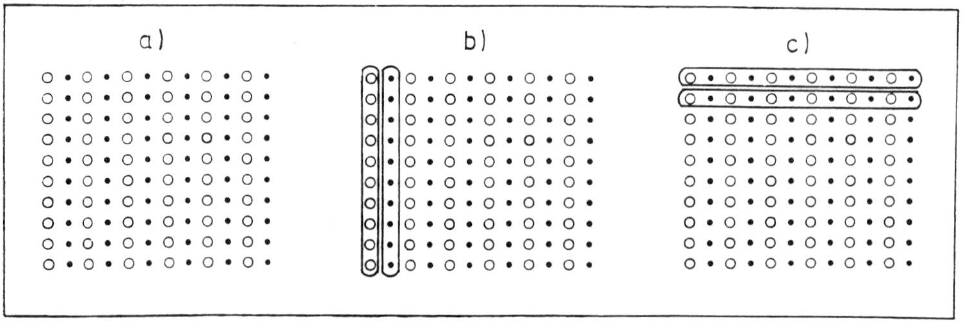

Figure 2.2. *Gestalt law of similarity. (a) Stimulus display: pattern of points. Columns are perceived as in (b) but not lines as in (c). [(a) from Wertheimer, 1923, p. 309. © 1923 Springer; reprinted with kind permission.]*

In the *law of similarity*, the properties of individual elements that facilitate a grouping are inspected more closely. The law states that there is a preference for perceiving individual elements that possess a common property (e.g. the same brightness or color) as a group. Figure 2.2 illustrates this principle: the observer sees black and white columns (and not, for instance, lines). According to Wertheimer, it is not absolutely necessary for individual elements to possess an identical property in order to be perceived as a group (e.g. the property 'red') . It is sufficient for certain individual elements to have sufficiently similar properties (e.g. different but nonetheless always red hues) as long as they differ sufficiently from other individual elements (e.g. those with blue hues)

In contrast to the laws of proximity and similarity, the *law of good Gestalt* or *Prägnanz* refers to stimulus configurations of class 2. If we look at these stimuli, we find line configurations that segment the stimulus display into specific subsections or areas (Figure 2.3). The lines form the borders between these specific areas, while the content of the areas themselves does not differ (in our figures, for example, they are all white). Strictly speaking, such figures no longer belong to the topic addressed in this chapter: they are stimuli that do not display any texture, and this chapter is concerned exclusively with textured stimuli and the mechanisms that could serve to detect (nonexistent) borders between differently textured areas. In stimulus configurations like those shown in Figure 2.4, the borders between the individual areas are nonetheless given explicitly by the border lines. To complete the picture, some Gestalt laws that refer to these stimuli will be mentioned briefly.

Figure 2.3 shows a typical stimulus display for demonstrating the effect of the law of good Gestalt: one sees individual lines that intersect. However, the question is: Which parts of lines are joined together perceptually and form the specific continuation? Wertheimer answers this question by naming several factors that could lead to a good Gestalt: these include closure, symmetry, internal balance and good continuity. Without wishing to go into these factors in any detail, one further figure should illustrate the law of good Gestalt: Figure 2.4a displays a hexagon that is duplicated unchanged in Figure 2.4b–f. In Figure 2.4b–d, an observer will be unable to rediscover the hexagon (or only with a lot of effort). Additional lines confront the observer with new good Gestalts. This is not the case in Figure 2.4e, f, in which the new lines do not impair the perception of the hexagon.

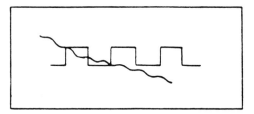

Figure 2.3. *Law of good Gestalt (law of continuous curve). [From Wertheimer, 1923, p. 323, Fig. 16, modified. © 1923 Springer; reprinted with kind permission.]*

All the above-mentioned Gestalt laws have referred to static stimulus presentations. The *law of common fate* refers to the phenomenal impression that arises when parts of a stimulus presentation undergo a common alteration (e.g. displacement, rotation). These parts are then perceived as a group, as a subgroup of the whole stimulus display.

In the presentation of individual Gestalt laws, we sometimes find, at least in the work of Wertheimer, attempts to specify these laws mathematically. These include, for example, the attempt to operationalize the concept of 'proximity', or the statement that a good curve should also be easy to describe in mathematical terms. However, Gestalt psychologists were not particularly interested in mathematical models. They placed much more emphasis on the phenomenal description of

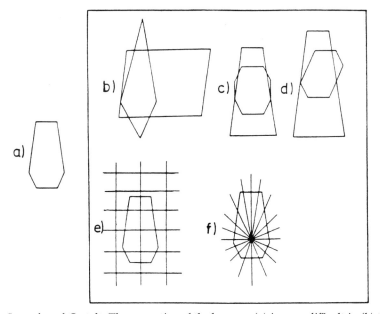

Figure 2.4. *Law of good Gestalt. The perception of the hexagon (a) is more difficult in (b) to (d). The lines added directly to the hexagon confront the observer with new good Gestalts. This does not occur in (e) and (f). [From Wertheimer, 1923, p. 328, Figs. 38–43, modified. © 1923 Springer; reprinted with kind permission.]*

perceptual impressions. This is evident when looking at Wertheimer's (1923) vivid descriptions of phenomenal impressions in the perception of Gestalts: 'Initially, the relationships are grasped as a whole; they are there' (p. 346). Subsections stand out; observers are often uncertain about the precise structure of these areas. The impression is simply that the subsection 'stands out' (p. 346). This perception is very stable and explicit. The 'relationships between fixation point, eye movements, attentional attitude, and distribution of attention' (p. 339) are irrelevant. It is not just that perception of the Gestalt remains unaffected by the specific current relationships between these factors, but, in contrast, eye movements and so forth are determined secondarily by the actual stimulus constellation.

Although the major heuristic value of the Gestalt laws cannot be doubted, the Gestalt psychologists were unable to specify their laws in sufficient detail to permit a strict test (insofar as this was in any case their intention).

2.2 Statistical Theory

Extensive research on visual segmentation only started up again in the 1960s under the strong influence of the work of Julesz and his coworkers (Julesz, 1962, 1975; Julesz et al., 1973). It is probable that this work was stimulated to a large extent by advances in the digital computer and the new possibilities of generating stimuli on cathode-ray tubes (see, for example, Green, 1963; Green, Wolf and White, 1959; Julesz, 1960). This frequently found close link between the current state of computer technology and progress in research on the visual system has been pointed out once more in an impressive article by Uttal (1986).

The innovation at the end of the 1950s resulted from the new ability to generate artificial textures in the digital computer. This procedure has two significant advantages: (1) The stimuli generated in this way can be described precisely by their underlying algorithm; and (2) such stimulus presentations ideally do not contain any structures with which subjects are familiar (familiarity cues). This makes it possible to ensure that the intended study of elementary organizational structures on 'early' stages of visual information processing remains uninfluenced by the involvement of 'higher' concept-driven processing.

The first textures studied by Julesz were synthesized by varying the probability that a certain point (pixel) within the texture would display a preset brightness (stochastic textures). Figure 2.5 presents an example of such a texture published by Julesz (1962). It is composed of points that are either black or white, that is, there are no intermediate grays. This frequently studied special case of a texture with only two levels of brightness is commonly called a binary texture.

As can be easily seen when looking at Figure 2.5, a vertical (rather fuzzy) border seems to run through the texture. When generating the picture, the probability that, for example, black would be selected for any random point is set somewhat higher on the left-hand side than the probability for black on the right-hand side. Specifically, the algorithm used to generate the texture in Figure 2.5 stipulates that each point on the left-hand side of the texture will be presented as black with a probability of 5/8, and thus, as it is a binary texture, as white with a probability of 3/8; while the right-hand side of the texture has the opposite probability distribution. The result of this manipulation is that the luminance integrated over a larger area of texture on the right-hand side is higher than that on the left-hand side. In

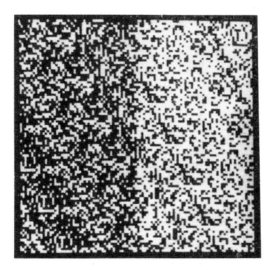

Figure 2.5. *Textures with different first-order statistics. The probability that a white point will be selected is higher on the right-hand side. [From Julesz, 1962, p. 85, Fig. 3. © 1962 IEEE, New York; reprinted with kind permission.]*

the terminology of Julesz, the two halves of the picture differ in the *first-order statistics* generated within their borders. Of course, various first-order statistics can also be generated for nonbinary textures, that is, textures with several shades of grey. As in the binary textures, the characteristic difference in first-order statistics in nonbinary textures is also a difference in mean luminance.

However, Julesz and his coworkers have not just studied textures with varying first-order statistics but have also extended their studies to textures with higher-order statistics. Initially, they particularly focused on textures with varying *second-order statistics*. In these textures, first-order statistics are constant, that is, the textures cannot be segmented on the basis of mean differences in luminance. Figure 2.6 presents an example of such a texture.

As Figure 2.6 shows, despite the lack of differences in luminance, two separate subtextures are perceived. The difference built into the two textures is as follows: in the smaller texture in the bottom right-hand corner of the stimulus display, the brightness values of the individual points making up the pattern are statistically independent from each other. However, this is not the case in the larger texture: here, there is a higher probability that two neighboring points possess the same brightness value within individual lines than within columns. In specific terms, the probability that a random point will have the same brightness as its right-hand neighbor is set at $P = 0.75$. This leaves a residual probability that two neighboring points will differ in brightness of $P = 0.25$. No restrictions are made for probabilities in columns. Through the above-random juxtaposition ($P = 0.75$) of points of equal brightness, this manipulation produces horizontal stripes in the larger subtexture that are not present in the smaller subtexture. It seems that the human visual system can use this difference to efficiently segment the two subtextures. With reference to the subjective perception that arises, Julesz (1962) has also labeled

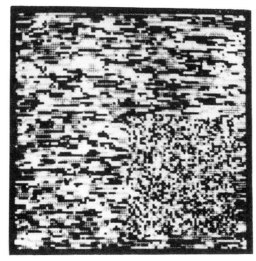

Figure 2.6. *Textures with different second-order statistics. First-order statistics are identical in both parts of the texture. [From Julesz, 1962, p. 85, Fig. 5. © 1962 IEEE, New York; reprinted with kind permission.]*

Figure 2.7. *Textures with different third-order statistics. First- and second-order statistics are identical in both parts of the texture. [From Julesz, 1975, p. 37, Fig. bottom left. Reprinted with kind permission of the author.]*

this difference in the second-order statistics as a difference in the *granularity* of the textures generated.

   In general terms, first-order statistics determine the probability with which a ring that is randomly 'thrown' onto a texture will circumscribe a certain grey value. Second-order statistics define the probability with which the ends of 'needles' of varying length and orientation, that are placed in randomly selected positions on a texture, take specific grey values. In a series of further studies, Julesz and coworkers have shown that textures with identical first- and second-order statistics that only differ in higher-order statistics can no longer be segmented preattentively (for a summary, see Julesz, 1975). Figure 2.7 presents an example of a texture in which

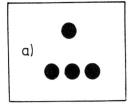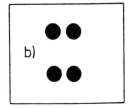

Figure 2.8. *Texture elements that generate textures with identical third-order statistics. [From Julesz, 1975, p. 41, Fig. top right. © 1975 Scientific American. Reprinted with kind permission of the author and the German publisher: Spektrum der Wissenschaft Verlags-GmbH, Heidelberg.]*

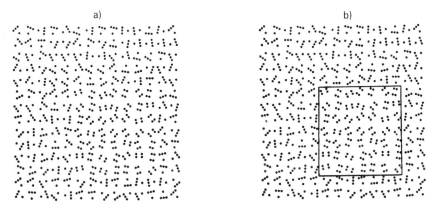

Figure 2.9. *Textures that contain the scaled-down texture elements from Figure 2.8; they therefore exhibit identical third-order statistics both within and outside the framed area. [From Julesz, 1975, p. 41, Fig. center left and bottom left. Reprinted with kind permission of the author.]*

the left- and right-hand halves vary in that different third-order statistics have been used to generate them. However, first- and second-order statistics remain the same.

Figure 2.7 shows that the two halves of the texture can no longer be segmented perceptually. This apparent inability of the human visual system to detect third- and higher-level statistics in textures preattentively has become known as the 'Julesz conjecture'. It has also been demonstrated for textures composed of texture elements that in themselves vary greatly in appearance (Julesz, 1975). Figure 2.8 shows two such texture elements that are relatively different in appearance and that can be used to generate textures with identical second-order statistics but different third-order statistics. As Figure 2.9 shows, a preattentive segmentation of the subtextures generated with texture element (a) or (b) is not possible.

2.3 Local Segmentation Theories

In the years that followed, however, the appropriateness of the Julesz conjecture was increasingly challenged by a rising number of contradictory findings (see, for example, Caelli and Julesz, 1978; Caelli, Julesz and Gilbert, 1978; Diaconis and

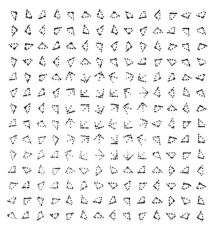

Figure 2.10. *Three examples of textures with identical second-order statistics. Despite the agreement in second-order statistics, preattentive segmentation can be observed. [From Caelli, Julesz and Gilbert, 1978, p. 202 (Fig. 1c); p. 203 (Fig. 3c); p. 206 (Fig. 7c). © 1978 Springer; reprinted with kind permission.]*

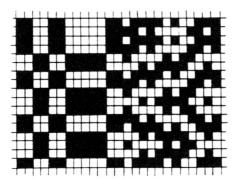

Figure 2.11. *Textures with identical third-order statistics in the left- and right-hand halves of the texture. In contradiction to the Julesz conjecture, preattentive segmentation occurs. [From Julesz, Gilbert and Victor, 1978, p. 138, Fig. 3. © 1978 Springer; reprinted with kind permission.]*

Freedman, 1981; Julesz, Gilbert and Victor, 1978). These findings are based on textures with identical second- and even third-order statistics that nonetheless can be segmented preattentively.[2] Figure 2.10 presents three textures reported by Caelli, Julesz and Gilbert (1978) in which a smaller texture in the middle of a larger surround is segmented perceptually although both textures have identical second-order statistics.

Figure 2.11 presents an example of two segmented textures with identical third-order statistics. The left-hand subtexture clearly differs from the right-hand one.

These counterexamples finally led Julesz to drop his original concept that focused on describing larger texture areas with the aid of statistics. Instead, he now started to search for *local* details in textures that could be decisive for preattentive texture perception. He presented his ideas on this within the framework of texton theory (Julesz and Bergen, 1983). At approximately the same time, Treisman (1982; Treisman and Gelade, 1980) published her feature-integration theory, and Beck (1982; Beck, Prazdny and Rosenfeld, 1983) the theory of texture segmentation. All three theories represent attempts to specify the local texture properties that lead to a perceptual segmentation of stimulus displays. The following presents a brief description of the common conception underlying these three approaches. Then, the ways in which they differ will be discussed, and, finally, we will consider how useful they are for explaining perceptual segmentation processes.

2.3.1 The Common Concept Underlying Local Segmentation Theories

The common concept underlying local theories can be outlined as follows: they assume that local texture properties are detected by so-called feature detectors; different distributions of these texture properties on the surface of the stimulus determine how well the stimulus display can be segmented perceptually.

---

[2]Because of the principles underlying their construction, textures with identical higher-order statistics also have identical statistics on all lower orders.

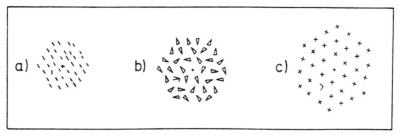

Figure 2.12. *Textures with Julesz' 'textons': (a) blobs; (b) terminations; (c) crossings. [(a) from Bergen and Julesz, 1983, p. 858, Fig. 3c. © 1983 IEEE. (b) from Julesz and Bergen, 1983, p. 1624, Fig. 4c. © 1983 AT and T. All rights reserved. (c) from Julesz and Bergen, 1983, p. 1636, Fig. 13b. © 1983 AT and T. All rights reserved. All figures reprinted with kind permission of the publishers.]*

Grain Size of the Analysis: Local Approach

As reported above, these theories attempt to detect local properties in the stimulus that influence texture segmentation. This differentiates them from the statistical theory of Julesz (1962), in which statistical probability relationships of grey value distributions are observed across the entire stimulus surface. This difference is also illustrated by the type of stimulus display used in most studies. Statistical theory studies generally use displays like that in Figure 2.6: pixel by pixel, the grey value is defined according to set probability rules, and 'quasi-random' patterns arise. In studies performed in the context of local theories, it is not pixels but individual, so-called texture elements that are defined, for example, certain letters. These elements are arranged on the stimulus display, and all the elements together form the texture (see Figure 2.12). In local theories, individual texture elements are subjected to a more detailed inspection. The texture elements are analyzed in order to find those features that influence the perceptual segmentation of the stimulus display. As will be shown below, the theories differ in the precision with which they report which stimulus features determine segmentation. One feature that all three theories consider to be relevant in this context is, for example, 'orientation'.

Feature Detectors

It is assumed that the human visual system contains specialized neurons that vary in their sensitivity to different stimulus features. So-called 'feature detectors' are discussed frequently in this context. Assumptions on the existence of feature detectors are supported by physiological findings. For example, cells have been reported that seem to be sensitive to orientation, size, stereoscopic depth, color or direction of movement (Cowey, 1979, 1985; Zeki, 1978, 1981).

Density Differences Lead to Segmentation

Texture area A stands out from area B when a different density of one or more stimulus features is to be found in A compared with B. This is the general description of the condition under which perceptual segmentation occurs. However, it has to be noted that most studies only make statements on a special case of this general principle. Most findings refer to stimulus displays in which a specific feature is present in area A of the stimulus display but not in area B. Gradual differences in density are not operationalized and hence not tested.

In summary, we can state that the elements that make up each texture play a central role in local segmentation theories: these theories search for those features that are the input information for the segmentation mechanism and thus determine the perceptual segmentation of the stimulus display. It is precisely at this point, when specifying which stimulus features are possibly effective here, that the three theories differ. This will be explained briefly below.

2.3.2 Differences Between Local Segmentation Theories

Type and Number of Critical Stimulus Features
The critical stimulus features are defined on different levels in the theories presented here. On the one hand, the texture elements themselves are the focus of attention (Julesz) and, on the other hand, the focus is on the features of these texture elements (Treisman).

Julesz talks about so-called 'textons' in his texton theory. He views these as specific texture elements or parts of these texture elements. Julesz and Bergen (1983) have assumed that segmentation phenomena can be described sufficiently by the following three textons (Figure 2.12). These are: (1) 'blobs', for example, ellipses, rectangles, or lines. These blobs have specific features such as color, orientation, length and width. Textons also include: (2) 'terminators,' that is, ends of lines. An arrow has three terminators, whereas a triangle has none. Finally, Julesz introduces: (3) 'crossings' as textons, that is, the complete intersection of two lines and the resulting cross.

Thus, Julesz considers that the critical stimulus features in perceptual segmentation processes are either texture elements (textons) possessing specific critical features (e.g. blobs with a specific orientation, color, etc.) or texture elements that are present or absent (e.g. terminators, crossings). As he specifies precisely three textons, texton theory is very easy to work with. However, this also makes it easy to disconfirm, as will be shown further below.

Treisman takes a somewhat different approach in her feature-integration theory. In this theory, the number of critical stimulus properties remains open. Although she tries to determine these critical properties, she does not commit herself *a priori* to a set list but lets the actual findings decide which stimulus properties should be added to the list and which should be dropped. She labels the critical stimulus properties 'features'. In principle, these are not the texture elements themselves (e.g. lines) but rather the properties of these texture elements (e.g. orientation). These features are encoded by the visual system separately from their respective texture elements.[3]

Treisman and coworkers have published a series of studies that test the segmentation effect of various features (Treisman, 1982; Treisman and Gelade, 1980; Treisman and Gormican, 1988; Treisman and Paterson, 1984; Treisman and Schmidt, 1982; Treisman and Souther, 1985; Treisman, Sykes and Gelade, 1977). Features found to be involved in perceptual segmentation include, for example, color, brightness, orientation and curvature. Additions have been made to this list of critical features over time. These include line length, closure and line ends (see Treisman and Gormican, 1988; Treisman and Souther, 1985).

---

[3]It is often impossible to determine whether a theoretical approach makes a clear separation between bearers of features (e.g. a line) and features themselves (e.g. the orientation of this line).

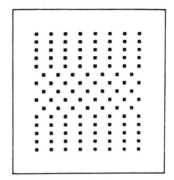

Figure 2.13. *Demonstration of Beck's higher-order texture elements. Individual texture elements (here, rectangles) are linked perceptually to higher-order texture elements (here, vertical and diagonal lines). [From Beck, Sutter and Ivry, 1987, p. 300, Fig. 1.* © *1987 Academic Press; reprinted with kind permission.]*

Hence, we can state that although Treisman has focused attention on the features of texture elements and does not – in contrast to Julesz – view texture elements to be relevant in themselves, both theoretical approaches nonetheless focus on the individual texture elements. This approach of searching for critical features on the level of the individual texture elements can also be found – in principle – in Beck's textural segmentation theory. Like Treisman and Julesz, Beck also assumes that features are extracted from stimulus displays with the help of feature detectors. However, he is not primarily concerned with compiling a complete list of these features. His approach focuses far more on his concept of 'higher-order textural elements' (Beck, Prazdny and Rosenfeld, 1983) that will be discussed briefly in the following.

Higher-order Texture Elements
Beck has suggested that individual texture elements (e.g. lines) can be joined together perceptually to form higher-order textural elements. Figure 2.13 illustrates the concept of higher-order textural elements: in the upper and lower thirds of the figure, the observer 'sees' vertical structures; the structures in the center are perceived to be more diagonal. These vertical and diagonal structures correspond to higher-order textural elements as defined by Beck. As Figure 2.13 also shows, these textural elements can possess features such as length and orientation. These features of higher-order textural elements do not have to correspond to the features of the individual texture elements.

Beck, Prazdny and Rosenfeld (1983) have postulated that factors such as the 'proximity' and 'similarity' of the individual texture elements can influence their perceptual grouping and thus the perception of higher-order textural elements. Their findings support this assumption and link up with the Gestalt laws of proximity and similarity (Wertheimer, 1923) discussed above.

Beck assumes that not only individual texture elements and their properties but also higher-order textural elements and their features can have a significant impact on segmentation performance. This makes one interesting addition to the determinants of segmentation performance that will be discussed below.

2.3.3 Summary Discussion of Local Segmentation Theories

How well do these local theories explain findings from studies on texture segmentation? We will analyze this question in three steps. First, it will be shown that the most parsimonious theory (texton theory) is not sufficient to explain certain findings. Second, it will be shown that critical features should not be sought just on the level of individual texture elements (texton theory and feature integration theory). Finally, a third step will discuss a fundamental problem in local theories.

Are Three Textons Sufficient?

Of the three local theories presented here, texton theory (Julesz and Bergen, 1983) seems to be the most parsimonious as it postulates that three textons are sufficient to explain perceptual segmentation processes. However, this parsimony also makes it vulnerable, as, for example, Enns (1986) and Nothdurft (1990, 1991) have been able to show. They have presented evidence that a slight alteration of the texture elements without modifying the critical textons can influence texture segmentation. We shall demonstrate this effect briefly with stimulus displays used by Enns (1986).

Enns (1986) presented his subjects with four stimulus displays. Figure 2.14 shows two stimulus displays that support the assumptions of texton theory. In Figure 2.14a, a rectangular area of elements without terminators is segmented from a background of elements with three terminators (0:3). In Figure 2.14b all texture elements possess two terminators (2:2). Here, in agreement with texton theory, no area is segmented. Figure 2.15 shows slightly modified displays. The segmentation effect begins to invert: texture (a) seems to be relatively homogeneous, while a subtexture is segmented (admittedly, not very strongly) in texture (b). This effect is obtained without making any changes to the critical textons of the texture elements: as in Figure 2.14, the ratio of terminators in the texture elements is 3:0 in texture (a) and 2:2 in texture (b).

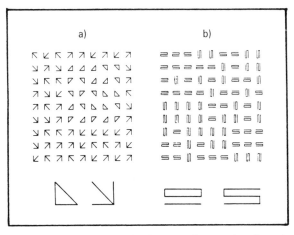

Figure 2.14. *Stimulus display that refutes Julesz' texton theory. The effect of terminations (see text for explanation). [From Enns, 1986, p. 143, Fig. 1A and B. © 1986 the Psychonomic Society, Inc.; reprinted with kind permission of the publisher and author.]*

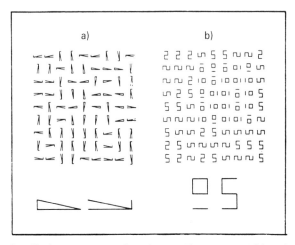

Figure 2.15. *Stimulus displays constructed analog to Figure 2.14. Although no modifications are made to terminations, segmentation performance changes (see text for explanation). [From Enns, 1986, p. 144, Fig. 2A and B. © 1986 The Psychonomic Society, Inc.; reprinted with kind permission of the publisher and author.]*

Several alternative explanations have been offered for this finding (for more details see Enns, 1986; Nothdurft, 1990, 1991). We shall sketch one of these alternatives here. It is conceivable, and Nothdurft (1991) provides empirical evidence in support of this, that the texton that is viewed as being critical (in our example, the end of a line) is not the texton that has been responsible for the texture segmentation from the very beginning. The stimulus modification may then have affected this 'previously disregarded' texton and caused a change in segmentation performance.

It can certainly be stated that the list of textons proposed in texton theory is in need of modification or expansion, as Enns (1986) has also noted. This brings us closer to Treisman's feature integration theory; her list of critical features is open to modification in line with new findings. Nonetheless, it has to be noted that such a procedure makes it very difficult if not completely impossible to test a theory.

Are Texture Elements and Their Features Sufficient?

Both texton theory and feature integration theory consider that the critical features for the perceptual segmentation of stimulus displays are to be found in the individual texture elements. In many cases, this approach may suffice; however, difficulties arise when trying to explain the following findings.

It has been shown that varying the spatial arrangement of individual texture elements in the stimulus display has a significant impact on the ability to segment textures, although the texture elements themselves remain unaltered. Increasing the density of texture elements can facilitate perceptual segmentation (e.g. Kehrer, 1989; Meinecke, 1989; Nothdurft, 1985) . This effect is shown in Figure 2.16. It has also been demonstrated that introducing 'jitter' (the random variation of the position of the texture elements within a certain grid) can impair segmentation performance (e.g. Gurnsey and Browse, 1989; Nothdurft, 1990, 1991) . However, varying the spatial arrangement of texture elements has no effect on individual texture elements

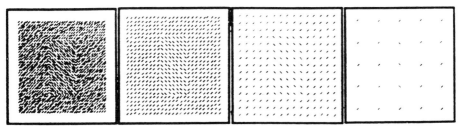

Figure 2.16. *Variations of the density of texture elements and modification of the perceptual impression according to Nothdurft (see text for explanation). [From Nothdurft, 1990, p. 300, Fig. 4d. © 1990 The Royal Society of London; reprinted with kind permission.]*

or their features, so that, at least in terms of texton theory or feature integration theory, segmentation should remain unaffected by such a variation.

The concept of higher-order texture elements developed within Beck's textural segmentation theory can be applied here. As Figure 2.13 has shown, stimulus displays can be constructed in which areas segment because the otherwise identical texture elements differ in the way they are arranged within the areas. According to Beck, neighboring texture elements are linked together perceptually according to their specific allocation. The observer then perceives higher-order textural elements, in this case: structures varying in orientation (vertical versus diagonal). Beck considers that these orientation differences in higher-order textural elements cause the texture segmentation.

In summary, we can state that, in addition to texture elements and their features, other aspects of the stimulus configuration, such as higher-order textural elements, should also be considered when searching for the critical stimulus properties of texture segmentation.

A Fundamental Problem

Although local theories of texture segmentation have been well received, we cannot disregard the fact that they exhibit one disadvantage compared with statistical theory: they are very much less precise. While the proponents of statistical theory tried to make the properties of textures accessible to mathematical description, local theories have returned to concepts permitting a broad scope of interpretation. We shall take the terminator concept as an example. The above-mentioned local theories postulate that two textures will always stand out from each other when they differ in the number of terminators within their texture elements (see, for example, Julesz and Bergen, 1983). But what is a terminator? For the domain of binary textures with their strong contrasts, it may seem possible to provide a reasonably satisfactory answer to this question. But what are terminators in natural contexts with their many shades of grey, sometimes weak contrasts, and lines of differing width (if it is at all possible to define what a line is)?

At this point, all the previously mentioned local segmentation theories reveal an important weakness: the possibilities of testing their range of validity are limited. All evidence presented by their supporters refers to artificial and mostly binary textures into which specific features have been built. If such manipulations prove to have something to do with segmentation, it is concluded that the visual system being studied possesses corresponding feature *detectors*. However, testing this assumption on a larger set of different textures is problematic, as testing by eye has to be used to decide to what extent and in what distribution these textures contain specific features. Estimating the content and density of features can be thoroughly difficult, particularly in *natural* textures when these are richly structured and reveal fine differences in brightness and fuzzy contours.

Local segmentation theories should not be discussed any further in this context without presenting some basic findings and considerations on the coding of visual information that have had a marked influence on research into the functions of the visual system. These are findings that support the assumption that the visual systems of mammals possess specialized subsystems that are capable of detecting *periodic structures* in the retinal image. These findings have led to far-reaching speculations on the possible functional value of such subsystems in the encoding of the retinal image, that is, the transformation into an internal representation.

3   THE ENCODING OF IMAGES

3.1   Spatial Frequency Channels

The studies presented below were suggested by an article written by Schade (1956). This article reports experiments in which sinusoidal gratings were used as stimulus configurations. A sinusoidal grating consists of alternating light and dark stripes. It arises when the luminance of, for example, a computer monitor, is modulated sinusoidally in one direction (at 90 degrees to the stripes) and is held constant orthogonal to this (in the direction of the stripes). One particular advantage of sinusoidal gratings is that the contrast between the light and the dark stripes and the density of their sequence (spatial frequency) can be varied without having to change the mean luminance of the total configuration. This maintains the human (or animal) subject's visual system in a constant adaptation state.

3.1.1   Findings

One of the findings demonstrated by Schade (1956) was that sensitivity to contrast in the human visual system depends critically on the spatial frequency generated in the stimulus. However, this finding initially received very little attention. It was only taken up again in the mid-1960s and confirmed and extended in both the human domain (Bryngdahl, 1966a, b; Campbell and Robson, 1964, 1968) and in the behavior of retinal ganglion cells in cats (Enroth-Cugell and Robson, 1966). These replications and extensions of Schade's (1956) findings led, in turn, to a great number of further studies. These are summarized by, for example, Graham (1981) and Shapley and Lennie (1985).[4] In all, findings show that there can be hardly any

---

[4]Detailed findings are reported in, for example: Bradley, Switkes and De Valois (1988); Burbeck (1988); Campbell, Cooper and Enroth-Cugell (1969); Campbell, Nachmias and Jukes (1970); Carpenter and Ganz (1972); Chua (1990); De Valois, De Valois and Yund (1979); Fiorentini and Berardi (1981); Glezer, Shcherbach and Gauzel'man (1979); Greenlee and Breitmeyer (1989); Harwerth and Levi (1978); Heeley (1987); Hirsch and Hyltton (1982); Kroon, Rijsdijk and van der Wildt (1980); Kroon and van der Wildt (1980); Lupp, Hauske and Wolf (1976); Maffei and Fiorentini (1973); Mayer and Kim (1986); Musselwhite and Jeffreys (1985); Phillips and Wilson (1984); Regan (1983); Regan and Regan (1988); Rudd (1988); Sagi and Hochstein (1984, 1985); Savoy and McCann (1975); Skrandies (1984); Wilson (1976).

doubt that the human visual system possesses individual, relatively autonomous *channels* that specialize in the detection of specific spatial frequencies.

3.1.2 The Fourier Transform

The detection of these spatial frequency channels has led to far-reaching speculations. For example, there has been conjecture that the human visual system is able to calculate two-dimensional *Fourier transforms* (see, for example, Ginsburg, 1984; Harvey and Gervais, 1978, 1981; Maffei, 1978; Maffei and Fiorentini, 1972, 1973; Mayhew and Frisby, 1978). This procedure is based on the fact that any number of images can be produced through the addition of suitable sinusoidal gratings. 'Suitable' means that each sinusoidal grating to be added must show a defined spatial frequency, phase position (relative position to each other), amplitude (intensity) and orientation (for details, see, for example, Weisstein, 1980). Conversely, Fourier's theorem states that any image can be decomposed into sinusoidal gratings (frequency dispersion).

The frequency dispersion of such images as arise in our normal surroundings nonetheless leads to a great number of sinusoidal gratings being necessary for their description; that is, natural images generally contain a great number of different spatial frequencies and orientations. In order to achieve the most comprehensible presentation of the outcome of dispersion, frequently two separate, in each case two-dimensional, spectra containing different kinds of information are calculated. One of these is the power spectrum.[5] The power spectrum represents each spatial frequency present in the image being analyzed according to its relative weight and its orientation as a column on a two-dimensional plane. Figure 2.17 shows such a plane in polar coordinates.

Each column, which can be conceived as being entered at any location in Figure 2.17, provides the following information:

(1) *The relative weight of the spatial frequency* represented: This information is represented by the length of the columns.
(2) *The height of the spatial frequency represented*: this information is given by the distance of the columns in question from the center (zero point) of the plane. Low spatial frequencies are found close to the zero point; higher frequencies are further in the periphery.[6]
(3) *The orientation of the spatial frequency represented*: this information is contained in the orientation of an imaginary line connecting the center of the plane to the spatial frequency column in question.

In summary, the power spectrum reports which spatial frequencies with which orientation and which relative weight are contained in the image being analyzed (detailed descriptions of power spectra can be found in, for example, Weisstein, 1980).

Information on the phase (i.e. the positions of the sinusoidal gratings relative to each other) of the spatial frequencies contained in the image being analyzed cannot

---

[5]The power spectrum is also called the energy spectrum. Some researchers also refer to the amplitude spectrum, which is simply the square root of the power spectrum.
[6]The cpd (cycles per degree), which is widely used as a unit in Anglo-American countries, has been adopted as a measure of spatial frequency.

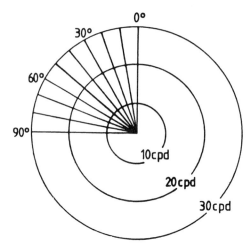

Figure 2.17. *Two-dimensional spectral level in polar coordinates.*

be derived from the power spectrum. This information is represented in the *phase spectrum*. Hence, without the information contained in phase spectrum, an image-retaining retransformation into the spatial domain is not possible.

3.1.3   Filter Operations in the Frequency Domain

Before evaluating the relevance of this approach to processes of perceptual organization, we must initially consider which advantages could be linked to the transformation of a (retinal) image from the spatial to the frequency domain. First of all, it has to be noted that a mathematically exact Fourier transform represents a linear (information-true) operation; that is, representations in spatial and frequency domains correspond in the sense that no information has been lost or gained in the transformation. Nonetheless, the two domains seem to differ in their suitability for representing certain properties of an image, as the explicitness with which these properties are represented in the two domains differs. As shown in the description of the power spectrum, periodic structures and orientations are properties of the image that stand out particularly in the frequency domain. This makes them easier to analyze and manipulate here than they would be in the spatial domain. The application of *filter operations* in the frequency domain can now emphasize or suppress these special image properties in a particularly simple way. In principle, two orthogonal filterings of the power spectrum are possible, as follows.

Frequency-specific Filtering
This filter operation is rotation-invariant; that is, it impacts on all orientations in the same way. By filtering out individual areas of the spatial frequency spectrum, certain properties of the image can be emphasized at the cost of others. For instance, higher spatial frequencies predominantly contain information about abrupt changes in the distribution of luminance within an image, such as those that can be elicited by object borders. In contrast, information on the broad, global structure of the

image can be taken from low spatial frequencies; fine details of the image are not represented in this frequency band.

Orientation-specific Filtering

This filter operation is size-invariant; that is, it extends across all the spatial frequencies contained in the image. One function of this operation could be the segmentation of pictorial information, and that always when dissimilar orientations dominate different areas of the image (see Daugman and Kammen, 1986) . The size of the elements of the image that contain information on the orientations is neglected in this filter procedure.

An important property of both of these filter operations is their position-invariance; that is, all areas of the image are equally affected by the filtering. The reason for this is that both filterings relate to the power spectrum. It is only in the power spectrum that information about the spatial frequencies and orientations contained in the image is so explicit that it can simply be filtered out. As already mentioned above, information can be drawn relatively simply from the power spectrum on, for example, whether the structuring of an image is coarser or finer (or both). However, the information contained in the power spectrum alone cannot determine *which* areas of the image this applies to. The situation is similar for individual orientations: although the power spectrum provides information on which orientations with which relative weight are contained in the image, it does not reveal *where* these orientations are to be found in the image.

This is also expressed in the so-called displacement theorem of the Fourier transform. This theorem states that a displacement (i.e. a change in the position) of an object within an image has no effect on the power spectrum. Such a shift is only registered in the phase spectrum. Hence, position information can only be obtained by referring back to the phase spectrum, as only the phase spectrum contains the information on the relative positions of all sinusoidal gratings needed to synthesize the original image.

3.1.4 Functional Value of Global Frequency Decomposition

From the end of the 1960s up to the middle of the 1970s, the dominant opinion in the literature was that spatial frequencies in some way formed the 'elementary particles' of visual perception (see Maffei, 1978; Maffei and Fiorentini, 1973; Pollen, Lee and Taylor, 1971). According to this concept, higher perceptual contents have to be synthesized from these elementary particles. This concept is confronted with at least three elementary difficulties:

(1) The functional purpose of spatial frequency channels remains unclear. Which pictorial information should be made explicit by the transformation and thus made available for easier further processing? As mentioned above, the information that can be taken from the power spectrum has only a very limited value as it does not contain any information on position. However, position information is only access-ible through recourse to the phase spectrum, with whose assistance the image has to be, so to speak, resynthesized. The question arises: What is gained through such a procedure? What is its value?

(2) If *all* visual impressions are actually synthesized from the activity of spatial frequency-specific channels, these channels must be extremely narrow-band, that is, highly selective. The reason for this is the high acuity in the fovea. Such a high resolution requires the activity of a large number of analyzers placed very closely together in the frequency domain. However, this contradicts available findings (see, for example, Wilson and Giese, 1977). Although an inspection of the literature reveals a fairly large variation in the number of frequency-specific channels assumed in various studies, this generally ranges from four (Graham, 1981) to eight (Watson, 1983) distinguishable channels, which is far too low a number.

(3) The two-dimensional Fourier transform is a 'global' operation; that is, its input information is a complete image. Hence, if a two-dimensional Fourier transform is actually performed during visual information processing, it should be possible to detect neurons within the visual system that can be triggered by light stimuli at any point in the retina, that is, whose 'catchment area' is the entire retina. However, as far as we know, no such neurons have been found up to now.

In summary, the observer is confronted with a somewhat curious picture at this stage: the multitude of research triggered by the highly acclaimed studies of, above all, Campbell and Robson (1968) and Enroth-Cugell and Robson (1966) leaves no serious doubt that there are spatial-frequency- and orientation-sensitive 'channels' in the visual systems of higher mammals and human beings. In addition, a reasonable amount is known about their number and properties. However, there is still uncertainty about their exact purpose.

3.1.5 Local Frequency Decomposition

Because of the above-mentioned difficulties involved in a global Fourier transform, another concept quickly gained in importance. This was suggested above all by findings on the reaction of receptive fields in the visual cortex of cats. The idea is based on a relatively coarse, *piece-by-piece* frequency decomposition (patch-wise Fourier analysis; see Glezer, Ivanoff and Tscherbach, 1973; Pollen, Lee and Taylor, 1971; Robson, 1975; for a more recent review, see De Valois and De Valois, 1988). The basic assumption is that there are functional subareas of the retina (receptive fields), and that these subareas are able to perform *local* frequency decompositions. This theory of local frequency decomposition has significant advantages. However, the complete extent of these advantages can only be understood when they are viewed against the background of a theoretical approach that has become particularly well known through the work of Marr (for a summary, see Marr, 1982) . This approach has criticized the scientific attitude to neurophysiology and psychophysics that dominated the early 1970s and has supplemented it with an additional concept. A crucial element of this new concept is the demand that more emphasis should be placed on ascertaining the *functional purpose* of specific *information processing strategies* in biological systems.

In the following, an attempt will be made to take into account Marr's comments and to consider the findings on the local frequency decomposition of the retinal image from a slightly different perspective. This perspective results from asking what functional purpose such a mechanism of local frequency decomposition could have. However, in order to pursue this question, it is first necessary to discuss some general considerations on the encoding of images.

3.2 Representation and Redundancy

An elementary problem in any image-processing system, be it biological or technical, concerns the system-internal representation of the image. The simplest method of transforming an image into a system-internal representation is the point-to-point method commonly used in nearly all technical systems. In this method, the activity of each photosensitive element is represented one-to-one in the system. Applied to biological systems, this would mean that each photoreceptor (at least on the level of the first layer of connections) is linked to exactly one nerve cell inside the system. However, such a method would be a very uneconomical way of dealing with the images that confront us in our natural environment. It would only be appropriate if white noise had to be transformed and represented. In white noise, the intensities of individual image points are statistically independent from each other. However, real images are characterized by a high level of correlation between neighboring points. In this case, high correlation means that there is a relatively high probability that neighboring points will have the same or similar brightness values. In other words, real images contain a large amount of *redundant* information. However, an effective representation should be cleared of redundancies to a large extent. This is the only way to optimally exploit limited resources (e.g. limited channel capacities). This idea was already formulated by Barlow in the early 1970s (e.g. Barlow, 1972).[7] Barlow considered that a functional goal of neural information processing should be to transform pictorial information into a system-internal representation based on the smallest possible number of active nerve cells without this leading to the loss of any important information. To achieve this goal, pictorial information has to be recoded in such a way that the highest possible proportion of redundant information is filtered out. How are such filters designed?

Because of the high correlation between neighboring points in natural images, these filters must first possess the following properties:

(1) They should not be restricted to the encoding of a *single* image point but should also take into account neighboring points that have a high probability of exhibiting a very similar luminance.
(2) They should be optimally adjusted to natural images, that is, they should economically encode those image structures that occur frequently in natural images.

In the following, two examples will be used to show that certain receptive fields found in the retina, lateral geniculate nucleus and visual cortex of mammals, are actually suitable for filtering out redundancies from images.

3.2.1 Contour Filters

The first example refers to receptive fields with concentrically arranged and antagonistically discharging areas (center-surround receptive fields; see, for example, Hubel and Wiesel, 1962; Kuffler, 1953). A three-dimensional presentation of the sensitivity function or weighting function of these fields looks like a Mexican

---

[7]The more recently published book *Vision: Coding and Efficiency*, edited by Blakemore (1990), once more impressively points out the particular importance of an efficient coding and representation of pictorial information in biological and technical systems.

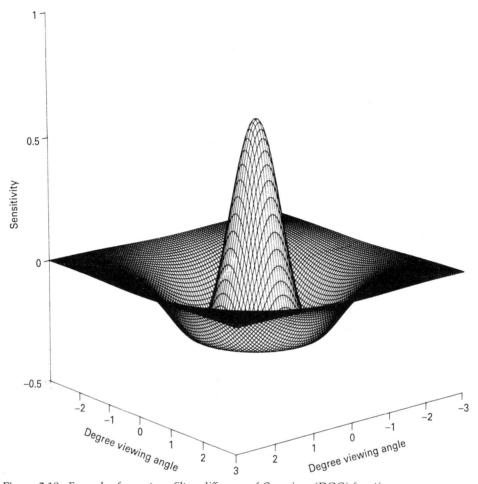

Figure 2.18. *Example of a contour filter: difference of Gaussians (DOG) function.*

hat (Marr, 1982). A Laplacian of Gaussian (LOG) operation (Marr and Hildreth, 1980) or a difference of Gaussians (DOG) (Heggelund, 1981; Rose, 1979; Wilson and Giese, 1977) is frequently used to provide mathematical descriptions of the empirically ascertained sensitivity properties of Mexican hats. Both functions (LOG and DOG) are very similar when suitable parameters are selected (Marr and Hildreth, 1980). Figure 2.18 shows such a function. It results from the difference between two three-dimensional gaussians in which the excitatory function has to have a larger amplitude but a smaller width than the inhibitory function.

The illumination of a receptive field that possesses the features presented in Figure 2.18 has the following effect: if a small point light is projected only onto the excitatory center of the field, this leads to an increase in the activity of the next layer of neural structures. A selective illumination of the inhibitory surround, in contrast, leads to an inhibition of the activity of these structures.

Encoding the retinal image with the help of Mexican hats leads to a reduction of the redundancy contained in the image, as the fields react particularly distinctively to *changes* (high information content) in the image (e.g. luminance edges), while homogeneous lighting (low information content) leads to much smaller reactions. This behavior is particularly apparent when the field is adjusted so that the effects of excitatory and inhibitory areas cancel each other out precisely. In this case the reaction of the field to homogeneous lighting is zero. However, if a discontinuity in luminance falls on the field (e.g. a contrast edge), its reaction is either larger than zero (if light falls on the center and shadow on part of the surround) or less than zero, that is, it drops below spontaneous activity (if light falls only on parts of the surround while the center remains in shadow).

3.2.2 Structure Filters

The second example of receptive fields that are able to filter out redundancy from images refers to orientation-sensitive structures like those already found by Hubel and Wiesel (1962) in the visual cortex of cats. While the contour filters presented in the prior section are able to reduce *first-order redundancies* (conditional probabilities in the distribution of the luminance of neighboring points without taking into account orientation), structure filters are applied to *second-order redundancies*. These redundancies arise from the fact that real images frequently depict objects with relatively straight borders and relatively constant surface properties. Redundancy arises because the probability that an object border continues in a specific direction without any major change of direction is higher, and hence easier to predict, than the probability that it will change direction continuously. The same argument can be applied to textured areas of images. As there is a relatively high probability that an area of the image with a certain texture also comes from the surface of a certain object, it is probable and hence predictable that the texture remains relatively constant over a certain area (as real objects have extension in space).

The redundancy-reducing effect of structure filters consists of their being very economical in encoding second-order redundancies. The mechanism of redundancy reduction leads to larger areas of an image made up of several image points being assigned to the activity of an individual cell. The level of this activity is determined by how far the section of the image projected on that filter agrees with its weighting function.[8] In turn, the weighting function is adjusted to particularly probable structures in natural images (straight edges, constant textures; see above). Hence, as a result of this presetting, particularly probable image structures are encoded into the reactions of only a few cells. To be able to perform the above-mentioned redundancy-reducing function, structure filters must demonstrate at least two properties:

(1) They must react selectively to specific spatial frequencies (in order to detect different periodic structures).
(2) They must respond to defined orientations (in order to be capable of signalling straight parts of the image).

Both these properties are met by a number of mathematical functions. For example, it has been proposed that contour filters should be relayed tandem-like,

---

[8]This description brings the structure filter conceptually very close to feature detectors as described by, for example, Selfridge (1959). A later section will show that, under certain conditions, structure filters can certainly be conceived as an operationalization of feature detectors.

one behind the other, to structure filters (Hawken and Parker, 1987; Marr and Hildreth, 1980; Watson, 1990). This procedure has the advantage that it presents a hierarchical structure, that is, 'simple' contour filters are used to construct more complex structure filters. Such a procedure is particularly economical (Nakayama, 1990; Rosenfeld, 1990). A further mathematical function that reacts sensitively to both spatial frequencies and orientations is the two-dimensional Gabor filter. This filter function has one significant advantage compared to all other functions. It will be reported in more detail below.

3.3   The Uncertainty Relation

Some time ago, two independent publications (Daugman, 1980; Marcelja, 1980) proposed a filter function for processing pictorial information originally developed for processing signals in the time and temporal frequency domain (radio signals; see Gabor, 1946) . This function (the Gabor function) is characterized by representing the best possible solution to the so-called uncertainty relation of the Fourier transform. When the uncertainty relation is applied to image processing, it states that there is an inevitable mutual dependence between the representation of an object in the spatial domain and in the frequency domain; that is, an object represented, for example, with high precision in the spatial domain leads to a blurred representation in the frequency domain and vice versa (for more detail, see Daugman, 1980, 1985). For example, a small point in the spatial domain has a very broad frequency spectrum, while a very broad sinusoidal grating in the spatial domain can be described with a single point in the frequency domain. Two-dimensional Gabor functions are characterized by the fact that the amount of space they occupy in *both* the spatial and frequency domains *together* is minimal.

This is relatively easy to illustrate: suppose that we intended to develop a spatial frequency filter with high selectivity, that is, a small bandwidth; and we wanted to do this without recourse to mathematical procedures. We could only achieve this goal by constructing a receptive surface with a great number of alternatingly excitatory and inhibitory areas. This receptive surface would then be at maximum excitation when illuminated with a pattern of stripes designed so that the light parts precisely cover the excitatory and the dark parts the inhibitory areas of the receptive surface. The frequency resolution of such a filter depends directly on the number of antagonistically connected areas: a high number leads to a high frequency selectivity (small bandwidth), while a small number of areas is linked to a broad bandwidth. The reason for this is that a small difference between the preferred frequency of the filter and the spatial frequency of the stimulus grating only becomes noticeable in the long run, as small deviations first have to add up to a larger error.

However, the number of antagonistically connected areas in this imaginary field simultaneously determines (when the preferred frequency is held constant) the extension of such a field: the greater the frequency selectivity (small bandwidth in the frequency domain), the larger the field in the spatial domain has to be. Conversely, a small field in the spatial domain leads to a poor selectivity for spatial frequencies (broad bandwidth in the frequency domain). This reciprocal, inevitable dependence between representations in the spatial and frequency domain is called the *uncertainty relation* of the Fourier transform.

Of course, the Gabor function is also unable to resolve the uncertainty relation; however, it does minimize the *shared* space taken in the spatial and frequency domains. This property of the two-dimensional Gabor function has been the major reason that it has received increasing interest in the field of visual research during the past 10 years (for an overview, see Daugman, 1983, 1984, 1985, 1988, 1989; Marcelja, 1980).[9] The reasons for this interest vary in nature; some will be discussed below.

3.3.1 The Fourier Transform and the Uncertainty Relation

First, we must discuss a question raised in the section on the Fourier transform that possibly can be answered by the uncertainty relation of the Fourier transform. This concerns the functional purpose of spatial frequency-specific channels and leads back to the findings on the local Fourier transform already mentioned earlier (Glezer, Ivanoff and Tscherbach, 1973; Pollen, Lee and Taylor, 1971; Robson, 1975). These findings report the presence of nerve cells in the visual cortex of cats that react when a sinusoidal grating with a specific spatial frequency and orientation is projected onto a *specific location* of the retina. If the *size* of this sinusoidal grating is varied, these cells track such a variation only up to a certain value. If the size of the grating is raised above this limit, the reaction of the cell remains asymptotic. As already described above, it was very soon realized that the bandwidths of the spatial frequency channels found prove to be relatively broad and only permit a coarse frequency decomposition.

Against the background of the uncertainty relation, this finding comes as no surprise, because the bandwidth of frequency-specific channels and the size of the receptive fields that cause the frequency decomposition have an inverse relationship: relatively small receptive fields necessarily result in broad bandwidths. In view of the uncertainty relation, the question raised above on the possible functional purpose of a local frequency decomposition should first be inverted: what would be the functional purpose of a global frequency decomposition (i.e. not local but extending across the entire retina)? The possible consequence of such a global frequency decomposition would without doubt be narrow-band filters, that is, a high frequency selectivity. Perhaps this would also permit a halfway exact Fourier transform. However, what would be gained by this? The uncertainty relation states that the price for this high frequency selectivity would be a very fuzzy representation in the spatial domain. What use can a system make of information that an object is represented *somewhere* in the retinal representation with a specific spatial frequency spectrum, even when the very precise spectrum reveals the identity of the object? Hence, if the visual system performs a frequency decomposition – and

---

[9]For further references, see Anderson and Burr (1989); Beck, Rosenfeld and Ivry (1989); Beck, Sutter and Ivry (1987); Bovik, Clark and Geisler (1990); Caelli and Moraglia (1985); Clark and Bovik (1989); Clark, Bovik and Geisler (1987); Dannemiller and Ver Hoeve (1990); Dobbins, Zucker and Cynader (1989); Field (1987); Fogel and Sagi (1989); Harvey Jr and Doan (1990); Heeley (1991); Jones and Palmer (1987); Kulikowski, Marcelja and Bishop (1982); Kulikowski and Vidyasagar (1986); Landy and Bergen (1991); Landy, Manovich and Stetten (1990); Malik and Perona (1990); Moraglia (1989); Pollen and Ronner (1981, 1983); Rubenstein and Sagi (1990); Sagi (1990); Sakitt and Barlow (1982); Stork and Wilson (1990); Sutter, Beck and Graham (1989); Toet and Koenderink (1988); Turner (1986); Victor (1989); Watson (1983, 1987); Watson, Barlow and Robson (1983); Webster and De Valois (1985); Wilson and Knutsson (1988); Young (1987).

in view of the findings reported above, there can be little doubt that it does–this frequency decomposition only makes sense when it is local and, hence, necessarily relatively coarse. This is the only way in which the representation in the spatial domain can have the necessary precision.

Against the background of these mutually conflicting demands for simultaneous, maximally focused representations in both the spatial and frequency domains given by the uncertainty relation, it does not appear to be improbable that an optimal solution to this problem has been sought during the course of evolution and perhaps has been found in the form of two-dimensional Gabor filters.

4   A MORE RECENT MODEL OF TEXTURE SEGMENTATION

4.1   Gabor Filters

Two-dimensional Gabor functions are composed of two, Gaussian shaped curves set at 90 degrees to each other. One of the two curves has a cosine-like modulation (Figure 2.19). They can be conceived as hypothetical structures of receptive fields.

The positive sections in Figure 2.19 correspond to the excitatory areas of the receptive field described by the function, while the negative sections stand for the inhibitory areas. Hence, when an excitatory area of the field is illuminated selectively, for example, with a small spotlight, activity increases; when an inhibitory area is illuminated, it decreases. When Gabor functions are applied as filters (Gabor filter), the cosine-like modulation generates a sensitivity for a specific spatial frequency. The reaction of the filter is namely at a maximum when it is illuminated with a grating that permits light to fall on the excitatory areas and shadow on the inhibitory areas. This is the case when the spatial frequency of the grating used for illumination and the preferred frequency of the filter are in agreement, and the grating is in the correct position. The grating is always in the correct position, that is, the one that triggers the maximum reaction, when it has a specific orientation and a specific phase position (shift in the direction of modulation) relative to the filter. The optimal orientation is given when the dark stripes of the grating lie longitudinally in the valleys of the filter and the light stripes illuminate the hills longitudinally. An illumination at 90 degrees to this preferred orientation has the same effect as an illumination with homogeneous light. The phase position is optimal when light stripes fall *only* on the hills and dark stripes *only* in the valleys. In addition, the strength of the filter's activity naturally also depends on the extent of the light contrast, that is, the *relative* difference in luminance between the light and dark stripes of the illumination grating. For the sake of simplicity, we will assume here that the *absolute* intensity of illumination has no effect on the reaction of the filter. This is always given when excitatory and inhibitory areas match each other in their antagonistic effect.

Hence, in summary, four parameters determine the reaction of the filter: contrast, spatial frequency, orientation and phase position. As these four parameters can vary independently, we are faced with the problem of the ambiguity of the filter reaction: if the activity of the filter changes, it cannot be decided unequivocally which parameter variation is responsible for this change. However, the ambiguity problem can be solved by introducing a *second* filter. This second filter must share the following features with the first one: (1) it must cover the same section of the

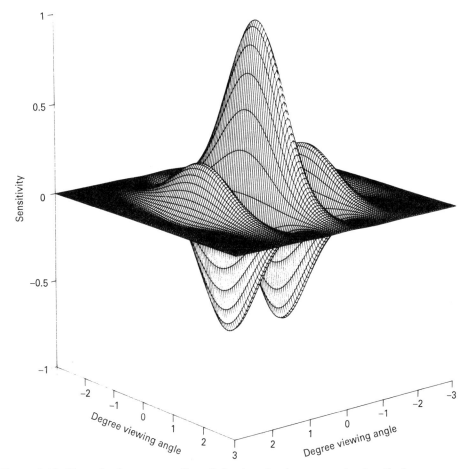

Figure 2.19. *Example of a structure filter: Gabor function (even, or cosine function).*

image; (2) it must have the same preferred frequency and preferred orientation; and (3) it must have a 90-degree phase shift to the first filter.

A Gabor filter with these properties is presented in Figure 2.20.

The first function, illustrated in Figure 2.19, is also called the even function or cosine function; and the second, shown in Figure 2.20, is the odd or sine function. At this stage, we will not derive why the ambiguities in the filter reaction can be overcome with a *pair* of filters. However, we shall refer to an article by Daugman (1988) that has demonstrated that an *image-retaining* transformation can be performed with the help of paired Gabor filters (see also Bovik, Clark and Geisler, 1990; Marcelja, 1980). Image-retaining means that an image is transformed through filtering into a Gabor representation and could finally be retransformed without any loss of pictorial information.[10] However, such an operation is only conceivable if all ambiguities in the filter reactions can be eliminated.

---

[10]Readers interested in a formal derivation will find further information in Bastiaans (1981).

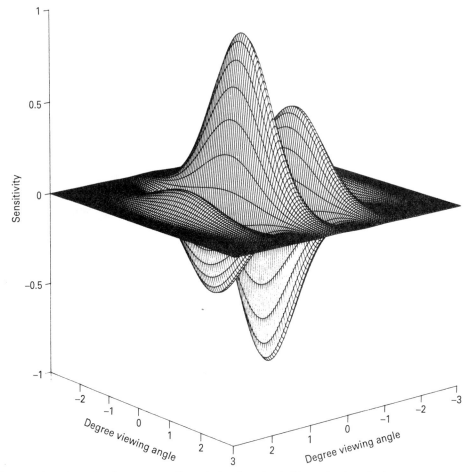

Figure 2.20. *Example of a structure filter: Gabor function (odd, or sine function).*

The possibility of being able to perform image-retaining transformations with the help of Gabor functions initially appears to contradict the arguments presented in the context of the Fourier transform. In section 2.4.2, we pointed out that an image-retaining Fourier transform would require a large number of frequency components placed very closely together. This holds at least for practically all real images. Against this background, it initially seems astonishing that the relatively coarse frequency decomposition obtained with Gabor filters can be image-retaining (see section 3.3 on the uncertainty relation). The reason for this is the local character of Gabor filtering, that is, the relatively small areas of an image to which the filter operations refer. The Fourier transform as discussed in section 3.1.1, in contrast, is a global filter operation involving the entire image. It follows that the outcome of the global Fourier transform is a spectrum containing the information on the entire image. However, a great number of single frequency components are required for a description of this complete image. Filtering an image with the help of local Gabor filters, in contrast, produces *several* spectra. The actual number is determined by the sizes and area of overlap of the filter systems applied. Hence, each individual Gabor filter covers only one section of the image; and a description of this section requires a smaller number of single frequency components than is necessary for the complete image.

The circumstance that fewer frequency components are required for a complete description (image-retaining synthesis) of a small section of the image than for the description of a larger section (or even the complete image) results from the linear (information-true) character of the Fourier transform pointed out above. Under the condition of a constant receptive sampling of the image to be filtered (given, for example, by the set retinal 'mosaic' of the photoreceptors), a smaller section of the image contains less information than the entire image; hence, fewer frequency components are necessary for its complete description. This becomes particularly apparent when we look at the *discrete* Fourier transform (Cooley and Tukey, 1965) that is always used when it is necessary to transform arbitrary signals, which cannot be described simply with mathematical formulae (e.g. real images), into the frequency domain. The discrete Fourier transform maximally provides just as many frequency components as sampling points from the spatial domain that enter into the transform. Under the given precondition of a set sampling grid, the number of scanning points will naturally be greater in a complete image than in a section of it. Hence, the transformation of the section of the image produces fewer frequency components than the transformation of the entire image.

Daugman (1988) has confirmed not only that an image-retaining transformation can be performed with Gabor filters but also, in addition, that real images[11] can be represented in Gabor space much more economically than with point-for-point encoding. This leads back to the original question on the functional purpose of a local frequency decomposition like the one that can be performed, for example, with two-dimensional Gabor functions. *One* function of this decomposition could be to extract second-order redundancies from the retinal image in order to make encoding as compact as possible. If this is actually true, it should be possible to confirm empirically that such transformations can also be performed by biological systems. This seems to be the case: in a series of studies, evidence was found that certain neurons in the visual cortex of mammals (simple cells) possess receptive fields that can be described very adequately with the properties of two-dimensional Gabor functions (Jones and Palmer, 1987; Kulikowski and Bishop, 1981; Kulikowski, Marcelja and Bishop, 1982; Mullikin, Jones and Palmer, 1984). Furthermore, Pollen and Ronner (1983) have reported that they were able to identify nerve cells in the visual cortex of cats with receptive fields that only differed from each other in a 90-degree phase shift. The existence of such cells is necessary in order to eliminate ambiguities (see above) in the reactions of single cells. Findings from psycho-physiological experiments indicate that Gabor-like receptive fields can also be found in the human visual system (Daugman, 1984; Sagi, 1990; Watson, Barlow and Robson, 1983; Webster and De Valois, 1985).

At this point, however, it has to be stressed that other weighting functions than those mentioned in this chapter have been proposed for both contour and structure filters. Nonetheless, they only deviate relatively slightly from those mentioned here (see, for example, Hawken and Parker, 1987).

---

[11] The actual image used was the well-known portrait of a woman wearing a hat (the so-called 'Lena picture').

The previous section viewed findings on local frequency decomposition from a particular perspective. This perspective focuses on image processing as an *information processing problem* and investigates the constraints that any system, regardless of what kind, has to consider when solving this problem. We focused on the restricted resources of such a limited system as *one* such constraint, and we then asked how the system-internal image representation can be coded as compactly as possible. It was shown that certain two-dimensional filters (DOG, Gabor) are suitable for reducing first- or second-order redundancies in the encoding of images and that, in this way, they lead to compact codes for system-internal image representation. In addition, empirical findings from neurophysiology and psychophysics have been reported that confirm that these filters can also be found in biological systems. In summary, this information suggests that redundancy-reducing, two-dimensional filters are involved in the processing of visual information.

4.2   Two-dimensional Filters and Segmentation

The following section will show that two-dimensional filters are not just suitable for generating representations of images with few redundancies but can additionally be used for the segmentation of pictorial information.

4.2.1   Contour Filters and Texture Segmentation

With regard to contour filters, it is apparent that this type of filter not only reduces redundancy but also segments, as it makes contrast edges explicit and thus makes it possible to separate areas of varying luminance. This permits a *segmentation* of pictorial information on the basis of differences in luminance. The next section shows that segmentation can also be performed with the help of structure filters. However, this segmentation process is not based on differences in luminance but on differences in the composition of textures.

4.2.2   Structure Filters and Texture Segmentation

The obvious correlations between Gabor filtering and the Fourier transform suggest that there might be a relationship between the filtering of visual input information by structure filters and perceptual segmentation processes. Both transforms convert an image from the spatial to the frequency domain. As already described in section 2.4.2, a representation in the frequency domain is particularly suitable for describing textures. With Gabor filters, it is very simple to determine, for example, the local periodic structure and orientation of areas of the image. Therefore, by comparing the activity of neighboring Gabor filters, it should be possible to trace local changes in these image properties and hence perceive probable texture borders. Such ideas have prompted researchers to test the ability of Gabor filters to segment textures in simulation studies on computer systems (Beck, Sutter and Ivry, 1987; Bergen and Landy, 1991; Bovik, Clark and Geisler, 1990; Clark and Bovik, 1989; Clark, Bovik and Geisler, 1987; Fogel and Sagi,1989; Sutter, Beck and Graham, 1989; Turner, 1986)

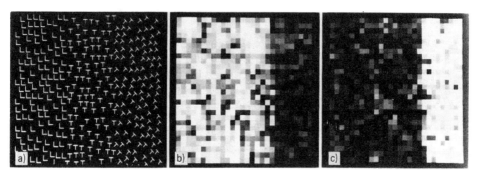

Figure 2.21. *(a) A texture first used by Beck (1966) to demonstrate the strong effect of orientation differences on segmentation. (b) Outcome of simulation when filters are used with only 0- and 90-degree orientation. (c) As (b), but now with 45- and 135-degree orientation. [From Turner, 1986, p. 76, Fig. 4. © 1986 Springer; reprinted with kind permission.]*

In general, the results of these simulation studies have been positive. We shall use the studies of Fogel and Sagi (1989) and Turner (1986) as examples and describe them in more detail, as both studies refer to psychophysiological findings that are considered to be particularly important in the field of texture segmentation. The goal of both studies was to use computer simulation to test how far certain textures used in psychophysiological experiments could be segmented with the help of Gabor filters in a way that is comparable to the performance of the human visual system. For this purpose, the textures to be segmented were first digitalized (all textures were exclusively binary) to enable their further processing on common computer systems. In a second step, the digitalized textures were either convolved (Fogel and Sagi, 1989) or cross-correlated (Turner, 1986) with a series of Gabor filters with different parameters. Both procedures (convolution, crosscorrelation), which will not be described in detail here (details can be found in, for example, Jähne, 1989, Rosenfeld and Kak, 1982), result in a value reporting the level of agreement between the characteristic of the filter mask (in this case, Gabor characteristic) and the area of the image it covers. A high level of agreement is always given when the light parts of the texture cover the areas of the Gabor filter that have an 'excitatory' effect and the areas of the filter mask with an 'inhibitory' effect remain unilluminated. In order to make the outcome of this operation visible, the calculated values of each filter activity were transformed into brightness values and presented together with the input texture. As a first example, Figure 2.21 presents the outcome of a computer simulation by Turner (1986).

Figure 2.21a shows a texture that was first used by Beck (1966) . A glance at this texture reveals the strong segmenting effect of differences in orientation. Although, in individual comparisons of the texture elements used, subjects estimate the similarity between a slanted and an upright T as being higher than the similarity between an upright T and an upright L, perceptual segmentation of textures composed of these letters shows a much clearer border between the slanted and upright Ts than between the upright Ts and the upright Ls. This finding on segmentation can be illustrated easily in the simulation with Gabor filters, as these are sensitive to orientation. This has been explained in detail in section 4.1. Figure

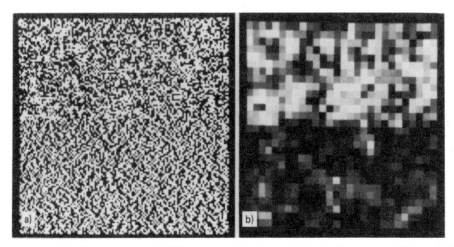

Figure 2.22. *(a) Julesz texture with different second-order statistics in the upper and lower half of the texture. (b) Outcome of simulation (90-degree filter orientation). From Turner, 1986, Fig. 6.* © *1986 Springer; reprinted with kind permission.]*

2.21b, c presents the values calculated in the simulation in the form of more or less gray squares, in which the light squares stand for a strong and the dark squares for a weak reaction of the Gabor filter covering the respective texture area. The preferred orientations for the Gabor filters used were set at 0 and 90 degrees to generate the reactions displayed in Figure 2.21b, and 45 and 135 degrees to generate the reactions in Figure 2.21c. The reactions of the single filters with a preferred orientation of either 0 and 90 degrees or 45 and 135 degrees were each added together and their sum was presented as a brightness value. The figures show that with the help of Gabor filtering it was possible to emphasize *specific local* orientations selectively. In Figure 2.21b these are 0 and 90 degrees; in Figure 2.21c, 45 and 135 degrees.

Figure 2.22 presents a further example of the successful use of Gabor filters to segment textures.

Figure 2.22 shows a 'Julesz texture' with different second-order statistics in its upper and lower regions. The difference is the result of random generation of the upper part of the texture compared with restricted randomness in the lower part. This restriction prevented more than four points in a line from having the same shade of gray. This manipulation leads to the generation of longer horizontal areas of the same shade of gray in the upper half of the texture than in the lower half. As Figure 2.22b shows, with the help of Gabor filtering, it was also possible in this example to transform this difference in second-order statistics into a difference in luminance, that is, a difference in first-order statistics. Of course, a precondition for a successful transform is the selection of suitable parameters for the Gabor filters. For example, only Gabor filters with a horizontal orientation preference were used to calculate Figure 2.22b. As the remaining parameters, such as preferred spatial frequency, extension in the spatial domain, and phase position are not important for the present argument, they are not illustrated here.

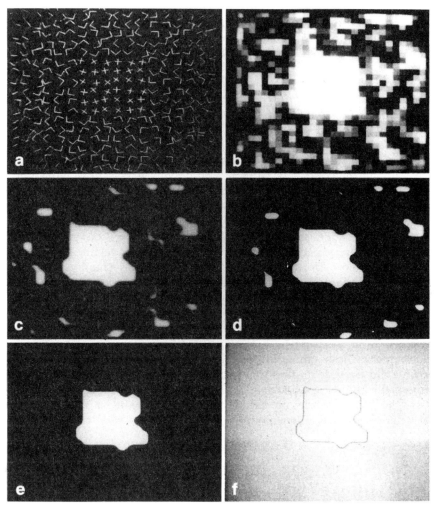

Figure 2.23. *(a) A texture as used by Bergen and Julesz (1983) to confirm the effect of crossings on segmentation. (b) Outcome of simulation with Gabor filters. (c)–(f) Additional computation steps to determine the boundary between target texture and ground texture (see text for explanation). [From Fogel and Sagi, 1989, p. 109, Fig. 7. © 1989 Springer; reprinted with kind permission.]*

Turner's (1986) simulation studies have shown that with the help of Gabor filtering, it is possible to reduce differences in second-order statistics by one order, that is, to differences in first-order statistics. However, Turner's studies do not show how this reduction can be used for a successful segmentation, that is, determination of borders between various texture areas. This is where the study by Fogel and Sagi (1989) comes in: as in Turner, the first stage of simulation was to perform a filtering of input information with the aid of Gabor filters. A good correspondence was found between simulation outcome (i.e. differences in luminance) and data from psychophysiological experiments. This validated and expanded Turner's findings (other textures were used). Beyond this, Fogel and Sagi traced the areas of higher Gabor activity (represented by higher luminance in a newly constructed image) on a second stage of processing with the aid of contour filters (LOGs) and segmented the texture by determining a border. Figure 2.23 presents each single stage of this calculation.

As Figure 2.23 shows, Fogel and Sagi's (1989) simulation calls for three further stages of processing in addition to the previously mentioned Gabor filtering (Figure 2.23b) and LOG filtering (Figure 2.23f). These are: a filtering out of higher spatial frequencies (Figure 2.23c), a threshold value calculation (Figure 2.23d) and the removal of small patches of noise (Figure 2.23e). These stages will not be reported in detail, as the present argument focuses on the successful processing of the input image with the help of Gabor filters. Our intention was to demonstrate that a texture that has been preprocessed with Gabor filters can be further processed in a way that finally produces a segmentation agreeing with that produced by the human visual system.

The studies of Fogel and Sagi (1989) and Turner (1986) have both shown that Gabor filtering can be used to perform a segmentation of textures by machine that corresponds to the performance of human subjects in psychophysiological experiments. These simulations used the type of artificial texture that is commonly used in experiments on perception. The simulation studies by Bovik, Clark and Geisler (1990), Clark and Bovik (1989) and Clark, Bovik and Geisler (1987) have confirmed beyond this that the principle of Gabor filtering can also be applied successfully to the segmentation of natural textures.

In summary, these simulation studies have shown that the principle of Gabor filtering could provide an important contribution to the segmentation of textures. Therefore, the following sections investigate whether correspondences can be found between the 'older' theories on texture perception presented at the beginning of this chapter and the 'newer' filter models.

5 SYNOPSIS: GABOR FILTERS AS A LINK BETWEEN GLOBAL AND LOCAL SEGMENTATION THEORIES

5.1 Gabor Filters and the Statistical Theory

As discussed above, most of the statistical theory proposed by Julesz and his colleagues in the 1960s and early 1970s (Julesz conjecture) is considered to be incorrect because of a series of contradictory findings. However, a not very well-known article by Gagalowicz (1981) has criticized the stimulus displays that were used to refute statistical theory. His criticism focuses on the algorithms used to generate textures with identical second- and third-order statistics. Contrary to the Julesz conjecture, these textures proved to be segmentable in psychophysiological experiments and finally led to the rejection of the Julesz conjecture. Gagalowicz (1981) has argued that:

(1) Textures could be *nonhomogeneous,* in that although they *retain the same* statistical properties *globally* (i.e. over a larger area), they simultaneously reveal *different* statistical structures on a *local* level (i.e. related to subareas).

(2) The textures in the examples used to refute the Julesz conjecture are thoroughly nonhomogeneous in this sense. Gagalowicz believes that these examples demonstrate the ability of the human visual system to detect preattentively not only global but also local differences in the statistical structures of textures.

It is therefore proposed that the Julesz conjecture should not be rejected too hastily. Instead, it should be modified to include not only the global structures of textures but also, in particular, local parts of them.[12] If we follow Gagalowicz's argument, then the examples used to refute the Julesz conjecture should be viewed with some skepticism, as we cannot rule out the possibility that the observed segmentation is based on a *local* comparison of subareas of nonhomogeneous textures. Should this prove to be true, the modified Julesz conjecture would then move much closer to Gabor filtering for the following reasons: It can be demonstrated that there is a close formal relationship between the second-order statistics contained in an image, the so-called autocorrelation function and the power spectrum of the Fourier transform.[13] The autocorrelation function will not be discussed here (details can be found in, for example, Uttal, 1975). Julesz (1981) himself has already pointed to this relationship. Against this background, the Julesz conjecture can be formulated as follows: A preattentive segmentation of textures is possible only when textures differ in their power spectra. Taking into account Gagalowicz's (1981) argument, this applies not only to textures as wholes but also to local sections of them. Accordingly, textures can always be segmented when their properties differ in the *local* power spectrum.

Indeed, the local power spectrum is very easy to determine with the help of Gabor filtering. The basis for this is the use of *pairs* of filters (sine and cosine filters) discussed above. Calculating the Pythagorean sum[14] of the reactions of these two filter systems leads directly to the value for the local power of a specific frequency and orientation. This procedure for determining the local power with the help of pairs of Gabor filters has been applied successfully in some of the above-mentioned simulation studies (Fogel and Sagi, 1989; Turner, 1986). In Turner's (1986) study, squares were not calculated to estimate the effectiveness of the procedure; only the absolute values of the filter reactions were added together. This leads to a lower segmentation performance. In one of his simulations, Turner (1986) was able to show that Gabor filters could be used to segment a texture with identical third-order statistics published by Julesz, Gilbert and Victor (1978) in a way that corresponds to human perception. This finding suggests that, in agreement with Gagalowicz (1981), *local* features in the texture statistics (Gabor filters are only sensitive to these) play a decisive role in the segmentation of textures.

In summary, it can be stated that ideas on the application of Gabor filters for the segmentation of textures fit very well with local statistical theory

---

[12] It should be pointed out here that, according to Gagalowicz, the local section of a texture may well contain several texture elements. This is in contrast to feature theories in which the analysis of a texture always refers to its constituent texture elements and their components.

[13] In very strict terms, this nonetheless only applies to binary textures. Detailed information on this can be found, for example, in Klein and Tyler (1986).

[14] That is, the squared and summed reactions of sine and cosine filters.

('Gagalowicz conjecture'). However, as discussed in more detail earlier, the Gagalowicz conjecture can be conceived as a modification of the Julesz conjecture. This gives clear parallels between statistical theory and the Gabor theory on texture segmentation. However, one advantage of the Gabor theory is that it names physiologically plausible mechanisms that can be used to carry out the necessary calculations.

5.2   Gabor Filters and Local Segmentation Theories

As the operations carried out with the help of Gabor filters refer to *local sections of the image,* as mentioned earlier, Gabor filters could also be understood as a possible operationalization of specific feature detectors. Nothdurft (1991), for example, has pointed out that the presence of terminators and crossings[15] in textures can be accompanied by a characteristic change in the local power spectrum (see also Turner, 1986). How the relationship between postulated textons and the corresponding properties of Gabor filters is formed in detail remains unclear because of insufficient data. However, findings reported by Fogel and Sagi (1989) suggest that the search for such relationships shows some promise of success, as their results reveal that Gabor filters respond sensitively to many texture features that have been identified as textons.

There also seems to be some promise that Gabor filters can be applied successfully to the detection of 'higher-order' texture properties. The studies of Beck, Sutter and Ivry (1987) and Sutter, Beck and Graham (1989) have both shown that texture segmentations can also be carried out with Gabor filters when the subtextures do not differ with respect to the *identity* of their texture elements but only in their *spatial arrangement*. An example of this type of texture has already been presented in Figure 2.13. It is obvious that segmentation cannot draw on differences in the texture elements in these kinds of texture, as these are identical across the entire texture. Segmentation can only occur when several individual texture elements combine to form 'higher-order texture elements' (Beck, Prazdny and Rosenfeld, 1983). This can be done with Gabor filters. As already demonstrated above (section 4.1), it is very simple to set the orientation, preferred frequency and size of Gabor filters. By suitably selecting these parameters (Sutter, Beck and Graham, 1989, have tested a total of 39 filter parameters), Gabor filters can be arranged so that those applied to the center of a texture react differently to those applied to the upper or lower parts. These different reactions make it possible to use Gabor filters to separate the three texture areas in a way that corresponds to human perception.

Sutter, Beck and Graham's (1989) study has also shown the limits of simple filter models like those presented in this chapter. These authors could describe only a *part* of their findings with a simple (linear) Gabor model. Another part of the data required an extension of the model. This extension anticipates a total of three, hierarchically arranged stages of information processing. On two of these stages (the first and third), linear filtering is performed with the help of two-dimensional Gabor functions. On the remaining intermediate stage, a *nonlinear* operation, which will not be explored any further here, is postulated. Sutter, Beck and Graham (1989) refer to the analog distribution of neurons in the visual cortex of mammals (simple

---

[15]Many studies treat 'terminators' and 'crossings' as 'textons'.

versus complex cells) and distinguish their nonlinear, three-stage conception from linear models by calling it a complex model.

At this point, it is necessary to emphasize explicitly that this chapter has focused primarily on *linear* filter models. However, neurophysiological findings indicate that there can be little doubt that *nonlinear* processing components are already effective at relatively early stages of visual information processing (see, for example, Glezer, Ivanoff and Tscherbach, 1973; Rose, 1979; Spitzer and Hochstein, 1985). Readers who are interested in formal models in this domain will find additional information in, for example, the more recent publications from Caelli (1988) and Caelli and Oguztoreli (1987).

If we compare the still small amount of data from simulation studies using Gabor filters with findings from psychophysiological experiments, there seems to be some justification for hoping that Gabor filters will help to bridge the gap between statistical theory and the feature theories of texture segmentation. In feature theories, such an approach may also lead to a much-needed specification of the feature concept.

ACKNOWLEDGEMENT

We wish to thank Janna Warnecke for her careful research into the literature on Gestalt laws.

REFERENCES

Anderson, S. J. and Burr, D. C. (1989). Receptive field properties of human motion detector units inferred from spatial frequency masking. *Vision Research,* **29,** 1343–1358.

Barlow, H. B. (1972). Single units and sensation: A neuron doctrine for perceptual psychology? *Perception,* **1,** 371–394.

Bastiaans, M. J. (1981). A sampling theorem for the complex spectrogram, and Gabor's expansion of a signal in Gaussian elementary signals. *Optical Engineering,* **20,** 594–598.

Beck, J. (1966). Effect of orientation and of shape similarity on perceptual grouping. *Perception and Psychophysics,* **1,** 300–302.

Beck, J. (1982). Textural segmentation. In J. Beck (Ed.), *Organization and Representation in Perception* (pp. 285–317). Hillsdale, NJ: Erlbaum.

Beck, J., Prazdny, K. and Rosenfeld, A. (1983). A theory of textural segmentation. In J. Beck, B. Hope and A. Rosenfeld (Eds), *Human and Machine Vision* (pp. 1–38). New York: Academic Press.

Beck, J., Rosenfeld, A. and Ivry, R. (1989). Line segregation. *Spatial Vision,* **4,** 75–101.

Beck, J., Sutter, A. and Ivry, R. (1987). Spatial frequency channels and perceptual grouping in texture segregation. *Computer Vision, Graphics, and Image Processing,* **37,** 299–325.

Bergen, J. R. and Julesz, B. (1983). Rapid discrimination of visual patterns. *IEEE Transactions on Systems, Man, and Cybernetics,* **13,** 857–863.

Bergen, J. R. and Landy, M. S. (1991). Computational modeling of visual texture segregation. In M. S. Landy and J. A. Movshon (Eds), *Computational Models of Visual Processing* (pp. 253–271). Cambridge, MA: MIT Press.

Blakemore, C. (Ed.). (1990). *Vision: Coding and Efficiency.* Cambridge: Cambridge University Press.

Boldt, M., Weiss, R. and Riseman, E. (1989). Token-based extraction of straight lines. *IEEE Transactions on Systems, Man, and Cybernetics,* **19,** 1581–1594.

Bovik, A. C., Clark, M. and Geisler, W. S. (1990). Multichannel texture analysis using localized spatial filters. *IEEE Transactions on Pattern Analysis and Machine Intelligence,* **12,** 55–73.

Bradley, A., Switkes, E. and De Valois, K. (1988). Orientation and spatial frequency selectivity of adaptation to color and luminance gratings. *Vision Research,* **28,** 841–856.

Bryngdahl, O. (1966a). Characteristics of the visual system: Psychophysical measurements of the response to spatial sine-wave stimuli in the photopic region. *Journal of the Optical Society of America,* **56,** 811–821.

Bryngdahl, O. (1966b). Perceived contrast variation with eccentricity of spatial sine-wave stimuli: Size determination of receptive field centres. *Vision Research,* **6,** 553–565.

Burbeck, C. A. (1988). Large-scale relative localization across spatial frequency channels. *Vision Research,* **28,** 857–859.

Caelli, T. (1988). An adaptive computational model for texture segmentation. *IEEE Transactions on Systems, Man, and Cybernetics,* **18,** 9–17.

Caelli, T. and Julesz, B. (1978). On perceptual analyzers underlying visual texture discrimination: Part I. *Biological Cybernetics,* **28,** 167–175.

Caelli, T., Julesz, B. and Gilbert, E. (1978). On perceptual analyzers underlying visual texture discrimination: Part II. *Biological Cybernetics,* **29,** 201–214.

Caelli, T. and Moraglia, O. (1985). On the detection of Gabor signals and discrimination of Gabor textures. *Vision Research,* **25,** 671–684.

Caelli, T. and Oguztoreli, M. N. (1987). Some task and signal-dependent rules for spatial vision. *Spatial Vision,* **2,** 295–315.

Calis, G. and Leeuwenberg, E. L. J. (1981). Grounding the figure. *Journal of Experimental Psychology: Human Perception and Performance,* **7,** 1386–1397.

Campbell, F. W., Cooper, G. F. and Enroth-Cugell, C. (1969). The spatial selectivity of the visual cells of the cat. *Journal of Physiology,* **203,** 223–235.

Campbell, F. W., Nachmias, J. and Jukes, J. (1970). Spatial-frequency discrimination in human vision. *Journal of the Optical Society of America,* **60,** 555–559.

Campbell, F. W. and Robson, J. G. (1964). Application of Fourier analysis to the modulation response of the eye. *Journal of the Optical Society of America,* **54,** 581.

Campbell, F. W. and Robson, J. G. (1968). Application of Fourier analysis to the visibility of gratings. *Journal of Physiology,* **197,** 551–566.

Carpenter, P. A. and Ganz, L. (1972). An attentional mechanism in the analysis of spatial frequency. *Perception and Psychophysics,* **12,** 57–60.

Chua, F. K. (1990). The processing of spatial frequency and orientation information. *Perception and Psychophysics,* **47,** 79–86.

Clark, M. and Bovik, A. C. (1989). Experiments in segmenting texton patterns using localized spatial filters. *Pattern Recognition,* **22,** 707–717.

Clark, M., Bovik, A. C. and Geisler, W.S. (1987). Texture segmentation using Gabor modulation/demodulation. *Pattern Recognition Letters,* **6,** 261–267.

Conners, R. W. and Ng, C. T. (1989). Developing a quantitative model of human preattentive vision. *IEEE Transactions on Systems, Man, and Cybernetics,* **19,** 1384–1407.

Cooley, J. W. and Tukey, J. K. (1965) . An algorithm for the machine calculation of complex Fourier series. *Mathematical Computing,* **19,** 297–301.

Cowey, A. (1979). Cortical maps and visual perception. The Grindley Memorial Lecture. *Quarterly Journal of Experimental Psychology,* **31,** 1–17.

Cowey, A. (1985). Aspects of cortical organization related to selective attention and selective impairments of visual perception: A tutorial review. In M. I. Posner and O. Marin (Eds), *Attention and Performance,* vol. 11 (pp. 41–62). Hillsdale, NJ: Erlbaum.

Dannemiller, J. L. and Ver Hoeve, J. N. (1990). Two-dimensional approach to psychophysical orientation tuning. *Journal of the Optical Society of America,* **7,** 141–151.

Daugman, J. G. (1980). Two-dimensional spectral analysis of cortical receptive field profiles. *Vision Research,* **20,** 847–856.

Daugman, J. G. (1983). Six formal properties of two-dimensional anisotropic visual filters: Structural principles and frequency/orientation selectvity. *IEEE Transactions on Systems, Man, and Cybernetics*, **13**, 882–887.

Daugman, J. G. (1984). Spatial visual channels in the Fourier plane. *Vision Research*, **24**, 891–910.

Daugman, J. G. (1985). Uncertainty relation for resolution in space, spatial frequency, and orientation optimized by two-dimensional visual cortical filters. *Journal of the Optical Society of America*, **2**, 1160–1169.

Daugman, J. G. (1988). Complete discrete 2-D Gabor transforms by neural networks for image analysis and compression. *IEEE Transactions on Acoustics, Speech, and Signal Processing*, **36**, 1169–1179.

Daugman, J. G. (1989). Entropy reduction and decorrelation in visual coding by oriented neural receptive fields. *IEEE Transactions on Biomedical Engineering*, **36**, 107–114.

Daugman, J. G. and Kammen, D. M. (1986). Pure orientation filtering: A scale invariant image-processing tool for perception research and data compression. *Behavior Research Methods, Instruments, and Computers*, **18**, 559–564.

De Valois, R. L. and De Valois, K. K. (1988). *Spatial Vision*. New York: Oxford University Press.

De Valois, K. K., De Valois, R. L. and Yund, E. W. (1979). Responses of striate cortex cells to grating and checkerboard patterns. *Journal of Physiology*, **291**, 483–505.

Diaconis, P. and Freedman, D. (1981). On the statistics of vision: The Julesz conjecture. *Journal of Mathematical Psychology*, **24**, 112–138.

Dobbins, A., Zucker, S. W. and Cynader, M. S. (1989). Endstopping and curvature. *Vision Research*, **29**, 1371–1387.

Driver, J. and Baylis, G. C. (1989). Movement and visual attention: The spotlight metaphor breaks down. *Journal of Experimental Psychology: Human Perception and Performance*, **15**, 448–456.

Enns, J. (1986). Seeing textons in context. *Perception and Psychophysics*, **39**, 143–147.

Enroth-Cugell, C. and Robson, J. G. (1966). The contrast sensitivity of retinal ganglion cells of the cat. *Journal of Physiology*, **187**, 517–552.

Field, D. J. (1987). Relations between the statistics of natural images and the response properties of cortical cells. *Journal of the Optical Society of America A*, **4**, 2379–2394.

Fiorentini, A. and Berardi, N. (1981). Learning in grating waveform discrimination: Specificity for orientation and spatial frequency. *Vision Research*, **21**, 1149–1158.

Fogel, I. and Sagi, D. (1989). Gabor filters as texture discriminator. *Biological Cybernetics*, **61**, 103–113.

Fox, J. and Mayhew, J. E. W. (1979). Texture discrimination and the analysis of proximity. *Perception*, **8**, 75–91.

Gabor, D. (1946). Theory of communication. *Journal of the Institute of Electrical Engineering*, **93**, 429–457.

Gagalowicz, A. (1981). A new method for texture fields synthesis: Some applications to the study of human vision. *IEEE Transactions on Pattern Analysis and Machine Intelligence*, **3**, 520–533.

Ginsburg, A. P. (1984). Visual form perception based on biological filtering. In L. Spillmann and B. R. Wooten (Eds), *Sensory Experience, Adaptation, and Perception* (pp. 53–72). Hillsdale, NJ: Erlbaum.

Glezer, V. D., Ivanoff, V. A. and Tscherbach, T.A. (1973). Investigation of complex and hypercomplex receptive fields of visual cortex of the cat as spatial frequency filters. *Vision Research*, **13**, 1875–1904.

Glezer, V. D., Shcherbach, T. A. and Gauzel'man, V. E. (1979). Are receptive fields of the visual cortex detectors of spatial frequency filters? *Neurophysiology*, **11**, 295–302.

Graham, N. (1981). Psychophysics of spatial-frequency channels. In M. Kubovy and J.R. Pomerantz (Eds), *Perceptual Organization* (pp. 1–25). Hillsdale, NJ: Erlbaum.

Graham, N. (1989). Low-level visual processes and texture segregation. *Physica Scripta*, **39**, 147–152.

Green, B. F. (1963). *Digital Computers in Research*. New York: McGraw-Hill.

Green, B. F. Jr, Wolf, A. K. and White, B. W. (1959). The detection of statistically defined patterns in a matrix of dots. *American Journal of Psychology*, **72**, 503–520.

Greenlee, M. W. and Breitmeyer, B. G. (1989). A choice reaction time analysis of spatial frequency discrimination. *Vision Research*, **29**, 1575–1586.

Grossberg, S. and Mingolla, E. (1985). Neural dynamics of perceptual grouping: Textures, boundaries, and emergent segmentations. *Perception and Psychophysics*, **38**, 141–171.

Gurnsey, R. and Browse, R. A. (1987). Micropattern properties and presentation conditions influencing visual texture discrimination. *Perception and Psychophysics*, **41**, 239–252.

Gurnsey, R. and Browse, R. A. (1989). Asymmetries in visual texture discrimination. *Spatial Vision*, **4**, 31–44.

Harvey, L. O. Jr, and Doan, V. V. (1990). Visual masking at different polar angles in the two-dimensional Fourier plane. *Journal of the Optical Society of America*, **7**, 116–127.

Harvey, L. O. Jr, and Gervais, M. J. (1978). Visual texture perception and Fourier analysis. *Perception and Psychophysics*, **24**, 534–542.

Harvey, L. O. Jr, and Gervais, M. J. (1981). Internal representation of visual texture as a basis for the judgment of similarity. *Journal of Experimental Psychology: Human Perception and Performance*, **7**, 741–753.

Harwerth, R. S. and Levi, D. M. (1978). Reaction time as a measure of suprathreshold grating detection. *Vision Research*, **18**, 1579–1586.

Hawken, M. J. and Parker, A. J. (1987). Spatial properties of neurons in the monkey striate cortex. *Proceedings of the Royal Society of London, B*, **231**, 251–288.

Heeley, D. W. (1987). Spatial frequency discrimination for sinewave gratings with random, bandpass frequency modulation: Evidence for averaging in spatial acuity. *Spatial Vision*, **2**, 317–335.

Heeley, D. W. (1991). Spatial frequency difference thresholds depend on stimulus area. *Spatial Vision*, **5**, 205–217.

Heggelund, P. (1981). Receptive field organization of simple cells in cat striate cortex. *Experimental Brain Research*, **42**, 89–98.

Hirsch, J. and Hyltton, R. (1982). Limits of spatial-frequency discrimination as evidence of neural interpolation. *Journal of the Optical Society of America*, **72**, 1367–1374.

Hubel, D. H. and Wiesel, T. N. (1962). Receptive fields, binocular interaction and functional architecture in the cat's visual cortex. *Journal of Physiology*, **160**, 106–154.

Jähne, B. (1989). *Digitale Bildverarbeitung*. Berlin: Springer.

Jáñez, L. (1984). Visual grouping without low spatial frequencies. *Vision Research*, **24**, 271–274.

Jones, J. P. and Palmer, L. A. (1987). An evaluation of the two-dimensional Gabor filter model of simple receptive fields in cat striate cortex. *Journal of Neurophysiology*, **58**, 1233–1258.

Julesz, B. (1960). Binocular depth perception of computer-generated patterns. *The Bell System Technical Journal*, **39**, 1125–1161.

Julesz, B. (1962). Visual pattern discrimination. *IRE Transactions on Information Theory*, **IT-8**, 84–92.

Julesz, B. (1975). Experiments in the visual perception of texture. *Scientific American*, **232**, 34–43.

Julesz, B. (1981). A theory of preattentive texture discrimination based on first-order statistics of textons. *Biological Cybernetics*, **41**, 131–138.

Julesz, B. and Bergen, J. R. (1983). Textons, the fundamental elements in preattentive vision and perception of textures. *The Bell System Technical Journal*, **62**, 1619–1645.

Julesz, B., Gilbert, E. N., Shepp, L. A. and Frisch, H. L. (1973). Inability of humans to discriminate between visual textures that agree in second-order statistics revisited. *Perception*, **2**, 391–405.

Julesz, B., Gilbert, E. N. and Victor, J. D. (1978). Visual discrimination of textures with identical third-order statistics. *Biological Cybernetics*, **31**, 137–140.

Katz, D. (1969). *Gestaltpsychologie*. Basel: Schwabe.

Kehrer, L. (1989). Central performance drop on perceptual segregation tasks. *Spatial Vision*, **4**, 45–62.

Klein, S. A. and Tyler, C. W. (1986). Phase discrimination of compound gratings: Generalized autocorrelation analysis. *Journal of the Optical Society of America A*, **3**, 868-879.

Klymenko, V. and Weisstein, N. (1986). Spatial frequency differences can determine figure-ground organization. *Journal of Experimental Psychology: Human Perception and Performance*, **12**, 324–330.

Koffka, K. (1935). *Principles of Gestalt Psychology*. London: Routledge and Kegan Paul.

Köhler, W. (1924). *Die physischen Gestalten in Ruhe und im stationären Zustand*. Erlangen: Verlag der philosophischen Akademie.

Köhler, W. (1933). *Psychologische Probleme*. Berlin: Springer.

Kroon, J. N., Rijsdijk, J. P. and Wildt, G. J. van der (1980). Peripheral contrast sensitivity for sine-wave gratings and single periods. *Vision Research*, **20**, 243–252.

Kroon, J. N. and Wildt, G. J. van der (1980). Spatial frequency tuning studies: Weighting prerequisite for describing psychometric curves by probability summation. *Vision Research*, **20**, 253–263.

Kuffler, S. W. (1953). Discharge patterns and functional organization of mammalian retina. *Journal of Neurophysiology*, **16**, 37–68.

Kulikowski, J. J. and Bishop, P. O. (1981). Fourier analysis and spatial representation in the visual cortex. *Experientia*, **37**, 160–163.

Kulikowski, J. J., Marcelja, S. and Bishop, P. O. (1982). Theory of spatial position and spatial frequency relations in the receptive fields of simple cells in the visual cortex. *Biological Cybernetics*, **43**, 187–198.

Kulikowski, J. J. and Vidyasagar, T. R. (1986). Space and spatial frequency: Analysis and representation in the macaque striate cortex. *Experimental Brain Research*, **64**, 5–18.

Landy, M. S. and Bergen, J. R. (1991). Texture segregation and orientation gradient. *Vision Research*, **31**, 679–691.

Landy, M. S., Manovich, L. Z. and Stetten, G. D. (1990). Applications of the EVE software for visual modeling. *Vision Research*, **30**, 329–338.

Lupp, U., Hauske, G. and Wolf, W. (1976). Perceptual latencies to sinusoidal gratings. *Vision Research*, **16**, 969–972.

Maffei, L. (1978). Spatial frequency channels: Neural mechanisms., In R. Held, H.W. Leibowitz, and H.L. Teuber (Eds), *Handbook of Sensory Physiology*, vol. 8: *Perception* (pp. 39–66). Berlin, New York: Springer.

Maffei, L. and Fiorentini, A. (1972). Processes of synthesis in visual perception. *Nature*, **240**, 479–481.

Maffei, L. and Fiorentini, A. (1973). The visual cortex as a spatial frequency analyser. *Vision Research*, **13**, 1255–1267.

Malik, J. and Perona, P. (1990). Preattentive texture discrimination with early vision mechanisms. *Journal of the Optical Society of America A*, **7**, 923–932.

Marcelja, S. (1980). Mathematical description of the responses of simple cortical cells. *Journal of the Optical Society of America*, **70**, 1297–1300.

Marr, D. (1982). *Vision*. San Francisco: Freeman.

Marr, D. and Hildreth, E. (1980). Theory of edge detection. *Proceedings of the Royal Society of London, B*, **207**, 187–217.

Mayer, M. J. and Kim, C. B. (1986). Smooth frequency discrimination functions for foveal, high-contrast, mid spatial frequencies. *Journal of the Optical Society of America*, **3**, 1957–1969.

Mayhew, J. E. W. and Frisby, J. P. (1978). Texture discrimination and Fourier analysis in human vision. *Nature*, **275**, 438–439.

Meinecke, C. (1989). Retinal eccentricity and the detection of targets. *Psychological Research*, **51**, 107–116.

Metzger, W. (1975). *Gesetze des Sehens* (3rd edn). Frankfurt: Kramer.

Moraglia, G. (1989). Visual search: Spatial frequency and orientation. *Perceptual and Motor Skills*, **69**, 675–689.

Mullikin, W. H., Jones, J. P. and Palmer, L. A. (1984). Periodic simple cells in cat area 17. *Journal of Neurophysiology*, **52**, 372–387.

Musselwhite, M. J. and Jeffreys, D. A. (1985). The influence of spatial frequency on the reaction times and evoked potentials recorded to grating pattern stimuli. *Vision Research*, **25**, 1545–1555.

Nakayama, K. (1990). The iconic bottleneck and the tenuous link between early visual processing and perception. In C. Blakemore (Ed.), *Vision: Coding and Efficiency* (pp. 412–422). Cambridge: Cambridge University Press.

Neisser, U. (1967). *Cognitive Psychology*. New York: Appleton-Century-Crofts.

Nothdurft, H. C. (1985). Sensitivity for structure gradient in texture discrimination tasks. *Vision Research*, **25**, 1957–1968.

Nothdurft, H. C. (1990). Texton segregation by associated differences in global and local luminance distribution. *Proceedings of the Royal Society of London, B*, **239**, 295–320.

Nothdurft, B.C. (1991). Different effects from spatial frequency masking in texture segregation and texton detection tasks. *Vision Research*, **31**, 299–320.

Olson, R.K. and Attneave, F. (1970). What variables produce similarity grouping? *American Journal of Psychology*, **83**, 1–21.

Oyama, T. (1986). The effect of stimulus organization on numerosity discrimination. *Japanese Psychological Research*, **28**, 77–86.

Phillips, G. C. and Wilson, H.R. (1984). Orientation bandwidth of spatial mechanisms measured by masking. *Journal of the Optical Society of America*, **1**, 226–232.

Pollen, D. A., Lee, J. R. and Taylor, J. H. (1971). How does the striate cortex begin the reconstruction of the visual world? *Science*, **173**, 74–77.

Pollen, D. A. and Ronner, S. F. (1981). Phase relationships between adjacent simple cells in the visual cortex. *Science*, **252**, 1409–1411.

Pollen, D. A. and Ronner, S. F. (1983). Visual cortical neurons as localized spatial frequency filters. *IEEE Transactions on Systems, Man, and Cybernetics*, **SMC-13**, 907–916.

Regan, D. M. (1983). Spatial frequency mechanisms in human vision investigated by evoked potential recording. *Vision Research*, **23**, 1401–1407.

Regan, D. M. and Regan, M. P. (1988). Objective evidence for phase-independent spatial frequency analysis in the human visual pathway. *Vision Research*, **28**, 187–191.

Robson, J. G. (1975). Receptive fields: Neural representation of the spatial and intensive attributes of the visual image. In E. C. Carterette and M. P. Friedman (Eds), *Handbook of Perception*, vol. 5: *Seeing* (pp. 81–116). New York: Academic Press.

Rose, D. (1979). Mechanisms underlying the receptive field properties of neurons in cat visual cortex. *Vision Research*, **19**, 533–544.

Rosenfeld, A. (1990). Pyramid algorithms for efficient vision. In C. Blakemore (Ed.), *Vision: Coding and Efficiency* (pp. 423–430). Cambridge: Cambridge University Press.

Rosenfeld, A. and Kak, A. (1982). *Digital Picture Processing*. New York: Academic Press.

Rubenstein, B. S. and Sagi, D. (1990). Spatial variability as a limiting factor in texture-discrimination tasks: Implications for performance asymmetries. *Journal of the Optical Society of America*, **7**, 1632–1643.

Rubin, E. (1921). *Visuell wahrgenommene Figuren*. Copenhagen: Gyldendalske Bogheandel.

Rudd, M. E. (1988). Quantal fluctuation limitations on reaction time to sinusoidal gratings. *Vision Research*, **28**, 179–186.

Sagi, D. (1990). Detection of an orientation singularity in Gabor textures: Effect of signal density and spatial-frequency. *Vision Research*, **30**, 1377–1388.

Sagi, D. and Hochstein, S. (1984). The contrast dependence of spatial frequency channel interactions. *Vision Research*, **24**, 1357–1365.

Sagi, D. and Hochstein, S. (1985). Lateral inhibition between spatially adjacent spatial-frequency channels? *Perception and Psychophysics*, **37**, 315–322.

Sakitt, B. and Barlow, H. B. (1982). A model for the economical encoding of the visual image in cerebral cortex. *Biological Cybernetics*, **43**, 97–108.

Savoy, R. L. and McCann, J. J. (1975). Visibility of low spatial-frequency sine-wave targets: Dependence on number of cycles. *Journal of the Optical Society of America*, **65**, 343–350.

Schade, O. H. (1956). Optical and photoelectric analog of the eye. *Journal of the Optical Society of America*, **46**, 721–739.

Selfridge, O. (1959). *A Paradigm for Learning. Symposium on the Mechanization of Thought Processes*. London: HMSO.

Shapley, R. and Lennie, P. (1985). Spatial frequency analysis in the visual system. *Annual Review of Neuroscience*, **8**, 547–583.

Skrandies, W. (1984). Scalp potential fields evoked by grating stimuli: Effects of spatial frequency and orientation. *Electroencephalography and Clinical Neurophysiology*, **58**, 325–332.

Smits, J. T. S., Voss, P. O. and Oeffelen, N.P. van (1985). The perception of a dotted line in noise: A model of good continuation and some experimental results. *Spatial Vision*, **1**, 163–177.

Spitzer, H. and Hochstein, S. (1985). A complex-cell receptive-field model. *Journal of Neurophysiology*, **53**, 1266–1286.

Stork, D. G. and Wilson, H. R. (1990). Do Gabor functions provide appropriate descriptions of visual cortical receptive fields? *Journal of the Optical Society of America, A*, **7**, 1362–1373.

Sutter, A., Beck, J. and Graham, N. (1989). Contrast and spatial variables in texture segregation: Testing a simple spatial-frequency channels model. *Perception and Psychophysics*, **46**, 312–332.

Toet, A. and Koenderink, J. J. (1988). Differential spatial displacement discrimination thresholds for Gabor patches. *Vision Research*, **28**, 133–143.

Treisman, A. (1982). Perceptual grouping and attention in visual search for features and for objects. *Journal of Experimental Psychology: Human Perception and Performance*, **8**, 194–214.

Treisman, A. and Gelade, G. (1980). A feature-integration theory of attention. *Cognitive Psychology*, **12**, 97–136.

Treisman, A. and Gormican, S. (1988). Feature analysis in early vision: Evidence from search asymmetries. *Psychological Review*, **95**, 15–48.

Treisman, A. and Paterson, R. (1984). Emergent features, attention and object perception. *Journal of Experimental Psychology: Human Perception and Performance*, **10**, 12–31.

Treisman, A. and Schmidt, H. (1982). Illusory conjunctions in the perception of objects. *Cognitive Psychology*, **14**, 107–141.

Treisman, A. and Souther, J. (1985). Search asymmetry: A diagnostic for preattentive processing of separable features. *Journal of Experimental Psychology: General*, **114**, 285–310.

Treisman, A., Sykes, M. and Gelade, G. (1977). Selective attention and stimulus integration. In S. Dornič (Ed.), *Attention and Performance*, vol. VI (pp. 333–361). Hillsdale, NJ: Erlbaum.

Turner, M. R. (1986). Texture discrimination by Gabor functions. *Biological Cybernetics*, **55**, 71–82.

Uttal, W. R. (1975). *An Autocorrelation Theory of Form Detection*. Hillsdale, NJ: Erlbaum.

Uttal, W. R. (1986). Special issue computers in vision research. Introduction. *Behavior Research Methods, Instruments, and Computers*, **18**, 484–486.

Victor, J. D. (1989). Models for preattentive texture discrimination: Fourier analysis and local feature processing in a unified framework. *Spatial Vision*, **3**, 263–280.

Watson, A. B. (1983). Detection and recognition of simple spatial forms. In O.J. Braddick and A. C. Sleigh (Eds), *Physiological and Biological Processing of Images* (pp. 100–114). New York: Springer.

Watson, A. B. (1987). The cortex transform: Rapid computation of simulated neural images. *Computer Vision, Graphics, and Image Processing*, **39**, 311–327.

Watson, A. B. (1990). Algotexture of visual cortex. In C. Blakemore (Ed.), *Vision: Coding and Efficiency* (pp. 393–410). Cambridge: Cambridge University Press.

Watson, A. B., Barlow, H. B. and Robson, J. G. (1983). What does the eye see best? *Nature*, **302**, 419–422.

Webster, M. A. and De Valois, R. L. (1985). Relationship between spatial frequency and orientation tuning of striate-cortex cells. *Journal of the Optical Society of America, A,* **2,** 1124–1132.

Weisstein, N. (1980). The joy of Fourier analysis. In C.S. Harris (Ed.), *Visual Coding and Adaptability* (pp. 365–380). Hillsdale, NJ: Erlbaum.

Wertheimer, M. (1923). Untersuchungen zur Lehre von der Gestalt, II. *Psychologische Forschung,* **4,** 301–350. (See a condensed trans. in W. Ellis (1950). *A Source Book of Gestalt Psychology,* Sel. 5. New York: Humanities Press.)

Wilson, H. R. (1976). The significance of frequency gradients in binocular grating perception. *Vision Research,* **16,** 983–989.

Wilson, H. R. and Giese, S. C. (1977). Threshold visibility of frequency gradient patterns. *Vision Research,* **17,** 1177–1190.

Wilson, H. R. and Knutsson, H. (1988). Uncertainty and inference in the visual system. *IEEE Transactions on Systems, Man, and Cybernetics,* **18,** 305–312.

Wong, E. and Weisstein, N. (1983). Sharp targets are detected better against a figure, and blurred targets are detected better against a background. *Journal of Experimental Psychology: Human Perception and Performance,* **9,** 194–202.

Young, R. A. (1987). The Gaussian derivative model for spatial vision: I. Retinal mechanisms. *Spatial Vision,* **2,** 273–293.

Zeki, S. M. (1978). Functional specialization in the visual cortex of the rhesus monkey. *Nature,* **274,** 423–428.

Zeki, S. M. (1981). The mapping of visual functions in the cerebral cortex. In Y. Katsuki, R. Norgren, and M. Sato (Eds), *Brain Mechanisms of Sensation* (pp. 105–128). New York: Wiley.

Zucker, S. W. and Davis, S. (1988). Points and endpoints: A size/spacing constraint for dot grouping. *Perception,* **17,** 229–246.

Chapter 3
Stereoscopic Depth Perception

Martin Eimer
University of Munich

1 INTRODUCTION

When we open our eyes, we perceive objects in our surroundings; not only objects directly in front of us but also objects that may be a long distance away. Our visual system informs us about the localization of perceived objects in space, the distances between them, and their position relative to ourselves as observers: the visual world is three-dimensional. What at first appears to be a self-evident ability of the human visual system requires explanation when we realize that the image on the retina – as the first stage of visual information processing – is two-dimensional, that is, it contains no explicit information on the localization of objects in space. This leads us to ask in what way the visual system is capable of constructing representations of the perceived world in which the spatial disposition of distant objects is made explicit on the basis of the two-dimensional image on the retina.

One possible answer to this question is given by the geometry of visual perception processes: if an observer fixates a point in her surroundings, this point is imaged on the central fovea of the right and left retinas; that is, the area in which visual acuity is at its maximum. In this case, the images of the fixated point are located at *matching positions* on the left or right retina. However, in normal binocular vision, not all distal points are represented at matching positions on the retina. This is because the centers of the pupils of both eyes are generally separated by a distance of approximately 6–7 cm. Only points on a curved surface that links together the fixation point and the centers of rotation of both eyes (the *horopter*) project onto matching retinal positions. All remaining points of a perceived distal scene fall, in contrast, on noncorresponding positions on the retina. This relative deviation of the two monocular images of spatially distant points from the geometrically or anatomically corresponding positions on the retina is labeled *disparity*. The direction of disparity depends on the spatial position of the represented object relative to the fixation plane (Figure 3.1): points that are located beyond the horopter are displaced in a nasal direction in both eyes (crossed disparity). All points that are located closer to the observer than the momentary fixation point are displaced temporally (uncrossed disparity). The extent of these displacements of monocular retinal images depends on the spatial distance between the fixation plane and imaged point: the further an object is located in front of or behind the

Handbook of Perception and Action: Volume 1
ISBN 0-12-516161-1

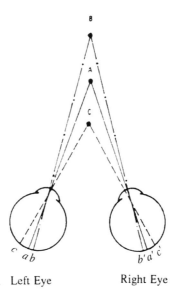

Left Eye   Right Eye

Figure 3.1. *The sign of binocular disparity depends on the location of distal points. The observer fixates point A, which is projected onto corresponding positions (a, a') in the left and right eye. Monocular images of a distant point (B) show crossed disparity (b, b'), for a point closer to the observer (C), retinal disparity is uncrossed (c, c'). [From Murch and Woodworth, 1978, p. 156.* © *1978 W. Kohlhammer, Stuttgart; reprinted with kind permission.]*

momentary fixation point, the larger will be the (uncrossed or crossed) disparity of its image.

Both the extent and the sign of the retinal disparity thus carry information about the localization of distal objects in space. The human visual system uses this information – as well as other information – in the course of constructing three-dimensional representations (*percepts*) of the perceived world. How this occurs – the question on the foundations of stereoscopic or binocular depth perception – is the subject of this chapter.

Which specific abilities must the human visual system possess in order to be able to draw on retinal disparity information about the spatial position of distal objects and to use this information in the construction of percepts? How can these abilities be described, and which mechanisms are they based on? In the search for answers to these questions, recent decades have seen important contributions from not only psychophysics and neurophysiology but also research on artificial intelligence. More than most of the other information-processing abilities, the study of stereo-scopic vision has become a multidisciplinary research field, in which different methods applied to explain the related questions and the empirical results of one discipline are also relevant for neighboring sciences.

Acknowledging this, the present review presents contributions to the explanation of stereoscopic depth perception from a psychophysical, neurophysiological and computational point of view. These contributions will be discussed in relation to the underlying issues raised by the study of stereoscopic vision. Section 2 presents a sketch of older theories on stereoscopic depth perception. In Section 3, a general description will be developed of the major information processing problems that the visual system has to solve when calculating spatial depth on the basis of retinal disparity values. Any theory of stereoscopic depth perception has to take these general constraints into account. Section 4 presents an influential recent model of the foundations of stereoscopic depth perception developed by David Marr – a theory that has been derived explicitly from the considerations presented in Section 3. This is followed by a discussion of some problems and extensions of Marr's model. Section 5 presents an alternative conception of stereoscopic vision: Grossberg's theory attempts to explain binocular depth perception within the context of a comprehensive model of human visual information processing.

2 HISTORY

Although the geometric factors that lead to the occurrence of binocular disparity and thus underlie the possibility of stereoscopic depth perception were broadly known in classical times and once again since the seventeenth century (see Wade, 1987), the experimental study of this phenomenon first began in the nineteenth century with the construction of the first functioning stereoscope by Charles Wheatstone (1838). Stereoscopes are used when two different stimuli (*half-images*) are each presented separately to one of the two eyes. This procedure should simulate disparity, as it is elicited by binocular viewing of spatially distant, distal objects.[1] Thus, in the stereoscopic presentation of the *line stereogram* in Figure 3.2a, the right-hand line is perceived to be diagonally behind the left-hand line. Figure 3.2b presents the correspondence between this stereogram pair and the distal configuration thus simulated.

Using the newly developed stereoscopic techniques, the nineteenth century saw the study of the effect of disparity values of varying magnitude on the perception of spatial depth. One of the first empirical findings was that half-images can only be integrated into a unified perceptual impression up to a certain maximum disparity value (Panum, 1858). If the disparity goes beyond a specific value labeled *Panum's fusional limit*, double images arise (*diplopia*)

The description of this maximum disparity value as a 'fusional limit' already suggests a certain conceptual model of the foundations of stereoscopic vision: the so-called *fusion theory* of stereoscopic perception assumes that binocular, three-dimensional perception is the result of a fusion of the right and left monocular retinal images. In order for the fusion process to take place at all, monocular images of distal objects that are not located on the horopter (i.e. retinal images that show a certain disparity) have to be matched to one another. After successful matching, disparity values and the spatial depth of objects can be calculated. A comparable conception of the mechanisms of stereoscopic vision can already be found in the work of Kepler (see Kaufman, 1974, pp. 265–266)

---

[1]There are different stereoscopic procedures for the monocular presentation of half-images (see Kaufman, 1974, pp. 269–275; Metzger, 1975, pp. 351–356). Wheatstone himself constructed a *mirror stereoscope* in which the stimuli located to the left and to the right of the observer are reflected by two mirrors. In this way they can be presented independently to each eye. Other variants are the *prism* and the *lens stereoscope*. In a more recent and more well-known method of stereoscopic presentation, the anaglyph procedure, one of the half-images is colored red and the other green. For an observer wearing a pair of glasses with one red and one green filter, the stereoscoplc effect occurs because either the green or the red half-image is filtered out.

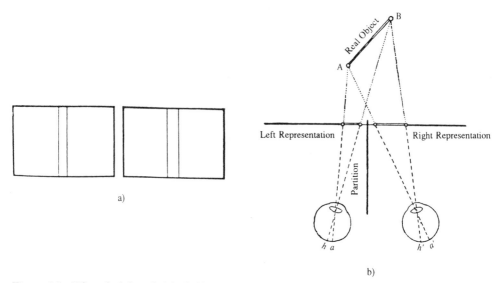

Figure 3.2. *When the left and right half-image of a line stereogram (a) are presented stereoscopically, the distal surface (A,B) is perceived (b). [From Metzger, 1975, pp. 351–352. © 1975 Kramer; reprinted with kind permission.]*

The general assumption of fusion theory – that spatial depth impressions result from the fusion of both retinal images – is, in itself, initially not very informative. In order to give a satisfactory explanation of stereoscopic depth perception, solutions must be proposed for two fundamental problems that arise as a consequence of the postulated binocular fusion process:

(1) *The matching or correspondence problem.* Sometimes there are a great number of possible matches of left and right retinal image points. How can the appropriate matches be determined in each case – how can false matches be avoided?

(2) *The calculation problem.* How is the spatial distance of distal points determined on the basis of a successful match of monocular images?

Older ideas on the fusion theory of stereoscopic vision frequently emphasize the calculation problem. For example, Hering (1868) suggested that a fixed 'depth value' is assigned to each individual point on the retina: in both eyes, this value is low in the temporal area and increases toward the nose. This assumption implies that the sum of the two monocular depth values must be identical for all distal points that fall on corresponding retinal positions (such as the fixation point). This does not hold for noncorresponding, that is, disparate images of distal points. According to Hering, the difference between the depth value of the fixation point and that of another, nonfixated point determines the perceived spatial depth of this second point. Today, Hering's theory is no longer accepted. One of the reasons for this is that it makes completely false predictions about monocular depth perception (Metzger, 1975, pp. 369–371)

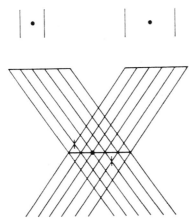

Figure 3.3. *The vertical positions of activated cells within a cortical network indicate the retinal disparity of monocular features. [From Kaufman, 1974, p. 280. © 1974 Oxford University Press; reprinted with kind permission.]*

Later attempts to solve the calculation problem (Boring, 1933; Charnwood, 1951; Dodwell and Engel, 1963) have postulated the existence of a retinotopically organized cortical network that links together neural channels originating from the retina. If a simple line stereogram (as in Figure 3.3) is presented and the two central points are fixated, the binocular disparity of matching left-hand and right-hand lines results from the localization of the cells within the network that are jointly activated by these lines. In the framework of this model, the existence of Panum's fusional limit is explained by the fact that only a limited area of retinal disparities can be assessed, because of the restricted number of available network nodes.

In order to solve the calculation problem, the visual system must already have found a solution to the correspondence problem: only if it is known which monocular representations of distal points have to be matched to each other can their respective binocular disparity be calculated and, on this basis, the spatial depth of distal points. In this sense, the correspondence or matching problem is more fundamental than the calculation problem – it is located at an earlier stage of visual information processing. More recent theories of stereoscopic depth perception take this into account: as will be shown in Section 3, this discussion focuses on possible solutions to the correspondence problem.

Alongside the fact that earlier versions of fusion theory were unable to provide any satisfactory explanations of the correspondence and matching problems, fusion theory is faced with a series of additional difficulties: for example, an impression of spatial depth is also gained when both monocular retinal images are not fused completely but a double image is perceived (Krekling, 1975; Ogle, 1953). Complete binocular fusion is clearly not a necessary condition for the occurrence of stereoscopic depth perception.

A further problem that a fusion theory of stereoscopic vision has to deal with is *Fechner's paradox* (see, for example, Hering, 1978). It was discovered that the luminance of the perceived world scarcely alters when one eye is closed and the amount of light entering the visual system is thereby reduced by one-half. This

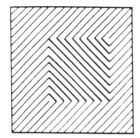 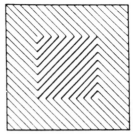

Figure 3.4. *Kaufman stereogram. [From Kaufman, 1974, p. 306. © 1974 Oxford University Press; reprinted with kind permission.]*

phenomenon has been investigated in a series of experiments: first, monocular light input is restricted with a filter. Then the eye that was previously covered with the filter is completely closed. It was found that the perceived luminance of the scenery increased markedly, although the sum of binocular light input had decreased as compared with the previous situation. Fusion theory, which postulates a simple summation of the features of both monocular retinal images in the fusion process, cannot explain this finding (Levelt, 1965)

Fechner's paradox increases the plausibility of one theoretical alternative to fusion theory: the *suppression theory* of stereoscopic vision. Suppression theory explains the unity of visual perceptual impressions by postulating that, at any point in time, one of the two monocular retinal images suppresses the other. Only the dominant image is further processed and forms the basis of a perceptual impression (Verhoeff, 1935) . At a later point in time, the relationship of dominance can reverse and the previously suppressed image can become dominant. Although this assumption of permanent binocular rivalry can be used to explain phenomena like Fechner's paradox, it does not provide a model of the foundations of stereoscopic depth perception. It fails to explain which functional relationship exists between the dominance of a monocular retinal image and the occurrence of an impression of spatial depth. In this context, one can even ask whether the suppression of a monocular retinal image is in any way incompatible with the process of stereoscopic vision: can the monocular information suppressed as a consequence of binocular rivalry in any way still be used for calculating spatial depth on the basis of binocular disparity values? Are not binocular rivalry and binocular depth perception mutually exclusive from the very start?[2] A stimulus pair (Figure 3.4) described by Kaufman (1974) shows that this is not the case. If this pair is presented through a stereoscope, one perceives a square hovering over the peripheral background. However, the diagonal lines that constitute the square are in a continuous state of binocular rivalry: at a given point in time, either the 45 degree or the 135 degree pattern of lines is dominant.

---

[2]The discussion on the contrast and possible functional relationships between stereoscopic depth perception, binocular fusion and binocular rivalry has regained in strength in recent years (Blake 1989; Blake and O'Shea, 1988; Timney, Wilcox and St. John, 1989; Wolfe, 1986, 1988).

A further model of the foundations of stereoscopic vision emphasizes the importance of *vergence movements*. As such, movements are elicited when an object has to be fixated that is located to one side or the other of the current fixation plane. The amount of change in the vergence angle contains information on the spatial depth of the fixated object. The *oculomotor theory* of stereoscopic vison assumes that the registration of the vergence angle and vergence movements is a major basis of binocular spatial vision. A similar idea had already been proposed by George Berkeley in 1709 (see Berkeley, 1910). In this context, Sherrington (1918) stressed the importance of processing afferent signals from the receptors to the extraocular muscles (inflow). Helmholtz (1866/1962), in contrast, considered efferent signals responsible for eliciting vergence movements (outflow) to be the relevant factor. Although current theories of binocular depth perception do not completely rule out the influence of a sensory registration of antecedents or consequences of vergence movements on the perception of spatial depth (see for example, Foley, 1978), this factor probably only plays a subordinate role: depth information derived from the registration of vergence movements can be effective solely for the localization of objects that are less than 3 m away from the observer (Gogel, 1977). Instead of assigning vergence movements and their registration a direct role in the calculation of spatial depth, the elicitation of these movements is currently viewed mainly as the consequence of a prior localization of distal objects on the basis of disparities. In this context, however, they might indeed play an important role in spatial perception (see Section 4).

None of the older concepts sketched above can offer a unified, comprehensive description of the foundations of stereoscopic vision. For this reason, there has been a long-lasting controversy on the issue of which of the proposed models provides the most appropriate description of the mechanisms underlying binocular depth perception (Kaufman, 1974, pp. 318–321)

In recent decades, not only psychophysical observations but also findings from other scientific disciplines have played an increasing role in research on binocular vision. Progress in research on the neurophysiological foundations of vision has led to a better understanding of the problems and mechanisms of stereoscopic depth perception. The same applies to the various projects aimed at constructing computer programs for the recognition of patterns or objects (*computer vision*). At present, most researchers favor modified versions of fusion theory. Nevertheless, elements of oculomotor theory and the suppression model have also found a place in these recent models. Some basic considerations underlying these recent models will be presented in the following section.

3 STEREOSCOPIC DEPTH PERCEPTION AS AN INFORMATION PROCESSING PROBLEM

One central problem facing fusion theory is the correspondence problem (see Section 2). How can it be ensured that, during binocular fusion, only such monocular features (or points) are matched to each other and fused that have been elicited by one single distal object (or one single distal point)? The correspondence problem arises in simple line stereograms but becomes very apparent in more

Figure 3.5. *Random-dot stereogram. [From Julesz, 1971, p. xi. © 1971 University of Chicago Press; reprinted with kind permission.]*

complex monocular stimuli. Figure 3.5 shows a random-dot stereogram (Julesz, 1960, 1971).[3] To compute the exact disparity value of individual, corresponding central squares, a great number of possible but false matches between these squares must be excluded. Experimental evidence demonstrates that this is possible: if the two random-dot patterns are presented through a stereoscope, a vivid impression of a central square hovering over the background is experienced after a short time.

How does the visual system solve the correspondence problem in this case? How are noncorresponding squares prevented from being matched to each other? One strategy could be to match only sufficiently similar monocular features. This proposal is based on the following idea: the deeper the processing of the two monocular retinal images before their binocular matching, the more dimensions are available for checking the similarity of features and, therefore, the simpler the solution to the correspondence problem. If binocular matching occurs between monocular images of the contours of two- or three-dimensional objects, there is scarcely any risk of false matches (Kaufman, 1974, pp. 283–284). Such a solution to the matching problem has already been proposed by Sherrington (1906). Gestalt psychology's conception of the existence of 'attractive powers' between similar monocular characteristics also suggests an extensive processing of monocular images (Metzger, 1975, p. 372)

However, Julesz's random-dot stereograms proved that this proposed solution to the matching problem did not fit the facts: observed in isolation, the two monocular patterns do not provide any information about possible spatial organizations. Nevertheless, stereoscopic presentation leads to a clear three-dimensional impression: in this situation, the visual system can evidently solve the correspondence problem without having performed an extensive perceptual analysis of the monocular image. Representations of complex object properties thus cannot be

---

[3]The random-dot stereogram in Figure 3.5 consists of copies of a random pattern of black and white squares in which a quadratic section in the center of one of the copies is shifted to the left. In the center of the other copy, this section is shifted to the right. The empty space created in this way is filled with a new random pattern. When both copies are presented stereoscopically, the centers of the monocular images are disparate: after successful binocular matching, this should evoke an impression of depth.

regarded as monocular matching partners. In contrast, the elements of the binocular fusion process are likely to be representations of relatively primitive distal features.

The findings from Julesz raise a series of new questions. First, the realization that the objects of the matching process must be comparatively simple features seems to have rendered a solution to the correspondence problem more difficult: the less differentiated the monocular elements matched to each other, the more demanding the task of differentiating correct from false correspondences. This particularly applies to random-dot stereograms: in contrast to simple line stereograms (see Figure 3.2a), in which competing matching possibilities are generally not present, a great number of contralateral image points are possible matching partners for each monocular image of a single square.

In the case of simple line stereograms, it is conceivable that the visual system uses a *local* matching strategy: for each monocular image point, a contralateral correspondence is sought without this process being influenced by the remaining, simultaneously occurring binocular matchings. In random-dot stereograms, such a strategy should be unsuitable because of the existence of a great number of competing matching possibilities. In this context, Julesz (1978) makes the distinction between local and global modes of stereoscopic depth perception: for random-dot stereograms, it is the *global* configuration of the stimulus pattern that has to be considered in the search for suitable binocular matches.[4] This does not mean that the binocular matching process takes place between complex, monocular features that have already been extensively processed, – as proposed by Sherrington. By describing this process as 'global', Julesz points to the fact that each local match between elementary, monocular features does not occur autonomously but influences – and is influenced by – other matches. The result of such an interaction of individual, binocular matchings should be an answer to the matching problem that is also coherent from a global perspective. The formulation of global strategies for solving the correspondence problem for Julesz's random-dot stereograms and other complex stimuli is the focus of a series of models of stereoscopic depth perception (see, for example, Julesz, 1986; Marr, 1982; Poggio and Poggio, 1984)

In order to be able to develop a theory of stereoscopic vision that is capable of explaining the occurrence of spatial impressions resulting from the presentation of random-dot stereograms, several fundamental questions have to be answered:

(1) How should we describe the monocular representations of distal features that are matched to each other? Could they be simple elements of the retinal image or are they rather later products of visual information processing?

(2) What are the single steps of the matching process? Which aspects are responsible for the fact that certain matches are realized (and thus viewed as correct) while others, in contrast, are rejected as false?

(3) How is the result of the matching process represented? How are binocular disparity values transformed into a representation of the perceived spatial depth of distal objects?

---

[4]Metzger makes a similar distinction (1975, pp. 371–372): he contrasts the 'atomistic' conception of the foundation of binocular matching processes with a 'holistic' conception. Within the holistic conception, binocular matching processes are held to be determined not only through comparisons between two single points but also through an evaluation of their embedment in a broader context.

Julesz's stereograms have shown that a successful binocular matching of mono-cular images in no way requires a previously completed perceptual segmentation of the visual input. Therefore, the processes that underlie such a matching might be assigned to an early stage of visual information processing. The first two questions raised above – on the nature of the monocular features matched to each other here, and the mechanisms of the matching process – could therefore be accessible to neuroanatomical and neurophysiological investigation. For these reasons, research on the functional organization of the optic nerve and the primary visual cortex is of major interest for the study of the foundations of stereoscopic vision. Some relevant findings from these studies will be presented in the next two sections within the context of contemporary theories of binocular depth perception.

Before findings from neuroanatomy and neurophysiology can be adequately evaluated, we must first ask which possibilities for the solution to the correspon-dence problem can in principle be conceived: how can acceptable matchings be differentiated from unacceptable ones? In order to formulate a general solution strategy and be able to test how far it is actually used in visual information processing, it is necessary – according to Marr (1982) – to develop a general descrip-tion of the determinants of the problem to be solved. This is done on the level of *computational theory* (Eimer, 1990, pp. 121–125). Here it is important to identify specific external 'constraints' – to specify general assumptions about the properties of the distal world whose correctness must be assumed when solving an informa-tion processing problem. Which assumptions could be relevant to the solution of the correspondence problem?

One central assumption results from the geometry of the optic apparatus: as the optical axes of both eyes are displaced in a horizontal but not in a vertical direction, it is guaranteed that also both monocular images of a distal point on the retina will only be displaced on a (more or less) *horizontal* axis. Put more precisely, they always lie on *epipolar* lines – the lines on which the projection plane and the image plane bisect (Dhond and Aggarwal, 1989, p. 1491).[5] For the process of binocular matching, this *epipolar line constraint* implies that only monocular features that lie on corre-sponding epipolar lines can be considered as candidates for the matching. This greatly reduces the number of matchings that have to be investigated.

Two further general assumptions that might be fundamental for any attempt to solve the correspondence problem are derived by Marr (1982, pp. 112–116) from considering the physical properties of distal objects. At a given point in time, each point on an object's surface has a unique spatial localization (*constraint of spatial localization*). In addition, distal surfaces are generally smooth; for this reason, sudden discontinuous changes in distance between surfaces of objects and the eyes rarely occur except at object boundaries (*continuity constraint*). However, this type of change frequently occurs at the boundaries of distal objects. These two assump-tions can now be used to specify several 'matching rules' that have to be taken into

---

[5]In the fixation of an infinitely distant point and the attendant parallel positioning of the eyes, the epipolar lines are horizontal and parallel to each other: only points with identical vertical positions can be matched to each other here. In all other cases, the orientation of the epipolar lines changes as a function of the respective angle of vision.

account when developing an algorithm for the solution of the correspondence problem:

(1) As the monocular features to be matched to each other are elicited by a common, single distal feature, they should be similar to each other. Only similar features can be considered as candidates for a match (*compatibility condition*).

(2) As the represented distal feature has a unique spatial localization, each left-hand monocular feature can only be matched to exactly one right-hand monocular feature and vice versa (*uniqueness condition*).[6]

(3) As distal surfaces are relatively smooth, the disparity values of neighboring points computed after binocular matching should always deviate only slightly from each other and change continuously across space (*continuity condition*). Binocular matches that lead to a discontinuous change in the disparity values of neighboring image points should therefore be rejected as false.

On the basis of these three matching rules, Marr (1982, pp. 114–115) has formulated his 'fundamental assumption of stereopsis': if a match between monocular features is possible that meets these conditions, this match can be regarded as appropriate. It can, in turn, serve as a basis for the calculation of binocular disparity values and the determination of the spatial distance of distal surfaces.

According to Marr (1982), formulating general assumptions about the constitution of the distal world and general conditions for the solution of an information processing problem on the level of 'computational theory' is necessary in order to be able to use these assumptions to develop plausible algorithms on a second level. The power of such algorithms to solve the information processing problem being studied will then show how far the considerations on the computational theory level apply and whether they are sufficient.

The question now arises whether the considerations presented in this section can be used to develop algorithms capable of solving complex binocular matching problems like those caused by Julesz's random-dot stereograms. This will be investigated in the following section.

4 RANDOM-DOT STEREOGRAMS AND THE CORRESPONDENCE PROBLEM IN BINOCULAR VISION

In order to define an algorithm to solve the correspondence problem, we first have to specify as precisely as possible the properties of the monocular features that have to be matched to each other. The earliest conceivable candidates for binocular

---

[6]However, this assumption does not apply without exception: the so-called *Panum's limiting case* is characterized by the fact that two distal points are located behind one another on the lines of sight of one eye (Kaufman, 1974, p. 290). For this eye, the more distant point is covered by the nearer one – only a single point is imaged on the retina. In the other eye, in contrast, both points are represented. Although a unique match is not possible here, the two points are perceived as differing in spatial depth (Marr, 1982, pp. 141–142; Mayhew and Frisby, 1981, p. 369).

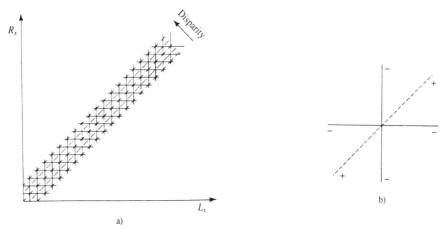

Figure 3.6. *(a) The nodes of this network represent possible binocular matches between left and right image features (L_x, R_x). (b) Excitatory $(+)$ and inhibitory $(-)$ connections between single nodes inside this network. [From Marr, 1982, p. 117. Reprinted from Marr and Poggio, 1976. © 1976 AAAS, Washington; reprinted with kind permission of the publisher and T. Poggio.]*

matching are single, retinal image points (*pixels*) or pixel patterns. Such a matching of features of retinal *grey-level images* (Marr, 1982) does not presuppose any previous processing of visual signals. Thus, for example, Sperling (1970) assumes in his cooperative model of binocular vision that disparity values are calculated on the basis of such grey-level images. However, it is now generally considered that the binocular matching of retinal image points offers no guarantee for an adequate solution to the correspondence problem. One reason for this is the fact that the spatial or structural features of retinal grey-tone values are not always highly correlated with specific properties of distal objects. There is, hence, considerable risk that their matching leads to the construction of spatially localized features for which there is no counterpart in the distal world (Marr, 1982, p. 105). For these reasons, it is better to look for the monocular matching partners on higher stages of visual information processing.[7]

Sperling's theory of stereoscopic vision encouraged the formulation of algorithms in which a solution of the correspondence problem for random-dot stereograms was sought in the cooperative–competitive interactions within a single network. The nodes of this network represent possible binocular matches (Dev, 1975; Marr and Poggio, 1976). Marr and Poggio's algorithm operates in a three-dimensional network: each level of this network is responsible for matching monocular representations of distal features located on one single horizontal line. One level of this network is presented schematically in Figure 3.6a. The values L_x and R_x represent the respective positions of the monocular images of distal features on the specific horizontal line: a node with the coordinates (L_x, R_x) is activated when

---

[7] Although Sperling's theory can be considered false on this point, other elements of his model remain influential: Sperling was one of the first to point out the special role of vergence movements in the binocular matching process (Sperling, 1970, pp. 467–477), and his considerations on the neurophysiological foundations of this process (Sperling, 1970, pp. 496–526) have also been influential.

a distal feature (here a black square as an element of a random-dot stereogram) is represented at positions L_x, R_x in both the left and the right eye. Each active node thus indicates one potential binocular match (up to a maximum possible disparity value indicated by the two outer diagonals in Figure 3.6a). In the presentation of a random-dot stereogram, numerous different binocular matches are imaginable; within the network, therefore, many nodes are at first activated simultaneously. The goal of the algorithm developed by Marr and Poggio (1976) must therefore be to lead the network to a final state in which all nodes representing an acceptable match between left and right monocular features have the value 1, while all remaining nodes take the value 0.

How can such a state be achieved? Drawing on the general considerations in Section 3, Marr and Poggio have defined the following rules of state transformation:

(1) The matching of monocular features must be unique: if a feature with the position $L_{x'}$ is matched to a contralateral feature with the position $R_{x'}$, a further matching of this very feature to another contralateral feature (that is to be found, e.g. at the position $R_{x''}$) should be excluded. In other words, for each position L_x or R_x, only one single node within the network should be active after the matching process is completed (and should thus represent the selected match). In Marr and Poggio's algorithm, this is achieved by nodes along each horizontal or vertical line inhibiting each other (Figure 3.6b): if a specific node is activated, this decreases the activity of all other nodes with an identical localization on the x- or y-axis.

(2) The local disparity values may not change discontinuously; the final and unique binocular matches should then be located roughly in a plane of constant disparity, that is, along one of the diagonals in Figure 3.6a. In the Marr–Poggio algorithm, this is realized by placing excitatory connections between all the nodes that lie on one diagonal (Figure 3.6b): the activation of a specific node thus leads to an increase in the activation value of all remaining nodes lying on the same diagonal.

The presentation of a random-dot stereogram initially activates a great number of nodes within this network. These active nodes then interact in the way described above. If the activity of one node passes a specific threshold after these interactions, then it is set to 1, otherwise it is set to 0. This completes one iteration of the matching algorithm. In the next step, the activated nodes once more interact according to the state transformation rules sketched above. Within a few steps of iteration, this cooperative algorithm generally finds the correct binocular matches for a random-dot stereogram.

However, the fact that the algorithm developed by Marr and Poggio (1976) produces an adequate binocular match in the case of random-dot stereograms in no way implies that the human visual system uses a comparable algorithm to solve the correspondence problem. A number of considerations actually question this assumption. It is to be doubted whether this algorithm would also find an answer to the correspondence problem under ecologically more realistic conditions: in a normal perceptual situation, the visual apparatus is confronted with complexly structured elements of the distal world that show a great number of small details. To be able to calculate the disparity values of distal surface points according to the Marr–Poggio algorithm, possible correspondences would have to be sought in a fine-grained network with an inconceivably large number of nodes. This would call for a great number of iteration steps and require more time – time that is not always available to the organism during confrontations with potentially threatening distal configurations.[8]

A further problem is that the algorithm described by Marr and Poggio does not consider the role of vergence movements. The function of eye movements for stereoscopic depth perception has been discussed since the beginning of experimental research on binocular vision. In recent times, the issue is being studied in experiments in which eye movements are neutralized by stabilizing the retinal image (for example, Fender and Julesz, 1967) or by using extremely short, tachistoscopic stimulus presentations (Julesz and Chang, 1976; Richards, 1977).[9] The general finding has been that binocular depth perception is strongly limited if eye movements are not possible: the area of fusible binocular disparity values is relatively narrow; absolute disparity values and thus the spatial depth of distal objects can hardly be determined.

A further psychophysical fact is the extreme plasticity of the binocular matching mechanism: for example, random-dot stereograms can still be fused when one of the two patterns is enlarged to a specific degree as well as when the spatial orientation of the elements to be fused or the strength of the contrast is varied (Julesz, 1971). Nonetheless, if the direction of contrast is inverted in one of the two patterns, binocular matching does not occur (Julesz, 1960). This plasticity of the matching process as well as its limits cannot be explained sufficiently by the algorithm developed by Marr and Poggio.

An additional, fundamental weakness of this algorithm is that it does not precisely specify the type of monocular features that have to be matched to one another. Therefore, better insights into the anatomic location and the neurophysiological foundations of the binocular matching process can hardly be obtained. However, exactly such issues are in the focus of attention in recent studies of stereoscopic vision, where neuroanatomical and neurophysiological findings are increasingly being considered. This particularly applies to attempts to find out which monocular features – beyond the gray-level values favored by Sperling – need to be considered as possible matching partners.

In this context, details on the functional anatomy of the retinogeniculate system become relevant: here we find retinal ganglion cells and cells of the lateral geniculate nucleus called *X cells*. These cells have almost circularly symmetric receptive fields that are composed of an excitatory center and an inhibitory periphery (*on-center*), or of an inhibitory center and excitatory periphery (*off-center*) (Kuffler, 1953). The presence of intensity differences at specific retinal locations leads to increased activity in specific X cells (Enroth-Cugell and Robson, 1966). Marr and Hildreth (1980) have described the activation of these cells as the result of a center-surround filtering process. During this process, locations on the retina

---

[8]Because of this need for the fastest possible spatial localization of distal objects, Marr suspects that iterative algorithms cannot be considered as a basis for human stereoscopic depth perception (1982, p. 107). In his opinion, 'one-shot' algorithms are more appropriate – procedures whose capability of producing binocular matches is not based on an iteration of elementary computations.

[9]The study by Fender and Julesz (1967) is also worth noting for another reason: they found that after successful fusion of a random-dot stereogram, the two monocular images on the retina could be pulled apart by a multiple of Panum's fusional area before double images were perceived. However, in order to refuse these images after binocular fusion had collapsed, they had to be brought back to approximately corresponding locations. This effect, labeled *hysteresis*, can be viewed as a manifestation of a primitive memory mechanism (Marr, 1982, pp. 126–127).

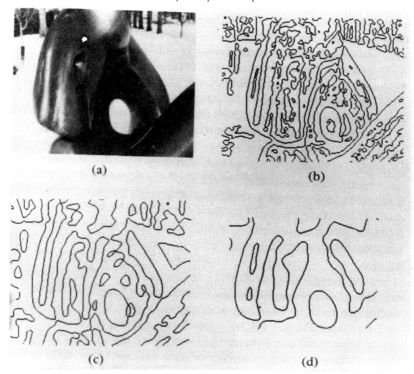

Figure 3.7. *Zero-crossing maps (b–d) for an image (a) that has been processed with filters of different scales: (b) fine; (c) medium; and (d) coarse. (From Marr, 1982, p. 69. Reprinted from Marr and Hildreth, 1980. © 1980 the authors; reprinted with kind permission of Ellen Hildreth.]*

are determined at which the registered light intensity undergoes maximum change.[10] Different retinal ganglion cells are sensitive to different spatial frequencies (De Valois and De Valois, 1988, pp. 88–89). Some respond solely to gradual changes in intensity (low spatial frequencies), others, in contrast, particularly to abrupt intensity changes (high frequencies). Marr and Hildreth (1980) suspect that these cells are organized in several autonomous center-surround filter systems (channels). Each of these channels is responsible for identifying changes in retinal intensity within a limited spatial frequency band (see also Marr and Ullman, 1981): a filter system that is set at low frequencies hence provides a coarse map of zero-crossings, while a filter system designed to register high frequencies can convey detailed information on local, closely demarcated changes in intensity. This relationship is illustrated in Figure 3.7: this presents different zero-crossing maps for an image (a) that is processed with: (b) a fine, (c) a medium, or (d) a coarse filter.[11]

---

[10]More precisely, *zero-crossings* in the second derivative of local retinal intensity changes are determined. Zero-crossings mark those points within the retinal image at which the activity of the receptor cells changes most strongly (Marr, 1982, pp. 54–60).

[11]The frequency specificity of these channels depends on the size of the retinal receptive fields of the X cells: the lower the average extension of the receptive fields, the higher, in general, the preferred spatial frequency.

Zero-crossings form an initial, primitive representation of the features of monocular retinal images; they are therefore the most peripherally located candidates for
binocular matching. But single zero-crossings only represent small, spot-like retinal
changes and not yet larger, oriented retinal intensity differences (contours, edges,
lines, etc.). To derive such representations, neighboring X cells, whose receptive
fields cover a specific, oriented retinal area, must be connected. Coordinated
activity of these groups of cells could then indicate the existence of an oriented
intensity change in this retinal area (Marr and Hildreth, 1980, pp. 208–209). When
looking for monocular features, whose disparity is calculated by the visual system
and transformed into information on the spatial distance between neighboring
distal surface points, such oriented 'zero-crossing segments' might be considered
as likely candidates.

Marr (1976, 1982) has postulated further steps in the processing of the retinal
image that follow the registration of oriented zero-crossing segments and finally
result in a first representation of the structural features of the retinal image (border
areas, lines, edges, textural changes, etc.) on various levels of spatial resolution.
Elements from this representation (*primal sketch*) could also be considered as
possible matching partners within the computational mechanisms that find a
solution to the correspondence problem.

With reference to these considerations on the functional anatomy of the visual
pathway, Marr and Poggio (1979) have formulated a second, noncooperative
algorithm for solving the correspondence problem. In this algorithm, the monocular
matching partners are singular zero-crossings. The problem of false matches is
minimized by matching zero-crossings separately within each frequency-specific
channel system. The lower the number of to-be-matched zero-crossings and the
greater the average interval between them, the lower is the risk of a false match and
the greater the range of disparity within which a search can be made for binocular
correspondences. As described above, channels sensitive to low spatial frequencies
provide coarse, less-detailed zero-crossing maps. Within channel systems that are
specialized to higher frequencies, maps are generated that include a much larger
number of zero-crossing segments (Figure 3.7). From this fact, Marr and Poggio
(1979) have derived the following general matching strategy: first, zero-crossings
from channels with low optimal spatial frequency are tested within a broad range
of possible disparity values. If two zero-crossings correspond, they are matched to
each other. On this basis, a first, approximate disparity value is calculated and
vergence movements may be elicited. These movements reduce the absolute
disparity to such an extent that fusion can now take place between zero crossings
from less coarse maps. After further vergence movements (disparity reductions),
zero-crossings from high-resolution channel systems can finally be matched to each
other. In this way, disparity values and the corresponding distances of distal
surface points can be precisely determined.

Whether this second algorithm can be successful in avoiding false binocular
matches between zero-crossings clearly depends on the distance between zero-
crossings after center-surround filtering of the retinal image within different
frequency-specific channel systems (Figure 3.8): for each entry in the zero-crossing
map of the left retinal image (L), a search has to be made within the right map for
a corresponding zero-crossing (R) within a specific area of disparity w. If the
probability is high that an additional, noncorresponding zero-crossing (a false

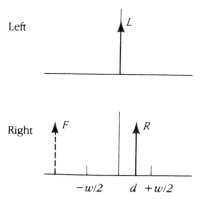

Figure 3.8. *False binocular matches can be avoided if false targets (F) for a left monocular zero-crossing (L) regularly occur outside the disparity interval w. Within this interval, R is the only candidate for binocular matching. [From Marr, 1982, p. 139, top left. Reprinted from Marr and Poggio, 1979; with kind permission of Tomaso Poggio.]*

target such as F in Figure 3.8) is present in this area, the matching problem could not be solved unambiguously.

How high is the probability of false targets? The center-surround filter systems postulated by Marr and Hildreth (1980) can be roughly regarded as bandpass filters. It can be demonstrated that the interval between single zero-crossings of a signal processed by bandpass filters generally does not drop below a certain minimum. The size of this minimal interval can be calculated (Marr, 1982, pp. 135–140): if the matching mechanism is restricted to checking a disparity interval in which the probability that two zero positions with the same sign occur together is sufficiently low, false matches are hardly to be expected.[12]

A series of computer simulations (Grimson, 1981a, b) have shown that Marr and Poggio's (1979) algorithm is capable of solving the matching problem for random-dot stereograms as well as for some natural visual stimuli. Nonetheless, the decisive question remains whether a similar algorithm actually underlies human stereoscopic depth perception. This can be studied by deriving specific empirical hypotheses from Marr and Poggio's (1979) considerations. They claim, for example, that the maximum fusible disparity value for each frequency-specific channel system is a function of the width of its receptive fields (or its preferred spatial frequency) – the greater this width (the lower the optimal spatial frequency), the broader the area of disparity is within which monocular features (zero positions) can be unambiguously matched to each other.

How can this hypothesis be tested? It is known that the average width of the receptive fields of cortical neurons increases as a linear function of retinal eccentricity: in the foveal area, it is low; in the periphery, receptive fields are many times larger (Hubel and Wiesel, 1974; van Essen, Newsome and Maunsell,

---

[12]The size of this disparity area (w) naturally varies with the spatial resolution capacity (i.e. the size of the receptive fields) of each filter system.

1984). Accordingly, cortical cells sensitive to high spatial frequencies generally possess receptive fields that are localized in foveal areas (Tootell et al., 1982).[13] Thus, the disparity interval within which successful matches can take place (Panum's fusional area) should increase with greater retinal eccentricity. This assumption has been confirmed (Mitchell, 1966; Ogle, 1964)

A more specific hypothesis, which can also be derived from Marr and Poggio's (1979) algorithm, states that there should be an approximately linear relationship between the spatial frequency of stimuli and the maximum disparity that can be coped with: low-frequency stimuli only activate low-resolution channels; high-frequency stimuli, in contrast, activate channels in which fine zero-crossing maps are generated. Thus, the extent of tolerable disparity should be high for low-frequeny stimuli. In contrast, small disparity values should be comparatively difficult to detect here – on the basis of coarse zero-crossing maps. The opposite would hold for high-frequency stimuli: highly disparate monocular stimuli should not be fusible, but fine differences in disparity should be detected. Although some experimental findings (Felton, Richards and Smith, 1972; Kulikowski, 1978; Levinson and Blake, 1979) suggest that these assumptions are at least partly correct, a series of other empirical findings make them more doubtful. Mayhew and Frisby (1979) have used filtered random-dot stereograms (stimuli in which all spatial frequencies except a small frequency band are eliminated) to study under which conditions two areas with different disparities can be discriminated. The disparity difference between the two areas was held constant at 2.6 min arc, while the absolute size of these disparities was varied between 0 min arc and approx. 20 min arc. To exclude the effect of eye movements, the stereograms were presented by a tachistoscope. Marr and Poggio's (1979) algorithm would predict that when low-frequency random-dot stereograms are presented, only channels sensitive to low frequencies would be stimulated. Under these conditions, areas with small absolute disparity values should not be discriminable. Mayhew and Frisby's results did not agree with this prediction: areas with small absolute disparity values could also be discriminated in low and medium spatial frequency stereograms (see also Julesz and Schumer, 1981).[14]

These and further findings (Mayhew and Frisby, 1981, pp. 370–376) dispute Marr and Poggio's (1979) view that the calculation of binocular disparities occurs independently and sequentially within single frequency-specific channels and generally depends on the possibility of vergence movements. For these reasons, Mayhew and Frisby (1981) have proposed a series of extensions to Marr and Poggio's (1979) model. They consider a binocular matching process based on an interaction between different, simultaneously active, frequency-specific channel systems (see Figure 3.9): in each channel it is checked whether a zero-crossing is

---

[13] Actually, the postulated linear relationship between the size of the receptive field of a cortical cell and its selectivity for a specific spatial frequency only holds with reservations. Cells that have the same optimal spatial frequency but differ in the width of their frequency bands often possess receptive fields with completely different diameters (De Valois, Albrecht and Thorell, 1978; De Valois and De Valois, 1988, p. 99).

[14] In a tachistoscopic presentation of unfiltered random-dot stereograms (Mayhew and Frisby, 1979, Exp. IIa), in which vergence movements were not possible, it was found that subjects were able to discriminate areas of different disparity within a broad range of absolute disparity values (up to a limit of approx. 13 min arc).

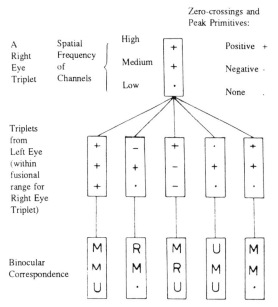

Figure 3.9. *In the model of Mayhew and Frisby, the binocular matching process is based on simultaneous comparisons within different frequency-specific channels (top and middle row). The bottom row shows the results of these comparisons. [From Mayhew and Frisby, 1981, p. 378. © 1981 Elsevier Science, reprinted with kind permission.]*

present in a specific retinal location and which sign (light–dark or dark–light) it possesses. The result of these simultaneous monocular measurements is presented in Figure 3.9 (top) in a simplified form as a triplet. To be able to determine the contralateral retinal position at which the feature to be matched is located, this data pattern is compared with several neighboring triplets that are recorded in the other eye within a limited disparity range (Figure 3.9, center). If the agreement between these signal patterns is sufficiently high (Figure 3.9 bottom right), binocular matching occurs.

Using a computer simulation of their algorithm, Mayhew and Frisby (1981) demonstrated that this parallel operation of several frequency-specific channels often excluded the binocular matching of false targets. They could determine correct matches between monocular features even under conditions in which Marr and Poggio's (1979) algorithm fails.

Alongside indicating the role of a simultaneous activity of different channel systems for binocular fusion, Mayhew and Frisby (1981) have extended Marr and Poggio's considerations in another way: they argue that, in addition to zero-crossings, other elementary monocular features (such as the maxima or minima of a filtered signal) could be used as binocular matching partners. They have also shown that the risk of false binocular matchings can be reduced when, in cases of doubtful matches between individual zero-crossings, the neighboring zero-crossing pattern is taken into account. It can be tested whether a pair that has been matched locally proves to be a constituent of a spatially continuous, oriented structure. According to Mayhew and Frisby (1981), the figural continuity of larger-scale zero-crossing segments is an additional important criterion for finding an adequate solution to the correspondence problem.

Despite these additional proposals, the considerations of Mayhew and Frisby (1981) and Marr and Poggio (1979) are closely related: both assume the simplest monocular features (zero-crossings, maxima or minima within the filtered gray-level image) as matching partners; operations within or between frequency-specific channel systems play a decisive role in both. As in the prior theories from Sperling (1970) and Marr and Poggio (1976), both models characterize the basic mechanism within stereoscopic depth perception as the calculation of a great number of local disparity values for retinal image points.[15] Such a small-scale, regular image pattern is particularly evoked by random-dot stereograms. This underlines the influence the work of Julesz has had on the Sperling–Marr–Mayhew–Frisby tradition,but does not reveal how far the algorithms postulated within this framework can also be regarded as a suitable basis for stereoscopic depth perception in natural contexts.

5 VISUAL SEGMENTATION AND STEREOSCOPIC VISION: GROSSBERG'S THEORY

An alternative to the models presented in the previous section has been put forward by Stephen Grossberg (1983, 1987b; Grossberg and Marshall, 1989). In contrast to the considerations in the Sperling–Marr tradition, in which the ability of stereoscopic depth perception is regarded as a more or less autonomous module that can be studied in broad isolation from all remaining aspects of visual information processing, Grossberg assumes that this ability is realized by subsystems within the human visual apparatus that simultaneously carry out a series of other visual functions. For this reason, Grossberg's ideas on the mechanisms of stereoscopic vision can be understood only within the framework of his more comprehensive conception of the foundations of visual information processing (Grossberg, 1987a, b). In the following, the basic principles of Grossberg's theory of stereoscopic vision will be sketched. His general ideas on the nature of visual information processing will be discussed only to the extent that they are necessary for an understanding of his theory of binocular depth perception.

Grossberg criticizes algorithms that try to determine the spatial position of distal surfaces on the basis of a great number of local disparity calculations. According to him, these algorithms are confronted with fundamental problems – problems that point to the need for a fundamentally different model of stereoscopic depth perception. These difficulties become clear in various perceptual situations: imagine an observer who fixates a homogeneous rectangle that is placed in front of a uniform background. How can the spatial depth of the rectangle be determined stereoscopically? Because all monocular image points from inside the rectangle are practically identical, an unambiguous calculation of binocular disparity for single image points based on local binocular matches is not possible here. Correct matches can be identified only in the area of the discontinuous boundaries between figure

---

[15]This view can also be found in Marr's description of the initial representation of the spatial features of distal surfaces: the $2\frac{1}{2}D$ sketch (Marr, 1982, pp. 277–279). According to Marr, the spatial depth or the orientation of *singular surface points* is separately represented.

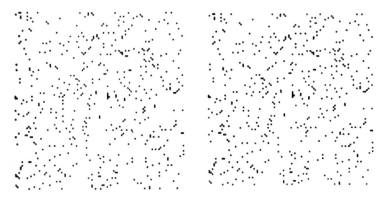

Figure 3.10. *Random-dot stereogram that includes only 5% black dots. [From Julesz, 1971, p. 122.* © *1971 University of Chicago Press; reprinted with kind permission.]*

and background. Nevertheless, one does not just perceive isolated object boundaries localized in space, but rather continuous distal surfaces located at a specific distance (Grossberg, 1987b, p. 126): how does perception of depth occur for the uniform, inner area of the square?

A similar problem arises in relation to one of the random-dot patterns presented by Julesz (1971) (Figure 3.10): although only 5% of the total area in this pair of stimuli is covered with black squares, stereoscopic presentation creates the impression that a central square hovers over the background of the image. In this case, not only the few black squares but also the total white area in the middle of the stereogram is perceived to be spatially displaced. Is it plausible to assume, in line with Marr and Poggio, that local disparity values are calculated for both the black and the white spots in the center of the stereogram, or does this phenomenon require a fundamentally different explanation?

Problems do not only arise when an observer perceives homogeneous distal surfaces, they also arise when a smooth object surface is textured (Grossberg, 1983, pp. 632–633): near the fixation point, disparity is minimal. With increasing retinal eccentricity, its value increases. Nevertheless, one perceives a *planar* surface and not, for example, a surface that curves toward the observer at the periphery. And why does the perceived spatial orientation of planar surfaces not change with every change in the direction of fixation?[16]

These considerations generally suggest that stereoscopic depth perception cannot be based merely on local computations of correspondences between small-scale monocular features. Can an alternative conceptualization of the foundations of stereoscopic depth perception be put forward? Grossberg suggests that the construction of a three-dimensional representation of distal surfaces (3-D *representation of form-and-color-in-depth*) results from the interaction of two visual subsystems. Stereoscopic depth perception occurs when the *boundary contour (BC) system* and the *feature contour (FC) system* interact.

---

[16]In this context, Grossberg (1987b, p. 127) points to the fact that, under certain conditions, perceived distance actually can vary with the location of fixation.

Which functions do these two subsystems serve within the framework of Grossberg's conception of visual information processing? What is their role in the construction of three-dimensional perceptual impressions? These questions will now be addressed.[17]

The primary function of the FC system is to convey information on the color and brightness of distal surfaces. The so-called *featural filling-in* for single elements of the visual world is controlled by such information.[18] As a result of these filling-in processes, representations of spatially localized and structured, perceptually segmented and colored distal surfaces arise.

This process of featural filling-in is set in motion by signals that are generated by the second subsystem, the BC system. The primary function of the BC system is to segment the visual input – to identify edges, corners or object boundaries and to separate differently textured surface areas. The borderlines conveyed by such segmentation processes also control the spatial expansion of the filling-in processes that occur in the FC system.

According to Grossberg, another important function of the BC system is the stereoscopic calculation of spatial depth – more precisely, the construction and binocular matching of monocular features as well as the subsequent determination of disparity values. How does this process take place within the BC system?

As described in Section 3, the first task of any theory of stereoscopic depth perception is to specify the monocular features that are matched to each other. Grossberg suggests that these features are boundaries that are constructed in the course of segmentation processes within the BC system (Figure 3.11): oriented changes in retinal intensity are registered by cells whose receptive fields are extended along their axis of symmetry. Two of these receptive fields are sketched in the lower part of Figure 3.11. Cells with such receptive fields react to vertically oriented retinal intensity changes (either from light to dark or from dark to light). Such cells are sensitive to both the orientation and the direction (or phase) of retinal contrasts, and can thus be compared to representations of 'oriented zero-crossing segments' postulated by Marr (see Section 4). They might be identical to cortical *simple cells* that have been described by Hubel and Wiesel (1962). Simple cells are phase- and orientation-specific cells in the primary visual cortex.

According to Grossberg, pairs of simple cells converge on cells of another type that indicate the amount and orientation but no longer the direction of retinal contrasts. This is the level of cortical *complex cells* (Hubel and Wiesel, 1962). Like simple cells, complex cells are orientation-specific but do not possess a preferred phase (De Valois, Albrecht and Thorell, 1982; De Valois and De Valois, 1988, pp.

---

[17]In this paper, only a short overview on the basic features of Grossberg's theory can be given. A more detailed introduction to the functions of the BC and FC systems can be found in Grossberg (1987a, pp. 90–93).

[18]Grossberg considers models that describe the first step of visual information processing as a frequency-specific filtering of the retinal image with a subsequent calculation of zero-crossings (e.g., Marr and Hildreth, 1980) as insufficient. Only a small part of the information that is implicitly contained in the retinal image, namely, information on the *localization* of retinal intensity changes, is determined by these procedures. In contrast, information on other relevant retinal features, such as the intensity or the frequency of the light falling on both sides of the detected discontinuities, is ignored (Grossberg, 1983, pp. 633–634). In Grossberg's model, the extraction and further processing of this type of information is the main function of the FC system.

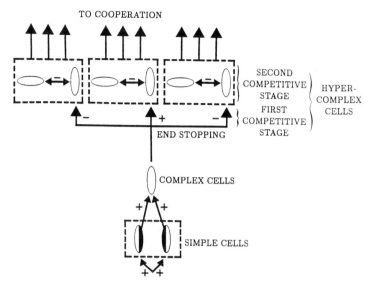

Figure 3.11. *Schematic model of processing stages within the boundary contour system. [From Grossberg and Marshall, 1989, p. 32. © 1989 Pergamon Press; reprinted with kind permission.]*

102–109). Like the retinogeniculate X cells mentioned in Section 4, both simple and complex cortical cells are characterized by their sensitivity to specific spatial frequency bands (De Valois and De Valois, 1988, pp. 119–128). This fact plays a decisive role in Grossberg's theory of stereoscopic depth perception.

The principal claim in Grossberg's model of binocular vision is that disparity values are computed at the stage where complex cortical cells become activated by simple cortical cells. To evaluate the empirical support for this assumption, we must first briefly discuss the different stages of information processing within the BC system (Grossberg, 1987a, pp. 93–102).

In this system, the registration of oriented, retinal contrasts through simple and complex cells is followed by two competitive stages and one cooperative stage. The common goal of these processes is to develop an unambiguous and complete reconstruction of distal contours that may not or only partly be present in the retinal image. In the first competitive stage, complex cells influence the activity of so-called *hypercomplex cells* – cells that also represent localization and orientation of retinal contrasts. Hypercomplex cells whose localization and orientations correspond to those of active complex cells are activated. Those hypercomplex cells that signalize the existence of contrasts with corresponding orientations but with spatially displaced retinal positions are, in contrast, inhibited (Figure 3.11, center).

In the second competitive phase, hypercomplex cells compete for the highest possible activation values with other hypercomplex cells representing retinal contrasts at the same position but with another orientation: an active hypercomplex cell with vertical orientation inhibits a cell that represents horizontally oriented contrasts at the same location (Figure 3.11, top). In contrast, if the vertical cell is inhibited, this leads to the activation of a horizontally oriented hypercomplex cell with the same localization. The goal of these two competitive processes is to synthesize so-called *end-cuts* and thus mark those contour boundaries beyond which the featural filling-in processes within the FC system should not go (Grossberg, 1987a, pp. 94–96). In addition, both competitive processes interact with a third, cooperative–competitive process of boundary completion. During this process, spatially extended, continuous segmentations are generated, reconstructed, or completed in order to complement the frequently incomplete retinal information (Grossberg, 1987a, pp. 97–98).

Grossberg believes that the process of binocular matching of monocular features is to be located on the level of complex cells – that is, before the beginning of the previously described competitive phases. He supports this hypothesis with a series of psychophysical phenomena that have been detected in the study of binocular rivalry processes. One of these is the previously mentioned case of the Kaufman stereogram (see Figure 3.4) . The depth impression generated by this stereogram points to the successful completion of a binocular matching process: the monocular features matched here are apparently (virtual) borderlines separating the patterns with different orientations. According to Grossberg, the early processes within the BC system described above are responsible for generating such borderlines. From the fact that the presentation of a Kaufman stereogram leads to the perception of an area that hovers over the surface of the image, Grossberg concludes that binocular matches must have occurred within the framework of these processes (Grossberg, 1987b, p. 120).

Within the area that hovers above the surface of the image, a permanent rivalry between the two monocularly presented, perpendicularly oriented line patterns can be observed. This phenomenon provides additional information on the time point when the monocularly controlled visual information processing turns into a binocularly controlled process. According to Grossberg (1987b, pp. 120–121), the rivalry between the displaced monocular line patterns can be traced back to the processes located on the second competitive stage (Figure 3.11, top): hypercomplex cells representing the same position but perpendicular orientations of contrasts compete here. Binocular rivalry can be traced back to the fact that, at a given point in time, hypercomplex cells with a certain orientation gain the upper hand and corresponding line completion processes are introduced.[19] To explain why monocular representations of two perpendicular line patterns are able to compete at this point, the second competitive stage within the BC system must be considered as binocular.

Another type of binocular rivalry suggests that the influence of binocular input on processes within the BC system might be placed at an even earlier stage. Figure 3.12 presents two stereogram pairs introduced by Kulikowski (1978), the upper pair consisting of two vertical sinusoidal gratings with a low spatial frequency whose phases are displaced at 180 degrees. The lower pair consists of vertical bar gratings with the same phase displacement. In this second pair, not only low spatial frequencies but also additional, higher frequency components are present. During stereoscopic presentation, a unified impression of depth is generated in the first case, whereas in the bar stereogram this impression of spatial depth is accompanied by binocular rivalry between the high-frequency components (the corners) of the two single patterns.

---

[19]Additional assumptions are necessary in this context to explain the changes between rival percepts that are characteristic for binocular rivalry phenomena (Grossberg, 1987b, pp. 123–124).

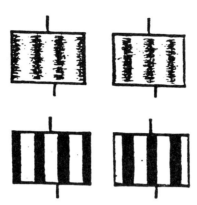

Figure 3.12. *Kulikowski stereograms. [From Grossberg and Marshall, 1989, p. 33.* © *1989 Pergamon Press; reprinted with kind permission.]*

How can this phenomenon be explained? First, it provides further support for the existence of multiple, frequency-specific channels: stimuli with a low spatial frequency can be matched to each other at relatively high disparity values, while this is not possible for higher frequencies (in the bar stereogram). Binocular rivalry arises here. The high-frequency components of the Kulikowski bar stereogram compete with parallel but disparate features from the other eye. In Grossberg's model, this type of binocular competition is located on the first competitive stage (Figure 3.11). According to Grossberg, the Kulikowski stereogram confirms that this stage is already controlled by binocular input (Grossberg, 1987b, pp. 121–122).

Grossberg concludes that complex cortical cells, whose activity triggers the various stages of competitive and cooperative interactions within the BC system, already contain binocular input. This hypothesis is confirmed by empirical findings (see, for example, Poggio *et al.*, 1985) on the binocularity of complex cells. Complex cells receive their input from monocular cortical simple cells (see above). The fusion of the information from both eyes (and the accompanying possibility of computing retinal disparity values) might therefore occur during the activation of complex cortical cells by simple cells.

What could this process look like? In which way can disparity information be made explicit through the activation of complex cells by cortical simple cells? To be able to follow Grossberg's considerations in this context, it is necessary to take another look at the functional organization of the visual cortex: monocular simple cells with corresponding receptive fields in the left or right eye are organized in so-called *hypercolumns* in the primary visual cortex (Hubel and Wiesel, 1979). A cortical hypercolumn consists of a group of simple cells that are sensitive to different orientations, contrast directions or spatial frequencies in a specific area of the right or left retina (De Valois and De Valois, 1988, pp. 135–143). Spatially corresponding information from each eye is located at neighboring positions in the visual cortex. An oriented contrast at identical positions on the left and right retinas should consequently lead to increased activity of two closely neighbored simple cells. However, as the receptive fields of monocular simple cells overlap, the presence of this contrast does not lead to an isolated reaction of two monocular simple cells but to a graded activity in a series of neighboring cells within the system of cortical hypercolumns.

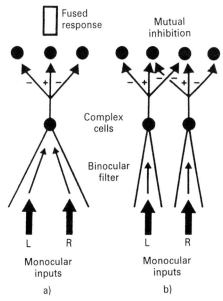

Figure 3.13. *A single, low-frequency specific complex cell can fuse disparate monocular input (a),
while the same input leads to an activation of two separate, high-frequency specific complex cells (b).
[From Grossberg, 1987b, p. 122. © 1987 The Psychonomic Society; reprinted with kind permission
of the publisher and author.]*

In what way does the activity of simple cells organized in hypercolumns contain
information about the extent of retinal disparity? In this context, it has to be recalled
that both simple and complex cells differ with regard to their preferred spatial
frequency band (see above). Like Marr, Grossberg sees a close connection between
the frequency specificity of cells involved in binocular fusion and the breadth of the
area of disparity values that can be fused: in the case of the Kulikowski bar
stereogram, low-frequency components can be matched binocularly, while high-
frequency components cannot – despite identical disparity. This phenomenon is
illustrated in Figure 3.13: a complex cell that is sensitive to low-frequency stimuli
is activated by two disparate monocular signals (Figure 3.13a). In contrast, the
identical signal pattern activates two independent, neighboring complex cells, as
long as these are specialized on higher spatial frequencies (Figure 3.13b). This can
lead to the formation of binocular rivalry on the following stages of processing.

The monocular signals presented in Figure 3.13 are transmitted by cortical
simple cells organized in hypercolumns. In order to explain the relationship
between the frequency specificity of cortical cells and the maximal fusible disparity
value, the connections between simple and complex cells have to be described in
more detail.

First of all, the question arises how the activities of neighboring simple cells
change when binocular disparity increases. While oriented contrasts that fall on
corresponding retinal positions (zero disparity), or are only slightly displaced,
activate only a rather narrowly restricted area of cortical simple cells in neighboring
hypercolumns, this activity pattern becomes wider with higher disparity. The

pattern of activity of cortical simple cells thus carries not only information on the localization and orientation of a retinal contrast but also information about the extent of the disparity and thus about the spatial location of the distal feature responsible for this contrast. How, then, can this information be made explicit during the activation of complex cells?

Grossberg (1987b, pp. 132–143) attempts to answer this question by presenting a network in which the functional connections between the levels of monocular simple cells (F_1) and binocular complex cells (F_2) are modeled – a network that should agree with the anatomical relationships in the primary visual cortex (Figure 3.14). The relationship between the frequency specificity of individual simple cells and their connection pattern with cells on the level F_2 plays a decisive role here: monocular simple cells sensitive to high spatial frequencies can only activate a few, closely neighboring complex cells on the upper level in the network. Simple cells that are specialized for low spatial frequencies are different: these cells are linked to a broad array of cells on level F_2.

It follows from this construction principle that the maximum interval between active simple cells on the F_1 level, that will lead to an activation of a common complex cell, varies as a function of the frequency specificity of the simple cells involved. Simultaneously active simple cells, which possess large receptive fields and are thus sensitive to low spatial frequencies, can therefore still activate common complex cells if their distance is relatively large. In contrast, simple cells specialized for high spatial frequencies and which possess small receptive fields on the retina, must be close neighbors, so that their signals can converge on individual complex cells (Grossberg, 1987b, pp. 141–143; Grossberg and Marshall, 1989, pp. 35–36). In the first case, oriented contrasts with relatively high disparity values (leading to broadly distributed activity patterns of neighboring simple cells in cortical hyper-columns) can lead to a unified reaction on the complex cell level, while, in the second case, such a pattern of activity would lead to the activation of independent complex cells. The general scheme of the relationship between the frequency sensitivity of cortical cells and the width of their fusional areas illustrated in Figure 3.13 could be implemented by the type of network architecture postulated by Grossberg (Figure 3.14).

Those complex cells that are specialized for high spatial frequencies and are connected with a narrow area of cortical simple cells only receive binocular input when the disparity of oriented contrasts is small. On the other hand, complex cells with low frequency preferences will also be activated by monocular input with larger disparity. This permits an initial, approximate determination of the actual disparity of the representations of oriented retinal contrasts. To determine a more precise value, it is nonetheless necessary to calculate the exact extent of the disparity *within* the single frequency-specific cell systems: the mere fact that certain complex cells have received binocular input while others have not is no longer a sufficient basis. If the pattern of activity of simple cells in neighboring hyper-columns contains precise information on the extent of retinal disparity, this information should be retained and made explicit on the level of complex cells. How this might be achieved by their specific network (Figure 3.14) is described in detail by Grossberg and Marshall (1989, pp. 35–39)

In what way does the calculation of exact disparity values within the BC system lead to the construction of spatially localized percepts? Grossberg assumes that the filling-in processes realized by the feature contour system can be triggered after

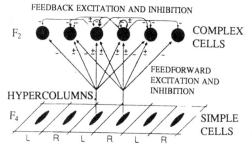

Figure 3.14. *Schematic model of connections between the level of simple cells organized in hypercolumns (F₁) and the complex cell level (F₂). [From Grossberg and Marshall, 1989, p. 31. © 1989 Pergamon Press; reprinted with kind permission.]*

successful binocular matching of single, oriented contrasts or larger line segments within the BC system. The FC system takes the disparity values of these features into account when constructing percepts: a surface circumscribed by boundaries with close to equal disparity is therefore perceived as being level. But if contrasts and boundaries are registered that vary in their disparity values, the corresponding surface will appear to be curved.

Grossberg's theory on the foundations of stereoscopic vision differs on several points from the approaches presented in Section 4. While in the second algorithm by Marr and Poggio, the calculation of the spatial depth of distal surfaces was based on a large number of independent local disparity measurements, Grossberg has integrated binocular fusion processes into a comprehensive model of perceptual segmentation of visual input. The competitive and cooperative mechanisms within the BC system that serve as the basis for visual segmentation, contour generation and contour completion already operate on the basis of binocular input. This means that possible, false binocular matches of oriented contrasts on the level of the complex cells might be identified and eliminated during these later processing stages. For this reason, the problem of avoiding incorrect matches of monocular features – focus of the considerations presented in Section 4 – plays no such central role in Grossberg's model. By adopting Grossberg's model of an interaction between the BC system (in which the localization, orientation, extension as well as the extent of the disparity of distal contours is determined) and the FC system (in which spatially localized percepts are constructed on the basis of this information through filling-in processes), it might be possible to avoid some of the difficulties discussed at the beginning of this section – difficulties created by approaches in which strictly local calculations of disparity values serve as the basis for computing spatial depth.

CONCLUDING REMARKS

What general judgement can be made on our current understanding of stereoscopic depth perception? How has the description of the underlying mechanisms changed since the early days of research on binocular vision? In which areas has progress in knowledge been particularly great? And in what way can the questions and problems for which no satisfactory solution has been found as yet be answered in the future?

In general, it can be stated that today, unlike in the days of Sherrington or Koffka, the binocular matching process is almost exclusively located on a very early stage of visual information processing. Decisive evidence for this view grew out of the random-dot stereogram experiments developed by Bela Julesz that have convincingly proved that binocular fusion processes occur without the possibility of a previous perceptual segmentation of the monocular input. The monocular matching partners involved in this process are therefore assumed to be correspondingly elementary features: while Grossberg locates them on the level of cortical simple cells, Marr and Poggio have looked for the biological counterparts of zero crossings in the retinogeniculate system. If the similarity of monocular features should be a decisive criterion for their binocular matching – as postulated in many theories of stereoscopic vision – this should only involve similarities on elementary dimensions (e.g. the orientation, phase or spatial frequency of retinal contrasts). If the features to be matched are elementary, correspondences between higher-stage properties (e.g. the form or color of object surfaces) should play no role in the initial binocular matching processes.

However, if this process occurs between the most simple, unstructured monocular features, one has to ask how it can possibly lead to a coherent result in a global sense. This problem, which was already articulated many years ago by Julesz with his demand for a global model of stereoscopic depth perception, is a focus of the current theoretical discussion on the mechanisms of binocular matching. Networks have been proposed in which individual matching processes do not proceed independently but influence one another in complex ways. With the aid of such interactions, these networks should be able to calculate consistent and globally acceptable solutions to specific binocular matching problems.

In this context, the interaction between cognitive-psychological theories and findings from the neurosciences is of ever-increasing importance. Current network models of the mechanisms of stereoscopic vision are much more concerned with being biologically plausible than their predecessors from the early 1970s – much more account is taken of the functional and anatomical properties of the human visual system. Growing knowledge on the neuronal foundations of visual information processing makes it highly probable that fundamental revisions of our current models of stereoscopic depth perception will be necessary in the future.

REFERENCES

Berkeley, G. (1910). *An Essay Towards a New Theory of Vision*. New York: Dutton (original work published 1709).

Blake, R. (1989). A neural theory of binocular rivalry. *Psychological Review*, **96**, 145–167.

Blake, R. and O'Shea, R. P. (1988). 'Abnormal fusion' of stereopsis and binocular rivalry. *Psychological Review*, **95**, 151–154.

Boring, E. G. (1933). *The Physical Dimensions of Consciousness*. New York: Century.

Charnwood, J. R. B. (1951). *Essay on Binocular Vision*. London: Hutton.

Dev, P. (1975). Perception of depth surfaces in random-dot stereograms: A neural, model. *International Journal of Man-Machine Studies*, **7**, 511–528.

De Valois, R. L., Albrecht, D. G. and Thorell, L. G. (1978). Cortical cells: Bar and edge detectors, or spatial frequency filters? In S. J. Cool and E. L. Smith (Eds), *Frontiers in Visual Science* (pp. 544–556). New York: Springer.

De Valois, R. L., Albrecht, D. G. and Thorell, L. G. (1982). Spatial frequency selectivity of cells in macaque visual cortex. *Vision Research,* **22,** 545–559.

De Valois, R. L. and De Valois, K. K. (1988). *Spatial Vision.* New York: Oxford University Press.

Dhond, U. R. and Aggarwal, J. K. (1989). Structure from stereo: A review. *IEEE, Transactions on Systems, Man, and Cybernetics,* **19,** 1489–1510.

Dodwell, P. C. and Engel, G. R. (1963). A theory of binocular fusion. *Nature,* **198,** 39–40, 73–74.

Eimer, M. (1990). *Informationsverarbeitung und mentale Repräsentation.* Berlin: Springer.

Enroth-Cugell, C. and Robson, J. G. (1966). The contrast sensitivity of retinal ganglion cells of the cat. *Journal of Physiology (London),* **187,** 517–522.

Felton, T. B., Richards, W. and Smith, R. A. (1972). Disparity processing of spatial frequencies in man. *Journal of Physiology (London),* **225,** 349–362.

Fender, D. and Julesz, B. (1967). Extension of Panum's fusional area in binocularly stabilized vision. *Journal of the Optical Society of America,* **57,** 819–830.

Foley, J. M. (1978). Primary depth perception. In R. Held, H. W. Leibowitz and H. L. Teuber (Eds), *Handbook of Sensory Physiology,* vol. 8: *Perception* (pp. 181–214). Berlin, New York: Springer.

Gogel, W. C. (1977). The metric of visual space. In W. Epstein (Ed.), *Stability and Constancy in Visual Perception: Mechanisms and Processes* (pp. 129–182). New York: John Wiley.

Grimson, W. E. L. (1981a). A computer implementation of a theory of human stereo vision. *Philosophical Transactions of the Royal Society (London),* B, **292,** 217–253.

Grimson, W. E. L. (1981b). *From Images to Surfaces: A Computational Study of the Human Early Visual System.* Cambridge, MA: MIT Press.

Grossberg, S. (1983). The quantized geometry of visual space: The coherent computation of depth, form, and lightness. *Behavioral and Brain Sciences,* **6,** 625–692.

Grossberg, S. (1987a). Cortical dynamics of three-dimensional form, color, and, brightness perception, I: Monocular theory. *Perception and Psychophysics,* **41,** 87–116.

Grossberg, S. (1987b). Cortical dynamics of three-dimensional form, color, and brightness perception, II: Binocular theory. *Perception and Psychophysics,* **41,** 117–158.

Grossberg, S. and Marshall, J. A. (1989). Stereo boundary fusion by cortical complex cells: A system of maps, filters and feedback networks for multiplexing distributed data. *Neural Networks,* **2,** 29–51.

Helmholtz, H. von (1866/1962). *Handbuch der physiologischen Optik.* Leipzig, Hamburg: Voss. [transl. 1962: *Treatise on Physiological Optics.* New York: Dover.]

Hering, E. (1868). *Die Lehre vom binokularen Sehen.* Leipzig, Hamburg: Voss.

Hering, E. (1878). *Zur Lehre vom Lichtsinn.* Wien: Gerold.

Hubel, D. H. and Wiesel, T. N. (1962). Receptive fields, binocular interaction and functional architecture in the cat's visual cortex. *Journal of Physiology (London),* **160,** 106–154.

Hubel, D. H. and Wiesel, T. N. (1974). Uniformity of monkey striate cortex: A parallel relationship between field size, scatter, and cortical magnification factor. *Journal of Comparative Neurology,* **158,** 295–306.

Hubel, D. H. and Wiesel, T. N. (1979). Brain mechanisms of vision. *Scientific American,* **241,** 150–163.

Julesz, B. (1960). Binocular depth perception of computer-generated patterns. *Bell System Technical Journal,* **39,** 1125–1162.

Julesz, B. (1971). *Foundations of Cyclopean Perception.* Chicago: University of Chicago Press.

Julesz, B. (1978). Global stereopsis: Cooperative phenomena in stereoscopic depth perception. In R. Held, H. W. Leibowitz and H. L. Teuber (Eds), *Handbook of Sensory Physiology,* Vol. 8: *Perception* (pp. 215–256). New York: Springer.

Julesz, B. (1986). Stereoscopic vision. *Vision Research, 26,* 1601–1612.

Julesz, B. and Chang, J. J. (1976). Interaction between pools of binocular disparity detectors tuned to different disparities. *Biological Cybernetics, 22,* 107–120.

Julesz, B. and Schumer, R. A. (1981). Early visual perception. *Annual Review of Psychology, 32,* 575–627.

Kaufman, L. (1974). *Sight and Mind.* New York: Oxford University Press.

Koffka, K. (1935). *Principles of Gestalt Psychology.* New York: Harcourt Brace.

Krekling, S. (1975). Depth matching with visible diplopic images: Stereopsis or vernier alignment. *Perception and Psychophysics, 17,* 114–116.

Kuffler, S. W. (1953). Discharge pattern and functional organization of mammalian retina. *Journal of Neurophysiology, 16,* 37–68.

Kulikowski, J. J. (1978). Limit of single vision in stereopsis depends on contour sharpness. *Nature, 275,* 126–127.

Levelt, W. J. M. (1965). *On Binocular Rivalry.* The Hague: Mouton.

Levinson, E. and Blake, R. (1979). Stereopsis by harmonic analysis. *Vision Research, 19,* 73–78.

Marr, D. (1976). Early processing of visual information. *Philosophical Transactions of the Royal Society (London), B, 275,* 483–524.

Marr, D. (1982). *Vision.* New York: Freeman.

Marr, D. and Hildreth, E. (1980). Theory of edge detection. *Proceedings of the Royal Society (London), B, 207,* 187–217.

Marr, D. and Poggio, T. (1976). Cooperative computation of stereo disparity. *Science, 194,* 283–287.

Marr, D. and Poggio, T. (1979). A computational theory of human stereo vision. *Proceedings of the Royal Society (London), B, 204,* 301–328.

Marr, D. and Ullman, S. (1981). Directional selectivity and its use in early visual processing. *Proceedings of the Royal Society (London), B, 211,* 151–180.

Mayhew, J. E. W. and Frisby, J. P. (1979). Convergent disparity discriminations in narrow-band-filtered random-dot stereograms. *Vision Research, 19,* 63–71.

Mayhew, J. E. W. and Frisby, J. P. (1981). Psychophysical and computational studies towards a theory of human stereopsis. *Artificial Intelligence, 17,* 349–385.

Metzger, W. (1975). *Gesetze des Sehens* (3rd edn). Franfurt: Kramer (Original work published 1936).

Mitchell, D. E. (1966). Retinal disparity and diplopia. *Vision Research, 6,* 441–451.

Murch, G. M. and Woodworth, G. L. (1978). *Wahrnehmung.* Stuttgart: Kohlhammer.

Ogle, K. N. (1953). Precision and validity of stereoscopic depth perception from double images. *Journal of the Optical Society of America, 43,* 906–913.

Ogle, K. N. (1964). *Researches in Binocular Vision.* New York: Hafner.

Panum, P. L. (1858). *Physiologische Untersuchungen über das Sehen mit zwei Augen.* Kiel: Schwers.

Poggio, G. F., Motter, B. C., Squatrito, S. and Trotter, Y. (1985). Responses of neurons in visual cortex (VI and V2) of the alert macaque to dynamic random-dot stereograms. *Vision Research, 25,* 397–406.

Poggio, G. F. and Poggio, T. (1984). The analysis of stereopsis. *Annual Review of Neuroscience, 7,* 379–412.

Richards, W. (1977). Stereopsis with and without monocular cues. *Vision Research, 17,* 967–969.

Sherrington, C. S. (1906). *The Integrative Action of the Nervous System.* London: Constable.

Sherrington, C. S. (1918). Observation on the sensual role of the proprioceptive nerve supply of the extrinsic ocular muscles. *Brain, 41,* 332–343.

Sperling, G. (1970). Binocular vision: A physical and a neural theory. *American Journal of Psychology, 83,* 461–534.

Timney, B., Wilcox, L.M. and St John, R. (1989). On the evidence for a 'pure' binocular process in human vision. *Spatial Vision, 4,* 1–15.

Tootell, R. B. H., Silverman, M. S., Switkes, E. and De Valois, R. L. (1982). Deoxyglucose analysis of retinotopic organization in primate striate cortex. *Science, 218,* 902–904.

Van Essen, D. C., Newsome, W. T. and Maunsell, J. H. R. (1984). The visual field representation in striate cortex of the macaque monkey: Asymmetries, anisotropies, and individual variability. *Vision Research, 24,* 429–448.

Verhoeff, F. H. (1935). A new theory of binocular vision. *Archives of Ophthalmology, 13,* 151–175.

Wade, N. J. (1987). On the late invention of the stereoscope. *Perception, 16,* 785–816.

Wheatstone, C. (1838). Contributions to the physiology of vision. I. On some remarkable, and hitherto unobserved, phenomena of binocular vision. *Philosophical Transactions of the Royal Society (London), 123,* 371–394.

Wolfe, J. M. (1986). Stereopsis and binocular rivalry. *Psychological Review, 93,* 269–282.

Wolfe, J. M. (1988). Parallel ideas about stereopsis and binocular rivalry: A reply to Blake and O'Shea (1988). *Psychological Review, 95,* 155–158.

Chapter 4

Neural Networks and Visual Information Processing

Werner X. Schneider

Ludwig-Maximilians-University, Munich

1 INTRODUCTION

Around 1950, experimental psychology saw the establishment of an approach that has tried to understand basic cognitive processes of perception, memory, problem solving or attention as information processing (Anderson, 1983; Broadbent, 1958; Lachman, Lachman and Butterfield, 1979; Neisser, 1967; Newell and Simon, 1972). This idea was put into concrete forms by comparing the cognitive apparatus with von Neumann's digital computer, the concept that nowadays forms the basis of every personal computer. It is not surprising, therefore, that constructs such as 'limited capacity canal' (Broadbent, 1958), 'short-term store' (Atkinson and Shiffrin, 1968), or 'production system' (Anderson, 1983) have found their way into the formulation of models.

Since the beginning of the 1980s, an alternative approach to the modeling of information processing has been gaining in influence. Instead of using the 'model' of the conventional digital computer, attention has been focused on the processing properties of the central nervous system, more specifically, the functions of interacting nerve cells.[1] Information processing is conceived as a combined activity of many, relatively 'dumb' neuron-like processing units that work in a highly parallel and distributed manner. Models constructed within this approach are labeled 'neural' or 'connectionist networks' (Feldman and Ballard, 1982; Grossberg, 1988) – some authors call it PDP (parallel distributed processing – or neurocomputational models (Rumelhart, McClelland and The PDP Research Group, 1986; Schwartz, 1990). Their field already covers large parts of the domain of experimental psychology, such as visual attention (Goebel, 1993; Phaf, van der Heijden and Hudson, 1990), motor control (Bullock and Grossberg, 1988) classical conditioning (Grossberg and Levine, 1987; Sutton and Barto, 1981), categorization and memory processes (Knapp and Anderson, 1984; McClelland and Rumelhart, 1986); word

---

[1]Initial work on this alternative approach can already he found in the 1940s (see, for example, Hebb, 1949; McCulloch and Pitts, 1943). However, after a relatively short heyday (Rosenblatt, 1958; Widrow and Hopf, 1960), the approach disappeared again at the end of the 1960s (partially due to Minsky and Papert, 1969). For a review of the history of neural networks, see Anderson and Rosenfeld (1988); Arbib (1987), Grossberg (1988) and Rumelhart, McClelland and The PDP Research Group (1986).

Handbook of Perception and Action: Volume 1
ISBN 0-12-516161-1

recognition (Grossberg and Stone, 1986; McClelland and Rumelhart, 1981) or early visual perception (Bridgeman, 1971; Daugman, 1988; Finkel and Edelman, 1989; Grossberg and Mingolla, 1985a, b).

The goal of this chapter is to present and discuss the neurocomputational approach in the field of vision or visual information processing. This explains which basic components are used in the construction of neural networks, how they explain experimental findings and functions, as well as how they can be tested and evaluated.

Sections 2 and 3 address these issues by describing two networks that refer to a common phenomenon: the generation of illusory contours. The first network, from Finkel and Edelman (1989), possesses a relatively clearly structured basic design and will be used to explain the fundamental principles of neurocomputation. It also has the advantage that its psychological competence has been supported by a series of computer-simulated illusory contour phenomena (e.g. the Kanizsa square). The second neural network (Grossberg, 1987a; Grossberg and Mingolla, 1985a), which also addresses illusory contours, has a more complex construction that is also more difficult to describe. The 'pioneering character' of this network for the field of vision is that its design is based on ideas and findings from experimental psychology and neurobiology as well as on computational considerations. Section 3 concludes with a brief and selective review of the current state of neurocomputation (1990) in the field of visual information processing.

The fourth and final section discusses the advantages and problems of the neurocomputational approach. This discussion focuses on one point that has been discussed frequently by supporters and critics: namely, how neural networks can and should be tested and evaluated as models that explain psychological phenomena. This question will be answered by discriminating between behavioral (psychological) validity and architectural validity. Behavioral validity refers to the ability of a network to behave in an analogous way to psychological findings. Computer simulation is the preferred means of testing this validity. Architectural validity concerns the plausibility of the functional and mechanistic assumptions of a network architecture. A central issue related to this discrimination is how far experimental psychological and neurobiological findings should provide necessary constraints for testing and evaluating a network.

2   NEURAL NETWORKS, ILLUSORY CONTOURS, AND FINKEL AND EDELMAN'S (1989) MODEL

Since as far back as the turn of the century, illusory contours have been among the classic research topics in the psychology of perception (Coren, 1972; Ehrenstein, 1941; Gregory, 1972; Halpern and Salzman, 1983; Kanizsa, 1955; Kellman and Shipley, 1991; Petry and Meyer, 1987; Schumann, 1900). Figure 4.1 presents a well-known example: the so-called 'Kanizsa square' (Kanizsa, 1955).

The 'illusory' white square, perceived as being slightly brighter than its background, forms a complete figure, although no differences in luminance or any other property (e.g. color, texture) can be measured physically along the contours of the square between the 'Pac-man' figures.

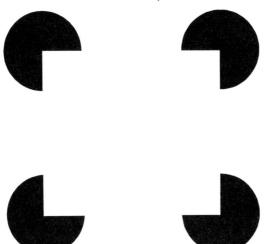

Figure 4.1. *A Kanizsa square.*

Such phenomena are particularly interesting when modeling networks, because they permit an unequivocal operationalization of the intended information processing performance and, hence, 'psychological validity'. A neural network has to compute an output pattern with illusory contours from input patterns without these contours. However, whether the neural network does this in a plausible way, that is, delivers a satisfactory explanation, additionally depends on the compatibility of the structure and dynamics of the network with relevant findings from experimental psychology, neurobiology and computational considerations. This point will be discussed in detail in the fourth section on advantages and problems.

Finkel and Edelman's neural network (1989; see also Finkel, Reeke and Edelman, 1989; Pearson, Finkel and Edelman, 1987) can, like any other network, be viewed as an information processing system. In such systems, be they neural networks or digital computers, a discrimination can be made between a functional and a mechanistic level of analysis (theory). Functional theory predominantly specifies the information processing tasks or information processing functions of the system, that is, it defines what should be computed, while mechanistic theory states how these tasks are computed.[2] Both theories together specify the architecture of a network model.

The network approach proposes a new conceptualization of mechanistic theory, namely, to model information processing as parallel and distributed processing with many and relatively dumb neuron-like computation elements. What this

---

[2]Functional theory may remind some readers of Marr's (1982) 'computational theory', and mechanistic theory of a combination of his 'algorithmic' and 'implementational' theories. This is not the place for an appropriate explanation of the differences between Marr's conception and the one expounded here (see, also Kosslyn and Maljkovic 1990). However, two aspects should he mentioned briefly: (1) unlike Marr (1982, p. 332), both the functional and mechanistic theories should be subject to experimental psychological and neurobiological tests; and (2) both theories should be developed interactively, although they can be conceptually separated.

means should be explained in a first step with Finkel and Edelman's (1989) neural network model. The functional theory will be described first and then the mechanistic theory.[3]

2.1 Functional Theory

The first stage in analyzing a network is to describe its functions or tasks. This involves reporting what the network computes on the basis of what. In more precise terms, it is necessary to describe what output information is computed on the basis of what input information. Hence, functional theory requires a statement on the pattern of input–output transformations. If a larger network is concerned, then the major functions assigned to the neural network as a whole can be decomposed into several subfunctions. This functional decomposition is continued until the subfunctions and, hence, the necessary input–output transformations cannot be decomposed any further. The neurocomputational operationalization of the individual subfunctions forms the content of the mechanistic theory (Section 2.2). This should be described as an information processing 'stage'.[4] Hence, the stages compute that which is given by the subfunctions.

Before functional decomposition can be performed, the tasks assigned to the particular system as a whole have to be described. In the visual system, this probably involves the computation of useful aspects of the world such as shapes of objects, their surface properties (e.g. color), their motions (e.g. trajectories) and their spatial relationships (e.g. relative locations in space; see DeYoe and van Essen, 1988; Felleman and van Essen, 1991; Livingstone and Hubel, 1988; Marr, 1982). The input for these computations are two activity patterns (two eyes) each containing approximately 130 million photoreceptors that specify information on retinal position (x, y), eye (left, right), wavelength and time.

Among these many subfunctions of the visual system, Finkel and Edelman (1989) have selected three for their network that refer to the computation of the attributes 'directions of motion', 'normal object contours' (two-dimensional shape) and 'occlusion contours'. Occlusion contours are the contours of an overlapping object that border on the overlapped object. Figure 4.5 (on page 114) presents an example in which the occlusion contours are marked in bold. It could also be said that occlusion contours are those contours behind which other objects presumably continue.

According to Finkel and Edelman (1989), the mechanism that computes occlusion contours is the same as the one that generates illusory contours (like the Kanizsa square in Figure 4.1), although the occlusion function is viewed as primary. If the visual system computes illusory contours then, according to this idea, it signals 'incorrect' occlusion contours.

Finkel and Edelman (1989) have decomposed the function of occlusion contours

---

[3]For clarity, functional theory will be introduced before mechanistic theory. Section 4 argues that such a sequence should not determine the construction of theory. Instead, an interactive construction of both theories is proposed.

[4]The 'stage' concept should not imply a strictly serial, hierarchical processing that continuously passes on discrete codes as is usually the case in cognitive psychology (Miller, 1988; Sanders, 1980; Theios, 1975).

into four subfunctions (Figure 4.2) Each of these subfunctions is defined by a specific subtask within the computation of occlusion contours. These are described briefly below. As Figure 4.2 shows, three further subfunctions are assumed that are summarized under the function 'local orientations'. This is: from the input pattern which represents a strongly simplified retinal distribution of luminance, an output pattern has to be computed that specifies the orientation of the local contrasts in that distribution (e.g. the edges of objects).[5]

Hence, the complete functional decomposition of Finkel and Edelman's (1989) network designates seven subfunctions.[6] These will be sketched briefly before discussing their empirical support. The first subfunction 'preprocessing' is specified as follows. From the input pattern, which should represent the absolute values of the retinal luminance distribution in a strongly simplified way, an output pattern is computed that only continues to represent changes in luminance. In the Kanizsa square, such changes in luminance occur at the edges of the 'Pac-man' figures. The second subfunction determines – as its name already suggests – the spatial orientation of luminance changes (or contrasts) that are computed locally, that is, for each 'retinal' position. The accompanying mechanism is explained in Section 2.2. The third subfunction requires these locally oriented contrasts to be filtered: the only contrasts that remain represented are those that cover a minimal spatial region, that is, lines of a minimal length. Very small luminance regions (such as very short lines) are eliminated at this stage. This function is relevant for the 'direction of motion' function that will not be discussed in this chapter.

The next four subfunctions (Figure 4.2) concern the actual computation of occlusion contours and illusory contours. At this stage, I shall give only a brief list of the four functions without defining their content and decomposition. They will be explained in detail when describing the mechanistic theory in Section 2.2, which presents Finkel and Edelman's (1989) idea on the generation of occlusion contours. The first subfunction of occlusion computation ('line terminations') computes – on the basis of the output of the prior stage ('filtered local orientations') – the ends of oriented contrasts or oriented lines by representing the direction of the termination (e.g. 'westward' line terminations). The next subfunction changes the representation of line terminations by combining adjacent orientations (e.g. 0 to 45 degrees, 45 to 90 degrees) to form a 'coarser' category with a larger bandwidth (0 to 90 degrees) and is labeled 'wide angle line terminations'. The third subfunction of the occlusion computation generates from line terminations local occlusion cues to mark occlusion boundaries. The last subfunction computes occlusion contours from the occlusion cues that may eventually correspond to illusory contours.

---

[5]If one is primarily interested in occlusion or illusory contours, is it really necessary to consider this 'local orientation' function and its functional decomposition? The answer is 'Yes.' To describe the occlusion function or its subfunctions, it is necessary to specify the input information that is determined by the output of previous 'local orientation' stage. This output cannot be a representation of the retinal luminance distribution, but – if one follows the functional decomposition – information that has already been further processed and that specifies the filtered local orientations.

[6]The seven subfunctions are arranged in serial and hierarchic sequence. This is not typical of either neural networks in general or of Finkel and Edelman's (1989) complete network, which cannot be described here for lack of space. Besides further functions, it designates additional, not-yet-serial processing that arises through a 'particular' form of feedback ('reentry').

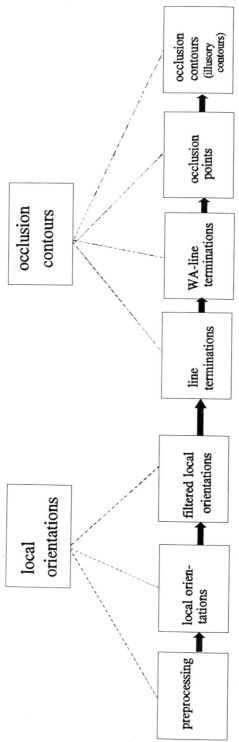

Figure 4.2. A functional decomposition of Finkel and Edelman's (1989) network.

Is there empirical support for the functional assignments described above? The assumption that the computation of object contours (shapes) – be they occlusion contours or normal contours – is preceded by stages of processing that compute the local orientations of local contrasts (e.g. edges) is shared by nearly all theories of early visual information processing (Grossberg and Mingolla, 1985a; Marr, 1982). One of the reasons why this hierarchical sequence is generally accepted – besides computational considerations – is the neurophysiological findings of Hubel and Wiesel (1962, 1977; see also De Valois and De Valois, 1988; DeYoe and van Essen, 1988; Felleman and van Essen, 1991) obtained from the cortex of cats and apes. These findings (Hubel and Wiesel, 1962) have shown that those nerve cells that probably perform the computation of local orientations are to be found already in the earliest part of the visual cortex, namely in V1 (or area 17). Cells that are sensitive to more complex stimulus properties (such as the length or end of lines), in contrast, are found in later, hierarchically 'higher' cortical areas such as V2 or other parts of area 18 (Hubel and Wiesel, 1965). Besides these neurophysiological data, there are also psychophysiological findings which suggest the existence of the 'local orientations' function (De Valois and De Valois, 1988). Particularly relevant for Finkel and Edelman's (1989) assumption, that local orientations are computed before occlusion contours or illusory contours, are findings from van der Heydt, Peterhans and Baumgartner (1984). By measuring single-cell activity in rhesus monkeys, these authors have shown that cells in V2 react to illusory contours, while the corresponding cells in V1, in contrast, only react to normal oriented contours.

A further subfunction supported by neurophysiological and psychophysiological data is preprocessing. For example, nerve cells in the lateral geniculate nucleus reveal the necessary tranformation properties (De Valois and De Valois, 1988).

2.2 Mechanistic Theory

The mechanistic theory – the actually new and specific aspect of the neural network approach – provides the neurocomputational specification of the functional theory. It determines how the individual functions are computed and thus how the processing stages are conceived.

In the following, three of the seven subfunctions or processing stages in Finkel and Edelman's (1989) network are explained. These refer to the computation of 'local orientations', 'occlusion cues' and 'occlusion contours' (illusory contours). Beforehand, the basic elements of neurocomputation on which each network is based have to be described. These are the so-called 'units' that are sometimes also labeled nodes. These units are the basic computation elements of each neural network. They are related to the functional properties of neurons (this aspect is addressed in Section 4.2). The task of a unit is to receive 'activation', to transform it and to pass it on. The level of a unit's activation determines to what extent this unit reflects the informational state that it represents. For example, activated units on the input layer of the 'local orientations' processing stage represent a distribution of changes in luminance. This is a local representation, that is, each activated unit stands for a luminance change at one 'retinal' position or input pattern region. This describes a general principle of representation in neural networks, namely, to present informational states (e.g. local luminance changes) in the form of activation

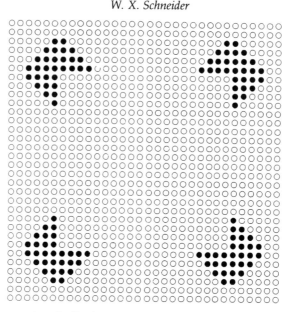

Figure 4.3. *A representation of a Kanizsa square on a 'retinal' input layer with 32 × 32 units.*

patterns. The input pattern that the network receives can only represent the retinal pattern of activity in an extremely simplified form. Hence, for example, differences in processing between the center and the periphery of the retina are not considered (Dowling, 1987).

In networks, functionally equivalent units are packed together in so-called layers. Simply structured processing stages mostly consist of two layers: an input layer and an output layer. The two-dimensional input layer for computing orientation in Finkel and Edelman's (1989) network is presented in a simplified form in Figure 4.3. The 32 × 32 units in this input layer or more precisely their activation pattern represent the luminance distribution of the Kanizsa square in Figure 4.1. Activated units are symbolized by dark circles and nonactivated units by light circles.

Computation in the sense of neurocomputation now means that units pass on their activation selectively to other units. This 'flow' of activation occurs across so-called 'connections'. Should two units or their informational states influence each other, then there has to be a connection between these units otherwise no activation could flow between them. Two classes of connection can be distinguished: 'excitatory' and 'inhibitory'. Excitatory connections are those that contribute to an increase in the activation of the receiver unit, while inhibitory connections lower activation. The size of an activation flow across a connection depends on its 'weight': the greater the weight of a connection, the more activation flows across it.

What determines the size of a unit's activation at a specific point in time? In many neural networks, this is given by three parameters: (1) the activation of the unit at a prior point in time; (2) activation through inputs from other units[7]; and (3) a decay term that regulates the necessary decline in activation. How these par-

---

[7]Self-referring connections are also possible, that is, after a certain lapse of time, a unit re-enters suprathreshold activation back to itself.

ameters are computed varies from network to network. In Finkel and Edelman (1989), there is a strong simplification because the momentary activation depends only on the input, while Grossberg and Mingolla (1985a) take all three parameters into account (see Section 3.2).

It is also a common practice to assign threshold values to units. A unit only passes activation on to other units when its momentary activation has gone beyond a threshold. If input is not high enough, activation remains subthreshold. Furthermore, minimum and maximum activation values have often been specified.

An important feature of neural networks that cannot be discussed here because of lack of space is their ability to learn (see, for example, Hanson and Burr, 1990). In principle, learning is based on the modification of the weights between units and thus on the modification of the flow of activation.

2.2.1   The Computation of 'Local Orientations'

How can units that represent specific informational states and exchange activation across connections perform such tasks as the computation of local orientations? This question requires a recourse to the functional theory in which the type of information is defined that specifies input and output patterns. In the case of the local orientations subfunction, the input pattern represents a two-dimensional distribution of luminance changes, while the output pattern should additionally contain the orientation of these local luminance changes (contrasts). However, how can this input–output transformation be performed? The answer lies in the structure of the connections between layers of units and the activation rules of the units – it is these that principally determine the information processing performance.

Two features characterize connections on the second network stage of Finkel and Edelman (1989):

(1) The input layer contains 32 × 32 units (see Figure 4.3) that are linked to a 32 × 32 unit output layer both topographically (i.e. retaining spatial relations) and unidirectionally (i.e. from one sender unit to one receiver unit and not in the other direction). The topographical assignment principle also applies to all further stages. If these were the only connections and high, suprathreshold input activation were present, then the pattern of input activation would transfer exactly to the units of the output layer and no transformation would occur.

(2) Therefore, each unit on the output layer additionally has a specific substructure of connections to the units of the input layer that refer to a small input region of the 32 × 32 layer. In line with its neurobiological counterpart, this substructure is called a 'receptive field' (Martin, 1991). It is responsible for the actual computation. Figure 4.4 presents such a substructure schematically.

For clarity, only one of the 32 × 32 units of the output layer and 25 of the 32 × 32 units of the input layer are portrayed. Nineteen of these input units connect with the output unit, which can be labeled the target unit. A '+' in the unit means that its connection with the output unit is excitatory, while a '−' signals an inhibitory connection. Such a receptive field with 3 excitatory and 16 inhibitory connections exists for each unit of the output layer, so that the fields overlap on the input layer.

W. X. Schneider

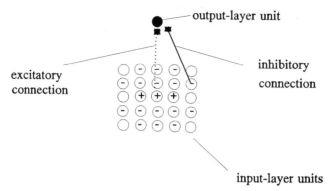

Figure 4.4. *Finkel and Edelman's (1989) network: a receptive field for computing orientation.*

The receptive field displayed in Figure 4.4 is sensitive to horizontally oriented contrasts or luminance changes. This means that the output (or target) unit receives suprathreshold activation when appropriately activated, that is, by a correctly positioned horizontal contrast. How is the activation of such an output unit computed? It is necessary to know the weights of the connections and the processing rules. Finkel and Edelman (1989) set the weights of excitatory connections at $+7$ and those of inhibitory connections at -2. The input to a target unit a_i (receiver unit) is now computed from the sum of the products between the activations of the sender units a_j and the weights of the connections w_{ij}:

$$a_i = \sum_{j=1}^{M} a_j w_{ij}$$

If we assume, for simplicity's sake, that an activated unit has an activation value of 1 and a nonactivated unit an activation value of 0, then we can compute what happens when all units of the receptive field are activated. The total activation of the target unit would then be negative, that is, below threshold (the threshold is 0), because the total value of the negative inhibitory input exceeds the total positive excitatory input:

$$a_i = 16 \ (1 \times -2) + 3 \ (1 \times +7) = -11$$

If, in contrast, the input pattern were to cover only the center and the lower (or upper) part of the units – one could also say the field would only be half filled with a horizontally oriented pattern – then a suprathreshold activation of the output unit would arise:

$$a_i = 3 \ (1 \times +7) + 8 \ (1 \times -2) + 8 \ (0 \times -2) = +5$$

A vertically oriented input pattern that only covers half of the field would, in contrast, lead once more to no positive activation:

$$a_i = 2 \ (1 \times +7) + 1 \ (0 \times +7) + 10 \ (1 \times -2) + 6 \ (0 \times -2) = -6$$

Hence, a receptive field for the computation of orientation, as proposed by Finkel and Edelman (1989), produces a suprathreshold output only when (1) a part of the units (field) are activated, that is, luminance contrast is present; and (2) the contrasts have the same orientation as the longitudinal axis of the field, that is, lie in the direction of the relative slope of the elongated, excitatory (and inhibitory) field area. The field displayed in Figure 4.4 is sensitive to horizontal contrasts. If the field is rotated by 90 degrees, then only vertical contrasts would generate a suprathreshold output.[8]

For each retinal position, Finkel and Edelman (1989) provide four different output units that each represent complementary orientations (vertical, horizontal and the two diagonals) and thus have different receptive fields. These four output units lie in four separate sublayers that are each characterized by their orientation and naturally also contain 32×32 units per sublayer. Hence, for each 'retinal' input region, computations are performed simultaneously in independent sublayers to see whether the orientation to be represented is present or not. One could talk about parallel and distributed processing.

In summary, the processing stage for the computation of local orientations consists of four separate layers of output units that represent complementary orientations. These are connected to an input layer in the form of receptive fields. The flow of activation, that is, the computation performance is determined by these substructures.

As far as empirical confirmation is concerned, the proposed structure of the receptive field (e.g. type and relative number of connections) can be traced back to a physiological model presented by Hubel and Wiesel (1962) that has been used to explain findings on the activity of single cells in the visual cortex of cats. Furthermore, the topographical or retinotopic organization between the layers or units of the processing stages can also be demonstrated within area 1 of the visual cortex (V1; see, for example, Tootell *et al.*, 1982).

2.2.2 The Computation of 'Occlusion Cues' and 'Occlusion Contours' (Illusory Contours)

Finkel and Edelman (1989) – as already pointed out above – understand occlusion contours as those contours (borders) of an object that cover another object. In Figure 4.5, these contours are marked as bold lines.

In formal terms, occlusion contours are defined not only by the presence of contrasts (e.g. lines) that end along the occlusion boundary but also by the absence of contrasts that go beyond this boundary (Figure 4.5). The computation of such occlusion contours is based on the previous computation of 'local cues for occlusion contours' (small circles in Figure 4.5) on the 'occlusion cues' stage. Occlusion cues that mark the terminations of occlusion contours simultaneously form the basis for generating illusory contours.

How are occlusion cues computed? A first step must be – just as in every other network stage – to specify the input pattern. This carries information on oriented and directed line terminations or contrast terminations (small rectangles made up of dashed lines in Figure 4.5 in which the direction of termination

---

[8]However, strictly speaking, the sensitivity of a field does not just relate to a single orientation value but also to a range of orientations (in this case, with a maximum deviation of 45 degrees) that can still generate suprathreshold outputs.

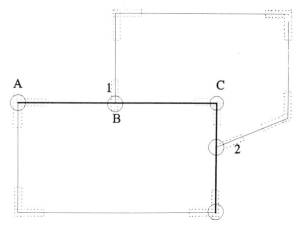

Figure 4.5. *Occlusion contours (bold lines).*

is coded as a geographical direction (e.g. eastward line termination). The reason for
this representation is that occlusion cues and occlusion contours are always present
at the terminations of contrasts or lines. Hence, the task of the 'occlusion cues' stage
is to select those line terminations out of the input pattern that correspond to
occlusion cues and thus mark the terminations of occlusion contours.

How can such occlusion cues be determined from the many line terminations?
Finkel and Edelman (1989) propose that a line termination has to meet two
conditions in order to be classified as an occlusion cue: (1) it must obviously border
on a line that could correspond to the occlusion contour – the orientation of the
termination should be orthogonal to the orientation of the line; and (2) at least two
further line terminations with the same orientation but opposing direction must
border on this line. For example, if the line terminations that mark the boundaries
of the overlapping object or the occlusion contour have a southward direction
(points A and C in Figure 4.5) then the line termination that marks the boundaries
of the overlapped object must have the opposing northward direction (point B).

A processing stage that meets the two above-mentioned conditions for ascertaining occlusion cues needs to have a relatively complex receptive field structure.
Figure 4.6 presents a highly schematized version that displays only one output unit
and a few connections to the input unit. For a specific retinal position, this output
unit can signal an occlusion cue that refers to an occlusion line (contour) with a
certain orientation (e.g. vertical).[9] Through its receptive field structure, the output
unit is connected to those input units that form a straight line with corresponding
positions (A and A′ in Figure 4.6) of 2 × 32 units in each of the two sublayers.[10] The
orientation of these straight lines, which potentially form an occlusion contour, is
orthogonal to the orientation of the represented line terminations (e.g. horizontal).
Because for each output unit a 2 × 32 unit-wide line is assumed in the input layer

---

[9]Analogous to the previous stages, occlusion cues and occlusion contours are computed separately
according to orientations (vertical, horizontal and the two diagonals) in the four sublayers.
[10]Naturally, the input unit that corresponds in position to the output unit is also part of these straight
lines.

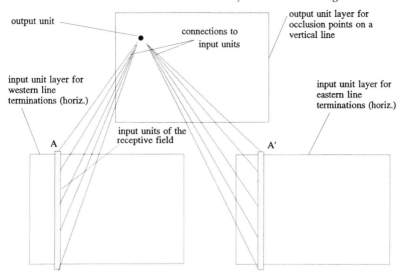

Figure 4.6. *Finkel and Edelman's (1989) network: the field structure for computing occlusion points.*

(within each orientation- and direction-specific sublayer), this receptive field construction requires a great number of connections between input and output layers.

When does such a straight-line receptive field deliver a suprathreshold output that represents an occlusion cue? To manage this, the output unit must receive not only activation from the retinally corresponding input unit but also simultaneous activation from at least two further input units that have to originate from the two straight lines that correspond in position (sublayers). One could say that the output units on this level act as logical 'AND-gates' for input from the two substructures (straight lines).

In the final network stage, occlusion contours are generated from occlusion cues. The functional principle is that an occlusion boundary is always drawn between two occlusion cues with the same orientation when they lie on one line.[11] The occlusion contours marked in bold in Figure 4.5 are computed in this way.

Next, the Kanizsa square (Figure 4.1) is used to explain how the machinery described above computes illusory contours. The input pattern on the level of occlusion cues is dealt with first. As described above, this represents information on the 'retinal' position, orientation and direction of line terminations. For the Kanizsa square, some of this input information is represented schematically in Figure 4.7. This concerns horizontal westward and eastward terminations (lines terminating in a circle) that are assigned to the straight-line receptive field (A and A') of the two output units. In addition, the outline of the Kanizsa input pattern is also drawn in Figure 4.7.

Two units are displayed on the output layer. Their receptive fields are similar and cover the straight lines A and A'. For the case presented here, both of these output units are activated above threshold because both straight-line receptive fields signal two horizontal westward and eastward line terminations.

---

[11] Finkel and Edelman (1989) provide very little information on this process.

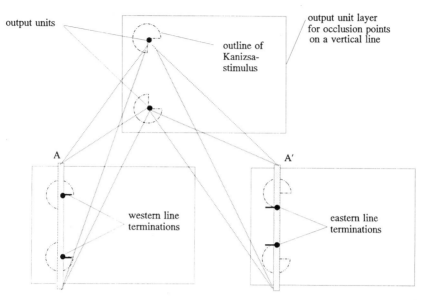

Figure 4.7. *Finkel and Edelman's (1989) network: the computation of 'occlusion points' in the Kanizsa square (illusory contours).*

On the next and final processing stage, occlusion cues that lie on one straight line (potential occlusion contour) are combined, so that complete contours arise. For the example in Figure 4.7, this means that the left-hand, vertical illusory contour in the Kanizsa square is generated. The right-hand vertical contour and the two horizontal contours are generated in the same way.

In a series of computer simulations, Finkel and Edelman (1989) have confirmed that the processing stages sketched above are actually capable of successfully generating illusory and occlusion contours. Both the Kanizsa square and several other figures that generate illusory boundaries in humans were used as input patterns. The same set of parameters (e.g. thresholds, activity maxima, etc.) was used every time. For the simulated examples, the output pattern revealed not only the illusory contours at the required position (e.g. the Kanizsa square) but also no additional contours that are not present in human perception. Hence, the network can be assigned 'behavioral validity' – a concept that is described in more detail in Section 4.

As far as empirical support for the architecture of the four stages of occlusion computation is concerned, Finkel and Edelman (1989) have remarked that their line termination stage or its units bears certain similarities to so-called 'end-stop cells' in V1 (Gilbert, 1977). Evidence in support of parts of the proposed structure of the occlusion cue or occlusion contour stage is provided by the previously mentioned work of von der Heydt, Peterhans and Baumgartner (1984). A further finding in this work has shown that those cells in V2 that are sensitive to illusory contours increase their firing rate only when both parts of the stimulus necessary to induce the illusory contour are present. Therefore, we can talk of a field structure in the sense of a logical AND-gate.

It should also be mentioned that Finkel and Edelman's (1989) complete network covers nine further processing stages.[12] Some contribute to the computation of directions of motion; others have the task of resolving conflicts between contradictory processing outcomes. Such conflicts occur when several parallel processing stages (e.g. direction of motion and wide-angle line terminations) deliver their output to one individual stage (e.g. occlusion contour). Furthermore, feedback loops (re-entry) are also stipulated in order to be able to eliminate, for example, local cues signaling false occlusions.

3 GROSSBERG AND MINGOLLA'S (1985a) NEURAL NETWORK 'FACADE' AND ILLUSORY CONTOURS

In a series of publications since the beginning of the 1980s, Grossberg and colleagues (Grossberg, 1983, 1987a, b; Grossberg and Mingolla 1985a) have presented a neural network architecture for 'early' – sometimes also called pre-attentive – visual information processing. The range of experimental psychological and neurobiological findings includes phenomena and functions from the perception of motion, brightness, color, form, texture and depth (Cohen and Grossberg, 1984; Grossberg, 1983, 1987a, b, 1991; Grossberg and Marshall, 1989; Grossberg and Mingolla, 1985a, b; Grossberg and Rudd, 1989; Grossberg and Todorovic, 1988). Grossberg (1990) has labeled the complete network architecture used to explain these diverse phenomena, 'FACADE' theory ('*form-and-color-and-depth*' theory).[13]

3.1 Functional Theory

The functional decomposition of FACADE assumes three interrelated main functions (Grossberg, 1983, 1987a, b; Grossberg and Mingolla, 1985a, b; Grossberg and Todorovic, 1988). The first function consists – analogous to Finkel and Edelman (1989) – in a kind of preprocessing of the 'retinal' input pattern, that is, a computation of a distribution of luminance differences or changes from a two-dimensional distribution of absolute luminance values (Grossberg and Todorovic, 1988). This preprocessed activation pattern is then used – according to the description of the second function – to compute a three-dimensionally organized form

---

[12]The total number of units is approximately 222 000 and the total number of connections approximately 8.5 million. This makes it one of the largest networks to be simulated to date (1990).

[13]From its origins (Grossberg, 1983) up to the present (Grossberg, 1991), FACADE theory has been expanded by a great number of points and even modified in parts. My review is based mainly on Grossberg and Mingolla (1985a) and Grossberg (1987a). The network architecture presented in these articles that is related to the present topic (the occurrence of illusory contours) has nonetheless remained largely unchanged.

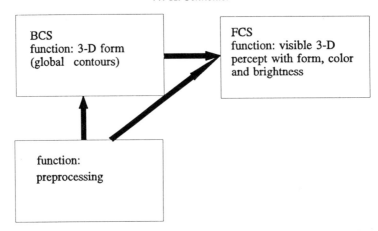

Figure 4.8. *Grossberg and Mingolla's (1985a) network: FACADE and its systems. BCS, boundary contour system; FCS, feature contour system.*

(shape) representation of the world without, however, already representing color and brightness. Nonetheless, the outcome of this processing (three-dimensional object boundaries) is not visible but only defines the input pattern for the third in the series of main functions (Figure 4.8). This function computes a percept that forms the basis of conscious representation and specifies information on brightness, color and three-dimensional form. This requires an additional input pattern besides the output pattern of the form function, whose generation is assigned to the preprocessing function. This second input pattern contains information on brightness and color contrasts. On the basis of Land's (1977) findings, Grossberg and Mingolla (1985a) have argued that color and brightness values are computed only from information that comes from contrasts.

The authors label the processing system of the second function the 'boundary contour' system (BC) and the system of the third function as the 'feature contour' system (FC; Figure 4.8). In simplified terms, the BC system computes, something like the 'external outlines' of objects (shapes) in the world, while the FC system uses this as a basis to fill in color and hence make objects visible.

A characteristic feature of the work of Grossberg and his colleagues is the effort to underpin the functional decomposition with experimental findings from psychology and neurobiology. For example, they justify discriminating a BC and an FC system by referring to a perceptual experiment described by Yarbus (1967). The results of this experiment have shown that when the contours of a colored object are stabilized with respect to the retina, that is, the internal computation of these contours is prevented, the colors flow out beyond the object and render it invisible. Contours seem to possess a barrier function for a process of 'filling in' with color (Grossberg and Mingolla, 1985a).[14]

---

[14]More recently, Paradiso and Nakayama (1991) and Ramachandran and Gregory (1991) have been able to find further experimental psychological evidence in support of the discrimination between the BC and the FC systems. Neurobiological data also suggest a similar discrimination, namely, between the color-sensitive 'blob-thin-stripe' system (FC system) and the form-sensitive 'interblob-pale-stripe' system (BC system) (De Yoe and van Essen, 1988; Livingstone and Hubel, 1988; Zeki and Shipp, 1988).

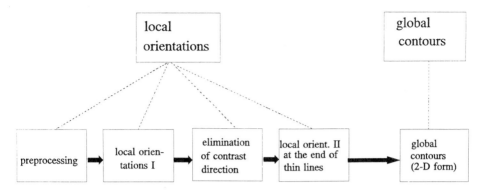

Figure 4.9. *A functional decomposition of Grossberg and Mingolla's (1985a) BC system.*

The BC system is also given the task of generating illusory contours. Although the FC system is required to make these contours visible, the relevant computation of the course of the contours occurs in the BC system. With this assumption, Grossberg and Mingolla (1985a) disagree with Finkel and Edelman (1989), who assign illusory contours to the occlusion contour function. Although the BC system implies three-dimensional form computation (Grossberg, 1987b; Grossberg and Marshall, 1989), the following presentations will be restricted to the two-dimensional case. A presentation of the computation of the dimension of depth is not necessary for the generation of illusory contours and would go beyond the range of this chapter.

As in Finkel and Edelman (1989), form computation is once more divided into two functions (Figure 4.9). The first function is defined by the fact that local orientations have to be computed for contrasts, while the second function is assigned the task of using the output pattern of the first function to generate global two-dimensional contours that correspond to forms.

Further functional decomposition of the first function leads to four subfunctions (Figure 4.9). The first subfunction of preprocessing has already been described above and is almost identical in content to Finkel and Edelman's (1989) preprocessing function. A further similarity in functional decomposition is given in the function of local orientations. Once more, the task is to determine the local orientation of contrasts. However, unlike Finkel and Edelman (1989), the output pattern still carries information on the direction of contrast, that is, on whether a light–dark or dark–light contrast is present. The next subfunction is characterized by an output pattern that no longer carries any information on direction of contrast. The authors account for this subfunction by pointing out that contours of an object can be generated by alternating light–dark and dark–light crossings. Therefore, this information should not play any role in the generation of contours and can be eliminated.[15] Neurophysiological findings on 'simple' and 'complex' cells in the sense of Hubel and Wiesel (1962)

---

[15]Naturally, this information on direction of contrast is indispensable within the FC system. The direct connection between preprocessing and the FC system contributes to this, so that the elimination of direction of contrast in the BC system has no effect on perceived brightness.

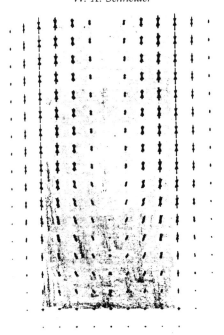

Figure 4.10. *An output pattern on the stage of 'local orientations I'. [From Grossberg and Mingolla, 1985a. © 1985 The American Psychological Association; reprinted with kind permission of the publisher and Stephen Grossberg.]*

are consistent with this proposal: the former are sensitive to direction of contrast but not the latter.

The assumption underlying the fourth subfunction 'local orientations II' demonstrates a further feature of the way in which Grossberg and Mingolla (1985a) perform their functional decomposition, namely, they do not develop functional and mechanistic theory in sequence (top-down) but in parallel and interactively.[16] This has the following implications for the fourth subfunction: previous subfunctions or the processing stages assigned to them do not deliver any clear orientations at the ends of thin lines. Figure 4.10, which is taken from Grossberg and Mingolla (1985a), illustrates this graphically.

The figure presents the output of the second subfunction. The size of the activations of the 'orientation' units is symbolized by the length of the lines, while the slope of the lines represents the orientation. The gray background represents the 'thin' lines. The size of the receptive fields exceeds the breadth of the input end and contains 16 × 8 units (see also Figure 4.11). On the one hand, it is conspicuous in Figure 4.10 that sometimes several orientations or representative units are activated per network position, and one orientation is frequently dominant (e.g. on the elongated edges of the line), that is, it indicates the highest activation value. On the other hand, at the end of the line, it can be seen that scarcely any orientation units are activated above threshold. If this representation of local orientations were

---

[16]Marr (1982), in contrast, proposed that functional (computational) theory should be developed independently from mechanistic (algorithmic and implementational) theory.

the basis of a subsequent global contour generation process (content of the fifth subfunction), then no clear contours could be computed at the ends of thin lines (smaller than the field size), and the form representation would be incomplete at these positions.[17] The subfunction of 'local orientations II' is postulated to prevent this. Its task is to construct unequivocal orientations of contours (in this case, input regions) in regions of input that are smaller than the field size (e.g. the ends of thin lines). The existence of such a subfunction is also supported by psychophysiological data on hyperacuity that show that subjects are capable of discriminating patterns that are below the size of the fields involved (Badcock and Westheimer, 1985).

The assumption of the fifth and final subfunction derives from the need to construct an output pattern from the local orientations at the fourth stage that represents coherent and complete contours or two-dimensional forms. Given appropriate 'retinal' input (e.g. the Kanizsa square in Figure 4.1), this should also contain illusory contours.

3.2 Mechanistic Theory

The description of Grossberg and Mingolla's (1985a; Grossberg, 1987a) mechanistic theory should begin on the unit level with the description of an activation equation. This is followed by a short digression into the structure of the receptive fields for the computation of local orientations I, before then describing the processing levels that are actually relevant for understanding how illusory contours arise. This involves the stages local orientations II and global contours.

Grossberg and Mingolla's (1985a) equation for computing the momentary unit activations of the preprocessing unit can be viewed as typical of many types of network. It is related to the properties of the membrane equation of a standard neuron and can be written as the following differential equation:

$$dx/dt = -Ax + (B - x)e(t) - (x + D)i(t)$$

In a discrete form, the equation can be interpreted as follows. The change in activation Δx of a preprocessing unit after the time period Δt is composed firstly, of a decay term A that determines how strongly the prior activation x is obliged to decline in Δt, secondly of an excitatory input e, whose impact depends on x and a maximum activation B, and, thirdly, of an inhibitory input i, whose impact is also determined by x and a minimum activation D.

Grossberg and Mingolla's (1985a; Grossberg, 1987a) stage 'local orientations I' is similar to the construction of the receptive fields for computing orientation ('local orientations' stage) in Finkel and Edelman (1989) (see Figure 4.5). As mentioned above, the decisive difference is that the receptive field is additionally sensitive to direction of contrast, that is, it can discriminate whether a light–dark or a dark–light contrast is present. Figure. 4.11 contains a schematized representation of such a field with 16 × 8 units.

---

[17] As Grossberg and Mingolla (1985a) emphasize, incomplete contours in the BC system would have drastic consequences for further processing, because the coloring process in the FC system (filling-in) requires complete boundaries. Otherwise, 'outflow catastrophes' would occur as described in Yarbus (1967).

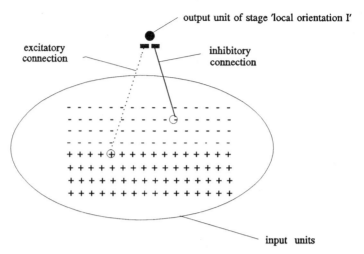

Figure 4.11. *Grossberg and Mingolla's (1985a) network: a receptive field for computing 'local orientations I'.*

It only remains to be added that, besides the findings from Hubel and Wiesel (1962), psychophysiological data on texture perception or texture discrimination (Sutter, Beck and Graham, 1989; see also De Valois and De Valois, 1988) are also compatible in major points (e.g. nonlinear filtering) with the field structure proposed by Grossberg and Mingolla (1985a; Grossberg, 1987a).

3.2.1   The Stage 'Local Orientations II': Computation of Orientations at the Ends of Thin Lines

The argument for the existence of the stage 'local orientations II' introduced above was as follows: in input pattern regions, that are smaller than the field size (e.g. at the ends of thin lines), orientation units produce no unequivocal and distinct response. In other words, for these regions (line ends), only very weakly differing orientations or even no orientations at all, are signaled. If, for example, a line end covers 6 units and the field size is 16×8 units – as in Figure 4.11 – then for those units whose positions represent the end of the line, various orientations will simultaneously be activated relatively weakly or not all (Figure 4.10). In order to nonetheless signal orientations for such regions of the input pattern that are spatially smaller than the field size, and thus to be able to generate boundaries at the end of thin lines, further processing is necessary.

Grossberg and Mingolla (1985a) introduce the fourth level of processing for this. It consists of two different substructures. The first substructure[18] relates to the connections between input unit and output unit, while the second substructure concerns a case that has not been presented here before: namely, connections between output units. The first substructure – unlike previously described struc-

---

[18]The authors call this a 'first competitive stage', while the second substructure is called 'second competitive stage' (Grossberg and Mingolla, 1985a). Pooling to one subfunction or stage of processing is motivated by the fact that both substructures combined perform one function; namely, the generation of orientations at the end of thin lines.

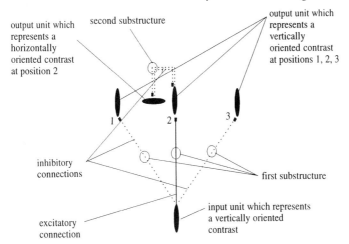

output unit which represents a horizontally oriented contrast at position 2

second substructure

output unit which represents a vertically oriented contrast at positions 1, 2, 3

inhibitory connections

first substructure

excitatory connection

input unit which represents a vertically oriented contrast

Figure 4.12. *Grossberg and Mingolla's (1985a) network: the field structure on the 'local orientations II' stage.*

tures – does not have convergent connections between input and output units (e.g. the receptive field for local orientation I computation) but divergent connections. As Figure 4.12 shows, the input units (e.g. for vertically oriented contrasts at a particular position) have excitatory connections with those output units at corresponding positions (with the same orientation) as well as inhibitory connections with the directly neighboring output units with the same orientation (vertical), although these connections are less strongly weighted. The complete substructure contains further excitatory and inhibitory connections that have been dropped for clarity of presentation.

However, at the end of thin lines, not only sufficient activations of contrasts should be computed but also, from among the units that represent the same 'retinal' position, but complementarily oriented contrasts, the unit that most closely reflects the states in the world (orientation of the line ends) should receive the highest activation value. Therefore, in the second substructure on the fourth processing stage, output units with the same 'retinal' position but different orientations are coupled horizontally and competitively (Figure 4.12). If, for example, a unit that represents the orientation X (e.g. vertical) receives excitatory activation, this leads to an inhibitory input to the unit in the same position that represents an orientation Y that is orthogonal to X, (horizontal). Due to the lateral coupling in Grossberg and Mingolla's (1985a; Grossberg, 1987a) fourth stage, the inhibition of one unit causes the disinhibition of another coupled unit (same position but orthogonal orientation).[19] The authors also talk about a 'push-pull opponent process' (Grossberg, 1980).

How the two substructures on the fourth stage compute orientations at the end of a thin vertical line in which the end is below the threshold of the field size should be explained in the following. The description starts on the third processing stage (Figure 4.10). For a thin vertical line, it designates a relatively strong output for

---

[19]The mechanism for this proposed by the authors, a dipole field (Grossberg, 1980, 1987a) cannot be described here because of insufficient space. It includes a discrimination between 'on' and 'off' units.

units positioned along the middle of the line that signal vertically oriented contrasts. For units from positions at line ends, output is increasingly weaker, so that horizontal or other orientations are only represented weakly, if at all.

On the fourth processing stage, this activation profile remains the same for the output units on the middle of the line. They continue to have a relatively strong output. However, a notable change occurs in output units at the end of the line that represent a vertical orientation: although these line-end units receive only weak excitatory activation from line-end input units with corresponding position – only low input in the receptive fields – they simultaneously receive, because of the first substructure (Figure 4.12), a relatively high inhibitory input from the units positioned more toward the middle. Their fields signal a strong and high-contrast input and thus produce a relatively large output.

Because of the simultaneous involvement of the second substructure with its horizontal connections, the activity pattern of the first substructure is once again changed in two ways. First, the difference in activation of units for vertical orientation positioned in the middle increases compared to units with complementary orientation. Second, and this is decisive for the formation of appropriate orientations at thin line ends, the inhibition of units for vertical orientation positioned at line ends leads to a disinhibition of units for horizontal orientation in corresponding positions. Global cooperative processes, which will be presented in the next section, can compute a horizontal boundary at the line end from the representation of these disinhibited oriented contrasts. Figure 4.13 shows a computer-simulated output of the fourth processing stage for an input pattern that – as in Figure 4.10 – has no orientations at line ends.

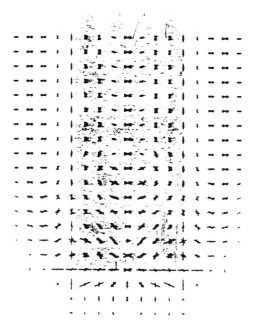

Figure 4.13. *An output pattern on the 'local orientations II' stage. [From Grossberg and Mingolla, 1985a. © 1985 The American Psychological Association; reprinted with kind permission of the publisher and Stephen Grossberg).]*

Grossberg and his colleagues (Grossberg and Marshall, 1989; Grossberg and Rudd, 1989) argue that the hypercomplex cells with end-stopping properties postulated by some physiologists (Gilbert, 1977; Hubel and Wiesel, 1965) provide neurobiological support for the existence of the first substructure. The neurobiological correlate of the second substructure could be a part of the 'hypercolumns' (Hubel and Wiesel, 1977).

3.2.2   The Computation of Global Boundaries and Illusory Contours

The preceding four processing stages transform a quasi-retinal input pattern to such an extent that several units are activated per retinal position. Each unit represents different and complementarily oriented contrasts, while one of these units has the highest activity value. As the example of an activation profile in Figure 4.13 shows, this does not produce any global and sharp contours in the output pattern that go beyond individual positions and represent the final outcome of form processing.

The generation of such two-dimensional boundaries (shapes) requires a further processing stage. This has the additional task of compensating for incompletions and breaks in the course of contours such as those induced by, for example, the blind spot on the retina.

The description of the fourth network stage and its output pattern (see, for example, Figure 4.13) raises the question why several units are frequently activated per retinal position that each necessarily represent different orientations. Why is output not shaped so that only one 'successful' orientation per position is signaled? The answer is because the activation of several orientation units for each retinal position increases the probability of being able to draw coherent and sharp boundaries. If only one orientation per position were to remain as local output, it would scarcely be possible to signal continuously the same orientations along the positions of a contour in the slightly distorted retinal inputs that frequently arise in natural environments. This would lead to the generation of mostly fuzzy boundaries.

The presentation of the fifth processing stage of global boundary computation introduces a new type of network mechanism: in addition to the forward flow of activations on all prior stages (feedforward), it postulates a backward flow (feedback). As in the framework of a serial feedforward architecture, the usual equation of the input pattern with the first layer of units (input units) and of the output pattern to the second layer of units (output units) is no longer adequate in such a stage construction. Units on the first layer of the fifth stage receiving input from the previous fourth stage are the same units that generate output. The units on the second layer receive activation from the first layer and then feed it back to the first layer. To avoid confusion when referring to different units, first-layer units on the fifth stage will be labeled 'HC units' in line with the neurobiological model of hypercomplex cells (Hubel and Wiesel, 1965). The second-layer units will be labeled 'bipole units' as suggested by Grossberg (1987a). Bipole units receive feedforward activation, compute it in a particular way (see below) and return the outcome as feedback to the HC units (first-layer). Figure 4.14, which is explained below, illustrates this graphically.

The function of the bipole-unit layer is to influence the units on the HC layer, that is, their activation patterns in such a way that, for each position, only such

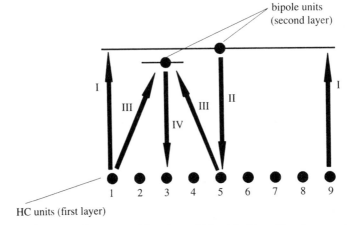

Figure 4.14. *A cooperative–competitive loop. [Adapted from Grossberg and Mingolla, 1985a.* © *1985 The American Psychological Association; reprinted with kind permission of the publisher and the authors.]*

orientations remain activated that lead to coherent, completed and sharply emerging boundaries. Bipole units 'fire' – in the simplest case – only when they simultaneously – like a logical AND-gate – receive input from two HC units. The two HC units must represent spatially adjacent retinal positions and the same orientation. One could also say that a bipole unit has to signal two nonidentical points on a straight line with a specific orientation. For a further understanding of the computation of global boundaries, it is necessary to recall the argument used for the fourth processing stage above: the output pattern of this stage designates several activated units with complementary orientations for each retinal position. For this reason, there is a high probability that a bipole unit – with given contrast state (e.g. object boundaries in the world) – generates an output triggered by the activation of two HC units. Then, from all the activated HC units assigned to these two retinal positions, which each represent different orientations in pairs, there should be two HC units that show the same orientation and are connected with the corresponding bipole unit.

How these bipole units can generate a longer and complete (break-free) global boundary will now be explained by describing the 'cooperative–competitive loop' (CC loop; Grossberg and Mingolla, 1985a) of the fifth stage. This will refer to Figure 4.14.[20]

The figure relates to the case of a boundary with gaps. It shows two activated HC units with the same orientation that are separated by seven further weakly activated units corresponding to intermediate retinal positions. The starting point of the CC loop is the receptive field of the middle bipole unit (above position 5). It is activated when the outer HC units (positions 1 and 9) transmit input (processing step I in Figure 4.14). In the next step, this bipole unit sends feedback to a spatially

---

[20]For clarity and because of the shortage of space, a simplified version of the fifth stage is presented here. Neither on and off-units as part of the bipole field (fourth-stage output units) nor the more detailed structure of the feedback connections can be explained here (see Grossberg, 1987a; Grossberg and Mingolla, 1985a).

intermediate HC unit (with the same orientation) – in the present example, to the fifth unit (step II). With this top-down activation, which intervenes in the fourth processing stage, the unit that has the same orientation as the bipole unit can compete successfully with other units with complementary orientation on position 5. Although the other units may also have received feedback from their bipole units, this must have been weaker, so that the difference between their activation and the activation of the unit with the preferred orientation should have increased. Hence, the CC loop also strengthens contrast. In a further processing step (III), the dominant position-5 HC unit together with the unit on the extreme left (position 1) sends output to a further bipole unit in the middle that has a smaller receptive field. This bipole unit, in turn, has a top-down effect (IV) on an intermediate HC unit (position 3) that also receives additional input and can thereby dominate units with other orientations. CC loop processing continues until a complete and coherent boundary is generated. If processing is completed and a nonzero equilibrium activity pattern has been established, then the activity pattern that represents coherent contours will be passed on to the FC system.

Hence, the CC loop also has temporal components. Thus, the final boundaries that provide the basis for visibility in the FC system do not arise immediately but only after completion of the CC loop. Without completed boundaries, no features can be generated in the FC system, and visibility is not given. If the BC system receives several different inputs in rapid sequence, then later input can disturb the as yet incomplete boundary completion process (CC loop) for the prior input and impede its visibility. Phenomena such as metacontrast (Breitmeyer, 1984), in which a second stimulus makes an immediately preceding stimulus invisible, are introduced by Grossberg (1987a) as experimental support of such a process.

The CC loop provides a functional computation principle that can bring about a decision among locally competing states (e.g. competing orientations per position) using globally directed, long-range processes. The authors also talk about an 'on-line statistical decision machine' (Grossberg, 1987a) that transforms 'analog' representations of the first two processing stages into a more 'structural and digital' representation. In neurophysiological terms, the authors (Grossberg, 1987a) assign the assumed bipole units to cortical area V2 (a part of area 18), which is supported by the findings from van der Heydt, Peterhans and Baumgartner (1984) described in Section 2.

Now how does this fifth processing stage compute illusory contours? Analogous to the description of Finkel and Edelman's (1989) network, the example of the Kanizsa square should be considered. The starting point is the output pattern of the previous fourth stage. It should have contained a two-dimensional representation of oriented contrasts reflecting the boundaries (edges) of the four Pac-man figures. For the purpose of graphic illustration, in Figure 4.15 the representational format of the vertical lines in Figure 4.13 is applied to the Pac-man figures of the Kanizsa square. Units representing oriented contrasts along the object boundaries of the four Pac-man figures should show a similar 'noisy' activation pattern. Figure 4.15 provides a highly simplified schematic description of this case. It refers to the horizontal illusory contours between the two upper Pac-man figures in the Kanizsa square.

Figure 4.15a shows the output pattern of stage 4. Only the oriented contrast units are depicted that refer to positions along the two horizontal outlines (contrasts) of the Pac-man figures. For better spatial correspondence, the other outlines of the Pac-man figures are also sketched. The lower part (Figure 4.15b) shows the

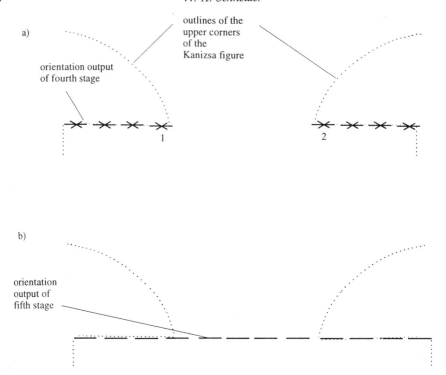

Figure 4.15. *Grossberg and Mingolla's (1985a) network and illusory contours. (a) A fourth-stage output pattern (without illusory contours); (b) A fifth-stage output pattern (with illusory contours).*

fifth-stage output pattern that arises after the CC loop has transformed the fourth-stage activation pattern. Illusory and real contours are symbolized by the horizontal dashes that form a line with breaks. A precondition for the generation of such an output pattern is that the receptive fields of the bipole units extend so far in space that they simultaneously receive input from the two HC units localized in the far right of the left-hand Pac-man figure (point 1 in Figure 4.15) and in the far left of the right-hand Pac-man figure (point 2). If the CC loop functions in the way described above, then, initially, the unit with the same orientation that lies in the middle between the two points 1 and 2 should receive feedback from the corresponding bipole unit before, in further cycles, the other units with the same orientation also receive stronger activation. At the same time, feedback leads to units with the correct orientations dominating each retinal position.

3.3 A Selective Overview of Neural Networks in the Field of Visual Information Processing

The presentation of Finkel and Edelman's (1989) and Grossberg and Mingolla's (1985a) models for generating illusory contours should exemplify the construction and functions of neural networks. Before discussing the general problems and advantages of such an approach, a brief and selective overview of further phenomena in the field of visual information processing that have already been modeled with neurocomputation (1990) should be given. Compared with other areas in experimental psychology (e.g. memory or language production), the construction and testing of neural networks is relatively advanced here. This is probably because vision is a field in which an enormous interdisciplinary database has grown (De Valois and De Valois, 1988; DeYoe and van Essen, 1988; Humphreys and Bruce, 1989; Livingstone and Hubel, 1988; Metzger, 1975; Prinz, 1983; Schiffman, 1990; Spillmann and Werner, 1990; van der Heijden, 1991).

For the two-dimensional segmentation of visual input (Beck, 1982; Julesz, 1975; Kehrer and Meinecke, this volume), a series of other neural networks have been developed in addition to the BC network from Grossberg and colleagues and Finkel and Edelman's (1989) network. Daugman (1988) has presented a network that performs local orientation computations with a neural 'implementation' of Gabor filters. Kienker *et al.* (1986) have presented a connectionistic network that focuses on a simple figure-ground segmentation.

Network architectures for the analysis of moving stimuli (Sekuler *et al.*, 1990) have also been developed by, for example, Grossberg and Rudd (1989; Grossberg, 1991). Ballard (1986) and Zipser and Andersen (1988) have studied how neural networks can be used to perform transformations between various coordinate systems that underlie visual information processing.

Up to now, far fewer network models have been presented in the field of 'late' as compared with 'early' vision. For the field of object recognition and object classification (Biederman, 1987; Hoffmann, this volume; Marr, 1982; Treisman, 1988) neural network models have been presented by, for example, Ballard (1984), Carpenter and Grossberg (1987) and Poggio and Edelman (1990). How perceptual information interacts with verbal knowledge (word recognition) is the subject of the interactive activation model of McClelland and Rumelhart (1981) as well as the model from Grossberg and Stone (1986). Also, a series of models have already been presented that refer to the mechanism of visual attention, which possibly has a decisive function for many of the visual issues mentioned above (Phaf, van der Heijden and Hudson, 1990; Sandon, 1990).

This selective overview should be concluded with an interesting and very promising extension of the repertoire of neurocomputational processing principles based on the work of von der Malsburg (1981, 1990; von der Malsburg and Schneider, 1986). The basic idea is that units (or groups of units) do not just code information through their level of activation (in neural terms, the strength of their firing frequency) but also through the temporal structure of changes in their activation. This implies that the activations of units are not constant over time but change, for example, oscillate periodically over time (e.g. in the form of a sine oscillation). With such units, information can be coded not only through the size of their activation but also through their temporal coherence. This means the following: those units that represent a common content oscillate (change their activity) in phase,[21] while those units that do not represent related contents do not do this. The fact that such a coding is possible and functions has since been demonstrated in a

---

[21]Oscillation is not necessary for temporal coding, but only synchronized neuronal activity (bursts) that might occur aperiodically.

series of studies from the field of segmentation. The corresponding networks (e.g. von der Malsburg and Schneider, 1986) produce a coherent representation of the features of an object as an output pattern, that is, they reveal phase-locked oscillations of the corresponding unit activations. Neurophysiological support for the existence of such temporal coding schemes has been provided by the detection of stimulus-dependent and phase-locked neural oscillations of neurons in cortical area V1 in cats (Eckhorn *et al.*, 1988; Gray *et al.*, 1989; Singer, 1990).

4 PROBLEMS AND ADVANTAGES OF THE NEUROCOMPUTATIONAL APPROACH: VALIDITY ISSUES AND PSYCHOLOGICAL THEORIZING

The purpose of the two previous sections is to illustrate what is hidden behind the label 'neural networks' and how they can be used to explain findings and functions in vision. This section considers the advantages and problems involved in such neurocomputational explanations. The discussion should be focused on the issue of how neural networks can be validated and evaluated. An answer must be provided in such a way that it is appropriate to judge the most diverse networks with the same measuring instrument. A conceptual framework for this purpose should be introduced that distinguishes between the 'behavioral' or 'psychological validity' and the 'architectural validity' of a network.

The first validity criterion asks to what extent neural networks behave in an analogous way to psychological (behavioral) findings. For example, are the two networks from Finkel and Edelman (1989) and Grossberg and Mingolla (1985a; Grossberg, 1987a) capable of computing illusory contours for those input conditions that also must be present in human perception (e.g. the Kanizsa square)? The answer to this question reveals a decisive advantage of the network approach, namely, the ability to test the described information processing (input–output transformations) explicitly and precisely with the help of computer simulations.

The second criterion, architectural validity, refers to whether a network computes psychological performance in a plausible way. To answer this question, it is necessary to test to what extent the proposed network architecture, that is, its functional and mechanistic theory, agrees with empirical findings. This particularly involves a discussion of which classes of neurobiological data are relevant for architectural validation. This set of questions also includes the previously disregarded issue of the relationship between units and neurons.

4.1 Behavioral Validity and Computer Simulation

Behavioral or psychological validity can be ascertained by testing whether the neural network behaves in a manner analogous to available psychological findings – one could also talk about 'psychological competence'. For the models from Finkel and Edelman (1989) and Grossberg and Mingolla (1985a; Grossberg, 1987a), which aim to explain the phenomena of illusory contours, this means the following: under input conditions in which human subjects report illusory contours (e.g. the Kanizsa square), they should also generate such contours. Vice versa, if subjects do not see any illusory contours, the network output pattern should not show any either.

On the basis of this research logic, Finkel and Edelman (1989) tested their network under a series of different input conditions with the help of computer simulation. As input patterns, they used not only a series of displays that elicit illusory contours in human beings (e.g. the Kanizsa square) but also displays in which no illusory contours are found. Test output corresponded to psychological findings on human beings. For Grossberg and Mingolla's (1985a; Grossberg, 1987a) model, such tests have not yet been published. The simulations presented by the authors only refer to the generation of the ends of thin lines as well as some textural segmentations (Grossberg and Mingolla, 1985b)

A major criterion for the behavioral validity of a neural network is how many experimental findings can be simulated when the set of parameters (weights, thresholds, etc.) remain constant.[22] The more findings and functions of a domain (e.g. form perception) that can be 'replicated' (simulated) successfully through neurocomputation, the higher the behavioral validity of the network.

Usually, computer simulations are applied to test behavioral validity. They simultaneously reveal one of the strong points of neural networks: one is not just dependent on verbal argumentation in order to show that the network can actually explain the findings and functions, that is, can actually compute the necessary input–output transformation. In addition, simulation helps to detect problems in the internal consistency of a model that remain hidden in mere descriptions of activation equations or in verbal specifications.

A further advantage of neural networks is that not only content-specific in-put–output transformations (e.g. illusory contours) can be used to test their behavioral validity: the processing time of the network from scanning the input pattern to computation of the intended output pattern can also be assessed as a dependent variable. This idea is based on the assumption that the flow of activation between units or layers that serves the computation of specific functions requires time – just as the spread of generator and action potentials between neurons in real brains takes time. Grossberg and Mingolla's (1985a; Grossberg, 1987a) fifth process-ing stage, or the competitive–cooperative loop, is particularly appropriate for illustrating this. Before this loop generates a complete contour as an output pattern, activation must have 'flowed' several times between the two layers on the fifth stage (see Section 3.2.2).

Hence, as a dependent variable, the processing time of a network is then an indispensable measure when findings on reaction times have to be explained, and this variable has been assessed frequently in experimental cognitive psychology (Lachman, Lachman and Butterfield, 1979; Luce, 1986; Neisser, 1967; Posner, 1978). In this case, testing behavioral validity requires a comparison of the pattern of reaction times found empirically with the time that the network requires to achieve the endstate (e.g. to generate an open reaction). Using this 'logic', Phaf, van der Heijden and Wolters (1990) have been able to show that their neural network for

---

[22]Nonetheless, there are good reasons why it has to be possible to alter experiment-specific and learning-dependent parameters.

visual attention can successfully simulate reaction time data from almost a dozen experiments.

A prerequisite for testing behavioral validity is that the neural network should compute stable output activation patterns in a consistent way. If, for example, feedback loops are entered into a network then, under certain conditions, unwanted, unstable, continuously changing states can arise. Appropriate modification of the architecture can make this behavior disappear once more, and the intended input–output transformation (e.g. contour completion) will occur. In order to be able to judge and actively avoid such cases for specific classes of network architecture, mathematical analyses of the possible activation states are both necessary and helpful (Cohen and Grossberg, 1983; Grossberg, 1988; Hopfield, 1982).

4.2 Architectural Validity, Neurobiological and Experimental Psychological Findings

Behavioral validity, which can be tested successfully with computer simulation, is only a necessary but in no way a sufficient condition for being able to state that a network provides a satisfactory explanation. Empirical tests of architectural validity, that is, of the functional and mechanistic assumptions underlying the network architecture, are also required. How could such a test be designed? To which aspects of a network should it refer? These questions will be answered by returning to the previously introduced distinction between functional and mechanistic theory.

The highest priority in architectural validation should be given to functional theory. Functional theory is seen not only in the decomposition into subfunctions but also in the specification of the input–output pattern transformations of these subfunctions, that is, in the specification of the information with which the network should compute. If these aspects of a neural network are incompatible with psychological or neurobiological findings, then the network has to be rejected as a model of information processing even if the test of behavioral validity has been successful. For example, if findings show that illusory contours are computed independently from occlusion contours, then Finkel and Edelman's (1989) network would have to be rejected. The same would apply to Grossberg and Mingolla (1985a) if the opposite case were 'true' and illusory contours actually were to depend on the computation of the occlusion boundaries.

If the functional theory is valid, then the next step is to test mechanistic theory. This calls for a discrimination between at least two levels: the lower level of mechanistic theory refers to single units and connections; the upper, to individual processing stages or the structures that define them (e.g. receptive fields).

As far as the lower level of mechanistic theory is concerned, an issue will be considered first that has been ignored up to now: How do structural and dynamic aspects of the units relate to that which they model: neurons? The first step toward an answer is to list the general and relatively broadly generalizable properties of a 'standard' neuron. The standard neuron exhibits an input section that consists of tree-like dendrites; a central 'computation unit', the soma; and an output section composed of an axon (Kandel, 1991). The output unit of one neuron (axon) is connected to the input unit of another neuron (dendrite), normally over an electrochemical 'device'—the synapse whose equivalent is the weight of a connection. Communication between neurons is linked to the spread of potential changes in which the signal generally moves along axons in the form of a transient, electrical, all-or-nothing signal labeled action potential. Its counterpart is the activation flow between units. Depending on their input and their momentary activity state, neurons respond by changing the frequency of the action potentials. Input from many excitatory neurons (e.g. pyramidal neurons in the cortex) leads to an increase in the action potential frequency in the receiver neuron, while input from inhibitory neurons (e.g. smooth stellate neurons) contributes to a reduction in the firing rate.

These general structural and dynamic similarities between units and neurons are taken into account in most neural network models. However, there are also further empirically demonstrated and more specific properties of nerve cells that complicate the picture and make it seem problematic to equate units too rashly with neurons (Crick and Asanuma, 1986; Kandel, Schwartz and Jessell, 1991). These neurobiological 'complications' include, for instance, the morphological and physiological properties of single neurons (Kandel, Schwartz and Jessell, 1991; Koch and Segev, 1991), the distribution and geometry of neuronal connection patterns (see, for example, Braitenberg and Schütz, 1991), or the temporal fine-structure of neuronal signaling (see, for example, Abeles, 1991).

How far such neurobiological knowledge about neurons and their connections can apply as a test criterion of the lower stage of mechanistic theory depends on the organizational stage of the central nervous system on which the phenomenon to be explained is located.[23] If the phenomenon to be explained is located on a relatively 'low' stage of the central nervous system, as found, for example, in findings on the synchronized stimulus-dependent oscillations of neural activity in the visual cortex of cats, then a unit-to-neuron (or -to a group of neurons) assignment is plausible and, correspondingly, detailed empirical constraints have to be used as test criteria for the mechanistic theory of such networks (König and Schillen, 1991; Wilson and Bower, 1991). If one is interested in phenomena in the higher stages of organization, which are typically of a psychological nature (e.g. letter recognition), then it is unclear whether the units used in such networks relate to neurons. Instead, such units, or the informational states they represent, could be conceived more easily as relatively complex bundles of neurons—which can, in turn, be modeled as neural networks—and their activation pattern. It would then be more meaningful for the mechanistic theory on the lowest stage to assume dynamics and structure of units are only roughly similar to real neurons and their interactions, maybe only in the general features mentioned above. The disadvantage that accompanies this possibility is evident: one loses—at least, at present—the

---

[23] As our knowledge about the organizational stages of the central nervous system (or corresponding functional theory) is very sparse and often speculative, given the current state of neurobiology and psychology, we can make only a rough separation extending from the level of synapses, across feature maps, up to highly complex systems such as the one for language production (Churchland and Sejnowski, 1988)

possibility of applying neurobiological findings to the design of the lower level of the mechanistic theory of such networks[24] in a plausible way and the possibility of being able to test the theory empirically. The risk of producing theories with incorrect basic assumptions (e.g. on the coding and passing on of activation), which will be overtaken by advances in knowledge, is then particularly high.

The second and upper stage of mechanistic theory refers to the structure and dynamics of the processing stages and their interconnection. The grain sizes of analysis are then no longer properties of individual units but their connections to functional computation units as represented by, for example, receptive field structures. The stage of 'computing local orientations' represents a field construction in both Finkel and Edelman (1989) and Grossberg and Mingolla (1985a; Grossberg, 1987a) that is largely compatible with a series of neurophysiological and experimental psychological findings (Hubel and Wiesel, 1962; Sutter, Beck and Graham, 1989). Furthermore, both research teams have implemented a strict topographic or retinotopic classification into the stages of their networks, for which there is also – at least for early visual processing (e.g. in V1) – support (Tootell *et al.*, 1982).

If the previous arguments on the validation of a neural network are summarized and arranged in order of priority, the highest priority should be assigned to behavioral validity. Only when computer simulations have ensured that the network behaves in a way similar to relevant psychological findings, can the architectural validity be analyzed in a next step. The suitability of the functional theory in the light of empirical data is then a prerequisite for an adequate test of the mechanistic theory, which, in turn, has two stages. The lower stage refers to individual units and their connections, while the upper stage involves the relationship of units to processing stages. To what extent the lower stage is compatible with neurobiological findings on individual nerve cells depends on the organizational stage of the central nervous system on which the finding or function to be explained is located. If these are 'low' stages, then comparisons of units with specific properties of neurons (or groups of similar neurons) are thoroughly appropriate. For findings on 'higher' stages, the unit–neuron relationship is unclear, and a powerful neurobiological test is not possible. The lower stage of mechanistic theory then remains broadly untestable – given the present state of knowledge in this domain.

4.3 On the Role of Neural Networks in the Formulation of Psychological Theories

The discussion on validation and evaluation has only provided implicit information on whether neural networks are necessary or superfluous for formulating theories in psychology. Two critical arguments should be discussed in this context. The first maintains that neurobiological findings are irrelevant to psychology and, hence, the neurocomputational approach they have inspired is also irrelevant, while the second argument questions the promise of the network approach (Massaro, 1988).

---

[24]Frequently, such networks, which refer to high-stage phenomena and only seek a loose relationship to neurobiology, are not labeled 'neural networks' but 'connectionistic networks'.

Supporters of the first argument frequently claim that the task of psychological researchers is to specify functional theory, while mechanistic theory, the actual domain of neurocomputational language, is uninteresting and irrelevant to this. Hence, functional relationships or decompositions should be generated without worrying on this level of analysis about which methods the brain uses to compute these functions. This stage can be developed at a later date and only concerns mechanistic implementation. This argument is based on the assumption that because functional and mechanistic theory can be separated conceptually, it follows that an appropriate functional theory should be developed independently from mechanistic theory. There is no logical necessity for this conclusion.[25] However, the search for suitable decompositions and assignments should, in contrast, gain decisively when the basic principles of mechanistic theory provided by neurocomputation are also taken into account, and this information is used to constrain the working space of functional theories. If we look at the development of theory formulation in the field of early vision, then we can confirm a clear increase in the acceptance of the idea that functional and mechanistic theories are interwoven (Schwartz, 1990).

The second counterargument that has to be discussed comes from a recent criticism of the network approach published by Massaro (1988). The central criticism is that neural networks are 'too powerful to be meaningful'. Massaro (1988) demonstrates this by presenting three connectionistic models of a central psychological function, namely, perceptual categorization. These are three variants of a three-layer network with 31 units that have arisen through different learning procedures, thus differing in the patterns of connections between their units. In the simulation of networks created in this way, it can be shown that with corresponding learning (modification of the weights of the connections) while retaining the same basic construction (three layers, but different connections!), very different and also meaningless input–output transformations are possible. Massaro concludes from this finding that networks are too powerful to be meaningful for psychological model formulation. This conclusion is based on a fundamental misunderstanding: just because 'meaninglessness' (e.g. psychologically inappropriate output) can be formulated in an information processing language, it does not follow that the language itself is meaningless. It only reveals the possibilities that are hidden within this language. If Massaro's (1988) 'research logic' were to be transferred to physics, then a differentiated and powerful mathematical apparatus would have to be rejected because, besides very promising formalizations, it also permits the formulation of physical meaninglessness.

The power of a language also does not say anything about the possibilities of testing it empirically. If the arguments in the previous sections are recalled, it should be evident that it is particularly the neuro-computational framework – in contradiction to Massaro's (1988) belief – that offers a very wide range of possibilities of performing empirical tests that can be applied at important points. This becomes particularly clear when the above-mentioned test requirements are considered, namely, testing the psychological validity of a network through simulation; and testing its architectural validity, that is, the assumptions of both functional and

---

[25]Churchland and Sejnowski (1988) as well as Kosslyn and Maljkovic (1990) have expressed a similar opinion.

mechanistic theory (with its two stages), by confrontation with empirical findings. This provides far more opportunities of being able to solve the unfortunate problem of the underdetermination of models and theories than are usually found in conventional psychological theories.

ACKNOWLEDGEMENTS

I wish to thank Heiner Deubel, Martin Eimer, Rainer Goebel, Robert Koch, Cristina Meinecke, Friederike Schlaghecken-Heid and, in particular, Wolfgang Prinz for helpful comments and criticism as well as Peter Eckert, Petra Ibach-Graß, Anna Ruppl, and Heidi John for their comments on style and for proof reading. Above all, I wish to thank Jonathan Harrow for the translation work.

REFERENCES

Abeles, M. (1991). *Corticonics. Neural Circuits of the Cerebral Cortex.* Cambridge: Cambridge University Press.

Anderson, J. A. and Rosenfeld, E. (1988). *Neurocomputing.* Cambridge, MA: MIT Press.

Anderson, J. R. (1983). *The Architecture of Cognition.* Cambridge, MA: Harvard University Press.

Arbib, M. A. (1987). *Brains, Machines, and Mathematics.* New York: Springer.

Atkinson, R. C. and Shiffrin, R. M. (1968). Human memory: A proposed system and its control processes. In K. Spence and J. Spence (Eds), *The Psychology of Learning and Motivation: Advances in Research and Theory,* vol. 2 (pp. 89–195). New York: Academic Press.

Badcock, D. R. and Westheimer, G. (1985). Spatial location and hyperacuity: The centre/surround localization contribution function has two substrates. *Vision Research,* **25,** 1259–1267.

Ballard, D. H. (1984). Parameter nets. *Artificial Intelligence,* **22,** 235–267.

Ballard, D. H. (1986). Cortical connections and parallel processing: Structure and function. *The Behavioral and Brain Sciences,* **9,** 67–120.

Beck, J. (1982). Textural segmentation. In J. Beck (Ed.), *Organisation and Representation in Perception* (pp. 285–317). Hillsdale, NJ: Erlbaum.

Biederman, I. (1987). Recognition-by-components: A theory of human image understanding. *Psychological Review,* **94,** 115–147.

Braitenberg, V. and Schütz, A. (1991). *Anatomy of the Cortex: Statistics and Geometry.* Berlin, New York: Springer.

Breitmeyer, B. G. (1984). *Visual Masking: An Integrative Approach.* New York: Oxford University Press.

Bridgeman, B. (1971). Metacontrast and lateral inhibition. *Psychological Review,* **78,** 528–539.

Broadbent, D. E. (1958). *Perception and Communication.* New York: Pergamon Press.

Bullock, D. and Grossberg, S. (1988). Neural dynamics of planned arm movements: Emergent invariants and speed–accuracy properties during trajectory formation. *Psychological Review,* **95,** 49–90.

Carpenter, G. A. and Grossberg, S. (1987). A massively parallel architecture for a self-organizing neural pattern recognition machine. *Computer Vision, Graphics, and Image Processing,* **37,** 54–115.

Churchland, P. S. and Sejnowski, T. J. (1988). Perspectives on cognitive neuroscience. *Science,* **242,** 741–745.

Cohen, M. A. and Grossberg, S. (1983). Absolute stability of global pattern formation and parallel memory storage by competitive neural networks. *IEEE Transactions on Systems, Man, and Cybernetics,* **13,** 815–826.

Cohen, M. A. and Grossberg, S. (1984). Neural dynamics of brightness perception: Features, boundaries, diffusion, and resonance. *Perception and Psychophysics,* **36,** 428–456.

Coren, S. (1972). Subjective contour and apparent depth. *Psychological Review,* **79,** 359–367.

Crick, F. H. C. and Asanuma, C. (1986). Certain aspects of the anatomy and physiology of the cerebral cortex. In J. L. McClelland, D. E. Rumelhart and the PDP Research Group (Eds), *Parallel Distributed Processing* (pp. 333–371). Cambridge, MA: MIT Press.

Daugman, J. G. (1988). Complete discrete 2-D Gabor transforms by neural networks for image analysis and compression. *IEEE Transactions on Acoustics, Speech, and Signal Processing,* **36,** 1169–1179.

De Valois, R. L. and De Valois, K. K. (1988). *Spatial Vision.* New York: Oxford University Press.

DeYoe, E. A. and van Essen, D. C. (1988). Concurrent processing streams in monkey visual cortex. *Trends in Neurosciences,* **11,** 219–226.

Dowling, J. E. (1987). *The Retina: An Approachable Part of the Brain.* Cambridge, MA: Belknap Press of Harvard University Press.

Eckhorn, R., Bauer, R., Jordan, W., Brosch, M., Kruse, W., Munk, M. and Reitboeck, H. J. (1988). Coherent oscillations: A mechanism of feature linking in the visual cortex? *Biological Cybernetics,* **60,** 121–130.

Ehrenstein, W. (1941). Über Abwandlungen der L. Hermann'schen Helligkeitserscheinung. *Zeitschrift für Psychologie,* **150,** 83–91.

Feldman, J. A. and Ballard, D. H. (1982). Connectionist models and their properties. *Cognitive Science,* **6,** 205–254.

Felleman, D. J. and van Essen, D. C. (1991). Distributed hierarchical processing in the primate cerebral cortex. *Cerebral Cortex,* **1,** 1–47.

Finkel, L. H. and Edelman, G. M. (1989). Integration of distributed cortical systems by reentry: A computer simulation of interactive functionally segregated visual areas. *The Journal of Neuroscience,* **9,** 3188–3208.

Finkel, L. H., Reeke, G.N. Jr, and Edelman, G.M. (1989). A population approach to the neural basis of perceptual categorization. In L. Nadel, L. A. Cooper, P. Culicover, and R. M. Harnish (Eds), *Neural Connections, Mental Computation* (pp. 146–179). Cambridge, MA: MIT Press.

Gilbert, C. D. (1977). Laminar differences in receptive field properties of cells in the cat's primary visual cortex. *Journal of Physiology,* **268,** 391–421.

Gray, C. M., König, P., Engel, A. K. and Singer, W. (1989). Oscillatory responses in the cat's visual cortex exhibit inter-columnar synchronization which reflects global stimulus properties. *Nature,* **338,** 334–337.

Gregory, R. L. (1972). Cognitive contours. *Nature,* **238,** 51–52.

Grossberg, S. (1980). How does a brain build a cognitive code? *Psychological Review,* **87,** 1–51.

Grossberg, S. (1983). The quantized geometry of visual space: The coherent computation of depth, form, and lightness. *Behavioral and Brain Sciences,* **6,** 625–692.

Grossberg, S. (1987a). Cortical dynamics of three-dimensional form, color, and brightness perception: I. Monocular theory. *Perception and Psychophysics,* **41,** 87–116.

Grossberg, S. (1987b). Cortical dynamics of three-dimensional form, color, and brightness perception: II. Binocular theory. *Perception and Psychophysics,* **41,** 117–158.

Grossberg, S. (1988). Nonlinear neural networks: Principles, mechanisms, and architectures. *Neural Networks,* **1,** 17–61.

Grossberg, S. (1990). A model cortical architecture for the preattentive perception of 3-D form. In E. L. Schwartz (Ed.), *Computational Neuroscience* (pp. 117–138). Cambridge, MA: MIT Press.

Grossberg, S. (1991). Why do parallel cortical systems exist for the perception of static form and moving form? *Perception and Psychophysics, 49,* 117–141.

Grossberg, S. and Levine, D. S. (1987). Neural dynamics of attentionally modulated Pavlovian conditioning: Blocking, interstimulus interval, and secondary reinforcement. *Applied Optics, 26,* 5015–5030.

Grossberg, S. and Marshall, J. A. (1989). Stereo boundary fusion by cortical complex cells: A system of maps, filters, and feedback networks for multiplexing distributed data. *Neural Networks, 2,* 29–51.

Grossberg, S. and Mingolla, E. (1985a). Neural dynamics of form perception: Boundary completion, illusory figures, and neon color spreading. *Psychological Review, 92,* 173–211.

Grossberg, S. and Mingolla, E. (1985b). Neural dynamics of perceptual grouping: Textures, boundaries, and emergent segmentations. *Perception and Psychophysics, 38,* 141–171.

Grossberg, S. and Rudd, M. E. (1989). A neural architecture for visual motion perception: Group and element apparent motion. *Neural Networks, 2,* 421–450.

Grossberg, S. and Stone, G. (1986). Neural dynamics of word recognition and recall: Attentional priming, learning, and resonance. *Psychological Review, 93,* 46–74.

Grossberg, S. and Todorovic, D. (1988). Neural dynamics of 1-D and 2-D brightness perception: A unified model of classical and recent phenomena. *Perception and Psychophysics, 43,* 241–277.

Halpern, D. F. and Salzman, B. (1983). The multiple determination of illusory contours: 1. A review. *Perception, 12,* 281–291.

Hanson, S. J. and Burr, D. J. (1990). What connectionist models learn: Learning and representation in connectionist networks. *Behavioral and Brain Sciences, 13,* 471–518.

Hebb, D. O. (1949). *Organization of Behavior.* New York: John Wiley.

Hinton, G. E., McClelland, J. L. and Rumelhart, D. E. (1986). Distributed representations. In D. E. Rumelhart, J. L. McClelland and The PDP Research Group (Eds), *Parallel Distributed Processing* (pp. 77–109). Cambridge, MA: MIT Press.

Hopfield, J. J. (1982). Neural networks and physical systems with emergent collective computational abilities. *Proceedings of the National Academy of Sciences, 79,* 2554–2558.

Hubel, D. H. and Wiesel, T. N. (1962). Receptive fields, binocular interaction and functional architecture in the cat's visual cortex. *Journal of Psychology, 160,* 106–154.

Hubel, D. H. and Wiesel, T. N. (1965). Receptive fields and functional architecture in two nonstriate visual areas (18 and 19) of the cat. *Journal of Neurophysiology, 28,* 229–289.

Hubel, D. H. and Wiesel, T. N. (1977). Functional architecture of macaque visual cortex. *Proceedings of the Royal Society of London, 198,* 1–59.

Humphreys, G. W. and Bruce, V. (1989). *Visual Cognition.* Hillsdale, NJ: Erlbaum.

Julesz, B. (1975). Experiments in the visual perception of texture. *Scientific American, 232,* 34–43.

Kandel, E. R. (1991). Nerve cells and behavior. In E. R. Kandel, J. H. Schwartz, and Th. M. Jessell (Eds), *Principles of Neural Science* (pp. 18–32). New York: Elsevier.

Kandel, E. R., Schwartz, J. H. and Jessell, Th. M. (1991). *Principles of Neural Science.* New York: Elsevier.

Kanizsa, G. (1955/1987). Quasi-perceptual margins in homogeneously stimulated fields. In S. Petry and G. E. Meyer (Eds.), *The Perception of Illusory Contours* (pp. 40–49). New York: Springer (original work published 1955).

Kellman, P. J. and Shipley, T. F. (1991). A theory of visual interpolation in object perception. *Cognitive Psychology, 23,* 141–221.

Kienker, P. K., Sejnowski, T. J., Hinton, G. E. and Schumacher, L. E. (1986). Separating figure from ground with a parallel network. *Perception, 15,* 197–216.

Knapp, A. G. and Anderson, J. A. (1984). Theory of categorization based on distributed memory storage. *Journal of Experimental Psychology*, **10**, 616–637.

Koch, C. and Segev, I. (1989). *Methods in Neuronal Modelling. From Synapses to Networks.* Cambridge, MA: MIT Press.

König, P. and Schillen, Th. B. (1991). Stimulus-dependent assembly formation of oscillatory responses: I. Synchronization. *Neuronal Computation*, **3**, 155–166.

Kosslyn, S. M. and Maljkovic, V. (1990). Marr's metatheory revisited. *Concepts in Neuroscience*, **1**, 239–245.

Lachman, R., Lachman, J. L. and Butterfield, E. C. (1979). *Cognitive Psychology and Information Processing: An Introduction.* Hillsdale, NJ: Erlbaum.

Land, E. H. (1977). The retinex theory of color vision. *Scientific American*, **237**, 108–128.

Livingstone, M. and Hubel, D. H. (1988). Segregation of form, color, movement, and depth: Anatomy, physiology, and perception. *Science*, **240**, 740–749.

Luce, R. D. (1986). *Response Times: Their Role in Inferring Elementary Mental Organization.* New York: Oxford University Press.

Marr, D. (1982). *Vision: A Computational Investigation.* New York: Freeman.

Martin, J. H. (1991). Coding and processing of sensory information. In E. R. Kandel, J. H. Schwartz, and Th. M. Jessell (Eds), *Principles of Neural Science* (pp. 329–339). New York: Elsevier.

Massaro, D. W. (1988). Some criticisms of connectionist models of human performance. *Journal of Memory and Language*, **27**, 213–234.

Maunsell, J. H. R. and Newsome, W. T. (1987). Visual processing in monkey extrastriate cortex. *Annual Review of Neuroscience*, **10**, 363–401.

McClelland, J. L. and Rumelhart, D. E. (1981). An interactive activation model of context effects in letter perception: Part 1. An account of basic findings. *Psychological Review*, **88**, 375–407.

McClelland, J. L. and Rumelhart, D. E. (1986). A distributed model of human learning and memory. In J. L. McClelland, D. E. Rumelhart and The PDP Research Group (Eds), *Parallel Distributed Processing* (pp. 170–215). Cambridge, MA: MIT Press.

McClelland, J. L., Rumelhart, D. E. and The PDP Research Group (1986). *Parallel Distributed Processing*, vol. 2. Cambridge, MA: MIT Press.

McCulloch, W. S. and Pitts, W. (1943). A logical calculus of the ideas immanent in nervous activity. *Bulletin of Mathematical Biophysics*, **5**, 115–133.

Metzger, W. (1975). *Gesetze des Sehens* (3rd edn). Frankfurt: Kramer.

Miller, J. (1988). Discrete and continuous models of human information processing: Theoretical distinctions and empirical results. *Acta Psychologica*, **67**, 191–257.

Minsky, P. and Papert, S. (1969). *Perceptrons: An Introduction to Computational Geometry.* Cambridge, MA: MIT Press.

Neisser, U. (1967). *Cognitive Psychology.* New York: Appleton-Century-Crofts.

Newell, A. and Simon, H. A. (1972). *Human Problem Solving.* Englewood Cliffs, NJ: Prentice Hall.

Paradiso, M. A. and Nakayama, K. (1991). Brightness perception and filling-in. *Vision Research*, **31**, 1221–1236.

Pearson, J. C., Finkel, L. H. and Edelman, G. M. (1987). Plasticity in the organization of adult cerebral cortical maps: A computer simulation based on neuronal group selection. *The Journal of Neuroscience*, **7**, 4209–4223.

Peterhans, E. and von der Heydt, R. (1991). Subjective contours – bridging the gap between psychophysics and physiology. *Trends in Neurosciences*, **14**, 112–119.

Petry, S. and Meyer, G. E. (1987). *The Perception of Illusory Contours.* New York: Springer.

Phaf, R. H. van der Heijden, A. H. and Hudson, P. T. (1990). SLAM: A connectionist model for attention in visual selection tasks. *Cognitive Psychology*, **22**, 273–341.

Poggio, T. and Edelman, S. (1990). A network that learns to recognize three-dimensional objects. *Nature*, **343**, 263–266.

Posner, M. I. (1978). *Chronometric Explorations of the Mind*. Hillsdale, NJ: Erlbaum.

Prinz, W. (1983). *Wahrnehmung und Tätigkeitssteuerung*. Berlin: Springer.

Ramachandran, V. S. and Gregory, R. L. (1991). Perceptual filling in of artificially induced scotomas in human vision. *Nature,* **350**, 699–702.

Rosenblatt, F. (1958). The perceptron: The probabilistic model for information storage and organization in the brain. *Psychological Review*, **65**, 386–408.

Rumelhart, D. E., McClelland, J. L. The PDP Research Group. (1986). *Parallel Distributed Processing,* vol. 1. Cambridge, MA: MIT Press.

Sanders, A. F. (1980). Stage analysis of reaction processes. In G. E. Stelmach and J. Requin (Eds), *Tutorials in Motor Behavior* (pp. 331–355). Amsterdam: North-Holland.

Sandon, P. A. (1990). Simulating visual attention. *Journal of Cognitive Neuroscience*, **2**, 213–231.

Schiffman, H. R. (1990). *Sensation and Perception*. New York: John Wiley.

Schumann, F. (1900). Beiträge zur Analyse der Gesichtswahrnehmung. Erste Abhandlung. Einige Beobachtungen über die Zusammenfassung von Gesichtseindrücken zu Einheiten. *Zeitschrift für Psychologie und Physiologie der Sinnesorgane*, **23**, 1–32.

Schwartz, E. L. (1990). *Computational Neuroscience*. Cambridge, MA: MIT Press.

Sekuler, R., Anstis, S., Braddick, O. J., Brandt, T., Movshon, J. A. and Orban, G. (1990). The perception of motion. In L. Spillmann and J. S. Werner (Eds), *Visual Perception: The Neurophysiological Foundations* (pp. 205–230). San Diego, CA: Academic Press.

Singer, W. (1990). Search for coherence: A basic principle of cortical self-organization. *Concepts in Neuroscience*, **1**, 1–26.

Spillmann, L. and Werner, J. S. (1990). *Visual Perception: The Neurophysiological Foundations*. San Diego, CA: Academic Press.

Sutter, A., Beck, J. and Graham, N. (1989). Contrast and spatial variables in texture segregation: Testing a simple spatial-frequency channels model. *Perception and Psychophysics*, **46**, 312–332.

Sutton, R. S. and Barto, A. G. (1981). Toward a modern theory of adaptive networks: Expectation and prediction. *Psychological Review,* **88**, 135–170.

Theios, J. (1975). The components of response latency in simple human information processing tasks. In P. M. Rabbitt and S. Dornič (Eds), *Attention and Performance*, vol. V (pp. 418–440). New York: Academic Press.

Tootell, R. B. H., Silverman, M. S., Switkes, E. and De Valois, R. L. (1982). Deoxyglucose analysis of retinotopic organization in primate striate cortex. *Science,* **218**, 902–904.

Treisman, A. M. (1988). Features and objects: The fourteenth Bartlett memorial lecture. *The Quarterly Journal of Experimental Psychology*, **40**, 201–237.

van der Heijden, A. H. C. (1991). *Selective Attention in Vision*. New York: Routledge.

von der Heydt, R., Peterhans, E. and Baumgartner, G. (1984). Illusory contours and cortical responses. *Science*, **224**, 1260–1262.

von der Malsburg, Ch. (1981). *The Correlation Theory of Brain Function* (Internal Report 81–2). Max Planck Institute for Biophysical Chemistry, Dept for Neurobiology, Göttingen, Germany.

von der Malsburg, Ch. (1990). A neural architecture for the representation of scenes. In J. L. McGaugh, N. M. Weinberger and C. Lynch (Eds), *Brain Organisation and Memory* (pp. 356–372). New York: Oxford University Press.

von der Malsburg, Ch. and Schneider, W. (1986). A neural cocktail-party processor. *Biological Cybernetics*, **54**, 29–40.

Widrow, B. and Hopf, M. E. (1960). *Adaptive Switching Circuits* (Stanford Electronics Laboratories Technical Report 1553-1). Stanford, CA: Stanford University.

Wilson, M. A. and Bower, J. M. (1991). A computer simulation of oscillatory behavior in primary visual cortex. *Neural Computation*, **3**, 498–509.

Yarbus, A. L. (1967). *Eye Movements and Vision.* New York: Plenum Press.

Zeki, S. and Shipp, S. (1988). The functional logic of cortical connections. *Nature,* **335,** 311–317.

Zipser, D. and Andersen, R. A. (1988). A back-propagation programmed network that simulates response properties of a subset of posterior parietal neurons. *Nature,* **331,** 679–684.

Chapter 5

Visual Processing and Cognitive Factors in the Generation of Saccadic Eye Movements

Heiner Deubel

Max Planck Institute for Psychological Research, Munich

1 INTRODUCTION

1.1 Eye Movements as Indicators of Cognitive Processes

Our everyday life activities are all accompanied by movements of the eyes. This coupling is so effortless that in most cases we are not even aware of the tight linkage between sensing, cognitive processing, locomotion and oculomotor performance. Whenever we move our body and head, these movements are almost perfectly compensated by eye movements, stabilizing the retinal image with respect to the visual environment. When we look at pictures and when we read, fast eye saccades scan the visual image. Even when we are thinking with eyes closed, or sleeping, the oculomotor system exhibits considerable activity.

This contribution will be concerned with exploring how peripheral vision is used to select a target and to direct the saccade, and how higher-level factors influence these processes. Indeed, for the fast saccadic eye movements visual stimulation forms the major source of information. In many situations, however, it seems that the scanning movements of the eyes are determined mainly by internal concepts and plans. This was demonstrated most outstandingly by Yarbus' investigations (Yarbus, 1967), which started in the early fifties. In his famous recordings he presented paintings to the human observer and analyzed the effect of different instructions on the preferred locations of fixations. It became clear that the scanpaths of the eye varied characteristically dependent on the question the observer tried to resolve. Yarbus (1967) suggested the idea that 'eye movements reflect human thought processes', which is where much of the interest of experimental psychology for eye movements originated.

Inspired by this idea, Noton and Stark (1971) investigated the sequence of eye saccades on drawings and even suggested that the exact order of saccades, at least when viewing familiar material, is guided completely by an internalized 'feature ring' representation of the visual stimulus. Similarly, Just and Carpenter (1976) analyzed eye fixations in mental rotation tasks with the idea that the eye fixates the referent of the symbol currently being processed. This and much other work was,

Handbook of Perception and Action: Volume 1
ISBN 0-12-516161-1

at least in part, based on the belief that eye movements may help us to understand higher psychological processes. (A thoughtful discussion on the validity of this hypothesis was presented by Viviani, 1990.)

On the other hand, in certain situations, eye movements have all the attributes of sensorimotor reflexes, for example when we perceive an object abruptly starting to move in the far retinal periphery. Before we think of it, our foveal gaze is locked on the target, and the eyes are stabilized on the object. While it is clear that scanning of pictures involves cognitive processing, this orienting reaction is commonly regarded as an automatic, reflex-like response driven by the stimulus ('bottom-up').

1.2   The Recent Historical Development of Eye Movement Research

Historically, the studies of the two components, bottom-up movement generation and top-down control, have evolved somewhat separately, as can be traced in separate lines of research in the short history of oculomotor research.

In the early days of modern human sciences, Donders (1847) and Helmholtz (1866) confirmed Listing's law of motion of the eye and intelligently discussed several problems still prevalent today in connection with eye movements. They were not yet aware of the existence of the distinct types of eye movements, however. Technological development was a major drive for further advance. The most important pioneer in modern eye movement research certainly was Dodge (Dodge and Cline, 1901). Using a photographic method for determining the dynamics of eye movements, he was the first to classify different types of human eye movements, distinguishing between the fast saccades and the slower movements such as pursuit. He also pointed out the importance of predictive capabilities and selective attention in eye movement control. Other earlier workers studied the characteristics of eye movements by the use of after-images (Barlow, 1952; Helmholtz, 1866).

A further important technical advance which triggered and determined future research was the development of the contact lens and of suction cap methods. By allowing devices such as mirrors to be firmly attached to the eye, experimenters could continuously record horizontal and vertical eye movements (Ditchburn and Ginsborg, 1953; Riggs and Ratliff, 1951; Yarbus, 1967). Later on, the basic idea of this method was taken and improved into the electromagnetic search coil technique (Robinson, 1963) which to this day is the most precise, frequently used recording technique. Finally, a method that achieves similar precision but is noninvasive is the 'Dual-Purkinje-image eyetracker', developed through several generations by the Stanford Research Institute (Crane and Steele, 1985); this provides an elegant method for measuring eye position with high spatial resolution and precision. These technological advances provided the basis for the precise measuring of oculomotor activity in everyday situations such as reading and performing various visual tasks.

As a consequence, much of the research of that time was engaged in studying the contribution of small eye movements to visual processing. This was gradually complemented by more psychologically oriented lines of research which centered around analyzing eye movements in complex tasks such as picture viewing, problem solving and reading (Just and Carpenter, 1976; Noton and Stark, 1971; Rayner, 1978; Yarbus, 1967).

A revolutionary step toward a better understanding of the informational basis of eye movement programming occurred in 1954 when two influential papers were published by Westheimer (Westheimer, 1954a, b). He proposed an analysis of oculomotor parameters in terms of linear models borrowed from control theory. From that time on, the servomechanic engineering approach became a major tool in the empirical analysis and theoretical description of oculomotor behavior and has preserved its theoretical prevalence until today (Becker and Jürgens, 1979; Deubel, Wolf and Hauske, 1984; Robinson, 1964, 1965, 1973; Young and Stark, 1963). Moreover, the system-analytical approach has also inspired and guided much of the recent neurophysiological work on eye movement generation. So, much effort was directed to the specification of the control signals to oculomotor neurons. Robinson's work over a long period (Robinson, 1964, 1975, 1981, 1982) has shown in an elegant way how the neural control signals are adaptively matched to the mechanical properties of the eye musculature. The way in which these signals are elaborated in the neural circuits of the brain stem is also well known (Fuchs, Kaneko and Scudder, 1985). Today the engineering approach is so well established that the presentation of physiological data usually comes along with their interpretation in terms of current, system-theoretical models of oculomotor control (Goldberg and Bruce, 1990; Scudder, 1988; van Gisbergen, Robinson and Gielen, 1981). In retrospect, it is safe to say that the rigorous application of system theory has been a major reason why the detailed understanding of oculomotor control has progressed ahead of the understanding of other sensorimotor systems.

A major reason for the applicability of the engineering approach to the analysis of the oculomotor system is certainly because the oculomotor system seems to be one of the simpler sensorimotor systems. The sensory stimuli to the system are normally well defined, and the response is relatively easy to access. Moreover, the hierarchical and modular organization of the system and the relatively simple physical properties of the plant (invariable inertia, 2–3 degrees of freedom) ideally lend the oculomotor system to analysis in terms of linear control theory.

1.3 Aim and Overview

Despite its indisputable success in helping to elucidate the basic properties of the peripheral motor and premotor eye movement system, the emphasis of the systems-analytical approach for more than 30 years has also led to the prevalence of a certain research strategy. A number of aspects of this development are significant and lend themselves to some criticism. First, because the physiology-backed system approach was most successfully applied in elucidating the functioning of the motor and premotor system, current oculomotorists are often rather narrow on the motor system. As a consequence, the role of *visual* processing is frequently perceived as of secondary importance. Second, the theoretical approach to the data was often characterized by the search for the most parsimonious model from control theory. This has led to a tendency to prefer extremely simple test stimuli and situations. The question then arises to what extent the experimental results are valid in more complex or even natural situations. Third, in order to avoid having to deal with phenomena that cannot be easily incorporated into simple models, experimenters have often vigorously tried to minimize the impact of *cognitive factors*, or even denied the effects of instruction, selection and voluntary effort.

These problems are where the interest of the present contribution originates. The chapter reviews empirical results concerning the programming of saccadic eye movements to visual stimuli appearing abruptly in the visual field. This means that the range of stimuli and experimental situations discussed will be limited to the rather simple, artificial ones which are traditionally ideally suited for the system approach. However, the aim will be to put more emphasis on the two aspects that, as suggested above, have been somewhat underrepresented in the mainstream of empirical work. These factors are the effect and function of first, sensory factors (i.e. visual processing) and second, higher-level components such as instruction, pre-knowledge, and learning. Taken together, the empirical results will suggest that oculomotor research should necessarily include the *concurrent* study of visual processing, cognitive factors and oculomotor performance as aspects of equal importance. Here the reader may object that, in the context of this book, he has expected to learn about *perceptual* processing rather than about oculomotor pro-gramming. However, this desire should be assuaged by a third central theme of this chapter which follows from the previous ones. Since, as will be demonstrated, perceptual processing is a major determinant of eye movement control, eye movement parameters form sensitive measures for the perceptual processing of various aspects of the retinal information. In other words, I will suggest that eye movements provide an elegant probe into visual functions. So, for example, evidence will be shown that characteristic properties of preattentional visual processing are reflected rather directly in saccadic response parameters.

Because this contribution is presented in the context of a handbook of *psychology*, the discussion will be centered on the only class of eye movement that is truly under voluntary control: the saccade. It should be mentioned, however, that there is accumulating evidence suggesting that in fact *all* types of eye movement are to various degrees subject to voluntary modification. Nevertheless, the saccadic system, fully developed only in the highest mammals, is certainly the most investigated candidate for the interaction of sensorimotor control and cognitive factors.

Saccades can also be elicited by and directed to auditory or tactile stimuli, or be made spontaneously or voluntarily in darkness, and they are made during sleep or for compensating defective vestibular function. Nevertheless, it seems clear that the major source of information for saccade control is *vision*. Accordingly, this presen-tation will be centered on emphasizing the variety in nature of the visual informa-tion that the saccadic system is confronted with, how various sensory aspects affect the saccadic response, and what this presumably tells us about how sensory information is processed to determine the motor reaction. Indeed, even when the scope is restricted to 'visual information' only, the sensory stimulus to elicit or guide a saccade may range from a few photons to the wealth of visual information present in pictures and in our normal environment. Following along this range will determine the outline of the paper.

After an introduction of the various types of eye movement and some basic findings on the saccade, the central Section 3 will be aimed at elucidating the way the information from a visual target is processed in order to provide a meaningful signal for saccadic eye movement control. The development of the argument will be, in a sense, *stimulus-driven*. So, I will start from the typical reduced laboratory situation of a dim stimulus within nothing else, then continue with moving and multiple targets, and finally end at scenes which include prominent background structure. This increasing complexity of visual stimulus structure is paralleled by the move from the artificial laboratory situation closer to more 'natural', ecological conditions, and this comes along with an increasing complexity of the underlying computational processes required.

Many facets of the oculomotor system cannot be covered by this overview, even when the scope of the chapter is limited to saccadic eye movements. For some of the vast and important work on the role of small, 'involuntary' saccades (microsaccades) during fixation the reader is referred to Ditchburn (1973) and Steinman and Levinson (1990). Also, the question of the spatial frame of reference will not be discussed, a simple retinotopic frame will be implicitly assumed (see Bridgeman, this volume) . Moreover, the physiological basis of saccades can be touched on only briefy. We will not consider saccades to stimuli of other than visual modalities, the interaction of saccades with other types of eye movements and eye movements during sleep. A number of recent reviews, however, provide excellent coverage of many of these aspects (Carpenter, 1988, 1991a; Hallett, 1986; Kowler, 1990; Wurtz and Goldberg, 1989).

2   EYE MOVEMENTS: EVOLUTION, FUNCTION AND PHYSIOLOGICAL BASIS

2.1   Evolution and Function of Eye Movements

Eye movements in humans are the sum of actions of subsystems that can be seen more clearly in animals with simpler oculomotor control. Therefore, tracing the evolution of the oculomotor system, together with theories of the function of eye movements, are basic steps that should precede attempts at data collection and interpretation. The purpose of this short excursion is to make clear that saccadic eye movements have evolved, late in evolutionary development, as 'voluntary' movements.

The oldest subsystem is the vestibulo-ocular reflex which is so basic that it remained essentially unchanged throughout the evolution of vertebrates (Walls, 1962). This reflex allows animals to see and move at the same time, by holding images still on the retina while the head is turning. The optokinetic system, found in all animals with a vestibular reflex, helps the vestibular system to move the eye when, due to self-motion, the entire visual world sweeps across the retinas. It seems clear that these basic reflexes do not serve to *move* the gaze with respect to the environment but rather to *stabilize* the retinal image during locomotion. The aspect of stabilization becomes increasingly important with the further development of visual capacities. Form perception deteriorates when retinal slip velocity exceeds rather low values (Carpenter, 1991b; Westheimer and McKee, 1975).

Further evolutionary pressure resulted when nature invented the fovea, which accompanied the trend to frontal eyes and stereopsis. The pursuit system developed to allow the eye to move in order to hold the image of an object on the primitive fovea, despite the conflicting input of the optokinetic system. Finally, the need arose not just to stabilize moving objects, but also to bring anything of interest from the periphery onto the fovea by means of a fast reorienting shift of the gaze. Shifting of the eye entails visual disturbances, and therefore nature has to make these shifts as short as it can. The resulting eye movements, the saccades, are actually very fast with velocities of more than $700 \deg s^{-1}$ in humans.

It becomes clear that the functional significance of saccadic eye movements is closely related to the anatomy of the retina. In humans, the foveola is a central region less than 0.5 degree of visual angle, densely packed with cone receptors. This overrepresentation of the foveal field is continued in the cortical visual areas (Rovamo and Virsu, 1979) providing high resolution and the capability for complex visual processing. Accordingly, target foveation is prerequisite to many aspects of form perception and object recognition. Foveation comes at the cost of reduced capacities for the remainder of the visual field; therefore, targets have to be carefully selected for their behavioral significance, requiring the visual awareness of the stimulus, attention and context-specific evaluations. The 'psycho-optic' reflex (Walls, 1962), the saccade, is essentially voluntary.

2.2   The Physiological Substrate of Saccadic Eye Movements

An excitingly rapid growth of knowledge of the neurobiology of eye movement generation has occurred in the past 30 years, which has advanced as the result of the fruitful combination of single cell recordings with behavioral studies and mathematical modeling. However, it also seems that while quite detailed understanding is now available for the brainstem generation of eye movements, the role and function of cortical and subcortical structures is still much less clear. The neural basis of the integration of attentional, higher-level processes remains especially opaque and subject to much current research.

This section presents a brief overview of the major neural structures involved in saccadic eye movement generation and their presumed functional significance. Figure 5.1 presents an anatomical schema of the important neural pathways involved. A full coverage of the neurobiology of saccadic eye movements can be found elsewhere (Wurtz and Goldberg, 1989).

2.2.1   Brainstem

The *motor part* of the saccadic system consists of the brainstem saccade generator and the oculomotor neurons, as well as the oculomotor plant – which is the aggregate of eyeball, eye muscles and the other tissues in the socket. The eye is rotated by three pairs of eye muscles each of which is innervated by a pool of *oculomotor neurons*. During fixation, the static discharge rate of the agonist motoneuron that holds the eye against the elastic forces is linearly related to gaze angle. During the rotation of the eye, a burst of action potentials in the neurons innervating the agonist muscle and a pause in the firing of antagonist motoneuron provide the high dynamic force – proportional to eye velocity – that is required to drive the eye against the viscous impedance of the oculomotor plant. Thus, saccade execution is accompanied by a *pulse-step pattern* of the firing rate in the motoneuron.

Oculomotor neurons are known to receive the pulse portion of their input from the *medium-lead burst neurons,* located in the paramedian pontine reticular formation

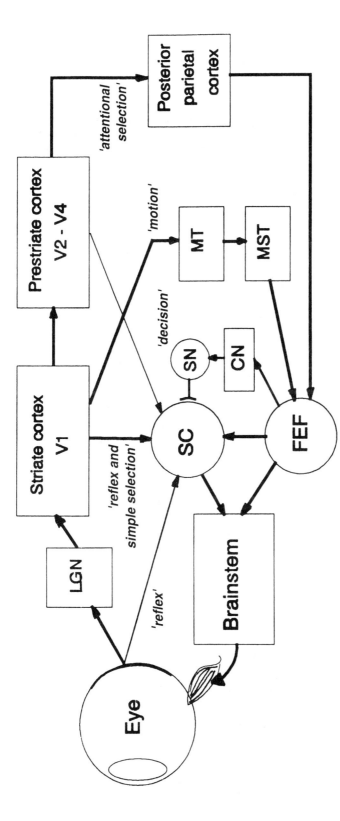

Figure 5.1. Schematic representation of the information flow in the neural structures contributing to saccade control. Pathways of presumably minor importance are indicated by the thinner connections. LGN, lateral geniculate nucleus; SC, superior colliculus; FEF, frontal eye fields; MT, middle temporal area; MST, medial superior temporal area; SN, substantia nigra; CN, caudate nucleus.

of the brainstem for horizontal saccade components, and in the mesencephalic reticular formation for the vertical components. The magnitude of the pulse compound is closely related to saccade velocity, saturating for saccades larger than 10 degrees. The position-related signals to the oculomotor neurons are thought to be provided by another group of cells found in the brainstem, the *tonic neurons*. It is suggested that these tonic signals are generated by a neural integration of the velocity code signaled by the medium-lead burst cells. Finally, the brainstem *omnipause neurons* exhibit a constant firing rate during fixation but cease firing completely during saccade execution. These neurons are probably involved in the suppression and/or release of saccadic eye movements.

It is important to note that in these brainstem areas eye movement parameters are largely *temporally coded*, i.e. eye velocity (and saccade amplitude) is determined by the *firing rate* of these neurons. In all other important centers that remain to be described, such as the superior colliculus and in the frontal eye fields, a *spatial code* prevails, i.e. saccade amplitude and direction are determined by *where* in a neural map activity resides. One of the most exciting puzzles of eye movement research that remains to be resolved is the question of where and how the transformation from the spatial to the intensity code, the 'spatiotemporal translation', is performed. So-called *long-lead burst neurons*, also found in the brainstem, are currently hypothesized to be involved in this process (Scudder, 1988).

Visual information can reach the brainstem oculomotor centers by at least four different possible routes, namely: (1) directly from the retina via the superior colliculus (SC); (2) via the lateral geniculate nucleus (LGN), the primary visual cortex (V1), and the superior colliculus; (3) via LGN, visual cortex, and the frontal eye fields (FEF); and (4) via LGN, striate, prestriate and parietal cortices and the FEF. Lesion studies with animals have shown that none of the three centers (visual cortex, superior colliculus and frontal eye fields) is indispensable for the production of target-elicited saccades. To eliminate such saccades totally, two separate pathways must be blocked (Mohler and Wurtz, 1977; Schiller, True and Conway, 1980). Human patients with damage to the visual cortical areas are able to make saccades to targets with reasonable accuracy even in regions of the visual field for which a cortical route is unavailable (Barbur, Forsyth and Findlay, 1988; Perenin and Jeannerod, 1975; Pöppel, Held and Frost, 1973; Zihl, 1980).

2.2.2   Superior Colliculus

The *superior colliculus* (SC) is perceived as the major relay station and as a prototypical example for an interface between sensory processing and movement generation. Animal studies consistently find that collicular lesions increase the latency of visually elicited saccades, and this has led to the suggestion that the most rapid target-elicited saccades are made through the collicular pathway (Fischer, 1987). Thus, it seems that the SC is mainly concerned with the automatic control of eye movements to visual stimuli and other simple orienting reactions, providing the control of the shortest latency saccades.

The SC consists of seven alternating fiber and cell layers which can be conveniently divided into the *superficial* and the *intermediate* and *deep* SC layers. The superficial layers receive retinotopic projections directly from the retina but also from the striate and prestriate visual cortex. The intermediate and deep layers show primarily motor-related activity; their cells discharge just before and during saccades. The intermediate layer connects to the pontine long-lead burst neurons.

The function of the SC has been extensively investigated by means of single cell recordings and electrical stimulation studies. It has been found that the visual fields in the *superficial layers* are organized in a well-defined, topographic manner. The cells seem to be nonselective for visual stimulus properties such as orientation, shape, and direction or speed of movement. On the other hand, about half of the neurons in the superficial layers exhibit an enhanced response to a visual stimulus only when it is going to be the target for a saccade. If a monkey attends to a stimulus without making a saccade to it, they show no enhanced response (for a review, see Sparks, 1986).

Cells in the *intermediate and deep* layers receive motor command-related input from the frontal eye fields but also modulatory input from the prestriate, middle temporal and parietal cortices. The cells exhibit large 'movement fields' in the sense that a specific population is active with saccades of specific magnitude and direction. Electrical stimulation elicits saccades at low current levels; the saccade vector depends on the site stimulated. Sensory and motor maps in the colliculus are in register: stimulation of a particular location of the SC brings the fovea into the receptive field area of the cells that had been activated electrically. The SC is inhibited by signals from the substantia nigra, which receives its input from the basal ganglia (Hikosaka and Wurtz, 1983). This gating pathway is important as a safeguard to prevent the system from saccading to just anything that appears in the visual field. It has been further suggested that SC activity is under attentional modulation from the parietal cortex, where neurons exhibit enhanced responses when the animal attends to the stimulus even without making a saccade to it.

2.2.3 Frontal Eye Fields (Area 8)

The *frontal eye fields* (FEF) share many properties with the superior colliculus, such as retinotopic mapping and the existence of both large visual receptive fields and motor-related movement fields. This suggests some redundancy in eye movement control and raises the question of the functional differences of both structures, which indeed turn out to be rather subtle. So, as opposed to the SC, the FEF neurons seem to be more engaged in the production of long-latency and memory-guided saccades and eye movements in free scanning.

Patients with FEF lesions make fast and accurate saccades to visual targets but have problems in saccading away from a visual stimulus (Guitton, Buchtel and Douglas, 1985). This is consistent with the view that the FEF also control the inhibition and release of saccades, via the substantia nigra and the SC. So, it now seems that the frontal eye fields are essential for the 'cognitively driven' aspects of saccades; without FEF, we would be left with the inevitability of a visuomotor reflex mediated by the SC.

2.2.4 Cortical Areas

Visual cortical areas involved in eye movement control include the striate cortex (V1), the prestriate cortex (V2–V4), the middle temporal and medial superior temporal areas (MT and MST), and the posterior part of the parietal association cortex (area 7). Electrical stimulation in all these areas leads to the elicitation of saccadic eye movements. Concerning the *striate and prestriate cortices* (*V1–V4*), there is no reason to ascribe specific oculomotor functions to them. Clearly the essential function of these stages is the analysis of the visual stimulus that is prerequisite to target selection, but this analytic information processing is probably identical for visual perception and oculomotor reactions. As will be emphasized below, this implies that properties of pre-attentive visual processing will be reflected in oculomotor reactions.

Since *MT and MST* are essential for processing information about target motion, they are most important for the generation of pursuit eye movements. As to saccades, they seem to provide signals for the predictive components of saccades to moving stimuli, at least in the monkey (Dürsteler and Wurtz, 1988).

The *posterior parietal cortex*, finally, is involved in complex aspects of sensorimotor integration, spatial aspects of object representation and selective visual attention. Neurons have retinotopic receptive fields and carry both visual sensory and visual memory signals. Most cells show enhanced activity to a visual stimulus when it becomes target for a saccade, particularly when the animal is highly motivated (Andersen, 1989). The findings suggest that the functional role of the posterior parietal cortex should be considered neither purely sensory nor strictly motor but rather one involved with sensorimotor integration, more specifically in transforming retinotopic visual signals to spatial and motor coordinate frames. Further, recent investigations (Duhamel, Colby and Goldberg, 1992) suggest that single neurons in monkey parietal cortex use information about intended eye movements to update the representation of visual space. The shift of the parietal representation of the visual world that precedes an eye movement may provide a dynamic link between successive retinal images, and allow the integration of visual information across saccades in order to grant a continuous representation of visual space.

From the concept of interacting and competing parallel pathways mediating the control of saccades, it is tempting to assign different functional aspects to the various control loops. The evidence presented seems to suggest that quite separate flows of information exist for the generation of involuntary, reflex-like movements versus voluntary saccades under attentional control. It is interesting to see how this dichotomy is reflected in the behavioral observations that will be reported in the following sections.

2.3   Saccades: Basic Parameters

In foveate animals and in humans, saccades serve to bring the images of objects of interest from the visual periphery onto the fovea. The subsequent fixation period then allows for closer scrutiny; accordingly, it is functionally important that the movement itself is as short (and, consequently, as fast) as possible. Saccades perfectly fulfil this requirement. They are the most rapid type of movement of the eye, reaching speeds of $700 \deg s^{-1}$ or more. Indeed, they are close to time-optimality in the sense that the saccadic system accelerates the eye at the maximum rate that is physically possible (Bahill, Clark and Stark, 1975). This acceleration is initiated by a pulse-like, high-frequency burst in the neurons that innervate the muscle fibers of the against eye muscles, driving the eyeball rapidly against the viscous forces. As a consequence, a large (20 deg) rotation of the eye can be as short as 60 ms – much too short a time for any guidance of the movement by means of continuous error feedback from the retina or from proprioceptors. Saccades must therefore be preprogrammed, producing, once initiated, stereotyped trajectories that are essentially predetermined by the magnitude and direction of the movement.

In this sense, the saccadic eye movement is an extremely simple response. For the purposes of this argument, this response may be adequately specified by just three measures: the instant of initiation and the amplitude of rotation of the eye in horizontal and vertical components. Although other aspects are of considerable interest (torsional components of movement: Ferman, Collewijn and van den Berg, 1987; variability in trajectory: Findlay and Harris, 1984; Smit, van Gisbergen and Cools, 1987), these may safely be ignored for the present purpose.

In the following, questions about, on the one hand, *when* a saccade is triggered and, on the other hand, *where* the eye comes to a rest will be treated separately, to a large degree. It will be demonstrated that this is not merely for descriptive convenience, but that there exists considerable evidence that the processes which decide when a saccade is elicited are indeed largely independent of the computational processes that determine saccadic landing position. Indeed, most models of saccade control also describe the saccadic system by specifying two distinct mechanisms. One mechanism generates a neural representation of the position to which the saccade is to be directed (the *where*-system), the other mechanism determines the moment of saccade occurrence by triggering the movement proper (the *when*-system).

3   THE SENSORY STIMULUS

3.1   Single-dot Stimuli as Targets for the Saccade

Let us start by considering a situation which is certainly among the extremely artificial ones, but nevertheless designates the experimental paradigm used most frequently in eye movement research of the past. Indeed, the majority of studies on saccade control in the past 35 years have been done in the typical, visually heavily impoverished laboratory environment. Typically, the subject is sitting, with head fixed, in darkness and is asked to direct the gaze to a single, tiny spot of light. After a delay, the fixation target disappears and is simultaneously replaced by the onset of an eccentric target. The subject is normally instructed to follow this 'target step'.

In this situation, the eye responds, after a latency period, with a saccadic eye movement (the 'primary saccade') that brings the fovea close onto the target. Remaining refixation errors are then eliminated, after a further latency period, by one or two 'corrective saccades'. Typical saccadic response patterns for a range of step sizes from 0.5 to 16 deg are given in Figure 5.2. There are at least four noteworthy aspects of this kind of response which shall be shortly discussed in the following:

(1) The *spatial precision* of the response which is high and insensitive to sensory stimulus parameters.
(2) The extent to which the *metrics* of the reaction can be influenced at a volitional level.
(3) The effect of *sensory parameters* on the latency of the reaction.
(4) The effect of *cognitive factors* such as preknowledge and selective attention on reaction time.

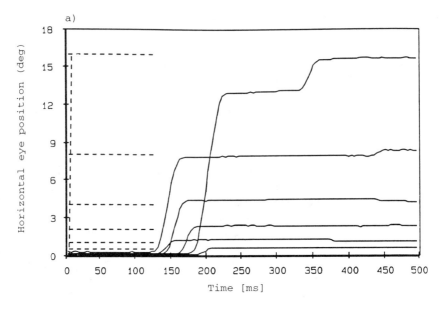

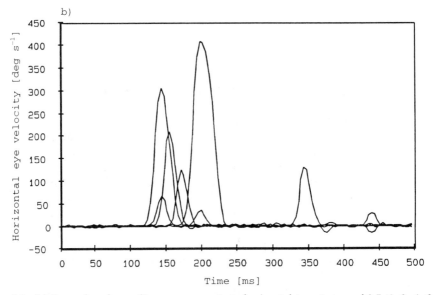

Figure 5.2. *(a) Examples of saccadic eye movements to horizontal target steps of 0.5, 1, 2, 4, 8 and 16 deg amplitude. Eye movements were registered with the scleral search coil technique. The figure illustrates the short reaction times and the stereotyped dynamics. (b) Horizontal eye velocity traces of these saccades.*

3.1.1 Spatial Precision

The first aspect concerns the spatial precision of the saccade and some systematic properties of the errors that occur. Saccades are amazingly precise as compared with other motor reactions: the absolute movement error is typically between 5 and

10% of saccade magnitude, with a tendency to undershoot the target (see below). Since humans mainly perform saccades smaller than 12 deg (Bahill, Adler and Stark, 1975), this accuracy suffices to hit most targets with the close foveal vicinity. The remaining error is then eliminated by 'corrective saccades'. It is clear-cut that the movement errors do not originate directly from limited *visual* processing capabilities, since the visual resolution in the central retina and in the periphery is much better than the precision of the saccades that are made to these areas. Therefore, the inaccuracy is probably caused by errors in motor programming or movement execution.

While pursuit performance responds to changes of contrast (Haegerstrom-Portnoy and Brown, 1979), saccadic accuracy is almost insensitive to large changes of the visual properties of the stimulus that elicits the eye movement. Indeed, the metrics of the saccade reaction to a small target are almost as stereotyped as its trajectory in the sense that response accuracy is, to a large extent, *invariant* with respect to intensity, contrast, color and presentation time of the stimulus. It seems that the only information that is extracted is distance and direction: the eye finds the target no matter what its sensory characteristics are. (It should be emphasized that, from a computational viewpoint, this kind of invariance is far from being a trivial problem.) So, while the rate of errors in triggering a saccade of correct *direction* is increased with stimulus luminance levels close to threshold, there is no marked increase of variability of response *magnitude* of correct direction saccades with reduced luminance or contrast of the stimulus (Hallett and Lightstone, 1976a, b; van Asten and Gielen, 1987). Further, accuracy and latency are not affected by stimulus duration (Hallett and Lightstone, 1976b). Thus, it seems that, as soon as the target is perceptually available, the sensorimotor system has no problem in assessing its spatial coordinates.

A puzzling feature of the response is that the errors remaining after the primary saccade are not symmetrically distributed around the target location. Rather, the saccades – at least when they are larger than about 5 deg – tend to systematically *undershoot* the target (Becker, 1972). This behavior entails the need for one or more additional correction saccades for precise foveation which seem to be controlled at an involuntary, unconscious level. These corrective saccades typically follow with latencies somewhat shorter than the primary saccade and are – as long as the error is not too large – based on visual feedback about postsaccadic refixation error (Deubel, Wolf and Hauske, 1982). So, for the final target acquisition, *visual* information is again essential.

There is suggestive evidence that saccadic undershooting represents a deliberate strategy of the oculomotor system (Deubel, Wolf and Hauske, 1986; Henson, 1978). *Why* saccades systematically fall short of the target remains a mystery. It has been argued that systematic undershooting behavior is more parsimonious in terms of energy expenditure and total time spent in the movement proper. Also, overshooting would entail a shift of the neural representation of the target into the opposite cortical hemisphere which could then require additional processing time as a result of information transfer through the corpus callosum. Moreover, it has been suggested that the typical undershooting of saccades originates from an unequal responsiveness of adaptive processes to overshoots versus undershoots (Deubel, 1991a, b).

These hypotheses are still mostly speculative in nature. Novel aspects may, however, become evident when saccadic behavior under more 'ecological' conditions will be investigated. Indeed, although undershooting is one of the few conspicuous imperfections of this otherwise machine-like reflex, its characteristics in a natural visual environment are still unclear. Indeed, saccadic errors become remarkably smaller with head-free conditions (Collewijn *et al.*, 1990) and are more accurate if directed to continuously visible targets within a structured visual context (Collewijn, Erkelens and Steinman, 1988a, b; Lemij and Collewijn, 1989). Further, statistical analysis with free scanning movements on pictorial material (in these unpublished investigations, the subjects had to evaluate the quality of video images) has failed to reveal the otherwise to-be-expected sequence of 'large saccade – small, short-latency correction'. Also, it is important to be aware that error correction in a visually highly complex scene requires some form of 'reassessment' of the target object appearing on a different retinal location after the primary saccade, a process that is somewhat equivalent to the well-known 'correspondence problem' in motion perception and stereopsis. Experimental evidence suggests that this type of correlation of presaccadic information with the postsaccadic foveal input for the programming of correction saccades may indeed exist (Deubel, Wolf and Hauske, 1984). It seems plausible that such a complex, predominantly *sensory* process is much more sensitive to eventual changes of the cortical hemisphere involved in the processing induced by overshooting. Again, the need for experimentation under more natural conditions becomes obvious.

3.1.2   Voluntary Control of Spatial Parameters of the Saccade

The second aspect concerns the extent to which this 'visual grasping reflex' is subject to immediate volitional modification. It is certainly not surprising that a subject can, with some effort, ignore the stimulus by suppressing his or her saccades to an appearing target. Also, observers may be asked to make a saccade of the target's eccentricity, but in the opposite direction of the target, or a saccade halfway to the target (Hallett, 1978). Interestingly, subjects manage to overcome this competition between foveation reflex and instruction after little training, producing saccades of low variability and relatively short latencies. This seems to suggest that the mapping from the sensory input onto the motor response can be 'rescaled' quickly at a volitional level, depending on instruction and situation. It is interesting to note, however, that some types of saccadic responses such as corrective saccades cannot be voluntarily suppressed, and the microsaccades occurring during fixation can be avoided only temporarily and with considerable effort. Also, it seems that the normal end-primary errors cannot be further reduced on the explicit instruction to be accurate, despite considerably longer latencies.

The 'anti-task' (Hallett, 1978) represents a prominent paradigm to investigate the effect of instructions on saccadic performance. In this paradigm, a stimulus appears abruptly with randomized timing, eccentricity and direction in the visual field. Upon target onset, the subject has to direct the gaze to a location at target eccentricity but *opposite* to the stimulus direction, thus driving the stimulus further into the retinal periphery. Although saccades are certainly optimized for foveation, it turns out that subjects have a good concept of goal position in these experiments, because the final end position of the eye (after an occasional corrective saccade) has been found to be amazingly close to the 'instructed' target position. This deliberate mislocalization occurs at the cost of increased reaction time, however.

These results are interesting since the ability to look away from a visually prominent object is an important aspect of voluntary behavior and is certainly of relevance for processes such as visual search and reading. Also, the data suggest that peripheral stages of the oculomotor system (such as sensory target localization) are shared for the foveation and the anti-task, while extra central decision processes are required for the latter. This paradigm may provide a means of attacking the question of when and how in the sensorimotor information flow higher-level decision processes can intervene. In this context, it should be mentioned that suppression of foveating saccades and the successful execution of the anti-task requires the frontal cortex, which is often rather silent in the 'normal' task (Guitton, Buchtel and Douglas, 1985).

3.1.3 Effect of Sensory Parameters on Saccadic Reaction Time

While precision is not very much affected by sensory stimulus properties and central factors, saccadic *latency*, however, is subject to considerable variation. For a given stimulus, latency depends on the subject, but also on factors like alertness, forewarning, attention, training and so forth. Indeed, somewhat unpleasantly, the major factor seems to be the subject. When no forewarning is provided, mean latencies to the onset of bright targets reported from different laboratories range from 150 ms to, more typically, 220 ms, but also up to 400 ms in some older reports. This large variability of saccadic latencies is somewhat puzzling. However, it turns out that saccadic latency also depends on sensory parameters such as intensity, color and form of the stimulus as well as the level of light adaptation. Of these factors, *luminance* is the major determinant.

With reduced illumination, latencies are increased. This is not too surprising, since with low luminance a longer waiting time is required to catch sufficient light quanta for perceptual processing. However, the effect is not very marked until luminance actually falls *below* foveal threshold. Many eye movement studies are performed with the adapted subject sitting in darkness. Wheeless (1967) demonstrated that in this situation the effect of stimulus luminance for a small saccade target can be nicely described by separate linear relationships, for scotopic and photopic vision, between the logarithms of latency and luminance. As can be seen from Figure 5.3 which presents saccadic reaction times as a function of target luminance, the scotopic and photopic ranges intersect at a luminance 0.5 log units below the foveal perceptual threshold, indicating the luminance value for the rod–cone transition.

A later detailed study by Doma and Hallett (1988) emphasized that Pieron's law, which has provided a useful quantitative description of manual reaction times and latencies of evoked potentials, also fits saccadic reaction time data reasonably well. Pieron's law relates the increase of reaction time from an asymptotic minimum to stimulus intensity I by an exponential function:

$$T - T_{\min} = kI^{-\beta}$$

where $T_{\min}$ is the minimum asymptotic latency for very bright stimuli and k is a constant specific for the scotopic and photopic mechanism. For perceptual and buttton-press tasks, β normally varies from 0.33 to 0.5, depending on the stimulus size.

Doma and Hallett's (1988) study demonstrated for saccadic eye movements that the asymptotic minimum latency is attained at 1.5–2 log units above foveal threshold. For the eye movement researcher this implies that stimuli should be well above this value in order to avoid interference from luminance effects. The study

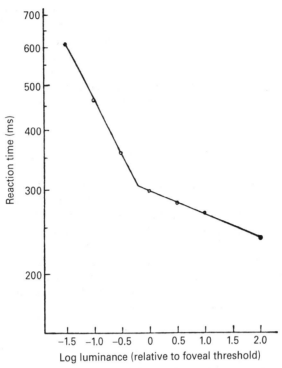

Figure 5.3. *Eye movement latencies to ± 6 deg horizontal target steps as a function of the luminance of the target (log–log plot). Target luminance is given relative to foveal threshold. [From Wheeless, 1967, p. 396. © American Institute of Physics; reprinted with kind permission.]*

also showed that, for pure cone and rod vision, the exponent β is close to 1 so the equation approaches a Bloch's law version of temporal integration for saccades. Under this condition, the amount of latency increase as a result of luminance reduction may be interpreted as a 'waiting time' or 'integration time', and the amount of light necessary to elicit a reaction can be estimated for rods and cones separately. (A detailed discussion of the role of temporal integration processes for visual perception is given by Reeves, this volume.) The experimental data revealed that for rod vision the saccadic threshold is close to the perceptual limit of about 100 photons; for the cones, however, saccadic threshold is *higher* by a factor of 5 than (foveal) cone perceptual threshold (while *perceptual* threshold in the periphery is *lower* by a factor of 2 than for foveal vision).

For photopic viewing conditions, latencies of saccades to equiluminant stimuli of different wavelengths differ. However, these differences disappear when the latencies are expressed as a function of Palmer's equivalent luminance (Palmer, 1966). (The Palmer transformation weights the relative contributions of rods and cones nonlinearly according to their sensitivities, as a function of adaptation level and field size.) This implies that, in the dark-adapted eye, saccadic latencies are essentially mediated by a luminance (achromatic brightness) mechanism. Rods can make a major input to the latencies of foveating saccades up to 1 log unit above cone threshold.

For other parameters, such as contrast and form, such detailed, quantitative analysis is still missing. The impression in general is that saccadic latencies can be well predicted from the known temporal properties of the retinal and afferent pathways, and are in correspondence with, for example, temporal summation in the transient and sustained channels. Indeed, in our laboratory, we have systematically observed longer latencies for stimuli with higher spatial frequencies. Van Asten and Gielen (1987) investigated to what extent the probability of eliciting a saccade to a stimulus depends on stimulus contrast and stimulus duration, for isochromatic and isoluminant stimuli. They used eccentric squares as stimuli for which they showed that the probability of eliciting a correct saccade and the probability of eliciting a correct psychophysical response depends on the contrast and the duration of the stimulus in a quantitatively identical way. In summary, there seems to be no reason to suppose that there are differences between the characteristics of the visual detection processes involved in psychophysical responses and those involved in the triggering of the saccadic response.

Saccadic latencies typically observed in laboratory situations are 180–250 ms. When no forewarning is provided, there are very few or no primary saccades with latencies shorter than 140 ms. The question has frequently been posed as to why the system is so slow while it has, in principle, the capability to react in half that time (see Section 3.1.4). However, it seems reasonable to assume that timing and metrical computation cannot be totally independent processes: timing has to consider the time requirements for metrical computation, i.e. a saccade should not be triggered *before* sufficient visual information is available for amplitude and direction computation. This rule predicts a covariation of, on the one hand, sensory stimulus aspects such as spatial frequency and complexity, and, on the other hand, saccadic latency. And indeed, it has been recently demonstrated that, when spatially more complex visual structures such as textures (see also Section 3.4) have to be successfully foveated, the additional processing requirements lead to a marked increase of saccadic reaction time, which is finally close to the 'normal' latency of saccades (Deubel and Frank, 1991). These findings offer a simple answer to the question posed above: the saccadic system may be adapted to performance in more complex sensory situations which demand delaying the response until information about texture borders becomes available. This implies that much of the saccade latency period in a reduced stimulus condition is the simple idling of a system which performs perfectly in a richly structured visual environment. Again, this emphasizes the importance of using more 'natural' conditions in eye movement research.

In summary, for weak stimuli, sensory parameters are the most relevant determinants of saccadic reaction time. However, even for bright targets, the oculomotor system normally does not perform at its limit: under specific conditions, much shorter latency periods suffice to bring the eye to the target. In the following, it will be demonstrated that manipulation of higher-level factors such as attentional processes can strip the processing delays down to their absolute minimum: the irreducible sensorimotor delay.

3.1.4 Effect of Higher-level Factors on Saccadic Reaction Time

Under specific conditions, saccadic latency can be reduced considerably to shorter and more consistent values. Higher-level factors such as preknowledge of target location, temporal forewarning, training and attentional factors have a marked effect on saccadic latency. This finding is a clear indication that the reaction is not reflexively evoked by the stimulus only, but also depends to some degree on preparative processes that occur before the stimulus appears.

Preknowledge of location where the target will appear reduces latency; hence Kowler, Martins and Pavel (1984) found that the latency for saccades to more probable locations was shorter. Accordingly, introduction of directional uncertainty (left/right) increases saccadic reaction time by about 20 ms. A further increase of the number of alternatives above two, however, does not lead to a further slowing of the reaction (Saslow, 1967a).

In contrast to directional uncertainty, the variation of target eccentricity does not affect the latency of the saccade. Further, the probabilistic structure of stimulus timing affects response latency: for repetitive target steps for which both the moment of occurrence and the direction and size can be predicted saccadic latency is frequently reduced to zero (Findlay, 1981a). Clearly, these responses are then completely anticipatory reactions.

Saccades show the conventional warning effects known from manual responses (Bertelson and Tisseyre, 1968). Any kind of warning signal that allows the subject to predict *when* the target step will occur may reduce latency by more than 80 ms (Ross and Ross, 1980). The most effective stimulus for speeding up the response, however, seems to be the extinction of the fixation mark well before the target appears. A number of investigations (Becker, 1972; Deubel and Frank, 1991; Deubel, Wolf and Hauske, 1982; Reulen, 1984a, b; Saslow, 1967b) have demonstrated that in this situation and under optimum conditions (bright target, direction known) the fastest nonanticipatory, stimulus-directed reactions that can be observed are as short as 80 ms for humans, and may be below 60 ms for rhesus monkeys (Schiller, Sandell and Maunsell, 1987). The latency values achieved in this paradigm are probably close to the propagation delays of the sensorimotor nervous system. Fischer and coworkers (Boch, Fischer and Ramsperger, 1984; Fischer and Breitmeyer, 1987; Fischer and Ramsperger, 1984) have provided the most extensive and detailed studies of these effects. They found that the extremely fast reactions, which they termed 'express-saccades', occur most frequently in a situation where the fixation point is removed 150 ms or so *before* the target comes on (the 'gap' paradigm), and where the area where the target will appear is not varied too much. As already demonstrated by Saslow (1967a), an extinction of the fixation point *after* target onset (the 'overlap' paradigm), on the other hand, leads to a marked slowing of the saccade reactions. Figure 5.4a, b shows stimulus and response sequences of the gap and overlap paradigms, and provides examples for typical saccadic latency distributions.

Fischer and colleagues argue that spatially selective attention plays a central role in determining the speed of response. They assume that directed spatial attention is normally locked onto the fixation point and inhibits the occurrence of express saccades. According to their model, the preparation of a saccade requires, as a first processing step, the 'disengagement' of attention from the fixation point, leaving the attentional system in a state termed 'free floating'. Disengagement of attention is a time-consuming process which, because of the early fixation offset, could be started and completed before target onset, resulting in a saving of processing time of the order of 70 ms. Several complementary investigations indeed have confirmed an important contribution of spatial attention to the occurrence of express saccades. Mayfrank *et al.* (1986), for example, conducted experiments in which they dissoci-

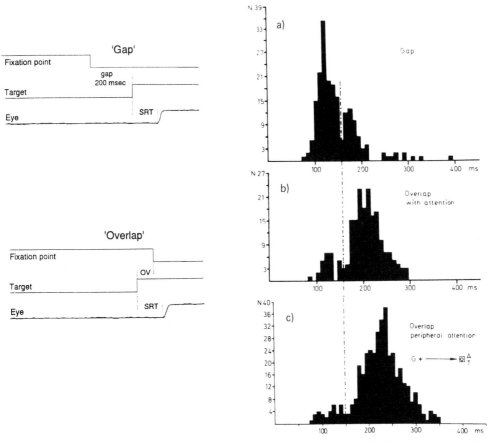

Figure 5.4. *Left: 'gap' and 'overlap' paradigms. Right: Distribution of saccadic latencies. (a) Saccadic reaction times (SRT) in a gap paradigm. The fixation point went off 200 ms before the saccade target was turned on. (b) Saccadic reaction times in an overlap paradigm where the subjects were instructed to attend to the central fixation point. (c) Saccadic reaction times in an overlap paradigm where the subjects were attending to a peripheral attention stimulus (A) that was located just above the saccade target (T) and remained visible. The subjects were required to keep their direction of gaze (G) in the middle of the screen without providing them with a fixation point. [Adapted from Fischer and Breitmeyer, 1987, pp. 75, 77. © Pergamon Press; reprinted with kind permission.]*

ated the direction of gaze from the direction of visual attention in space. It turned out that attention to a part of the visual field reduces the incidence of express saccades. Surprisingly, this was even found to be true when attention was cued to the saccade target location (Figure 5.4c). From these findings, Fischer and coworkers concluded that the engagement of attention, no matter where in the visual field, prevents express saccades. It is also worth noting that extended training has a strong effect on the occurrence of express saccades (Fischer and Ramsperger, 1986). Observations showed that, while some subjects are immediately able to produce express saccades, others require long training periods and still produce few of them. Also, expectations are important; hence, the occurrence of express saccades is markedly reduced when a small percentage of catch trials is introduced in the experimental sequence (Jüttner and Wolf, 1992).

Some workers also have provided tentative suggestions of the pathways that mediate express saccades. It is currently believed that the release of express saccades needs both an intact striate cortex (Boch and Fischer, 1986) and superior colliculus (Schiller, Sandell and Maunsell, 1987). In the primate visual system, the magnocellular pathway projects to both the superior colliculus and the visual cortex, and the fast magnocellular, cortico-collicular loop is deemed of essential importance for fast saccadic programming. However, it has also been demonstrated (Weber *et al.*, 1991) that express saccades can be elicited even by isoluminant, pure color contrast stimuli which are generally supposed to be mediated by the slower, parvocellular pathways.

The empirical findings on the reaction of the saccadic system to single steps of small targets as described in Section 3.1 may be summarized by saying that the oculomotor system responds to that type of stimulus in a rather stereotyped way, producing fast responses with high spatial accuracy. A closer look reveals that reaction time depends somewhat on sensory stimulus parameters, especially for weak stimuli. Both reaction time and spatial parameters are also very susceptible to volitional effort and attentional state.

3.2 Double Step Stimuli

It has been shown before that, when no forewarning is present, the reaction time of a saccade to the onset of a stimulus is normally more than 200 ms. Such a long time interval suggests that, before a saccade is elicited, substantial processing has taken place in the brain. What is the nature of the computation that occurs during that time? The previous paragraphs have demonstrated that approaching this question with the analysis of saccadic responses to single target steps is only of limited value. In order to provide a more detailed picture, it is necessary to break saccade computation down into a chain of several, more detailed processing steps. This problem may be approached experimentally by interrupting the ongoing computation by means of abrupt modifications of the visual input, at various times before the saccade occurs. The questions then arise, if and how parameters of the reaction under preparation are affected by the second, interfering stimulus. An experimental approach that has been frequently and successfully used for that purpose since its initial application by Westheimer (1954a) is the 'double step' paradigm. It is characterized by the target jumping twice before the primary saccade occurs.

From Westheimer's (1954a) findings and appreciating that some control process was in operation to prevent saccades occurring in too rapid succession, the suggestion arose of a 'sampled data' system. In its most extreme form (Young and Stark, 1962) the sampled data model assumed that the angle between the desired angle of gaze (the target position), and the actual eye position is sampled discretely every 200 ms. When this angle is sufficiently large, i.e. outside a postulated dead zone, a saccade results with a latency of 200 ms, i.e. at about the time of the next sample. Later, it became evident that a number of empirical findings were incompatible with the predictions of this model. For example, Wheeless, Boynton and Cohen (1966) showed that, when tracking targets that jumped twice with an interval between the jumps of 100 ms, 77% of saccades ignore the first target step and move straight to the position after the end of the second step. Such a result suggests that information about target behavior can influence a saccade if it occurs within 100 ms of its onset.

The empirical and theoretical work of Becker and Jürgens (1979) led to a thorough revision of thinking about the sensorimotor information processing in the saccadic system. They presented combinations of two horizontal target steps with interstep intervals ranging from 50 to 200 ms and amplitudes of between 15 and 60 deg. In most cases, therefore, the second, interfering target displacement occurs before the onset of the primary saccade. This type of paradigm and typical results are illustrated in Figure 5.5a. In a follow-up study, we (Deubel, Wolf and Hauske, 1984) used small and short, pulse-like target displacements before the saccade as test stimuli (Figure 5.5b). In contrast to the experiments with the large secondary steps, where the perturbing target shift frequently leads to a cancellation of the saccadic response, saccade initiation turned out to be less affected by these small, behaviorally insignificant stimuli. Another important study (Ottes, van Gisbergen and Eggermont, 1984) investigated more closely the effect of relative distance between the first and the second target location in the double step task.

From all of these studies it turned out that much of the variability that characterizes the responses can be accounted for by taking notice of the temporal interval between the perturbing target displacement and the onset of the first saccade. This interval is denoted by D in Figure 5.5. Both spatial end position and latency of the saccade may be affected by the interfering target displacement, however, in characteristically different ways. Depending on its relative size, the perturbing stimulus induces basically different effects, which led Ottes, van Gisbergen and Eggermont (1984) to postulate two different 'modes': one, in which *averaging* responses occur, and the other, in which a *bistable* response pattern prevails. The essentials of the findings may be summarized as follows:

(1) The *first mode* can be observed when the two locations stimulated are on the same side of the retina and are not too far apart (e.g. at 10 deg and at 15 deg eccentricity). In this case, the *amplitude* of the response is modified in a characteristic way.

(2) Under this condition, the amplitude can be modified by the sensory information from the second stimulus if it occurs as late as 70 ms before the saccadic reaction. It is interesting to note that a value of 70 ms is close to the estimated minimum propagation delays of the sensory (35 ms) and motor (25 ms) systems combined. This surprisingly short value indicates that the oculomotor system is prepared to take into account new visual information until the very latest possible moment before the onset of the movement.

(3) More surprisingly, if the target step or pulse occurs in an interval between approx. 70 and 180 ms before saccade onset, the saccade consistently lands *in between* the first and the final target location. This finding suggests that rather than using an instantaneous value of target position, a spatial *average* of target eccentricity is calculated within a particular *temporal window* before the saccade is taken. So, when the window includes the second target step, the window would include contributions from *both* target positions and thus arrive at an intermediate value for the saccade amplitude. This leads, with increasing D, to a systematic transition of the saccade end points between the two locations (this function was termed the 'amplitude transition function' by Becker and Jürgens, 1979). The temporal integration can thus account both for saccades directed to intermediate positions and also for the transition shown in the amplitude transition function.

(4) The *second mode* occurs when the presaccadic second target shift is large with respect to the first step, i.e. 10 and 30 deg, or shifts the target into the contralateral

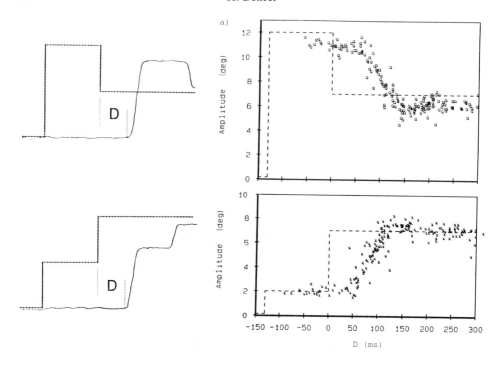

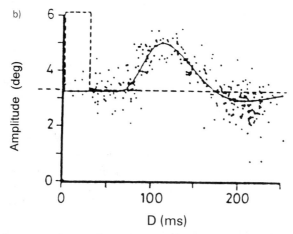

Figure 5.5. *(a) Left: target and eye position in two types of the double step paradigm. Right: saccadic reactions to double target steps. The data points represent the end positions of single primary saccades as a function of D, the interval between the occurrence of the second target displacement and the onset of the saccades. (b) Effect of impulse-like target displacements on saccade amplitude. The data points show the landing positions of single (corrective) saccades as a function of the time interval between the onset of the target displacement and the beginning of the saccades. [Adapted from Deubel, Wolf and Hauske, 1984, p. 59. © Elsevier; reprinted with kind permission.]*

retina. Instead of being directed to a spatial average, the saccade now is directed to one location or the other, depending on the specific timing. Also, the occurrence of delayed responses is markedly increased. In this case, therefore, mainly *timing* is affected. It is interesting to note that the timing of the saccade can be affected only until up to about 120 ms before saccade onset.

(5) Finally, it should be mentioned that Becker and Jürgens (1979) found an indication for the *parallel programming* of two successive saccades in different stages of the computation process. This was suggested essentially by the observation that the characteristics of the second saccade of a two-saccade response to a double step stimulus depends on the time between the second target step and the first response. These results also indicated that saccades may be programmed on the basis of extraretinal signals.

Several aspects of these findings are of considerable interest. It seems that the result of amplitude computation is independent of the absolute latency of the primary saccade to the first step and, moreover, the effect of the target displacement can be observed until up to 240 ms after its occurrence (Deubel, Wolf and Hauske, 1984). This suggests that amplitude computation is a process that runs continuously, independent of the decision of triggering a saccade. Also, for small target displacements, latency of the response does not covary with the amplitude value that is actually computed (Deubel, 1984). The latest point in time where saccade triggering is affected is earlier than the minimum modification time for amplitude. This result is an indication that the decision to elicit a saccade is accomplished *before* the amplitude computation is finished. Taken together, the findings suggest that the process that computes *where* a saccade is going to be directed to is, to a large degree, *independent* of and *parallel* to the process that decides *when* the movement should be elicited. While the process of amplitude computation shows the attributes of a machine-like, low-level process, the amount of susceptibility of the timing to the perturbations is much more vulnerable to instructions and expectations and exhibits considerable variability between subjects (Deubel, unpublished observations). This suggests that the observed behavior is another example of the interaction of the automatic and continuous computation of spatial values and higher-level decision processes that determine the initiation of the saccade.

Becker and Jürgens (1979) emphasized the integration process as involving *temporal* integration of the spatial error signal which somehow implies that it occurs essentially in the motor system where the signals that code motor coordinates are already available. However, in fact the computation involves a spatiotemporal integration since the parameter that is being integrated is the spatial target position. Moreover, data from our laboratory (for a review, see Becker, 1991) indicated that the reactions to double steps are sensitive to sensory stimulus parameters in a way which suggests that the spatiotemporal integration originates in the *sensory* rather than in the motor subsystem. The question arises whether 'spatial' and 'temporal' integration could be expressions of a single process; this is discussed in more detail in Deubel, Wolf and Hauske (1984). In this respect, further investigations are urgently needed.

A slightly different paradigm to be introduced in the next section shows clearly that spatial integration is an integral aspect of the programming of saccade amplitude. This comes from studies of saccades to targets which consist of two separate elements in neighboring positions (double targets). In this situation, the first saccade made is directed to an intermediate position between the targets. This observation, termed the 'center of gravity' effect or 'global' effect, forms the central aspect of the next sections. Again, it will turn out that the two components that constitute the leitmotif of this contribution, i.e. the roles of sensory processing and cognitive factors, are central to the better understanding of the empirical findings.

3.3 Double and Multiple Stimuli

All the experimental conditions described earlier are characterized by the presence of only a single target in the visual field at any moment. However, it is perfectly clear that in any but this highly artificial laboratory situation the observer has to *select* one object out of many potential targets for the next eye movement, or has to generate an internal 'plan' of the sequence of saccades in order to optimally scan a complex scene. Indeed, our subjective impression is that we can direct the gaze to any location in the visual field. Obviously, the decision of what in the field to look at next essentially includes cognitive-attentional processes, but may nevertheless be constrained by sensorimotor factors. Perceptual processes certainly provide the basic requisite information upon which cognitive-attentional processes function. The question thus arises to what extent 'physical' properties of the retinal input are determinants for target selection processes. In other words, how do size, shape, contrast, color, texture and transients determine the *salience* of one stimulus among others? This is an important aspect also for applied research, concerning fields such as advertising, the jet pilot scanning an instrument panel or the radiologist searching for lung tumors.

An experimental approach to these questions clearly requires a move from the previous situation to one where more than just one stimulus is present in the visual field, thus introducing the necessity for the subject to *decide* what to look at. The simplest of all configurations for the experimenter is a condition where not one, but *two* stimuli are simultaneously present in the visual field. This *double stimulation* or *double target* situation has indeed attracted much research effort in the past decade. Just as for the double step experiments, a number of studies have demonstrated that, when two stimuli are simultaneously present, the mode of interaction of both depends (as a major factor) on how far apart the stimuli are. There are again two modes which will be treated separately in the following.

3.3.1 Selection Among Stimuli that are Widely Separated

The first mode is shown most clearly when stimuli appear simultaneously in opposite hemifields. A typical paradigm of this type involves presenting the stimuli simultaneously, at a certain eccentricity, to the left and to the right of the fixation point. As expected, a bistable response occurs in this situation, i.e. the unbiased subject saccades to either one target or the other. When stimulus attributes are varied, it is reasonable to assume that the more salient target receives more spontaneous fixations. The double stimulation procedure can be thus used to obtain an operational measure of target salience or, more precisely, of the relative salience of one stimulus with respect to another.

The work of Lévy-Schoen (1969; Lévy-Schoen and Blanc-Garin, 1974) demonstrated that, in this case, the latency of the primary saccade was inflated by 30–40 ms with respect to the situation where only one target was presented. This increase may be attributed to the additional decision processes involved. Most subjects showed *a priori* bias, preferring one direction above the other. Of course, such a bias could also be installed voluntarily, upon instruction.

Findlay (1980) analyzed saccadic reactions in such a paradigm in more detail, varying aspects of visual stimulus properties such as proximity to the fovea, transient onset and spatial structure. He found that the most important variable that determines target salience is the proximity of the stimulus to the fovea. A second strong determiner of salience was the amount of transient stimulation. Comparison of the effect of homogeneous target disks in competition with grating patches suggested that spatial structure is of much less importance (this conclusion may be premature because the border of a homogeneous disk also provides a strong visual discontinuity of presumably high visual salience). The preliminary conclusion from this work was that saccades are activated by a 'transient mechanism, rather insensitive to spatial detail' (Findlay, 1981b).

3.3.2 Stimuli Close Together: The 'Global Effect'

The experiments mentioned above showed that when stimuli are presented in different retinal hemifields, no spatial interactions between the target positions occur, in the sense that the magnitudes of the responses are not affected. This picture changes dramatically when stimuli are presented sufficiently close together and without a too large directional separation. Under this condition, the bistable response pattern disappears and spatial integration effects become predominant.

Coren and Hoenig (1972) appear to be the first to have described that the presence of an additional visual stimulus (a 'distractor') inflates the precision with which saccades can be directed to a target. In their experiments, a red asterisk at 10 deg eccentricity was given as saccade target. Simultaneously with target onset, a black asterisk could also appear at various distances from the target. Although the subjects could easily discriminate the stimuli and were asked to ignore the distractor, saccadic magnitudes were nevertheless systematically affected. The authors described the observed tendency as the eye being drawn to the *center of gravity* of the total stimulus configuration. This important observation was not really appreciated by the eye movement researchers of that time. In the beginning of the 1980s, however, the paradigm witnessed considerable revival with several investigations demonstrating that the exact saccade landing position in between the targets depends systematically on various relative visual properties of the targets. For instance, if one target is made larger (Findlay, 1982), more intense (Deubel and Wolf, 1982; Deubel, Wolf and Hauske, 1984), is presented with higher contrast (Deubel and Hauske, 1988) or with a higher dot density (Menz and Groner, 1987), then the first saccade lands closer to this target.

Findlay (1982) varied the relative size of two spatially separated squares appearing in the near periphery as well as the distance between them. The general finding again was that saccades landed systematically at an intermediate position between the targets, with a tendency to be more attracted by the larger stimulus (Figure 5.6a). Since this result implies that the computation of the spatial parameters of the saccade uses the global stimulus configuration, Findlay (1982) termed this finding the *global effect*. He also was the first to notice that stimuli that are closer to the fovea receive a higher weight in spatial computation, i.e. for equally sized targets, the eye tends to land closer to the less eccentric stimulus.

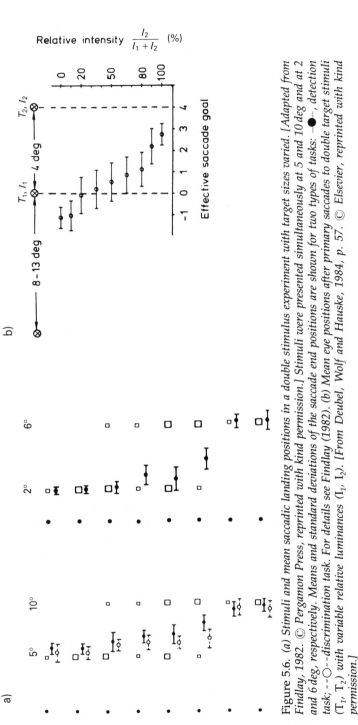

Figure 5.6. (a) Stimuli and mean saccadic landing positions in a double stimulus experiment with target sizes varied. [Adapted from Findlay, 1982. © Pergamon Press, reprinted with kind permission.] Stimuli were presented simultaneously at 5 and 10 deg and at 2 and 6 deg, respectively. Means and standard deviations of the saccade end positions are shown for two types of tasks: —●—, detection task; --○-- discrimination task. For details see Findlay (1982). (b) Mean eye positions after primary saccades to double target stimuli (T_1, T_2) with variable relative luminances (I_1, I_2). [From Deubel, Wolf and Hauske, 1984, p. 57. © Elsevier, reprinted with kind permission.]

Work in my laboratory (Deubel and Hauske, 1988; Deubel and Wolf, 1982; Deubel, Wolf and Hauske, 1984) has extended Findlay's basic observations. We varied the relative brightness of double dot stimuli and demonstrated that it is literally possible to steer the saccade end position between both targets, by adjusting the relative stimulus intensities (Figure 5.6b). It has been concluded that the saccade generating mechanism computes the center of gravity of the (physical) luminance distribution as the effective saccade goal.

It is important to note that, again, the findings suggest a dissociation into two distinct modes, depending on the *interstimulus spacing*. As for double steps, when the angular separation of the targets becomes too large, a *bistable* response pattern predominates. The range over which spatial integration occurs can be estimated by the target separation when effect breaks down. Ottes, van Gisbergen and Eggermont (1984) presented an example from a double target experiment where stimuli at 15 and 25 deg produced averaging responses while the combination of a 5 with a 35 deg eccentric target yielded a bistable response pattern. As a rough rule, the above findings and our own observations suggest that averaging occurs when the ratio of the eccentricity of the more eccentric target to the less eccentric target is 2 : 1 or less. When the targets are further apart, the saccade is directed to one stimulus or the other, but there is also an intermediate region where the saccade seems to be directed to one target but the end-point is still affected by the distractor. Also, averaging is not restricted to stimuli in the horizontal plane but is equally present for stimuli of moderate directional separation. Ottes, van Gisbergen and Eggermont (1984) demonstrated that two targets presented simultaneously at the same eccentricity anywhere in the visual field evoke a saccade directed to their common center of gravity provided their directional separation was 45 deg or smaller, i.e. was within an octant of the visual field. Again, more widely spaced stimuli usually led to saccades that were directed to one or the other stimulus, and less frequently in between the two.

The empirical findings suggest that widespread spatial integration is a fundamental characteristic of the pathways that mediate target-elicited saccadic eye movements: visual information covering a wide retinal area is integrated in the saccadic response. Also, it is important to note that the weight with which a stimulus is considered in this computation process is now determined by *sensory* attributes such as size and luminance. This has the important implication that the integration takes place at a stage in which visual parameters can still affect the coding of saccade metrics. This is a direct indication, therefore, that sensory processing forms an essential determinant of oculomotor control.

An implementation of the spatial averaging process is suggested by visual system physiology. It is known that the receptive fields in the superior colliculus and the frontal eye field are generally very large. It is possible that the spatial integration might arise from these large receptive fields and it has been suggested (Findlay, 1982) that they might correspond to low spatial frequency channels. Such an assumption would predict that dark and bright structures should cancel and, moreover, that higher spatial frequencies would not contribute to the computation of amplitude. This is not the case: by using combinations of lines of positive and negative contrast it has been demonstrated (Deubel and Hauske, 1988) that positive and negative contrasts summate rather than cancel each other, indicating the existence of an essential nonlinearity in the visual computation process. This is indicative of a crucial difference from the integration of luminance occurring in low spatial frequency channels: while filtering properties can be observed in parameters of the response, averaging itself seems to occur *after* some visual preprocessing in the afferent channels. The observation that saccadic averaging is also present with dichoptic double target presentation (Findlay, personal communication) is in accord with this assumption.

Another study demonstrated that the target weight depends critically on the spatial frequency content of the stimuli (Zetzsche, Deubel and Elsner, 1984) in a manner closely related to the modulation transfer function of the peripheral visual system (Koenderink and van Doorn, 1978; Rovamo, Virsu and Näsänen, 1978), indicating that indeed the full range of spatial frequencies that is perceptually available also contributes to saccade control. An interesting aspect of the aforementioned experiments is that properties of afferent, sensory processing seem to be directly reflected in parameters of the saccadic response. This observation leads to the idea that the saccadic response to spatial stimuli might allow the elucidation of properties of the sensory visual pathways; in other words, eye movements may serve as a 'probe' into visual processing. In this context, Deubel, Wolf and Hauske (1984) demonstrated that both the saccadic 'amplitude transition function' found in double step experiments (Becker and Jürgens, 1979; and Section 3.2), and the global effect shown in double target experiments are well in accord with the predictions of a model that assumes, in a first stage, a spatiotemporal filtering (in the sensory pathways) of the input signal and, in a second stage, the computation of saccadic magnitude and direction by means of a weighted averaging of the preprocessed, filtered signal. This suggests that the 'amplitude transition function' is simply the result of spatiotemporal filtering in the sensory visual pathways.

It is somewhat discomforting to see the above findings predict that saccades can be accurately directed to a target only if it stands in an isolated region of the visual field. This is in contrast to our everyday experience and, also, the eyes are certainly not 'locked' to the brightest spot in the field. How is it then possible to bring the eye to a stationary target along with distracting stimuli in the background? The next paragraph will reveal to what extent the global effect can be modified and overcome by deliberate strategies.

3.3.3   The Role of Volitional Control

The results presented above all emphasize the determining influence exerted by sensory factors in the spatial averaging involved in saccade control. On the other hand, saccadic eye movements are motor responses that can obviously be controlled at a volitional level. In fact, a criticism of the aforementioned experiments on spatial averaging has been that the role of *voluntary selection* of a target or an area in the visual field was not specifically controlled. As already addressed by Findlay (1981b) and Findlay and Crawford (1983), such a lack of clear instruction might have allowed the subject to develop deliberate strategies. This suggests that the directing of saccades to an intermediate position might reflect some strategy designed to optimize visual information intake, and the centering tendency might be just the expression of an effective visual search plan. However, the findings described earlier show that the saccade lands nearer to the target which should be the most visible. This is difficult to reconcile with such a strategic view.

On the other hand, it would be highly surprising to find that there is no room for voluntary target selection in the control of rapid saccades. In the case of pursuit movements, for example, it has been clearly demonstrated that pursuit targets can be deliberately 'selected': the presence of a prominent background has little influence on pursuit performance (Murphy, Kowler and Steinman, 1975). Indeed, it turns out that the automatic centering tendency for saccades is subject to modification by at least two measures: (1) by deliberately suppressing the visual grasp reflex and waiting for the target selection process to become more effective; and (2) by preknowledge and training. Both are indices of the involvement of additional, higher-level processes.

An effect of *latency* on the occurrence of averaging saccades was already noted by Findlay (1981b) and by Viviani and Swensson (1982). Later, Ottes, van Gisbergen and Eggermont (1985), in a more detailed study, also found strong effects of saccadic reaction time. These authors required subjects to saccade to a green target spot that was presented simultaneously with a red nontarget spot of the same (subjective) brightness. Target and distractor appeared at 20 deg eccentricity and at an angular separation of 30, 60 and 90 deg above and below the horizontal midline. The subjects were explicitly instructed to ignore the distractor. Because of the large angular separation and the differing colors, target and distractor were clearly discriminable perceptually. For the small angular separation (30 deg) the finding was that saccades with short latencies (less than 250 ms) landed in between the two stimuli, in conformance with the prediction of the center-of-gravity concept. However, with increased latency the probability of the subject saccading to the nontarget decreased, also resulting in less averaging saccades.

The response categories 'averaging' and 'bistable' are probably extremes in a continuum, with a gradual transition from one response type to the other. For short latency saccades, Ottes, van Gisbergen and Eggermont (1985) noted an amazing robustness of the averaging effect against volitional effort. They suggested that the fast averaging responses constitute the 'default option' of the saccadic response and described their observation in this way: '... if a preconceived strategy played any role in all of these experiments, it was essential to *avoid* rather than to *generate* averaging responses'. If required, subjects would have to overcome the default option by means of delaying the response. When the two targets appeared at the same angular direction but with different eccentricities (Ottes, van Gisbergen and Eggermont, 1984), weighting again occurred in favor of the small eccentricities: objects on the near side of the target clearly diminished saccade amplitude, while objects on the far side only slightly increased amplitude.

The effect of latency was further analyzed and confirmed by Coëffé and O'Regan (1987). In two experiments, they were able to demonstrate that the influence of nontarget stimuli on saccadic accuracy can be attenuated in two ways. The first is when the moment of saccade triggering is delayed and the second is when preknowledge about target location within the stimulus configuration is provided. In their first experiment, they delayed the subjects' responses by instructing them to saccade only when the central fixation mark went off. The data given in Figure 5.7 (solid curve) stem from a similar experimental approach where we required subjects to saccade, on an acoustic signal, to a previously presented target/nontarget configuration. The results confirm that saccade accuracy increases with longer processing delays, which means that the distracting effect can be compensated at the expense of reaction time. In their second experiment, Coëffé and O'Regan (1987) tested the effect of preknowledge of target location by means of blocked presentations; their data confirmed previous findings that preknowledge and extended

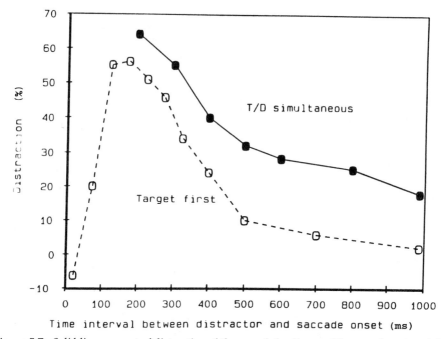

Figure 5.7. *Solid line: amount of distraction of the saccade landing position as a function of the time interval between the simultaneous onset of two spatially separated stimuli (a cross and a circle) and the initiation of the saccade. The subject was instructed to saccade to the circle on an acoustic 'go' signal. Dashed line: amount of saccade distraction caused by abrupt onset of a distractor at various time intervals before the saccade. Here the subject had to direct the gaze, on an acoustic 'go' signal, to a stationary target visible well before saccade onset.*

training produce some modification to the global effect (Findlay and Crawford, 1983).

Coëffé (1987) offered a conceptual model to account for these findings. Central to his concept is that while saccade computation is done automatically and continuously on the basis of the available information, it is also modulated from moment to moment by *attentional mechanisms*. More specifically, when the stimulus configuration appears in the periphery, spatiotemporal filtering in the early stages of the visual system allows only a crude, low spatial frequency version to be available at first, so the target cannot be distinguished from the nontargets. Some time later, the attentional focus has shifted onto the general region of the stimulus which is the center of gravity of the configuration. Higher spatial frequencies become available with time, allowing discrimination between target and distractors and entailing an increasing focusing of attention on the target location. The end-point being calculated at any moment is assumed to be the center of the attentional focus. Therefore, if a saccade is triggered early, it is directed to the global center of gravity of the configuration. If saccade triggering is delayed, however, it will be directed closer to the true target location.

Although this concept requires some qualification because of our finding that higher spatial frequencies are also considered in the computation of the fast, averaging saccades, the emphasis on the role of attentional processes in the selection of the target seems to be warranted. Nevertheless, the description given by Ottes, van Gisbergen and Eggermont (1985), that the global effect is the default option for the saccadic system, is also in accordance with the findings. For fast responses, the signal for saccades appears to integrate visual stimulation in an automatic and systematic way which does not differentiate between target and distractor (Ottes, van Gisbergen and Eggermont, 1985). The idea that the centering tendency constitutes the 'default' mode for fast responses that must be 'overcome' with directed effort has drawn some recent criticism, however. In fact, the extent to which saccades in the double stimulus situation are 'automatic' reflexes has been the subject of current passionate discussion between psychologists and system approach-oriented workers (see Kowler, 1990). In an approach somewhat similar to that of Ottes, van Gisbergen and Eggermont (1985), He and Kowler (1989) used a target/nontarget situation in which they varied the probability that the target appeared at a certain location. They found that the saccadic end-points were strongly biased toward the more probable location. If the target was to occur more likely in a rightward position, the saccades were directed further to the right. From these findings Kowler (1990) argued, somewhat polemically, that the global effect is not the result of a low-level, sensorimotor averaging mechanism, but rather is the reflection of higher-level plans and cognitive control. It is difficult to see how such an extreme position is warranted: in their experiments a situation was introduced in which the subject produced rather stimulus-independent, stereotyped and highly learned motor responses. Therefore, these findings rather suggest that a subject can, with effort, *ignore* certain aspects of the visual stimulus. Clearly, expectations can influence the saccade landing position, but they alone do not determine the reaction.

Nevertheless, ample empirical indication exists that the subject's expectations and knowledge of the range over which the targets will occur are reflected in the distribution of saccadic amplitudes. So, for example, Kapoula (1985) demonstrated that when targets are consistently presented in a certain range of eccentricity, the saccades to the near targets tend to overshoot and saccades to the far targets show a relative undershoot – the saccadic 'range effect'. Clearly, even in this extremely simple situation, the size of 'reflexive' saccades is not entirely predetermined by the location of the stimulus, but also depends on the task context.

Finally, Jacobs (1987) has added a somewhat alternative perspective, reinterpreting the global effect in terms of efficiency of oculomotor behavior. He put forward the view that a two-saccade strategy, consisting of a fast primary saccade and a second, corrective saccade, brings the eye onto the target much earlier than when precise foveation with a single saccade is achieved by sufficiently delaying the primary saccade. The global effect is thus interpreted as the result of an optimization strategy. This interpretation, however, has difficulty in accounting for the occurrence of the global effect in the presence of clearly discriminable, rather widely spaced target/nontarget configurations. Nevertheless, again this work emphasizes the possible role of 'deliberate strategies' in reflexive oculomotor control.

In summary, it has been demonstrated in this section that even the simplest reflex-like saccades are subject to higher-level influences. It may turn out that a clue to the somewhat contradictory positions pointed out above consists in a prominent detail which is characteristic of the experimental procedure. All the aforementioned experiments were performed under the condition of an abrupt, transient onset of the peripheral stimulus. Apart from the fact that the ecological validity of this situation is questionable, the effect of rapid appearance of the stimulus probably subserves the appearance of obligatory eye movements to the target location. This emphasizes the close linkage of saccades and selective visual attention, discussed in more detail in Section 4.1. This link is still not completely understood. It seems promising, therefore, to relate the findings to experiments on spatial attention. Indeed abrupt visual onsets seem, in a sense, unique for capturing visual attention (Jonides and Yantis, 1988). For example, Nakayama and Mackeben (1989) have demonstrated that transient visual cueing triggers a transient shift of focal visual attention to the cue. They suggested that this transient component was independent of the observer's prior knowledge of target position and was not subject to voluntary control.

In a related approach, I recently used a modified double target paradigm to investigate the effect of abrupt distractor onset on the saccadic reaction. In these experiments, subjects had to saccade, on an acoustic 'go' signal, to a target well visible 500–1000 ms before saccade onset. Shortly before the saccade triggering, a distractor could appear in the vicinity of the target. The data presented in Figure 5.7 (dashed curve) show that, although the subject had sufficient time for complete-ly preparing the saccade program, there is a strong, inevitable distracting effect due to nontarget onset. This demonstrates that – with transient stimulation – preknowl-edge and voluntary effort of the subject to ignore the distractor are *not* sufficient to elicit an accurate reaction: involuntary components prevail. Interestingly, the time course of the amount of distraction is very similar to the attentional effects determined by Nakayama and Mackeben (1989) in their psychophysical approach with peripheral cueing.

3.4 Stimuli Including Background Structure

The previous sections presented examples of the increasing amount of research work concerned with the reaction of the saccadic system to combinations of two or more, simultaneously presented, spatially well-separated targets. It became clear that the computation of saccadic direction and magnitude is based on the integra-tion of sensory information over a wide area, in which sensory stimulus properties are important determinants of the oculomotor reaction. Still, all of these experi-ments were conducted in the absence of background structure. Our natural environment outside the laboratory, however, is normally characterized by the presence of a many-faceted visual structure, everywhere in the visual field. Outside the laboratory, stimuli that are selected as targets may range from simple ones where mere detection might suffice (like a bird in the sky) to extremely complex visual arrangements (like the proverbial needle in the haystack). The question arises how, if the relatively simple spatial averaging mechanism demonstrated previously operates, perceptual processes could possibly cope with this situation, given that spatial integration occurs on an early representation of the visual signal.

With this step, a qualitative change occurs in the computational requirements to target finding. Stimuli normally do not stand in isolation, with the targets defined by their mere presence. Rather, objects are primarily defined by their *difference in visual structure* from the background. Successful foveation of an object in this situation should demand, as a first processing step, the segregation of a 'foreground' from the visual structure that constitutes the background, and this segregation must be based on information about luminance, contrast, color and form of object and background.

Inferentially, the sensorimotor system should be well able to find and follow objects that are distinct from the background by structural features rather than only by their global luminance characteristics. This concept requires that borders between different texture areas should form salient features for the oculomotor system and this has been investigated only recently in a series of experiments described in the next section.

3.4.1 Saccades to Texture Stimuli

For visual perception, it has been frequently demonstrated that a human observer has the ability to discriminate instantaneously between two surfaces that are identical in color or average luminance, but differ in small-scale luminance variations – what is generally called *texture*. A major contribution to the study of this type of early visual perception has come from the work of Bela Julesz. His research has been concerned with the segmentation of the visual scene on the basis of differences in visual characteristics, and particularly differences in microtexture. These studies have led to a large body of work on human texture discrimination (for reviews see Julesz, 1986; Julesz and Bergen, 1983; Kehrer and Meinecke, this volume). A basic assumption is that human vision operates in two distinct modes which are denoted 'preattentive vision' and 'attentive vision' (Neisser, 1967). According to the definition given by Julesz, preattentive visual processing allows the immediate, instantaneous discrimination of different texture areas. Julesz uses the term 'texton' to denote the micropatterns constituting textured areas. Preattentive vision reflects a system working in parallel over a large part of the visual field, acting almost instantaneously, and indicating *where* texton gradients occur. Attentive vision, on the other hand, involves a serial step-wise search by a small focus of attention. Attentive vision is required to determine *what* the targets are.

It is readily suggested that the essential functional role of preattentive vision is – through instantaneous texture discrimination – to direct focal attention to locations in the visual field where texture gradients occur, thus allowing subsequent analysis by the attentive system. This implies that preattentive texture processing should deliver essential signals for the guidance of the eye when viewing complex visual structures (Julesz, 1986). The question thus arises whether preattentive texture discrimination can immediately affect the signals relevant for saccadic eye movement control.

Recently, this hypothesis was tested by using stimuli where foreground/background segregation was a necessary prerequisite for saccadic programming (Deubel *et al.*, 1988). The work investigated the effect of texture-defined stimuli on saccades in a target/nontarget situation. As an example for a number of different textures used in the experiments, Figure 5.8a sketches a typical visual stimulus. The scene was composed of line elements of specific contrast and orientation. On appearance of the scene, the subject had to saccade from a fixation cross F to the elongated target structure T, which was in this case defined by elements with an orientation difference of 90 deg from the background structure. The histogram below is a representative distribution of the saccade landing positions. Our general finding

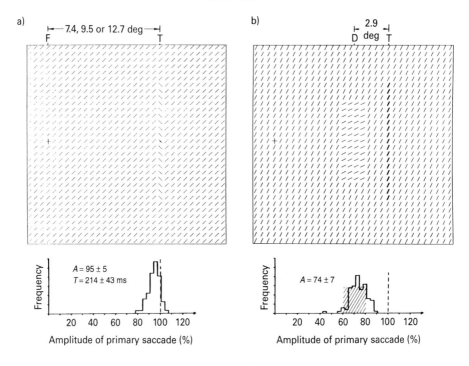

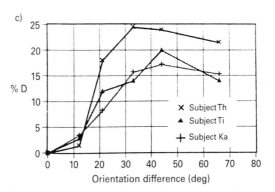

Figure 5.8. *Stimuli and distribution of saccadic landing positions from experiments with texture-defined stimuli. [Adapted from Deubel et. al., 1988.] (a) Upon appearance of the scene, the subject had to saccade from a fixation cross (F) to the elongated structure (T) defined by the element orientation difference with respect to the background structure. (b) Double stimulus experiment. The subject had to saccade to the elongated structure defined by the element luminance. Simultaneously, a texture-defined distractor (D) was presented. The distribution of the end position of the primary saccades reflects the saccade distraction that resulted from the texture patch. (c) Amount of saccade distraction as a function of the orientation difference between foreground and background elements for stimuli as shown in (b), given for three subjects.*

was that the subjects had no difficulties in performing this task. This is reflected in the high saccadic accuracy, i.e. low standard deviations of amplitudes, and in rather short saccadic latencies.

Figure 5.8b displays a stimulus scene from another set of experiments. Here, the target T was defined by its higher luminance compared with the background structure. Additionally, a distractor D is simultaneously present consisting of an area of line elements that differ from the background in their orientation. As can be seen from the accompanying histogram, the presentation of the texture-defined distractor embedded in a background structure leads to a distinct shift of the mean saccade landing position while the variability of the saccadic amplitudes essentially remains unaffected. Clearly, in this more complex stimulus situation also, the saccade landing position is constituted by some 'center of gravity' of target and distractor, as can be seen by the considerable shift of the distribution towards the distractor. It turns out that the amount of distraction is a function of the orientation difference between distractor (the foreground) and background structure (Figure 5.8c).

These findings have some implications for our concept of the role of visual preprocessing in saccade control. By introduction of the background structure a situation was obtained where the target is not defined by its mere presence, but rather by its structural difference with respect to the background. Clearly, this visually more complex situation does not restrain the oculomotor reaction: the high precision of the saccade is maintained and latencies are only slightly increased.

Most critically, areas with a texture that differs from the background can also act as distractors for saccadic eye movement, showing that spatial averaging in the sense of the center of gravity effect also occurs in the presence of background structure. It must be concluded that a considerable amount of sensory processing of visual information is involved in the programming of fast saccades. This processing segregates foreground objects from the background structure. Only then, at a subsequent stage, does spatial averaging occur on the preprocessed information to determine saccadic amplitudes. This means that texture gradients form highly important features for the amplitude computation process.

The fact that the weight of the distractor is found to be closely related to the orientation difference between background and foreground elements (Figure 5.8c) suggests that the salience of a stimulus in saccadic amplitude computation is a direct function of its *dissimilarity* to the background. Very similar conclusions can be drawn from the finding that local changes in spatial frequency also attract the eye (Deubel *et al.*, 1988). In this case, the salience of the distractor as reflected in its weight is a direct function of the spatial frequency difference between distractor and background.

Since the data reveal a continuous effect of target/background dissimilarity, this kind of experimental approach offers a novel methodological means to investigate the preattentive processing of complex visual signals. It is tempting to compare our results with data from experiments studying texture perception by conventional psychophysical approaches. Nothdurft (1985) quantitatively determined the discriminability of textures composed of oriented line elements very similar to the stimuli presented in Figure 5.8. Texture orientation difference, line length and element spacing were systematically varied. The results from these experiments indicated that texture discriminability is closely related to the orientation difference of related texture areas, in a quantitatively similar way as saccadic distraction is related to orientation difference. Together, these data represent another indication that processing of afferent signals may be identical for visual perception and oculomotor control (Zetzsche, Deubel and Elsner, 1984).

The global effect clearly represents some form of spatial integration. Findlay (1982) argued that averaging must arise because of the convergence of visual signals into a spatially integrative channel and suggested that a hypothetical correlate for such a channel might be a cell with a large receptive field. Cells with large receptive fields are indeed found in the superior colliculus and frontal eye fields, two brain centers involved in the control of saccadic eye movements. However, it now seems unlikely that any center of gravity calculation involving simple weighting of crude spatial information about the target elements could provide an appropriate signal for the texture-defined stimuli. The results suggest, rather, that spatial averaging as observed in the global effect occurs on a representation of the visual signal, which is already the result of complex visual preprocessing. Specifying the signal presented to the spatial integration stage has already involved extraction of orientation-specific information and comparison of this information across neighboring spatial regions. Obviously, the 'primal sketch' for saccade control consists of visual objects already segregated from the background structure. In this signal, surprisingly, texture changes and luminance changes appear to exert very similar influences as reflected in the data on latencies and amount of distraction.

In this sense, eye movements are immediate indicators of perceptual processes. The eye movement data presented above probably reflect a (genetically programmed?) hardwired property of the early visual system: an 'intelligent' processing which is optimized for effective perception. Since we further assume that eye movements are in a close relationship with visual selective attention, 'saccadic' salience as measured by means of saccadic eye movements in paradigms such as the double stimulus paradigm may provide a valuable, immediate observation of what in the visual world is salient, drawing attention. Thus, eye movement analysis may indeed provide a quantitative measure of early visual processing.

3.4.2   Implications for Neural Mechanisms of Target Selection

The finding that texture borders attract saccadic eye movements strongly supports the viewpoint that cortical pathways are involved in visually elicited saccades. The direct retinocollicular pathway is generally assumed not to exhibit selective properties to form aspects like orientation (Wurtz and Albano, 1980). The properties of collicular cells are rather nonspecific, showing most sensitivity to coarse, transient stimulation with large receptive fields (Goldberg and Wurtz, 1972; Sparks, 1986). The results from the texture experiments, however, show that the spatial signal for saccades is sensitive to the discrimination of texture areas defined by local orientation differences among small elements. It is therefore unlikely that the information about the locus of texture-defined targets is conveyed by the direct retinocollicular pathways. Retinal ganglion cells and cells of the lateral geniculate nucleus (LGN) also are most sensitive to differences in luminance and show no marked orientation selectivity. These neural structures may suffice to detect borders which are defined by a discontinuity in first-order statistics (equivalent to a luminance change). Striate cortex cells, on the other hand, show marked sensitivity to line orientation (Hubel and Wiesel, 1962). Thus, the striate cortex might detect differences in second-order statistics such as texture orientation differences as used in our experiments. In fact, Nothdurft and Li (1985) were able to demonstrate that responses of striate cortex cells of cats convey a representation of texture features defined by element orientation. In summary, the behavioral data presented here suggest strongly that a loop via the primary visual cortex is essential to account for the sensorimotor processing of more complex targets such as textures.

4 COGNITIVE FACTORS IN SACCADE GENERATION

The previous section reviewed some of the various effects that the sensory stimulus exerts on the generation of saccadic eye movements. In that sense, the major emphasis has been on the attempt to present and discuss the bottom-up (stimulus-driven) aspects of the sensorimotor transformation. Most of the work previously described is indeed characterized by the situation that, at a time unpredictable for the subject, a target or a stimulus pattern appears transiently, and the interest was specifically in the properties of the initial saccade. Certainly, again, this is far from the ecological situation where the eye scans a rather stationary scene in which objects only rarely appear or disappear completely. It is not surprising that, under more natural, static conditions, the effects of instruction, knowledge, context etc. seemingly predominate in the scanning pattern. This becomes especially clear in highly learned tasks such as reading. However, only a few studies exist that attempt to bridge the gap between the paradigms of stimulus elicitation and free scanning. At many places in the previous argument it became obvious that the understanding of all aspects of the response requires the consideration of higher-level factors. The last of the empirically oriented paragraphs will touch on a few examples of how the basic, experimentally oriented paradigms presented here may be supplemented by investigations specific to the role of higher-level processing.

The first aspect concerns the interaction with spatial attention. Attentional processes were invoked earlier to account for observations such as the occurrence of express saccades and target selection in double stimulus situations. Despite the obvious plausibility of a tight relationship between saccades and oriented attention, the exact nature of this link is still not clear. The next paragraph reviews some of the relevant empirical work that has been specifically aimed at these questions.

4.1 Saccadic Eye Movements and Selective Visual Attention

The modern prevalence of the functionalist approach that came along with the move from behaviorism to cognitive psychology has made 'attention' a central research objective of experimental psychology. Selective spatial attention is described as an alignment of processing capabilities with selective aspects of the sensory input, and has been demonstrated in well-known experiments showing that the precueing of a location in the visual field leads to a local advantage in reaction time and discrimination performance (Eriksen and Hoffman, 1973; Posner, 1980). This led to the establishment of the metaphor of a 'spotlight' or an 'attentional beam' to describe the effects of attentional selection.[1] The question soon arose as to what extent these shifts of the 'eye of the mind' can occur independently

---

[1]It should be mentioned, though, that the spotlight metaphor has a much longer history in psychology (see Helmholtz, 1866; James, 1890; Wundt, 1903.

of eye movements and vice versa. Today it seems to be well established that the focus of attention can be shifted about without any eye movements (Posner, Snyder and Davidson, 1980; Reeves and Sperling, 1986). Whether the inverse is true, however, i.e. whether the eyes could be moved to a visual target *without* an obligatory, concomitant shift of attention, is still an open question and there is indeed some suggestive evidence against this hypothesis.

Klein (1980) was among the first to attack this question directly. He used a paradigm where saccades were programmed to a location in the field while the subjects were also instructed to press a button on the appearance of a visual stimulus. The question was whether, on the one hand, saccadic reaction was speeded by the allocation of attention and, on the other hand, manual reactions were facilitated by a saccade directed to a target at the stimulus location. Neither effect was confirmed, and this result led Klein to conclude that the programming of saccades did not automatically compel a shift of attention. Several features of Klein's experiments, however, suggest caution in accepting these conclusions. For instance, his subjects had to perform a relatively difficult discrimination task which resulted in extremely long saccadic and manual reaction times. It may be argued therefore that the results cannot be generalized to conditions that involve normal, rapid reactions.

A somewhat different picture was indeed revealed from a number of follow-up studies. Remington (1980) conducted a series of detection experiments that analyzed, in more detail, the time course of the shifts of attention with saccades. Subjects were required to detect a 3 ms probe stimulus that appeared with various asynchronies with the onset of a saccade target. Locations of the saccade target and test stimulus were varied among four positions. The results showed that detection performance before and after the eye movement was best when cue position was also the saccade target position, suggesting that a shift of attention preceded the eye movement. He concluded that a peripheral cue summons both eye movement and attention, but that separate mechanisms may control the two movements. Shepherd, Findlay and Hockey (1986) later criticized that in the majority of these previous experiments attention could be automatically 'captured' by the onset of the peripheral stimulus and, therefore, the experiments could not distinguish between the effects caused by the stimulus and those that resulted from the eye saccades. Hence, in their study saccades were directed by a central arrow while spatial attention was manipulated by varying the probability of a test stimulus appearing at different allocations. It turned out that the manual reaction to the probe stimulus was facilitated when its location was at the same side as the saccade target, irrespective of the probability manipulation, suggesting that the effect of preparing a saccade was stronger than the effect of voluntary attentional allocation. From this, the authors concluded that it is not possible to make an eye movement without making a corresponding attentional shift.

In summary, the empirical evidence shows that the allocation of attention to a peripheral position can be facilitated by the programming of an eye movement to this position, and saccadic reaction times can be reduced by allocating attention to the target position. It may be tentatively suggested – although this suggestion is not yet based on decisive data – that shifts of attention form an obligatory part of the program for target-directed saccades. How tight this link actually is, spatially and temporally, remains to be investigated. It must be tested by concurrent measurements of saccades and perceptual attention whether or not the attended location is also the landing point of the saccade. Moreover, it would be important to see whether expressive properties of saccadic reactions, such as the amplitude transition in double step stimuli or the center of gravity effect, are also equivalently present in attentional control.[2]

4.2   Sequences of Saccades

Another important aspect that has not yet been covered by the previously described work concerns the question as to how much of the processes of target selection, amplitude computation and saccade triggering occurs on a fixation-to-fixation basis and how much is pre-planned. Since all necessary information is available at each fixation, saccades could indeed well rely on the target on the actual retinal pattern only. Zingale and Kowler (1987) approached this question by letting two subjects scan 1–5 stationary targets in sequence, which were located at the vertices of an imaginary pentagon. Essentially, the authors found that the latency of the first saccade in the sequence and the intersaccadic intervals of the following saccades depended on the number of items to be scanned; this is clearly not to be expected if saccades are programmed on a fixation-to-fixation basis. Similar observations were made by Inhoff (1986). Latency increased by approximately 20 ms per target to be scanned. Interestingly, the data were very similar when the targets were removed before the start of the scanning sequence, so that the saccades were to be directed to memorized target locations. From this, Zingale and Kowler concluded that the observed dependence of saccades on the sequence was not a result of the properties of the visual error signal. Rather, they suggested that before motor execution, organized plans for patterns of saccades are established in memory. After the plans have been built up, visual error signals may merely modify and elaborate the specific saccade parameters during the execution of the sequence. They linked their data closely to models of typing and speech production put forward by Sternberg *et al.* (1978) in which the plans for the execution of a sequence of motor responses are stored in memory before the sequence actually begins. In these models, response latency increases with sequence length because the information has to be retrieved by a serial memory search process.

   These findings seem surprising since it is not quite comprehensible why, while precise visual information is available, the saccadic system should rely on rather imprecise representations of spatial response structure in memory. Zingale and Kowler (1987), however, argue quite convincingly that if a patterned sequence of saccades is preplanned, its execution may proceed with relatively little effort, relieving attentional resources for the analysis of the contents of the scene. Also, they put forward that normally saccade sequences are accompanied by concomitant movements of the head, limbs and fingers, and a single central motor controller may sequence the disparate motor elements into a purposeful pattern of activity.

5   SUMMARY AND CONCLUSION

This chapter started with the question whether we should see saccades as voluntary motor activities or as reflexive reactions elicited and determined by peripheral stimuli. Empirical work has demonstrated how the saccadic response is determined

---

[2]The important role of selective spatial attention was also demonstrated for the control of vergence (Erkelens and Collewijn, 1991).

by both sensorimotor constraints and higher-level central processes. Indeed, apart from the properties of motor signal generation, it seems clear that eye movements can be understood only when both lower-level visual factors and cognitive, internal factors are taken into consideration. It has been shown that, when a single target is provided, saccadic *latency* depends on sensory factors such as luminance, contrast and color, and this becomes most pronounced at or below foveal threshold. However, for sufficiently bright targets, subjective factors become dominant, reflected in the strong effects of forewarning and spatial attention, and of the difference between individuals. *Spatial parameters* of saccadic reactions seem almost stereotyped in their precision, although of course the subject can voluntarily suppress the saccade, deliberately land short of the target or simply look in the opposite direction.

When more than one stimulus is present in the visual field, averaging responses aim at a local center of gravity of the preprocessed input (preprocessing may include preattentive figure/ground discrimination). On the other hand, *voluntary effort, preknowledge and training* may overrule this tendency, leading to accurate responses, at the cost of speed of response. Also, one probably cannot generalize immediately from the case of stimuli which appear suddenly in the visual field to the case of scanning of static pictures. Here it seems that averaging effects are, if present at all, rather small, indicating that transient appearance of the visual display could be a determining factor. This factor is also central in linking the saccadic program to involuntary shifts of attention. So, it is the case that neither the stimulus nor the observer completely determines the oculomotor reaction. Instead, we should 'regard the saccade as a key to unlock the interface between environment and cognition' (Findlay, 1992).

Further, the empirical evidence reviewed in this article emphasized that eye movement research should include careful study of the sensory processing in the visual system. Visual processing is an integral part of saccade control. Empirical observations that have been attributed to the motor part of the system can possibly be better understood when they are interpreted as an effect of the sensory processes. In other words, the oculomotor system should be seen less as a specific module for movement production, but rather – more holistically – as a representative example of a complete sensorimotor loop. In other words, concurrent study of visual processing, cognitive factors and oculomotor performance is required, and all three elements need to be included in a theory on how eye movements function in the natural world.

It also became clear that sensorimotor control in the saccadic system is based upon processes that are highly flexible, allowing 'switching' between different response modes dependent on the requirements given by the environment. A further complication arises from the fact that the eye movement proper changes the retinal input profoundly. This transient change affects vision and should be included in the interpretation of corrective saccades, scanning movements, visual search and reading data. Finally, we should never lose sight of the fact that the basic, and only, oculomotor function is that each eye be oriented optimally with respect to the object of current interest. This requires, in subsequent processing steps, the selection of the target among many potential targets, the computation of its spatial location and the generation of movement itself. Certainly, a central control is required for this purpose that interprets the many afferent and reafferent signals and organizes the 'orchestration' of eye movements, also taking into account other motor activities. It seems likely that gaze control has evolved as a holistic system rather than as separate subsystems with partial, and often conflicting, goals. The many facets of interaction will become clear only when the performance of the oculomotor system is observed in the complex environment that it is normally confronted with by nature.

REFERENCES

Andersen, R. A. (1989). Visual and eye-movement functions of the posterior parietal cortex. *Annual Review of Neuroscience,* **12,** 377–403.

Bahill, A. T., Adler, D. and Stark, L. (1975). Most naturally occurring eye movements have magnitudes 15 degrees or less. *Investigative Ophthalmology and Visual Science,* **14,** 468–469.

Bahill, A. T., Clark, M. R. and Stark, L. (1975). Dynamic overshoot in saccadic eye movements is caused by neurological control signal reversals. *Experimental Neurology,* **48,** 107–122.

Barbur, J. L., Forsyth, P. M. and Findlay, J. M. (1988). Human saccadic eye movements in the absence of the geniculo-calcarine projection. *Brain,* **111,** 63–82.

Barlow, H. B. (1952). Eye movements during fixation. *Journal of Physiology (London),* **116,** 290–306.

Becker, W. (1972). The control of eye movements in the saccadic system. In J. Dichgans and E. Bizzi (Eds), *Cerebral Control of Eye Movements and Motion Perception* (pp. 233–243). Basel: Karger.

Becker, W. (1991). Saccades. In R. H. S. Carpenter (Ed.), *Vision and Visual Dysfunction,* vol. 8: *Eye Movements.* Basingstoke: Macmillan.

Becker, W. and Jürgens, R. (1979). An analysis of the saccadic system by means of double-step stimuli. *Vision Research,* **19,** 967–983.

Bertelson, P. and Tisseyre, R. F. (1968). The time-course of preparation with regular and irregular foreperiods. *Quarterly Journal of Experimental Psychology,* **20,** 297–300.

Boch, R. and Fischer, B. (1986). Further observations on the occurrence of express-saccades in the monkey. *Experimental Brain Research,* **63,** 487–494.

Boch, R., Fischer, B. and Ramsperger, E. (1984). Express saccades in the monkey: Reaction times versus intensity, size, duration, and eccentricity of their targets. *Experimental Brain Research,* **55,** 223–231.

Carpenter, R. H. S. (1988). *Movements of the Eyes* (2nd edn). London: Pion.

Carpenter, R. H. S. (1991a). *Vision and Visual Dysfunction,* vol. 8: *Eye Movements.* Basingstoke: Macmillan.

Carpenter, R. H. S. (1991b). The visual origins of ocular motility. *Vision and Visual Dysfunction* vol. 8: *Eye Movements* (pp. 1–10). Basingstoke: Macmillan.

Coëffé, C. (1987). Two ways of improving saccade accuracy. In J. K. O'Regan and A. Lévy-Schoen (Eds), *Eye Movements: From Physiology to Cognition* (pp. 105–114). Amsterdam: North Holland.

Coëffé, C. and O'Regan, J. K. (1987). Reducing the influence of non-target stimuli on saccade accuracy: Predictability and latency effects. *Vision Research,* **27,** 227–240.

Collewijn, H., Erkelens, C. J. and Steinman, R. M. (1988a). Binocular coordination of human horizontal saccadic eye movements. *Journal of Physiology (London),* **404,** 157–182.

Collewijn, H., Erkelens, C. J. and Steinman, R. M. (1988b). Binocular coordination of human vertical saccadic eye movements. *Journal of Physiology (London),* **404,** 183–197.

Collewijn, H., Steinman, R. M., Erkelens, C. J., Pizlo, Z. and van der Stein, J. (1990). The effect of freeing the head on eye movement characteristics during 3-D shifts of gaze and tracking. In A. Berthoz, W. Graf and P. P. Vidal (Eds), *The Head–Neck Sensory Motor System.* New York: Oxford University Press.

Coren, S. and Hoenig, P. (1972). Effect of non-target stimuli on the length of voluntary saccades. *Perceptual and Motor Skills,* **34,** 499–508.

Crane, H. D. and Steele, C. M. (1985). Generation V dual-Purkinje-image eye-tracker. *Applied Optics*, **24**, 527–537.

Deubel, H. (1984). Wechselwirkung von Sensorik und Motorik bei Augenbewegungen. Eine kybernetische Beschreibung des visuellen Systems. Unpublished doctoral dissertation, Technical University of Munich, Germany.

Deubel, H. (1987). Adaptivity of gain and direction in oblique saccades. In J. K. O'Regan and A. Lévy-Schoen (Eds), *Eye Movements: From Physiology to Cognition* (pp. 181–190). Amsterdam: North Holland.

Deubel, H. (1989). Sensory and motor aspects of saccade control. *European Archives of Psychiatry and Neurological Sciences*, **239(N1)**, 17–22.

Deubel, H. (1991a). Adaptive control of saccade metrics. In G. Obrecht and L. W. Stark (Eds), *Presbyopia Research* (pp. 93–100). New York: Plenum Press.

Deubel, H. (1991b). Plasticity of metrical and dynamical aspects of saccadic eye movements. In J. Requin and G. E. Stelmach (Eds), *Tutorials in Motor Neuroscience* (pp. 563–579). Dordrecht: Kluwer.

Deubel, H., Elsner, T. and Hauske, G. (1987). Saccadic eye movements and the detection of fast-moving gratings. *Biological Cybernetics*, **57**, 37–45.

Deubel, H., Findlay, J., Jacobs, A. and Brogan, D. (1988). Saccadic eye movements to targets defined by structure differences. In G. Lüer, U. Lass, and J. Shallo-Hoffmann (Eds), *Eye Movement Research: Physiological and Psychological Aspects* (pp. 107-145). Göttingen, Toronto: Hogrefe.

Deubel, H. and Frank, H. (1991). The latency of saccadic eye movements to texture-defined stimuli. In R. Schmid and D. Zambarbieri (Eds), *Oculomotor Control and Cognitive Processes* (pp. 369–384). Amsterdam, New York: Elsevier.

Deubel, H. and Hauske, G. (1988). The programming of visually guided saccades. In H. Marko, G. Hauske and A. Struppler (Eds), *Processing Structures for Perception and Action* (pp. 119–132). Weinheim: Verlag Chemie.

Deubel, H. and Wolf, W. (1982). The programming of correction saccades by retinal feedback. *Investigative Ophthalmology and Visual Science*, **22** (Suppl), 86.

Deubel, H., Wolf, W. and Hauske, G. (1982). Corrective saccades: Effect of shifting the saccade goal. *Vision Research*, **22**, 353–364.

Deubel, H., Wolf, W. and Hauske, G. (1984). The evaluation of the oculomotor error signal. In A. G. Gale and F. Johnson (Eds), *Theoretical and Applied Aspects of Eye Movement Research* (pp. 55–62). Amsterdam, New York: Elsevier.

Deubel, H., Wolf, W. and Hauske, G. (1986). Adaptive gain-control of saccadic eye movements. *Human Neurobiology*, **5**, 245–253.

Ditchburn, R. W. (1973). *Eye Movements and Visual Perception*. Oxford: Clarendon Press.

Ditchburn, R. W. and Ginsborg, B. L. (1953). Involuntary eye movements during fixation. *Journal of Physiology (London)*, **119**, 1–17.

Dodge, R. and Cline, T. S. (1901). The angle velocity of eye-movements. *Psychological Review*, **8**, 145–157.

Doma, H. and Hallett, P. E. (1988). Rod cone dependence of saccadic eye-movement latency in a foveating task. *Vision Research*, **28**, 899–913.

Donders, F. C. (1847). Beitrag zur Lehre von den Bewegungen des menschlichen Auges. *Holländische Beiträge zu den anatomischen und physiologischen Wissenschaften*, **1**, 104–145, 384–386.

Dürsteler, M. R. and Wurtz, R. H. (1988). Pursuit and optokinetic deficits following chemical lesions of cortical areas mt and mst. *Journal of Neurophysiology*, **60**, 940–965.

Duhamel, J.-R., Colby, C. L. and Goldberg, M. E. (1992). The updating of the representation of visual space in parietal cortex by intended eye movements. *Science*, **255**, 90–92.

Eriksen, C. W. and Hoffman, J. (1973). The extent of processing of noise elements during selective encoding from visual displays. *Perception and Psychophysics*, **14**, 155–160.

Erkelens, C. J. and Collewijn, H. (1991). Control of vergence – gating among disparity inputs by voluntary target selection. *Experimental Brain Research*, **87**, 671–678.

Ferman, L., Collewijn, H. and van den Berg, A. V. (1987). A direct test of Listing's Law – II: Human ocular torsion measured under dynamic conditions. *Vision Research, 27,* 939–951.

Findlay, J. M. (1980). The visual stimulus for saccadic eye movements in human observers. *Perception, 9,* 7–21.

Findlay, J. M. (1981a). Spatial and temporal factors in the predictive generation of saccadic eye movements. *Vision Research, 21,* 347–354.

Findlay, J. M. (1981b). Local and global influences on saccadic eye movements. In D. E. Fisher, R. A. Monty, and J. W. Senders (Eds), *Eye Movements: Cognition and Visual Perception.* Hillsdale, NJ: Erlbaum.

Findlay, J. M. (1982). Global visual processing for saccadic eye movements. *Vision Research, 22,* 1033–1045.

Findlay, J. M. (1992). Programming of stimulus-elicited saccadic eye movements. In K. Rayner (Ed.), *Eye Movements and Visual Cognition.* New York: Springer.

Findlay, J. M. and Crawford, T. J. (1983). The visual control of saccadic eye movements: Evidence for limited plasticity. In R. Groner, C. Menz, D. F. Fisher, and R. A. Monty (Eds), *Eye Movements and Physiological Processes: International Views* (pp. 115–127). Hillsdale, NJ: Erlbaum.

Findlay, J. M. and Harris, L. R. (1984). Small saccades to double-stepped targets moving in two dimensions. In A. G. Gale and F. Johnston (Eds), *Theoretical and Applied Aspects of Eye Movement Research* (pp. 71–78). Amsterdam, New York: Elsevier.

Fischer, B. (1987). The preparation of visually guided saccades. *Review of Physiological and Biochemical Pharmacology, 106,* 1–35.

Fischer, B. and Breitmeyer, B. (1987). Mechanisms of visual attention revealed by saccadic eye movements. *Neuropsychologia, 25,* 73–83.

Fischer, B. and Ramsperger, E. (1984). Human express saccades: Extremely short reaction times of goal-directed eye movements. *Experimental Brain Research, 57,* 191–195.

Fischer, B. and Ramsperger, E. (1986). Human express saccades: Effects of randomization and daily practice. *Experimental Brain Research, 64,* 569–578.

Fuchs, A. F., Kaneko, C. R. and Scudder, C. A. (1985). Brainstem control of saccadic eye movements. *Annual Review of Neuroscience, 8,* 307–337.

Goldberg, M. E. and Bruce, C. J. (1990). Primate frontal eye fields. vol. 3: Maintenance of a spatially accurate saccade signal. *Journal of Neurophysiology, 64,* 489–508.

Goldberg, M. E. and Wurtz, R. H. (1972). Activity of superior colliculus cells in behaving monkey. vol. I: Visual receptive fields of single neurons. *Journal of Neurophysiology, 35,* 542–559.

Guitton, D., Buchtel, H. A. and Douglas, R. M. (1985). Frontal lobe lesions in man cause difficulties in suppressing reflexive glances and in generating goal-directed saccades. *Experimental Brain Research, 58,* 455–472.

Haegerstrom-Portnoy, G. and Brown, B. (1979). Contrast effects on smooth pursuit eye movement velocity. *Vision Research, 19,* 169–174.

Hallett, P. E. (1978). Primary and secondary saccades to goals defined by instructions. *Vision Research, 18,* 1279–1296.

Hallett, P. E. (1986). Eye movements. In K. R. Boff, L. Kaufman, and J. P. Thomas (Eds), *Handbook of Perception and Human Performance* (ch. 10). New York: John Wiley.

Hallett, P. E. and Lightstone, A. D. (1976a). Saccadic eye movements towards stimuli triggered by prior saccades. *Vision Research, 16,* 99–106.

Hallett, P. E. and Lightstone, A. D. (1976b). Saccadic eye movements to flashed targets. *Vision Research, 16,* 107–114.

He, P. and Kowler, E. (1989). The role of location probability in the programming of saccades: Implications for 'center-of-gravity' tendencies. *Vision Research, 29,* 1165–1181.

Helmholtz, H. von (1866/1962). *Physiological Optics.* New York: Dover.

Henson, D. B. (1978). Corrective saccades: Effect of altering visual feedback. *Vision Research, 18,* 63–67.

Hikosaka, O. and Wurtz, R. H. (1983). Visual and oculomotor functions of the substantia nigra pars reticulata. IV: Relation of substantia nigra to superior colliculus. *Journal of Neurophysiology*, **49**, 1285–1301.

Hubel, D. H. and Wiesel, T. N. (1962). Receptive fields, binocular interaction, and functional architecture in the cat's visual cortex. *Journal of Physiology*, **160**, 106–154

Inhoff, A. W. (1986). Preparing sequences of saccades under choice reaction conditions: Effects of sequence length and context. *Acta Psychologica*, **61**, 211–228,

Jacobs, A. M. (1987). On localization and saccade programming. *Vision Research*, **27**, 1953–1966.

James, W. (1890). *The Principles of Psychology*. New York: Dover.

Jonides, J. and Yantis, S. (1988). Uniqueness of abrupt visual onset in capturing attention. *Perception and Psychophysics*, **43**, 346–354.

Julesz, B. (1986). Texton gradients: The texton theory revisited. *Biological Cybernetics*, **54**, 245–251.

Julesz, B. and Bergen, J. R. (1983). Textons, the fundamental elements in preattentive vision and perception of textures. *Bell Systems Technical Journal*, **62**, 1619–1645.

Just, M. A. and Carpenter, P. (1976). Eye fixations and cognitive processes. *Cognitive Psychology*, **8**, 441–480.

Jüttner, M. and Wolf, W. (1992). Occurrence of human express saccades depends on stimulus uncertainty and stimulus sequence. *Experimental Brain Research*, **89**, 678–681.

Kapoula, Z. (1985). Evidence for a range effect in the saccadic system. *Vision Research*, **25**, 1155–1157.

Klein, R. (1980). Does oculomotor readiness mediate cognitive control of visual attention? In R. Nickerson (Ed.), *Attention and Performance*, vol. VIII (pp. 259–276). Hillsdale, NJ: Erlbaum.

Koenderink, J. J. and van Doorn, A.J. (1978). Visual detection of spatial contrast influence of location in the visual field, target extent, and illuminance level. *Biological Cybernetics*, **30**, 157–167.

Kowler, E. (1990). *Reviews of Oculomotor Research*, vol. 4: *Eye Movements and their Role in Visual and Cognitive Processes*. Amsterdam, New York: Elsevier.

Kowler, E., Martins, A. J. and Pavel, M. (1984). The effect of expectations on slow oculomotor control. IV: Anticipatory smooth eye movements depend on prior target motions. *Vision Research*, **24**, 197–210.

Lemij, H. G. and Collewijn, H. (1989). Differences in accuracy of human saccades between stationary and jumping targets. *Vision Research*, **29**, 1737–1748.

Lévy-Schoen, A. (1969). Détermination et latence de la reponse oculomotrice à deux stimulus simultanés ou successifs selon leur eccentricité relative. *L'Année Psychologigue*, **69**, 373–392.

Lévy-Schoen, A., and Blanc-Garin, J. (1974). On oculomotor programming and perception. *Brain Research*, **71**, 443–450.

Mayfrank, L., Mobashery, M., Kimmig, H. and Fischer, B. (1986). The role of fixation and visual attention in the occurrence of express saccades in man. *European Archives of Psychiatry and Neurological Sciences*, **235**, 269–275.

Menz, C. and Groner, R. (1987). Saccadic programming with multiple targets under different task conditions. In J. K. O'Regan and A. Lévy-Schoen (Eds), *Eye Movements: From Physiology to Cognition*. Amsterdam: North Holland.

Mohler, C. W. and Wurtz, R. H. (1977). Role of striate cortex and superior colliculus in visual guidance of saccadic eye movements in monkey. *Journal of Neurophysiology*, **40**, 74–94.

Murphy, B. J., Kowler, E. and Steinman, R. M. (1975). Slow oculomotor control in the presence of moving backgrounds. *Vision Research*, **15**, 1263–1268.

Nakayama, K. and Mackeben, M. (1989). Sustained and transient components of focal visual attention. *Vision Research*, **29**, 1631–1647.

Neisser, U. (1967). *Cognitive Psychology*. New York: Appleton-Century-Crofts.

Nothdurft, H. C. (1985). Sensitivity for structure gradient in texture discrimination tasks. *Vision Research*, **25**, 1957–1968.

Nothdurft, H. C. and Li, C. Y. (1985). Texture discrimination: Representation of orientation and luminance differences in cells of the cat striate cortex. *Vision Research,* **25,** 99–113.

Noton, D. and Stark, L. (1971). Scanpaths in saccadic eye movements while viewing and recognizing patterns. *Vision Research,* **11,** 929–942.

Ottes, F. P., van Gisbergen, J. A. M. and Eggermont, J. J. (1984). Metrics of saccade responses to visual double stimuli: Two different modes. *Vision Research,* **24,** 1169–1179.

Ottes, F. P., van Gisbergen, J. A. M. and Eggermont, J. J. (1985). Latency dependence of colour-based target versus non-target discrimination by the saccadic system. *Vision Research,* **24,** 826–849.

Palmer, D. A. (1966). A system of mesopic photometry. *Nature,* **209,** 276–281.

Perenin, M. T. and Jeannerod, M. (1975). Residual vision in cortically blind hemifields. *Neuropsychologia,* **13,** 1–7.

Pöppel, E., Held, R. and Frost, D. (1973). Residual visual function after brain wounds involving the central visual pathways in man. *Nature,* **243,** 295–296.

Posner, M. I. (1980). Orienting of attention. *Quarterly Journal of Experimental Psychology,* **32,** 3–25.

Posner, M. I., Snyder, C. R. R. and Davidson, B. J. (1980). Attention and the detection of signals. *Journal of Experimental Psychology,* **109,** 160–174.

Rayner, K. (1978). Eye movements in reading and information processing. *Psychological Bulletin,* **85,** 618–660.

Reeves, A. and Sperling, G. (1986). Attention gating in short-term visual memory. *Psychological Review,* **93,** 180–206.

Remington, R. W. (1980). Attention and saccadic eye movements. *Journal of Experimental Psychology: Human Perception and Performance,* **6,** 726–744.

Reulen, J. P. H. (1984a). Latency of visually evoked saccadic eye movements, I. Saccadic latency and the facilitation model. *Biological Cybernetics,* **50,** 251–262.

Reulen, J. P. H. (1984b). Latency of visually evoked saccadic eye movements, II. Temporal properties of the facilitation mechanism. *Biological Cybernetics,* **50,** 263–271.

Riggs, L. A. and Ratliff, F. (1951). Visual acuity and the normal tremor of the eyes. *Science,* **114,** 17–18.

Robinson, D. A. (1963). A method for measuring eye movements using a scleral search coil in a magnetic field. *IEEE Transactions of Biomedical Engineering,* **26,** 137–145.

Robinson, D. A. (1964). The mechanics of human saccadic eye movements. *Journal of Physiology (London),* **174,** 245–264.

Robinson, D. A. (1965). The mechanics of human smooth pursuit eye movement. *Journal of Physiology,* **180,** 569–591.

Robinson, D. A. (1973). Models of the saccadic eye movement control system. *Kybernetik,* **14,** 71–83.

Robinson, D. A. (1975). Oculomotor control signals. In G. Lennerstrand and P. Bachy-Rita (Eds), *Basic Mechanisms of Ocular Motility and their Clinical Implications* (pp. 337–374). Oxford, New York: Pergamon Press.

Robinson, D. A. (1981). The use of control systems analysis in the neurophysiology of eye movements. *Annual Review of Neuroscience,* **4,** 463–503.

Robinson, D. A. (1982). A model of cancellation of the vestibulo-ocular reflex. In G. Lennerstrand, D. S. Zee, and E. Keller (Eds), *Functional Basis of Ocular Motility Disorders* (pp. 5–13). Oxford: Pergamon Press.

Ross, L. E. and Ross, S. M. (1980). Saccade latency and warning signals: Stimulus onset, offset, and change as warning events. *Perception and Psychophysics,* **27,** 251–257.

Rovamo, J. and Virsu, V. (1979). An estimation and application of the human cortical magnification factor. *Experimental Brain Research,* **37,** 495–510.

Rovamo, J., Virsu, V. and Näsänen, R. (1978). Cortical magnification factor predicts the photopic contrast sensitivity for peripheral vision. *Nature,* **271,** 54–55.

Saslow, M. G. (1967a). Effects of components of displacement step stimuli upon latency for saccadic eye movement. *Journal of the Optical Society of America,* **57,** 1024–1029.

Saslow, M. G. (1967b). Latency for saccadic eye movement. *Journal of the Optical Society of America,* **57,** 1030–1033.

Schiller, P., Sandell, J. H. and Maunsell, J. H. R. (1987). The effect of frontal eyefield and superior colliculus lesions on saccadic latencies in the rhesus monkey. *Journal of Neurophysiology, 57*, 1033–1049.

Schiller, P. H., True, S. D. and Conway, J. L. (1980). Deficits in eye movements following frontal eye field and superior colliculus ablations. *Journal of Neurophysiology, 44*, 1175–1189.

Scudder, C. A. (1988). A new local feedback model of the saccadic burst generator. *Journal of Neurophysiology, 59*, 1455–1475.

Shepherd, M., Findlay, J. M. and Hockey, R. J. (1986). The relationship between eye movements and spatial attention. *The Quarterly Journal of Experimental Psychology, 38*, 475–491.

Smit, A. C., van Gisbergen, J. A. M. and Cools, A. R. (1987). A parametric analysis of human saccades in different experimental paradigms. *Vision Research, 27*, 1745–1762.

Sparks, D. L. (1986). Translation of sensory signals into commands for control of saccadic eye movements: Role of primate superior colliculus. *Physiological Review, 66*, 118–171.

Steinman, R. M. and Levinson, J. Z. (1990). The role of eye movement in the detection of contrast and spatial detail. In E. Kowler (Ed.), *Reviews of Oculomotor Research*, vol. 4: *Eye Movements and their Role in Visual and Cognitive Processes* (pp. 115–212). Amsterdam, New York: Elsevier.

Sternberg, S., Monsell, S., Knoll, R. and Wright, C. (1978). The latency and duration of rapid movement sequences: Comparisons of speech and typewriting. In G. E. Stelmach (Ed.), *Information Processing in Motor Control and Learning* (pp. 117–152). New York: Academic Press.

van Asten, W. N. J. C. and Gielen, C. C. A. M. (1987). Comparison between psychophysical and saccadic responses to near threshold visual stimuli. In J. K. O'Regan and A. Lévy-Schoen (Eds), *Eye Movements: From Physiology to Cognition* (pp. 152–153). Amsterdam: North Holland.

van Gisbergen, J. A. M., Robinson, D. A. and Gielen, S. (1981). A quantitative analysis of generation of saccadic eye movements by burst neurons. *Journal of Neurophysiology, 45*, 417–442.

Viviani, P. (1990). Eye movements in visual search: Cognitive, perceptual and motor control aspects. In E. Kowler (Ed.), *Reviews of Oculomotor Research*, vol. 4: *Eye Movements and their Role in Visual and Cognitive Processes* (pp. 353–393). Amsterdam, New York: Elsevier.

Viviani, P. and Swensson, R. (1982). Saccadic eye movements to peripherally discriminated visual targets. *Journal of Experimental Psychology: Human Perception and Performance, 8*, 113–126.

Walls, G. L. (1962). The evolutionary history of eye movements. *Vision Research, 2*, 69–80.

Weber, H., Fischer, B., Bach, M. and Aiple, F. (1991). Occurrence of express saccades under isoluminance and low contrast luminance conditions. *Visual Neuroscience, 7*, 505–510.

Westheimer, G. (1954a). The mechanism of saccadic eye movements. *Archives of Ophthalmology, 52*, 710–714.

Westheimer, G. (1954b). Eye movement responses to a horizontally moving stimulus. *Archives of Ophthalmology, 52*, 932–941.

Westheimer, G. and McKee, S. P. (1975). Visual acuity in the presence of retinal-image motion. *Journal of the Optical Society of America, 65*, 847–850.

Wheeless, L. L. (1967). Luminance as a parameter of the eye-movement control system. *Journal of the Optical Society of America, 57*, 394–400.

Wheeless, L. L., Boynton, R. and Cohen, G. (1966). Eye movement responses to step and pulse-step stimuli. *Journal of the Optical Society of America, 56*, 956–960.

Wundt, W. (1903). *Physiologische Psychologie*, vol. III (5th edn). Leipzig: Engelmann.

Wurtz, R. H. and Albano, J. E. (1980). Visual-motor function of the primate superior colliculus. *Annual Review of Neuroscience, 3*, 189–226.

Wurtz, R. H. and Goldberg, M. E. (1989). *Reviews of Oculomotor Research*, vol. 3:, *The Neurobiology of Saccadic Eye Movements*. Amsterdam: Elsevier.

Yarbus, A. L. (1967). *Eye Movements and Vision*. New York: Plenum Press.

Young, L. R. and Stark, L. (1962). A sampled-data model for eye tracking movements. *Quarterly Progress Report, Research Lab of Electronics MIT*, **66**, 370–384.

Young, L. R. and Stark, L. (1963). Variable feedback experiments testing a sampled data model for eye tracking movements. *IEEE Transactions on Human Factors in Engineering*, **1**, 38–51.

Zetzsche, C., Deubel, H. and Elsner, T. (1984). Similar mechanisms of visual processing in perception and oculomotor control. *Perception*, **13**, A16.

Zihl, J. (1980). 'Blindsight': Improvement of visually guided eye movements by systematic practice in patients with cerebellar blindness. *Neuropsychologia*, **18**, 71–77.

Zingale, C. M. and Kowler, E. (1987). Planning sequences of saccades. *Vision Research*, **27**, 1327–1341.

Chapter 6

Extraretinal Signals in Visual Orientation

Bruce Bridgeman

University of California, Santa Cruz

1 INTRODUCTION

Visual perception is not simply a matter of information flowing from the outside through the eyes into the brain. Perception can be passive only as long as it requires merely recognition of external events or patterns relative to one another. As soon as visual information is used for making judgements relative to the self, or if it guides behavior, information about the positions of the receptors in the world is needed. Receptor information and optic information can then be combined to determine the positions of objects relative to the self.

Information about the positions of visual receptors relative to the head and body might come either from mechanoreceptors in the muscles controlling the positions of the visual receptors (a proprioception or 'inflow' from the periphery to the brain), or from an internal monitoring of the innervations sent to those muscles (an efference copy or 'outflow' from the brain to the periphery). Matin (1972) used the term 'extraretinal signal' to describe information about visual receptor position coming either from inflow or from outflow.

This chapter reviews the relative contributions of oculomotor inflow and outflow to perception of location and to visually guided behavior, and then concentrates on the properties of outflow. Coverage is limited to translations of the visual array rather than rotations, and is largely confined to the horizontal dimension and to the fixed head, where there is no role for gravity receptors, head acceleration receptors and skeletal muscle proprioceptors. The literature citations are not exhaustive, but rather are selected to address specific questions about outflow and inflow.

The literature can be clarified by differentiating influences on perception and influences on visually guided behavior; there is now extensive evidence that these two visual functions are separately represented at some stages of visual processing and that they follow different rules (Bridgeman, 1981, 1986; Goodale *et al*, 1994; Paillard, 1987; Wong and Mack, 1981). Following the nomenclature of Paillard (1987), these will be called the *cognitive* and *sensorimotor systems*, respectively. The two systems have been applied in many contexts and given many different names. Seven sets of contrasting terms, along with their principal originators, are given in Table 6.1 – a 'Rosetta stone' of terms for the two branches of the visual system. It is not yet clear whether all of the sets refer to the same neurological machinery, for some of them address different aspects of behavior. However, all share a common

Handbook of Perception and Action: Volume 1
ISBN 0-12-516161-1

Table 6.1. A 'Rosetta stone' of terms for the two branches
of the visual system

Terms		Originator
Focal	Ambient	C. Trevarthen
Experiential	Action	M. Goodale
Cognitive	Motor	B. Bridgeman
Cognitive	Sensorimotor	J. Paillard
Explicit	Implicit	L. Weiskrantz
Object	Spatial	M. Mishkin
Overt	Covert	K. Rayner

distinction between on the one hand a uniquely spatial, generally unconscious, motor-oriented system, and on the other hand a more symbolic system, the contents of which are at least partially conscious, thus forming the basis for perception.

Several excellent recent reviews have touched on domains related to the subject of this chapter, although none concentrated on the contrasting roles of extraretinal signals in cognitive and sensorimotor function. Matin (1972, 1982, 1986) and Shebilske (1977) have reviewed visual localization and eye movements, while Anstis (1986) and Mack (1986) have covered visual motion. Grüsser (1986b) has reviewed experiments from his own laboratory on the problem. Holtzman and Sedgwick (1984) and Shebilske (1986) provide similar reviews of studies from their laboratories. Steinbach (1986) has reviewed eye muscle proprioception.

2 HISTORY

The first explicit formulation of efference copy ideas was by Bell (1823/1974) and Purkinje (1825a,b). Grüsser (1986a) reviews even earlier literature concerned principally with older Greek and Arabic ideas of energy emanating from the eye, that is not directly applicable to the concept of an internal copy of motor efference.

Both Bell and Purkinje based their conclusions on observations of the contrasting apparent motions of afterimages or of real images when the eye is pressed and when it is actively moved. An afterimage in darkness appears stationary if the eye is moved passively with an eyepress, but it appears to move with the eye during an active eye movement. Conversely, a real image appears to move during an eyepress, but the image remains fixed during a normal eye movement, a phenomenon termed 'space constancy'. (These observers assumed that the eye was passively moved during an eyepress with a real image. This assumption is incorrect under some conditions (Bridgeman, 1979), but the conclusions are still valid.) If afterimages appeared to move when eye position was changing, but nothing was changing on the retina, then only an extraretinal signal could be responsible. Bell and Purkinje assumed that the extraretinal signal was associated with an effort to move the eyes. Purkinje (1825a,b) went further to conclude from these observations that signals representing the gaze movements cancelled the image displacements on the retina, resulting in space constancy for natural images and apparent motions for afterimages. These early analyses were applied to perception but not to sensorimotor functions.

Hering (1861/1990) also assumed outflow to be responsible for these effects and further predicted that, if this analysis is correct, one should see compensations for all voluntary movements but not for involuntary ones (such as vestibular nystagmus). His extensive observations supported the analysis.

Helmholtz (1866/1962) elaborated these ideas with conclusions from observations by Albrecht von Graefe on neurological patients with eye muscle pareses, and in the process extended the outflow idea from perception to include sensorimotor coordination. Helmholtz used the concept of *Willensanstrengung* (effort of will) as a signal that compensates for image motions on the retina during active eye movements. A patient with a reduced motility of one eye muscle perceived targets in the field of the paretic muscle to lie further in the periphery than they really did (a cognitive effect), and also pointed further to that side than the target's actual position when attempting to point to the target (a sensorimotor effect).

In addition to the insights on patients, Helmholtz (1867/1925) gave four observations of normal function that supported a quasisensory aspect of oculomotor innervations: (1) apparent motion occurs when the eye is moved passively; (2) afterimages are spatially stable when the eye is moved passively; (3) displacement of the image is compensated in normal saccades; and (4) adaptation to displacing prisms transfers intermanually (adaptation to constant movement or displacement of the visual world persists when the movement or displacement ceases).

Mach (1906) explicitly postulated a neuronal copy of oculomotor efference, a signal that is fed back within the brain to sum algebraically with the retinal signal. Later, von Uexküll (1920, 1928) introduced a flow diagram to differentiate feedforward control and control by sensory feedback (Figure 6.1). He also differentiated outflow and inflow variations of internal feedback (Figure 6.2), foreshadowing later mathematical analyses of the concept. He proposed his model in the context of a distinction between a hypothesized *Merkwelt* (cognitive or perceptual world) and

a)

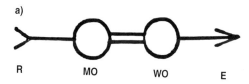

R   MO   WO   E

b)

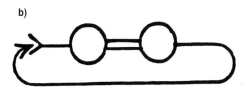

Figure 6.1. *Flow diagrams. Images are enlarged but unretouched reproductions from von Uexküli (1928) and are identical to the figures in von Uexküll (1920) except for the labels in the top diagram. (a) Generalized feedforward control. R, Receptor; MO, Merkorgan (perceptual organ); WO, Wirkorgan (motor organ; called Handlungsorgan (behavior organ) in von Uexküll, 1920); E, effector. (b) Feedback control of behavior by a servomechanism, such as control of birdsong. [© 1928 Springer; reprinted with kind permission.]*

a)

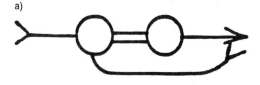

b)

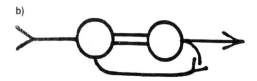

Figure 6.2. *(a) Control of behavior by proprioceptive feedback. Information from the effector is fed back to the perceptual organ to create a control loop that includes the state of the effector. (b) Control by efference copy. The efferent signal is fed back to the perceptual organ by splitting the signal; one copy goes to the effector, while another returns to the perceptual organ to complete a feedback loop. This is the first diagram incorporating modern ideas about efference copy. [From von Uexküll, 1928. © 1928 Springer; reprinted with kind permission.]*

Wirkwelt (motor world), anticipating the modern cognitive–sensorimotor distinction. Tantalizingly, von Uexküll provided no references and little evidence of how he arrived at these pioneering conceptions of biological information flow. External servocontrol (Figure 6.1b) is exemplified by a songbird whose song is disturbed if the bird cannot hear its own voice, but there are no examples for the remaining flow diagrams. The control in Figure 6.1b is likened to control of movement by the eye or by touch organs, that in Figure 6.2a to control by muscle sensations, and that in Figure 6.2b to control by internal goal states (*Richtungszeichen*).

2.1 Quantitative Theories

Modern interest in outflow was catalyzed by two papers published in 1950, each providing new experimental evidence, a control-theoretic interpretation and new terms for the signal. Von Holst and Mittelstaedt (1950) rotated the head of the fly *Eristalis* by 180°, which does not harm this species, and observed that the fly would circle indefinitely. They interpreted the behavior as a result of converting a normal negative feedback into a positive feedback by the head inversion, and coined the term *Efferenzkopie* (efference copy) to describe the postulated outflow signal. This seminal paper also distinguished *exafference*, change in retinal motion signals as a result of movement of objects in the world, from *reafference*, change in the motion signals resulting from movements of the organism. In these terms, the function of the efference copy is to distinguish exafference from reafference. Incidentally, the paper also showed that neck receptors in *Eristalis* did not affect the sense of the locomotion control loop.

Sperry (1950) made similar observations of circling in a fish with a surgically inverted eye, with a similar interpretation. The fish would circle indefinitely in one direction; but if the lights were turned off, circling would cease and activity would look relatively normal, thus excluding explanations based on brain or nerve damage. When light was restored, the fish might begin circling in the same or in the opposite direction, at random. Sperry introduced the term 'corollary discharge' to describe the internally monitored outflow signal. The discharge has the character of a *copy*, not of a mathematical corollary (Mittelstaedt, personal communication), so the terminology of outflow or efference copy will be used here.

3. EFFERENCE COPY IN COGNITIVE AND SENSORIMOTOR FUNCTION

The visual system has two kinds of jobs to do, which have been characterized as the 'what' and the 'where' functions. These two functions make different demands on an efference copy mechanism: the 'what' or cognitive function has no need of quantitative egocentered information about spatial localization, being concerned primarily with pattern recognition. Qualitative information about location may be adequate for this system, and there is abundant evidence that humans are not very good at quantitatively estimating distances, directions, etc. The 'where' or sensorimotor function, in contrast, needs quantitative egocentrically calibrated spatial information to guide motor acts.

The contrast between these two functions parallels a multiple representation in the primate cortex, where the visual world is represented in several topographic maps (Van Essen, Newsome and Bixby, 1982). This characteristic of the visual system raises a fundamental question: do all of these maps work together in a single visual representation, or are they functionally distinct? If they are distinct, how many functional maps are there and how do they communicate with one another? Because these questions concern visual function in intact organisms, they can be answered best with psychophysical techniques. Evidence reviewed here reveals that the multiple maps support at least two functionally distinct representations of the visual world in normal humans; under some conditions, the two representations can simultaneously hold different spatial values. The representations do not always function independently, however, but sometimes communicate with one another. Each of the two representations uses several of the physiological retinotopic maps; the representations may correspond to the temporal and parietal pathways of Mishkin, Ungerleider and Macko (1983).

Many experiments using a variety of methods have revealed that subjects are unaware of sizeable displacements of the visual world if they occur during saccadic eye movements (Bridgman, Hendry and Stark, 1975; Brune and Lücking, 1969; Ditchburn, 1955; Stark *et al.*, 1976; Wallach and Lewis, 1966). This implies that information about spatial location is degraded during saccades. There is an apparent paradox to this degradation, however, for people do not become disoriented after saccades, implying that spatial information is maintained. Experimental evidence supports this conclusion. For instance, the eyes can saccade accurately to a target that is flashed (and mislocalized) during an earlier saccade (Hallett and Lightstone, 1976a, b) and hand–eye coordination remains fairly accurate following saccades (Festinger and Canon, 1965). How can the perceptual information be lost while visually guided behavior is preserved?

Resolution of this paradox begins with the realization that the two kinds of conflicting observations use different response measures. The saccadic suppression of displacement experiments requires a nonspatial verbal report or button press, both symbolic responses. The behavior has an arbitrary spatial relationship to the target. Successful orienting of the eye or hand, in contrast, requires quantitative spatial information, defined here as requiring a 1:1 correspondence between a target position and a motor behavior, such as directing the hand or the eyes to the target. The conflict might be resolved if the two types of report, which can be labelled as cognitive and sensorimotor, could be combined in a single experiment. If two pathways in the visual system process different kinds of information, spatially oriented motor activities might have access to accurate position information, even when that information is unavailable at a cognitive level that mediates symbolic decisions such as button pressing or verbal response. The saccadic suppression of displacement experiments cited above address only the cognitive system.

3.1 Empirical Differentiations of Cognitive and Sensorimotor Function

In our first study on this problem (Bridgeman *et al.*, 1979), the two conflicting observations (saccadic suppression on the one hand and accurate motor behavior on the other) were combined by asking subjects to point to the position of a target that had been displaced and then extinguished.

A target was jumped 2°; on some trials the jump was detected, while on others the jump went undetected because of a simultaneous saccadic eye movement. As one would expect, when subjects were asked to point to the position of the now-extinguished target following a detected displacement, they did so accurately. Pointing was equally good, however, following an undetected displacement. It is as though we had asked the subjects where the target was, and they said 'on the left'; but when asked to point to it, they pointed to the right. It appeared that some information, perhaps from efference copy, was available to the motor system even when it was unavailable to perception.

This result implied that quantitative control of motor activity was unaffected by the perceptual detectability of target position. But it is also possible (if a bit strained) to interpret the result in terms of signal detection theory as a high response criterion for the report of displacement. The first control for this possibility was a two-alternative forced-choice measure of saccadic suppression of displacement, with the result that even this criterion-free measure showed no information about displacement to be available to the cognitive system under the conditions where pointing was affected (Bridgeman and Stark, 1979). The information was available to a motor system that controlled pointing but not to a cognitive system informing visual perception.

A more rigorous way to separate cognitive and sensorimotor systems was to put a signal only into the sensorimotor system in one condition and only into the cognitive system in another. We know that induced motion affects the cognitive system because we experience the effect and subjects can make verbal judgments of it. However, the above experiments implied that the information used for pointing might come from sources unavailable to perception. We inserted a signal selectivity into the cognitive system with stroboscopic induced motion (Bridgeman, Kirch and Sperling, 1981). A surrounding frame was displaced, creating the illusion that a target had jumped although it remained fixed relative to the subject. Target and frame were then extinguished, and the subject pointed open-loop to the last position of the target. Trials where the target had seemed to be on the left were compared with trials where it had seemed to be on the right. Pointing was not significantly different in the two kinds of trials, showing that the induced motion illusion did not affect pointing.

Information was inserted selectively into the sensorimotor system by asking each subject to adjust a real motion of the target, displaced in phase with the frame, until the target appeared to be stationary. Thus, the cognitive system specified a stable target. Nevertheless, subjects pointed in significantly different directions when the target was extinguished in the left or the right positions, showing that the difference in real target positions was still available to the sensorimotor system. The visual system must have picked up the target displacement, but not reported it to the cognitive system, or the cognitive system could have ascribed the visually specified displacement to an artifact of frame movement. Thus, a double dissociation occurred: in one condition an illusory target displacement affected only the cognitive system, and in the other a real displacement affected only motor behavior.

Dissociation of cognitive and sensorimotor function has also been demonstrated for the oculomotor system by creating conditions in which cognitive and sensorimotor systems receive opposite signals at the same time. Again, the experiment involved stroboscopic induced motion in an otherwise uniform field; a target spot jumped in the same direction as a frame, but not far enough to cancel the induced motion. The spot still appeared to jump in the direction opposite the frame, while it actually jumped a short distance in the same direction. At this point, the retinal position of the target was stabilized by feedback from a Purkinje image eye tracker, so that retinal error could not drive eye movements. Saccadic eye movements followed the veridical direction, even though subjects perceived stroboscopic motion in the opposite direction (Wong and Mack, 1981). If a delay in responding was required, however, eye movements followed the perceptual illusion, implying that the sensorimotor system has no memory and must rely on information from the cognitive system when responding to what had been present rather than what is currently present.

All of these experiments involve motion or displacement, leaving open the possibility that the dissociations are associated in some way with motion systems rather than with representation of visual location *per se*. A newer design allows the examination of visual context in a situation where there is no motion or displacement at any time during a trial (Bridgeman, 1989). The design is based on the Roelofs effect (Roelofs, 1935), a perceptual illusion seen when a static frame is presented asymmetrically to the left or the right of a subject's center line. Objects that lie within the frame tend to be mislocated in the direction opposite to the offset of the frame. For example, in an otherwise featureless field, a rectangle is presented with its right edge in the subject's median plane, so that the rectangle lies to the subject's left. Both the rectangle and stimuli within it will tend to be localized too far to the right.

In experiments using this effect, subjects first memorized five possible target positions 2° apart. Then they either guessed the position of a target or pointed to its position with an unseen pointer. All of the subjects revealed a Roelofs effect for the perceptual measure, judging the targets to be further to the right when the frame was on the left and vice versa. But only half of them showed the effect for pointing – the rest were uninfluenced by frame position in pointing, although their perceptual effects were as large as those of the other subjects.

In this experiment subjects pointed or judged immediately after stimulus offset. Reasoning that the delay in response might have caused some subjects to switch from using motor information directly to using information imported from the cognitive representation of visual space, we attempted to get all of the subjects to switch to using cognitive information. By delaying the response cue long enough, all subjects began showing a Roelofs effect in pointing as well as judging. Thus, like Wong and Mack's induced motion experiment reviewed above, this experiment showed a switch from motor to cognitive information in directing the pointing response, revealed by the appearance of a cognitive illusion after a delay.

The general conclusion from all of these experiments is that information about egocentric spatial location is available to the visual system even when cognitive illusions of location are present. The efference copy could provide the needed localization information to the sensorimotor system even while the cognitive system, relying on relative motion and relative position information, holds unreliable information about location.

4.   OUTFLOW VERSUS INFLOW

4.1   History

Outflow was the dominant candidate for extraretinal signals in the nineteenth century; even Hering (1868/1977), who disagreed with Helmholtz on so many other issues, agreed with him on this one. Growing knowledge of muscle receptors, however, led Sherrington (1898, 1918) to propose that proprioceptive inflow from the extraocular muscles was important. Several kinds of receptors are found in various mammalian eye muscles, including stretch receptors (Bach-Y-Rita and Ito, 1966) and palisade endings (Steinbach and Smith, 1981). Physiological recording shows that proprioceptive information reaches the superior colliculus (Donaldson and Long, 1980) and the visual cortex (Buisseret and Maffei, 1977) among other regions. The literature concerning the anatomy and physiology of oculomotor proprioceptors has been reviewed by Steinbach (1987).

Clearly, such an elaborate physiological system must have a functional role. The preponderance of psychophysical and behavioral evidence, however, implicates outflow rather than inflow as the signal used in perception and visually guided behavior. Following up on Helmholtz's observations, paralysis studies have implicated outflow rather than inflow in determining perceived position. During paralysis, subjects perceive motions of the world at the time of attempted eye movements despite lack of proprioceptive input (Brindley et al., 1976; Kornmüller, 1931; Siebeck, 1954)

A difficulty in interpreting such results arose with the finding that during complete paralysis, with no measurable eye or body movement, the jump of the world seems not to occur. Stevens et al. (1976) observed, however, although no jump was perceived at the time of an attempted saccade by a fully paralyzed subject, the world seemed to be in a different position when sustained eccentric gaze was (unsuccessfully) attempted. This result would be expected if efference copy provides information about position rather than motion of the visual world (see the discussion of efference copy dynamics, Section 5). In the presence of even a small motion transient under conditions of incomplete paralysis, the perceptual system accepts the retinally given transient as marking the location change that is specified by mismatch of efference copy and static retinal position. With complete paralysis there is no retinal motion transient and no time at which the changed efference copy can contribute to replacing previous spatial values: hence the ambiguity of the perception and the difficulty of reporting it accurately.

4.2 New Methods

Experiments using the method of pressing on the side or lower lid of the eye have clarified relative contributions of inflow and outflow signals under conditions where the two theories make different predictions. When a subject presses slowly on the side of one eye while the other is occluded, oculomotor stabilization systems maintain fixation on the current fixation point. As a result, the innervation to the eye changes, but the posture of the eye does not. This analysis has been supported by several kinds of experiments, using both infrared oculography (Stark and Bridgeman, 1983) and the search coil technique (Ilg, Bridgeman and Hoffman, 1989).

4.2.1 Slope Favors Outflow

If outflow determines visual localization, the amount of perceptual deviation should match the amount of the deviation in efference, which can be measured quantitatively by monitoring the position of the occluded fellow eye. Only one eye moves, but both receive an equal compensatory innervation to maintain the position of the viewing eye, and the compensatory innervation will equal the deviation of the occluded eye. If inflow determines localization in the monocular eyepress, however, the situation is different. The proprioceptive signals from the rotated, occluded eye and the pressed, fixating eye should sum: because the viewing eye's inflow does not change, perceptual offset should be one half of eye deviation, and the slope of a line relating eye deviation to perceptual offset should be 0.5 (Figure 6.3) However, the experimentally measured perceptual deviation is nearly as great as the eye deviation, implicating outflow (Stark and Bridgeman, 1983). Bridgeman and Fishman (1985) plotted magnitude of eye deviation against perceived deviation of a target, obtaining slopes near 1 (Figure 6.4).

4.2.2 Eyepress in Darkness

Another condition where inflow and outflow theories make different predictions concerns the control of eye movements. The experimental manipulation is an eyepress in complete darkness. Here, there is no target to stabilize the pressed eye, and the eye rotates passively in the orbit as Helmholtz and Purkinje would have predicted. The passive eye rotation should excite receptors in the extraocular muscles, and if inflow were having an effect these receptors should elicit reflex movements of both the pressed eye and the fellow eye.

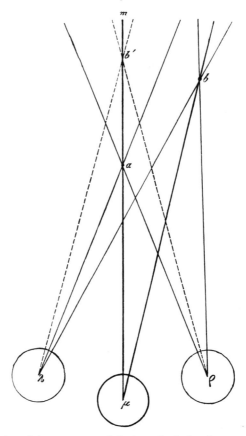

Figure 6.3. *Generalized view of the two eyes and the hypothetical cyclopean eye from below. Lambda: left eye. Rho: right eye. Mu: cyclopean eye, located on the Veith-Müller horopter, from which perceived direction can be calculated. Conjugate eye movement changes the point of fixation from b' to b, while vergence movement changes it from b' to a. Eyepress results in a deviation of outflow to both eyes, equivalent to changing fixation from b to b'. The pressed eye does not move, however, so that inflow signals correspond to a movement of the point of sight along the line b–lambda if the left eye is pressed. As a result, the average change in the binocular proprioceptive signal is half of the deviation of the moving eye. [From Hering, 1868. Translated version by Bruce Bridgeman. © 1977 Plenum Press, New York; reprinted with kind permission.]*

The fact that such movements of the fellow eye are not seen (Bridgeman and Delgado, 1984; Ilg, Bridgeman and Hoffman, 1989) demonstrates that proprioceptive inflow does not normally contribute to maintenance of eye posture. This observation does not rule out a contribution of inflow to other visual functions, however.

4.2.3 Voluntary Versus Involuntary Movement

A more fundamental problem with proprioception as the sole source of information about eye movements is that it responds equally for every type of movement. Every type of movement would enter the control loop, unless it is somehow compensated

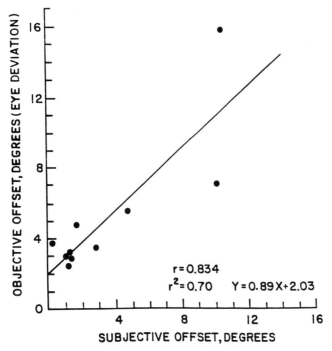

Figure 6.4. *Objective deviation of an occluded eye during monocular press on the viewing eye versus subjective deviation of a straight-ahead target. Each point represents one subject. A slope of near 1 implicates outflow as the chief source of information about eye position. (From Bridgeman and Fishman, 1985. © 1985 Psychonomic Society, Inc.; reprinted with kind permission of the publisher and B. Bridgeman.]*

before reaching the loop, and the system could not tolerate a voluntary change of eye position (Mittelstaedt, 1990). To compensate for the effects of movements, the system must compare the intent to move with the result of the movement; a mere record that a movement has occurred cannot differentiate voluntary from involuntary sources of the oculomotor innervation.

It is still possible that proprioception plays a role, for the tonus of the intrafusal fibers in the extraocular muscles may be different in darkness than in light. If this is so, the muscle receptors may be unable to respond to small amounts of stretch induced by the passive rotation (Matin, 1972). While this interpretation cannot be excluded by the present data, there is no direct evidence for it either. Because extraocular muscles remain active even in darkness, the most reasonable conclusion at present is that inflow plays no role in control of eye posture under these conditions.

4.2.4 Physiological Evidence

What then is the role of the proprioceptors? Current evidence implicates them in a low-level gaze stabilization system and assigns them a role in calibrating the system during development. In cats, cutting the proprioceptive fibers in the ophthalmic branch of the fifth nerve results in gaze instability when the animals are in darkness and cannot stabilize fixation with retinal feedback (Fiorentini and Maffei, 1977). The movements were very slow, the fastest being low-amplitude, nearly sinusoidal oscillations at about 0.6 Hz and the slowest being larger drifts at about 0.08 Hz. A similar intervention in rabbits results in large eye deviations during vestibular nystagmus, even while the unoperated contralateral eye shows normal fast phase beats of nystagmus and good positional control (Kashii *et al.*, 1989). Humans also show fixational instability in darkness, and are less accurate at judging their eye level without a visual context (Stoper and Cohen, 1986), suggesting (but not proving) that the mechanism is similar in humans.

Other evidence supports a developmental role for oculomotor proprioception. Hein and Diamond (1983) surgically interrupted inflow and showed deficits in visually guided behavior, but only in developing animals. The same interruptions in adult cats had no effect.

In summary, it seems that Ludvigh (1952) was right: proprioception is involved in a low-level servocontrol loop stabilizing eye position, once the direction of gaze has been determined by other influences and mechanisms.

4.3 Quantitative Comparisons

Advances in the eyepress method of altering the relationship between extraretinal signals and gaze pcsition have made it possible to perform a quantitative comparison of the roles of oculomotor inflow and outflow in the same experiment, although the comparison currently is limited to static conditions. The eyepress changes outflow because oculomotor innervation compensates for the eyepress, as reviewed above. The viewing eye's fixation remains constant.

Inflow also changes in this condition, however, because the occluded eye rotates, driven by the change in binocular innervation. Thus, we can define an 'outflow' condition which measures a combination of outflow and inflow. There is no way with the eyepress method to modify outflow without also affecting inflow.

A new manipulation can change inflow, without affecting outflow. In the same monocular viewing condition, pressing on the occluded eye results in a passive rotation. Since there is no retinal error signal in this case, there is no change in outflow, even though the occluded eye rotates along with its proprioceptors. This defines an 'inflow' condition. Bridgeman and Stark (1991) measured perceived target deviations and pointing biases in an unstructured visual field under inflow, outflow and control conditions, and the behavioral localizations were plotted against eye deviation for each subject. Gains (ratios of perceived target deviation to eye deviation) were 0.740 for the outflow condition and 0.128 for the inflow condition, with no statistically significant difference between perceptual judgement and open-loop pointing.

With quantitative measures of the slopes of the functions in both the inflow and the outflow conditions, one can calculate the physiological effects of the two sources of extraretinal information. To combine monocular and binocular effects, all signals are interpreted as influences on an imaginary cyclopean eye, equally affected by the two anatomical eyes according to Hering's law. We use the following nomenclature:

D_{ipsi},   experimentally measured outflow condition;
D_{contra}, experimentally measured inflow condition;

O, real efference outflow;
I, real proprioception inflow.

The outflow measure D_{ipsi} contains both an outflow component and half of the physiological inflow effect:

$$D_{ipsi} = O + I/2 \tag{1}$$

The inflow measure D_{contra} is half of the physiological effect, since only one eye is deviated:

$$D_{contra} = I/2 \tag{2}$$

Solving equation (1) for *O*, and changing signs because the perceptual effects are in the opposite direction from the eyepress, we obtain:

$$O = I/2 - D_{ipsi} \tag{3}$$

Substituting from equation (2) yields:

$$O = D_{contra} - D_{ipsi} \tag{4}$$

Solving equation (2) for *I* yields:

$$I = 2(D_{contra}) \tag{5}$$

Equations (4) and (5) can now be used to find the physiological effects of outflow and inflow. Substituting into equation (4):

$$O = 0.128 - 0.740 = -0.612$$

This is an estimate of the gain of efference copy. The gain is negative because the perceptual effects are in the opposite direction from the eyepress. Substituting into equation (5):

$$I = 2(0.128) = 0.256$$

This is an estimate of the effect of proprioception on perception when no visual context is present.

The resulting gains, 0.612 for outflow and 0.256 for inflow, sum to only 0.868, indicating an incomplete registration of eye eccentricity. It would seem that the total extraretinal signal fails to register the true deviation of the eyes from straight ahead. This is a counterintuitive and seemingly unsatisfactory conclusion. But other evidence suggests that the conclusion is correct.

Several studies provide evidence that static eye position is underregistered in a uniform visual field. The studies show remarkable quantitative agreement despite differences in method and range. In the study that most nearly matches the perceptual conditions of the eyepress experiments, Morgan (1978) measured an illusion of straight-ahead direction with eccentric gaze; she found that the perceived straight ahead deviated systematically in the direction of gaze. The gain of the illusion can be calculated from her paper as 0.128, so that the sum of outflow, inflow and illusion is 0.994. Hill (1972) used a different method, measuring apparent location of a fixated target when the eyes were deviated 30° left or right; converting again to units of gain calculated from the published results, the average magnitude of the apparent deviation from veridicality in Hill's subjects was 0.132. Despite the fact that the range of eye deviation used by Hill does not overlap that possible in eyepress experiments, the sum of the eyepress-determined extraretinal signals and the gaze direction illusion is 1.000, again in remarkable agreement with what the missing extraretinal signal component predicts. The exact summing of the components must be considered a lucky coincidence – neither Hill's data nor Bridgeman and Stark's can be trusted to three significant figures. Nevertheless, it seems that the issue of the relative roles of retinal signals and extraretinal signals, and of inflow and outflow, is settled at least for static eyes in uniform fields.

5   CHARACTERISTICS OF THE EFFERENCE COPY

We have learned a good deal about the efference copy and its accompanying mechanisms since the time of Helmholtz. Below are presented nine 'commandments' of efference copy (I haven't got as far as Moses yet!), characteristics that have been described or discovered mostly in the past forty years and whose implications remain incompletely worked through. Most of the remainder of this chapter will be an elaboration of the evidence supporting these nine commandments of efference copy and the methods used to study them.

   (1) An efference copy accompanies all voluntary eye movements and some involuntary ones, including pursuits, saccades and the fast phases of vestibular and optokinetic nystagmus.
   (2) The efference copy is not a simple branch of motor axons, for some eye movements that are not accompanied by an efference copy have the same dynamics as those that are.
   (3) The gain of the efference copy mechanism is less than 1.
   (4) Efference copy is supplemented by other mechanisms in achieving space constancy.
   (5) The efference copy branches from the motor system without taking account of oculomotor delays and kinematics.
   (6) Use of efference copy information is different for perception and for visually guided behavior.
   (7) The efference copy/space constancy system operates at low temporal frequency.
   (8) There is only one efference copy for both eyes, reflecting Hering's law.
   (9) Effect of the efference copy signal is subject to adaptation in direction as well as magnitude.

5.1   Methodology

In order to study the efference copy and to distinguish influences of proprioceptive inflow from influences of outflow, it is necessary to dissociate gaze angle from innervation. With such a dissociation, inflow will indicate the position of gaze while outflow indicates the innervation state. Psychophysical judgments and visually guided behavior can then determine what aspects of visual function are being driven by inflow and which by outflow.

Separating gaze from innervation has proved to be a difficult technical problem, and all of the methods used have some drawbacks. Here are the major methods:

(a) Clinical paralysis or paresis of extraocular muscles. The results first systematized by Helmholtz (1867/1925) include illusory motion of the visual field when attempting to look in the paretic direction, and 'past pointing' to targets in that direction.

(b) Paralysis of the body, including extraocular muscles, with curare or its synthetic analogs. Results are similar to (a), but they can be better quantified because both the innervation and the eye muscles remain normal. Only the neuromuscular junction is affected. The classic studies by Kornmüller (1931), Siebeck (1954) and Stevens *et al.* (1976) used this method. Matin *et al.* (1980, 1982) have made the most recent and most effective use of this method by manipulating both visual target and structure of the visual field and using several response measures. In these studies, all of the subjects were also coauthors of the papers.

(c) Retrobulbar injection of toxins can paralyze the extraocular muscles without body paralysis. Botulism toxin works well, and has the advantage (at least for the experimenter) of lasting several months, so that adaptation to the muscle paralysis can be studied. Grüsser (1985) used this method with a shorter-acting blocker to demonstrate that stimulation of an immobilized eye can lead, in the nonparalyzed fellow eye, to changes in optokinetic nystagmus, smooth pursuit and movement perception.

(d) The eye can be fixed mechanically by applying putty to the sclera and allowing it to dry (Mach, 1885/1959). The method has the disadvantage of being uncomfortable. Again, illusory movements of the visual field accompany attempted eye movements.

(e) The cornea can be anesthetized with local anesthetics and the sclera pulled with forceps. The method has the advantage that the eye can be passively rotated, while the above methods are limited to reducing the motor results of attempted eye movements. It is difficult to hold the eye completely fixed during attempted movements, however. Brindley and Merton (1960) showed with this method that there is no proprioceptive sensation in the human eye.

(f) Again with the cornea anesthetized, a suction contact lens can be applied. A small stalk on the lens can support weights to precisely define the external rotational force applied to the eye. With tiny pulleys, force can be applied in any direction. A specially made contact lens is required for each subject. Skavenski, Haddad and Steinman (1972) concluded from studies with this method that inflow does not affect perceived direction, but Gauthier, Nommay and Vercher (1990) have recently found small effects of inflow with a similar technique.

These methods have the drawback that they are not suitable for any but the most dedicated experimenters. This discourages use of naive subjects and limits the generalizability of the results. Two more recently developed methods of dissociating gaze position from innervation require no invasive physical or pharmacological intervention.

(g) Sustained eccentric gaze can adapt the oculomotor system, so that subsequent efforts to look to the adapted side are potentiated and efforts to look to the opposite side are inhibited. This phenomenon, the 'minor motor anomaly', has been used to assess the role of extraretinal information in everyday perceptual situations (Shebilske, 1986). However, it is difficult to quantify the amount of mismatch between innervation state and gaze direction with a measure that is independent of the experiment's dependent variables. The final method overcomes this difficulty.

(h) A sustained press with a finger on the outer canthus of a monocularly viewing eye will bias oculomotor outflow while the normal fixation stabilization mechanisms maintain gaze position directed at a visible target. In total darkness, the same maneuver results in a change in gaze position without a change in efference. A sharp tap on the eye can briefly rotate the eye without a concomitant change in outflow.

The oculomotor results of the eyepress have been consistently misinterpreted for centuries, beginning with Purkinje's (1825b) assumption that pressing on the side of the eye resulted in a passive eye movement. Helmholtz (1866/1962) made the same assumption, and the textbook analysis of the maneuver is that pressing results in apparent motion of the visual world because there is a passive eye movement without an accompanying command to move the eye.

The assumption of passive eye movement was based on two observations, both consistent with one another, but both flawed. The first observation is the apparent movement of the entire visual world during eyepress. This could be due to a perception of the change in oculomotor efference, which is interpreted as visual motion (Bridgeman, 1979). The second observation is that the eye of another person performing the eyepress maneuver appears to move. What the observer sees, however, is not a rotation of the eye but a lateral translation of the eye in the orbit. The eye is influenced by two rotational forces in opposite directions: one from the finger and an equal and opposite one from the extraocular muscles. Thus, the rotational forces cancel. But each of these influences also introduces a translational force in the medial direction, and both sum to move the eye several millimeters in the orbit. The translation has been measured experimentally by Stark and Bridgeman (1983). Since the cue that humans use to perceive fixation movements of the eyes of others is the amount of sclera visible on the two sides of the iris, the translational motion is misinterpreted as a rotation. The dynamics of oculomotor compensation for the eyepress are complex and have been worked out (Ilg, Bridgeman and Hoffmann, 1989). An extension of the eyepress method has been used recently to work out relative contributions of inflow and outflow under static conditions, as reviewed in Section 4.

5.2   Properties of Efference Copy

This section will consider in detail the nine 'commandments' listed on page 204.

(1) *An efference copy accompanies all voluntary eye movements and some involuntary ones, including pursuits, saccades and the fast phases of vestibular and optokinetic nystagmus.* When Helmholtz and his contemporaries discussed outflow mechanisms, they did not differentiate the signals accompanying different types of eye movement. Indeed, the primary distinction between saccadic and pursuit movements was first made decades after Helmholtz (1867/1925) had reviewed the area and developed his outflow-based concept of *Willensanstrengung*.

The types of eye movements accompanied by efference copy can be inferred from observations of which types are accompanied by spatial compensation (space constancy or a reduction of apparent concomitant movement in the direction of space constancy). Clearly, saccades are included in this category. Pursuit is also included, although there is evidence that the amount of outflow compensation in perception is less than the full extent or velocity of the movement (Festinger and Easton, 1974; Holtzman and Sedgwick, 1984); the system seems to assume a rather slow maximum sweep rate of about 1 deg s^{-1}.

Also included in the movements accompanied by efference copy are vergence movements. The observations supporting this inclusion are old ones, formalized by Hering (1868/1977) in his arguments for the binocular coordination of vergence. He observed an apparent movement of the world during monocular viewing when a subject changed accommodation between two objects overlapping each other along the line of sight of the viewing eye. Fixating a distant target with the right eye, for instance, the visual world seems to shift to the right when fixation is moved to an overlapping near target. The covered left eye, driven by accommodative vergence, moves inward along with the apparent movement. To assign this apparent movement to an outflow rather than an inflow, we must rely indirectly on the evidence cited above for outflow as the major contributor to perception and visually guided behavior for other types of eye movement. The lack of movement of the viewing eye implies stationarity of the target; only the movement of the covered eye can lead to movement sensations.

(2) *The efference copy is not a simple branch of motor axons, for some eye movements that are not accompanied by an efference copy have the same dynamics as those that are.* Efference copy does not extend to all types of eye movement. The contrast between compensated and uncompensated eye movements is particularly evident during vestibular nystagmus or optokinetic afternystagmus, when the world seems to glide smoothly in one direction. The sawtooth-like eye movement patterns of the nystagmus are characterized by alternating fast and slow phases, the fast phases having the dynamics of saccadic eye movements.

The slow eye movements of the nystagmus are not accompanied by an efference copy – otherwise the world would continue to appear stable as it does in a normal environment. In the natural world, the slow phase of nystagmus compensates for self-motion, while the fast phase is needed only for resetting the gaze position to allow further slow phases. The slow phase tracks a real-world event while the fast phase does not. Lack of compensation for slow phases of pursuit is not due to the dynamics of the movements, for pursuit movements of similar speed and duration are compensated.

Further evidence on this issue comes from observations of the apparent movements of afterimages, which complement the observations with natural images. During the nystagmus movements there is no apparent movement of an afterimage, as Hering (1861/1990) had already noted, indicating lack of compensation. A deviation of the afterimage to one side has been noted, however (Dittler, 1921). The deviation may be a direct result of vestibular influence on visual localization, rather than an effect of efference copy. It reverses direction when the phase of vestibular afternystagmus changes and is not influenced by the rhythmic repeating nystagmus movements.

The existence of eye movements unaccompanied by efference copy has important implications for the theory of visual localization. It means that the efference copy cannot literally branch from the efferent axons innervating the extraocular muscles. Rather, there must be a switch or branch earlier in the pathway that allows the efference copy to flow for some kinds of eye movements and not for others. The passage through this switch must be based on the normal ecological function of the eye movement, not on its dynamics or on the state of alertness of the observer.

(3) *The gain of the efference copy mechanism is less than 1.* Early theorists assumed that an efference copy would completely compensate for the sensory effects of receptor motion. Several investigators have found, however, that the gain of the efference copy is less than 1 for both saccades and pursuits – it compensates for somewhat less than the entire eye movement. The efference copy has turned out to be a complex set of internal brain signals described by many parameters; gain is only one of them, and is a useful quantity only in the context of other parameters such as temporal factors and type of eye movement. Still, it is useful to look at gain in order to obtain an initial impression about how much of perception and visually guided behavior can be assigned to efference copy.

In order to isolate the gain of the efference copy in an objective measure, the stimulus–motion/retinal–motion feedback loop must be opened. This is done most frequently by stabilizing the retinal image, either with an afterimage or with optical/electronic techniques that leave enough residual retinal motion to prevent image fading. With these techniques the effects of efference can be measured in isolation. Efference copy gain can be defined as the ratio of apparent target movement to eye movement when the target is stabilized on the retina and no other patterns are visible in the field.

The gain of efference copy during saccades can be calculated from the results of an afterimage study by Grüsser, Krizič and Weiss (1987). Subjects fixated a bright light to create a foveal afterimage in darkness, and then performed repeated saccades to alternate their fixations between two auditory targets. The dependent variable in the experiment was the subjects' estimates of the spatial separation of the resting points of the afterimage when the eye was in the left versus the right position. The perceived separation depended strongly on the frequency of the saccades, a result that will be important below; here, concern is with data at the slowest saccade rate: about one saccade every 667 ms. Subjects estimated position of the afterimage on each side with a pointer, so that this experiment measures the sensorimotor visual system.

For ten subjects, average separation of pointing estimations in the two positions was about 22° across saccades of 46°. These numbers cannot be used directly to calculate gain, however, because slope of the line comparing pointer positions with target separations using real light stimuli was only between 0.8 and 0.95. Using the center of this range as a correction factor, I calculate the gain of efference copy in this experiment to be 0.55. Extrapolation from the data of Grüsser, Krizič and Weiss (1987) indicates that gain might be slightly higher with longer intersaccadic intervals, but the intervals are already well within the frequency obtained in normal visual exploration, so that the natural system must function with gains in this range.

For pursuit eye movements the experiments are more complicated because there must be a stimulus for pursuit as well as an open-loop target. Recent data from Pola and Wyatt (1989) meet these requirements. These authors isolated extraretinal contributions to movement perception by presenting an outline square stabilized on the retina with a photoelectric eye movement monitor. Any apparent movement of the square must be the result of extraretinal influences such as efference copy because real motions on the retina are cancelled mechanically. To elicit smooth tracking eye movements, retinal slip was produced by stepping a bar back and forth within the square. The observer, attempting to fixate the bar, generated smooth pursuit movements because the bar did not move far enough from the fovea to elicit saccades. Apparent motions under the open-loop condition were compared with subsequent perceived motions under normal closed-loop conditions by a method of adjustment (a cognitive measure).

As was the case for saccades, the gain of efference copy in this experiment was strongly dependent on the frequency of oscillation of the bar (and of the pursuit eye movements). At the slowest oscillation frequency of 0.5 Hz, the average gain for three subjects was 0.79; it decreased to less than 0.4 at a frequency of 2 Hz. Pola and Wyatt model the transfer function as a moderately damped second-order system.

Earlier studies had also attempted to measure efferent contributions to motion perception during smooth pursuit, but did not have the methodological control of more recent studies. Dichgans, Körner and Voigt (1969), for example, compared speed of perceived motion during pursuit with perceived motion during fixation of an egocentrically fixed target. Perceived velocity was estimated with magnitude estimation techniques, applying an interval scale to what should be a ratio-scale measurement.

Even with these limitations, gain estimates of efference copy in pursuit were in the same range as those in more recent studies. The efferent:afferent ratio is given as 1:1.60 to 1.66, which works out to a gain of 0.63–0.60, within the range Pola and Wyatt (1989) found with more modern methods. Again, the calculated gain was sensitive to attentional and visual context parameters. Dichgans, Körner and Voigt (1969) review an extensive earlier literature that predominantly finds ratios of retinal perceived velocity to pursuit perceived velocity in the same range. Because calculated gain is sensitive to other parameters, it is best not to consider gain in isolation but rather in the context of a complete control system. Systematic variation in gain with changes in the visual task and context does have implications for the possible functions of efference copy, however.

During steady fixation, efference copy gain can be defined only for gaze positions deviating from primary position, for the gaze position is the denominator of the gain calculation and is 0 at primary position. Thus, the fixational gain can be measured as the ratio of the perceived deviation to the actual deviation of gaze from primary position. Most estimates of this gain confound inflow and outflow components of the extraretinal signal; an exception is the method of Bridgeman and Stark (1991), reviewed above, which revealed a gain of outflow amounting to 0.612.

(4) *Efference copy is supplemented by other mechanisms in achieving space constancy.* Since the classic conceptions of efference copy assumed that the compensatory outflow exactly equalled the change in retinal signal, there was no need for other mechanisms to supplement it. Teuber (1960) has named these theories 'cancellation theories'. There is a flaw built into them: it is the requirement that the efference copy must provide a perfect compensation for the retinal image displacement during an eye movement. The signal must support the introspection that the world does not seem to move in the slightest when the eye jumps. But all biological signals are noisy – they wander with time, they depend to some extent on state of arousal, health and nutrition, and they will vary slightly from one movement to the next. Further, the outflow signal is a prediction, a neural feedforward indicating not where the eyes are but where they ought to be. Thus, any change in motor

execution will also lead to mismatch between the change in retinal signal and the outflow that predicts its timing and extent. Further, if the gain of outflow ever became more than 1, the oculomotor control system would become unstable under some stimulus conditions and would be prone to ever increasing oscillations.

As these considerations imply, outflow does not do its work alone. Since its gain is less than 1, other mechanisms supplement outflow to achieve space constancy and to determine perceived visual direction. Bridgeman, Hendry and Stark (1975) argued that the finding of saccadic suppression of displacement, an increase in thresholds for detecting target displacements that occur during saccades, is inconsistent with the classic cancellation version of efference copy theory. If retinal movement were perfectly compensated by efference copy during a saccade, displacement detection thresholds should remain about the same during saccades as during fixation. Yet the thresholds reach as much as a third of the magnitude of a saccade and are 3–4 log units higher during saccades than during fixation.

The neural basis of this saccadic suppression of displacement may be an internal signal, a sort of qualitative efference copy that informs the system that any upcoming displacement is to be ignored (MacKay, 1973). This sort of signal would be inadequate to mediate cancellation, however. Since saccadic suppression can account for at best one-third of the retinal displacement signal removed from perception during a saccade, the qualitative MacKay efference copy would have to be supplemented by a quantitative signal, even if its gain were low.

Another line of research supporting the principle that efference copy cannot work alone is that of Matin et al. (1980, 1982), who decoupled efference copy from gaze position by using partial paralysis – subjects could still move their eyes, but the oculomotor gain was reduced by the paralytic agent. Breathing was still possible without artificial respiration. The major contribution of the Matin et al. studies to the paralysis literature was a systematic control over stimulus parameters as well as oculomotor gain.

For the purposes of this section, the most important contribution of these experiments was the definition of conditions under which visual context changed the role of efference copy in perception. Subjects sat with their heads pitched slightly back while directing their gaze to a set of illuminated points located at eye height in a normally illuminated room. Paralysis reduced the oculomotor gain, so that attempts to fixate away from primary position resulted in large deviations of the efference copy from true eye position in the orbit. Perception remained completely normal. When the room lights were extinguished, however, the illuminated points seemed to float down to the floor and remain there. With forward head pitch, perception was also normal in the light but the luminous points drifted upward in the dark.

Matin et al. (1982) explained these observations in terms of suppression of efference copy by information from the structured visual field. As long as room lights were on, retinal information dominated to inform the visual system that the luminous points were at eye height. Stark and Bridgeman (1983) have called this 'visual capture of Matin', a visual capture of the information potentially available in the efference copy. Without a structured visual field, however, efference copy is the only indicator of object position, and it gradually comes to dominate visual perception when a background pattern is removed. Matin et al. also measured visual–auditory spatial matching, finding that efference copy was changed even when, in the light condition, it had no effect on visual position perception.

Bridgeman and Stark (1981) and Stark and Bridgeman (1983) replicated this result using a press on the outer canthus or the lower lid of the eye to dissociate efference from gaze position. As noted earlier, the press results not in a passive movement of the eye, but in an active resistance to the press. As the finger presses harder and harder on the eye, the oculomotor fixation systems innervate the extraocular muscles more and more strongly to counter the effects of the press and maintain the visual target on the fovea. The result is a situation similar to paralysis: the efference to the eye changes but the image remains at the same position on the retina. The technique involves no drugs, it can be applied to naive subjects with some training, and control trials can be interspersed with experimental trials.

Using this technique, Stark and Bridgeman asked subjects to set a target to appear straight ahead with and without eyepress. Subjects sat in darkness with only a luminous target visible. During eyepress on the right eye, they set the target further to the left than they did during interspersed control trials. In a normal visual environment, however, straight-ahead settings were the same in experimental and control trials.

There are two ways to explain these results. The first is the visual capture of Matin theory, outlined above. The second theory is based on the idea that two oculomotor systems interact during normal fixation. The first, a phylogenetically old optokinetic system, stabilizes the visual world on the retina with a negative feedback. Spatial summation makes it most effective with very large, texture-rich environments. The second oculomotor system is the phylogenetically newer pursuit system found only in foveate animals. It works to stabilize targets on the fovea even if that requires working against the efforts of the first system (Post and Leibowitz, 1982, 1985). In the context of the paralysis or the eyepress experiments, the output of the first system (which is unregistered in perception) would hold fixation on the target with negligible additional pursuit innervation as long as the environment is illuminated. In darkness, however, only the pursuit system would be available to maintain fixation on the target, and its output, registered in perception, would be required to counter the effects of the paralysis or the eyepress (Bridgeman, 1986).

Either of these two theories can explain the results of the Matin *et al.* paralysis experiments or the Bridgeman and Stark eyepress studies. To establish which of them is correct, Bridgeman and Graziano (1989) explored a condition in which the two theories make different predictions. The experiment involved setting straight ahead with and without eyepress, when the target was presented against a number of backgrounds. A substantial effect was expected when the target was presented in a 180° blank field, and no effect was expected with a natural landscape background projected on the 180° screen. The deciding condition was a background with texture but no structure, a random-dot pattern or a repeating checkerboard. The visual capture theory predicts that subjects in this condition should behave as they do in the dark, because there is no visual structure to enable visual capture to be effective. The oculomotor theory, in contrast, predicts that subjects should behave as they do with the landscape background, because the texture provides contours that can stimulate the optokinetic system without the need for added pursuit innervation.

As expected, the deviations of experimental from control trials with no background were indistinguishable from the deviation of the efference copy, measured objectively for each subject in the occluded fellow eye. With the landscape background, this more sensitive experiment picked up some small deviations where none had been significant before, but they were very small – less than 1°. In the deciding condition, where the two theories make different predictions, the results came out exactly halfway between the predictions of the two theories.

Disliking what we interpreted as an inconclusive result, we repeated the entire experiment with different landscape and texture stimuli, a different method of measuring straight ahead, and experienced psychophysical observers instead of naive undergraduates. The results were exactly the same, except that all the deviations were scaled up. Perhaps the experienced observers were willing to press harder on their eyes than the undergraduates. Again, though, the result in the texture-only condition was exactly halfway between the magnitudes of results in the other two conditions.

The two theories are not mutually contradictory. Either each of them is equally important in determining visual direction, or there is a third as yet undiscovered theory that will explain all of the results.

(5) *The efference copy branches from the motor system without taking account of oculomotor delays and kinematics.* For perception during pursuit, the implications of this commandment include misperception of the motions of targets tracked against uniform fields. Under these conditions, information about the path of the moving target can originate only from efference copy. Now the target can be moved in such a way that the eye cannot follow it accurately, for instance with linear or angular accelerations that approach infinity (sudden stops or starts, or abrupt turns). If the efference copy could accurately track the angular and linear accelerations of the eye, perception would remain veridical. Since it cannot, the theory predicts illusions of motion.

This technique has been used to investigate a rebound illusion (Mack, Fendrich and Sirigatti, 1973): if a tracked spot suddenly stops, it seems to rebound sharply backward before coming to rest. Mack *et al.* explain the illusion by noting that the eye continues to move during a reaction time. During that time the image moves sharply backward on the retina. But because the central command to stop has already been given, the reafferent retinal motion is not countered by a change in efference copy and is perceived as real exafferent motion. Eye movement recordings showed that the amount of overshoot of the eye was commensurate with the perceived illusion.

Figure distortions during pursuit were extended to two dimensions by Festinger and Easton (1974), who had subjects track a target moving in a square path. Perceptual distortions occurred at the corners, commensurate with the inability to change tracking direction abruptly. The unforgiving visual system, not taking account of kinematic limitations of the oculomotor system, compared the abruptly changing oculomotor command with the wandering path on the retina, and a perception of pinching-in of the trajectory of the target resulted. Festinger and Easton also uncovered a paper with similar observations during tracking in a triangular path, by Fujii (1943). The Fujii paper had been previously unknown to workers in this field.

A spot describing a circle of constant size was used by Coren *et al.* (1975) to further test the dynamics of the Fujii effect. The circle was seen at the veridical size when the spot moved slowly. As it moved faster the circle appeared to become smaller, until the size passed a minimum and even faster spot movement resulted in a larger apparent size. At high speeds of spot movement, of course, tracking becomes impossible and a circle of the veridical size is seen again. The minimum was reached at rotational velocities of 1.13–1.73 Hz. This sort of target stimulus invites interpretation by the techniques of linear analysis.

A possible artifact of stimulation may explain why the circle appeared at the veridical size for very fast or very slow movements, in contradiction to the underperceptions described above and predicted by theory. The reasons for this may be related to the size of the uniform screen on which the target spot moved, and the possibility of comparing spot position to the edges of the screen. The Fujii effect is seen only on large uniform screens, certainly a stimulus of limited ecological validity. Texture in the background minimizes the effect.

(6) *Use of efference copy information is different for perception and for visually guided behavior.* The evidence for this statement comes principally from two lines of research. In both of them, cognitive and sensorimotor functions are clearly differentiated in a context where extraretinal and retinal information can be decoupled. One is the eyepress paradigm outlined earlier, in which efference can be separated from tonic gaze position. In the eyepress experiments of Bridgeman and Stark (1981) and Stark and Bridgeman (1983), three output measures were used: setting a point to appear straight ahead, pointing to a target and visual–auditory matching. In darkness, with only a point target visible, all three measures yielded biases with eyepress that were indistinguishable from the deviation of the occluded fellow eye. Thus, the subjective and the objective measures of efference copy were in agreement, and efference copy seemed to account for all of the results. In a structured visual field, however, perceptual estimates of target position were little changed with eyepress, while the pointing and visual–auditory matching measures continued to show a robust effect of modified efference. Thus, subjects could perceive the target to be in one location, but point to it in another. In perception, the efference copy signal was evaluated along with visual context, but the motor output relied only on efference copy and was little affected by context.

The second line of research in which efference copy influences cognitive and sensorimotor systems differently is complementary to the first. Rather than biasing efference copy and leaving visual context constant, this approach biases the visual context and leaves efference copy unchanged.

A design which highlights the contrast between cognitive and sensorimotor systems uses saccadic suppression of displacement to manipulate perceived visual context. This saccadic suppression phenomenon is a large increase in the threshold for detection of a target displacement if that displacement occurs during a saccadic eye movement. The research effort was born at a meeting of the Association for Research in Vision and Ophthalmology where the author showed that preservation of spatial values across saccades was poor (Bridgeman, Hendry and Stark, 1974). In the next talk, Peter Hallett (Hallett and Lightstone, 1974) showed that preservation of spatial values across saccades was excellent. The difference between the two contrasting experiments turned out to be the response measure: Hallett and Lightstone (1976a, b) had used an oculomotor looking response to determine available spatial information, while Bridgeman, Hendry and Stark (1975) had used a cognitive judgment of image displacement.

Hallett and Lightstone had asked subjects to look to the positions of targets flashed during saccades – a task which they could perform with impressive accuracy despite their poor ability to perceive the locations of the targets. The experiments have been criticized because only a few target locations, which subjects might have memorized, were available, but subsequent work (reviewed below) has found the conclusion of good spatial ability for motor measures to be valid. Bridgeman *et al.* had asked subjects to detect the displacement of a large visual context, finding that detection would fail even for very large displacements if the displacement occurred during a large saccade. A displacement of 4° could be missed if it occurred about 10 ms after the start of a large saccade.

The observations of good localizability during saccades with a motor measure and poor localizability with a cognitive measure were combined into a single experiment by Bridgeman *et al.* (1979). As reviewed in the introduction, these experiments showed that extraretinal information enabled subjects to perform motor tasks accurately even when perceptual illusions distorted the apparent positions of targets.

This conclusion was further explored by Wong and Mack (1981) who, as noted in the introduction, also found dissociations between perceived direction and the direction of oculomotor behavior. A complication in the results appeared if the saccade occurred after a delay. In this case, the saccade would follow the perceived direction. It is as though the sensorimotor system had only a short memory and after that time it had to use the less accurate spatial values preserved in the cognitive system.

The effect of delay on the switch from veridical tracking to perceptual illusion was also shown dramatically in a series of studies on perception during pursuit eye movements (Festinger, Sedgwick and Holtzman, 1976; Holtzman, Sedgwick and Festinger, 1978; Sedgwick and Festinger, 1976; reviewed by Holtzman and Sedgwick, 1984). In these studies, a subject tracked a horizontally oscillating target while another target moved obliquely above the first. The direction of oblique motion was misperceived because of induced motion. Now the subject made a saccade to the obliquely moving target and continued tracking. When the eye acquired this target, however, it was stabilized on the retina, so that any perceived motion must be due to efference copy. The eye tracked in the veridical direction, pulling the target along with it, until the target would have reversed its direction. Tracking also reversed, but now the eye moved in the perceived direction, rather than the one actually presented. During the whole period, the subject perceived motion in the original illusory direction.

It was as though a veridical efference copy could drive the eye until the direction reversal interrupted the process; then only cognitive information remained, and this was tracked. Importing the cognitive signal into the motor system brought the cognitive illusion of induced motion along with it. Manipulation of speeds and extents of motion showed that the motion reversal event, rather than the time delay, was crucial in the switch from sensorimotor to cognitive driving of pursuit.

Since these experiments involved stimulus motion or displacement at some point during each trial, there is a possibility that motion and position information are confounded in perception, making interpretation difficult. The experiments on the Roelofs effect reviewed in the introduction made it clear that the dissociation of pointing and perceptual judgment can occur even with completely static displays, where no visual motion occurs at any time during a trial.

From this evidence we can conclude that the efference copy, as a part of the motor system, has no information about visual context and is not affected by perceived visual illusions. It is only when efference copy information is unavailable to guide motor action that the cognitively based representation of visual space is pressed into service to guide behavior. Normally, with a visual world continuously present, efference copy guides motor behavior while perception uses efference copy in a much more limited way.

(7) *The efference copy/space constancy system operates at low temporal frequency.* This commandment again has two aspects, for pursuit and for saccadic eye movements. In the case of pursuit, Mack (1986) reviews evidence that pursuit eye movements are systematically underregistered in perception, an effect described quantitatively by Mack and Herman (1972). Both the velocity and the amplitude of the movements are underregistered.

The experiments are done with fixation targets moving against homogeneous backgrounds, however, a condition which may require less pursuit innervation than is normally necessary to move the eyes at a given velocity (it is assumed that the system calculates amplitude in this situation by integrating the velocity signal). In normal visual environments, the optokinetic system (described in (4) above) tends to hold the eyes in a fixed position relative to the background. A large pursuit innervation is necessary to overcome the optokinetic stabilization and enable the eyes to track a target accurately. In a homogeneous field, less pursuit innervation is necessary because there is no optokinetic influence to overcome. As a result, perceptions of motion velocity and amplitude are reduced.

The underregistration of pursuit does not explain a second phenomenon relating to slow efference copy dynamics: a failure of the oculomotor system to compensate for presses and releases of the eye by a finger at rates greater than about 1 Hz. If a monocularly viewing eye is pressed and released slowly, in the presence of a fixed visual context, it does not rotate. Rather, the fovea remains fixed on a target point and the oculomotor system actively adjusts the innervation needed to counter the finger press. As a result, the occluded fellow eye rotates in counterphase with the finger press (Ilg, Bridgeman and Hoffmann, 1989). As the press and release are performed more rapidly, however, compensation is no longer complete – the pressed eye begins to rotate too, so that both eyes are moving in counterphase. Finally, at the highest press–release frequencies, the fellow eye no longer compensates for the press (Figure 6.5).

This effect can be interpreted as a phase lag of attempted compensations for the retinal image motion induced by the eyepress. It could be related to the dynamics of spatial compensations observed for saccadic eye movements, but for the cognitive system rather than the sensorimotor system. Grüsser and Krizič (1984) measured spatial constancy in the apparent position of a foveal afterimage in darkness. At low frequencies of alternating saccades the afterimage seems to move with each saccade, corresponding to Ilg and coworkers' low-frequency condition, where the fellow eye deviates but the pressed eye does not. At intermediate frequencies the afterimage appears as two images, separated by less than the expected angle; this corresponds to Ilg and co-workers' intermediate frequencies of eyepress, where both the pressed eye and the fellow eye move. At Grüsser and Krizič's highest frequencies the afterimage appeared at a single point in space despite the saccadic alternation, replicating an earlier qualitative observation of Köllner (1923). This corresponds to Ilg and co-workers' highest frequencies, where the pressed eye deviates but the oculomotor system does not compensate with movements of the fellow eye.

Eyepress Dynamics

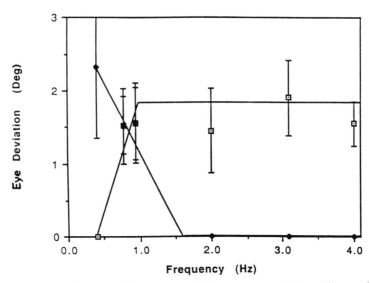

Figure 6.5. *Amount of deviation of (□) a pressed viewing eye and (■) a fellow occluded eye at a range of frequencies of eyepress. Movements of both eyes are measured simultaneously with binocular search coils. Data points within 0.1 Hz of each other are combined. Linear fits are made by eye for a constant slope portion at lower frequencies and a horizontal saturated portion at higher frequencies. More data are needed in the region between 1 and 2 Hz to determine precisely the highest frequencies of motor compensation for the eyepress. [Published in tabular form in Ilg, Bridgeman and Hoffmann, 1989, Fig. 5.]*

The parallel between Ilg, Bridgeman and Hoffmann's (1989) oculomotor results and Grüsser and Krizič's (1984) perceptual results suggests that the mechanisms that mediate motor compensation may also be influencing perceptual space constancy. Both space constancy and oculomotor compensation seem to be heavily damped.

The low temporal frequency of the efference copy system may explain several other results. The lack of compensation for the movements of optokinetic or vestibular nystagmus, for example, may be due not to their involuntary nature but simply to their high frequency. The low frequency characteristic might also be used to interpret a result of Honda (1984) that constant error in pointing to a target after successive saccades seems most correlated with the largest component saccade. The saccades in the cascade may come too quickly for all of them to be compensated properly.

(8) *There is only one efference copy for both eyes, reflecting Hering's law.* If the efference copy is a copy of oculomotor innervation, and Hering's (1868/1977) law states that there is only one control system innervating the two eyes, then there should be only one efference copy representing the innervation state of the double eye.

Evidence for this conjecture comes from observations of patients with one paralyzed eye: if the mobile eye is occluded and a target is presented to the paralyzed eye, movements of the occluded eye result in apparent movements of the target, even though neither the eye nor the target has moved. Similar observations have substantiated the effect in subjects paralyzed by retrobulbar block (Grüsser *et al.*, 1981).

A more quantitative support for a fused binocular efference copy comes from comparisons of retinal cyclorotary position (rotation of the eye about the line of sight as the axis) with the subjective vertical at eccentric gaze positions. Cyclorotary orientation at tertiary positions (not along a horizontal or vertical meridian from the primary fixation position) is given to a first approximation by Listing's law, but there are consistent differences from the predictions of the law, and the cyclorotary orientations of the two eyes are slightly different from one another at any given gaze position. Deviations of subjective vertical from cyclorotary position can be accounted for, if one assumes that target orientation is determined from the fused image of both eyes and that eye position is accounted for by an extraretinal signal common to both eyes (Haustein and Mittelstaedt, 1990).

That the efference copy is derived binocularly is also substantiated by experiments of Ono and Nakazimo (1977), who studied localization during asymmetrical convergence when a far target was obscured for one eye by a near target. They showed that visually guided saccades, presumably controlled by efference copy, were accurate even when position illusions were elicited in this way. Under these conditions, moving fixation from the near target to the far one results in an illusory movement of the far target, even though both targets are fixed in space. Yet the eye movement from one target to the other (involving both saccade and vergence components) remains accurate. So again, motor behavior remains accurate even when subjects are experiencing illusions of target location.

(9) *The efference copy signal is subject to adaptation in both direction and magnitude.* The initial evidence for this property of efference copy came from commonplace observations and clinical experience whose theoretical significance was not at first recognized. Initially there was the observation of adaptation to spectacle lenses that enlarge or reduce the size of the retinal image. At first, this leads to saccadic dysmetria as the new wearer of spectacles makes saccades to the location indicated by the previous retinal magnification, but soon the saccades adapt and reach their targets as they did before. The adaptation extends to both gain and direction and has been formalized in several elegant experiments (Deubel, 1987; Mack, Fendrich and Pleune, 1978; Wolf, Deubel and Hauske, 1984). In these experiments, a target is moved in a predictable way during a saccade, and subjects soon manage to capture the target in a single saccade despite the movement. The adaptation requires a change in the control signal, since the saccade controller is an open-loop feedforward system: once the movement begins, retinal input has no effect on its execution, and error feedback is useful only in planning subsequent saccades.

More important for the efference copy, perception adapts as well in these conditions, though to a lesser extent (Moidell and Bedell, 1988) . At first, the world seems to jump slightly with each saccade, if the discrepancy in gain is great enough, but soon everything appears normal again. The saccades have changed and the efference copy has changed to match them.

The perceptual adaptation has been quantified by measuring thresholds for detection of vertical motion after adapting to a target that moved vertically with each horizontal saccade (Fendrich, Mack and Pleune, 1977). The result was an increase of 7.8% in the threshold for detection of motion in the same direction as the target displacement, and a decrease of 6.4% for detection of motion in the opposite direction. The most reasonable interpretation of these perceptual changes is that there was a change in the evaluation of the efference copy signal.

Other work has further defined the flexibility of saccadic targeting and the accompanying efference copy. Shebilske (1981) reviews evidence that as little as 30 s of sustained deviation of gaze yields adaptation of visual direction. Subjects make errors in judgments of gaze direction and direction of visible objects (Craske, Crawshaw and Heron, 1975; Paap and Ebenholtz, 1976). The direction of the errors indicates that the baseline level of gaze control has shifted in the direction of the deviation. After a shift of gaze to the right, for instance, objects to the right of fixation are judged to be less eccentric than they were previously. Shebilske has used the term 'minor motor anomaly' to describe the phenomenon. If efference copy is important in establishing visual direction, the minor motor anomaly suggests that the efference copy has adapted in the direction of gaze over a very short time period. In the example of gaze deviation to the right, a subsequent straight-ahead fixation would induce a smaller-than-normal efference copy for targets to the right of fixation.

Clinical observations bear out the importance of adaptation. Patients suffering from the sort of oculomotor paresis that caught Helmholtz's attention complain of shifting visual fields, but after a few weeks the complaint goes away. The saccades have not changed, but the efference copy accompanying them has. A smaller adapted efference copy matches the smaller saccades, restoring perceived space constancy despite the saccadic dysmetria.

6   CONCLUDING REMARKS

The concept of oculomotor efference copy has come a long way in the past few decades. From a simple assumption about monitoring of eye innervation, the concept has grown to a family of related signals with varying gains, dynamics and access to perceptual and motor apparatus. A subdiscipline of the neurosciences has grown up around the concepts of feedforward monitoring of eye position, and it is tackling the many problems which the research to date has revealed. This chapter marks a start, not a finish, of that discipline.

REFERENCES

Anstis, S. M. (1986). Motion perception in the frontal plane: Sensory aspects. In K. R. Boff, L. Kaufman and J. P. Thomas (Eds), *Handbook of Perception and Human Performance*, vol. 1: *Sensory Processes and Perception* (pp. 16. 1–16.27). New York: John Wiley.

Bach-Y-Rita, P. and Ito, F. (1966). Properties of stretch receptors in cat extraocular muscles. *Journal of Physiology*, **186**, 663–688.

Bell, C. (1823/1974). In P. F. Cranefield (Ed.), *François Magendie, Charles Bell and the Course of the Spinal Nerves*, with the facsimile of Charles Bell's annotated copy of his 'Idea of a new anatomy of the brain'. Mt Kisco, NY: Futura.

Bridgeman, B. (1979). Adaptation and the two-visual-systems hypothesis. *Behavioral and Brain Sciences*, **2**, 84–85.

Bridgeman, B. (1981). Cognitive factors in subjective stabilization of the visual world. *Acta Psychologica*, **48**, 111–121.

Bridgeman, B. (1986). Multiple sources of outflow in processing spatial information. *Acta Psychologica, 63,* 35–48.

Bridgeman, B. (1989). Separate visual representations for perception and for visually guided behavior. In S. R. Ellis and M. K. Kaiser (Eds), *Spatial Displays and Spatial Instruments.* Moffett Field, CA: NASA (14.1-14.15).

Bridgeman, B. and Delgado, D. (1984). Sensory effects of eyepress are due to efference. *Perception and Psychophysics, 36,* 482–484.

Bridgeman, B. and Fishman R. (1985). Dissociation of corollary discharge from gaze direction does not induce a straight-ahead shift. *Perception and Psychophysics, 37,* 523–528.

Bridgeman, B. and Graziano, J. A. (1989). Effect of context and efference copy on visual straight-ahead. *Vision Research, 29,* 1729–1736.

Bridgeman, B., Hendry, D. and Stark, L. (1974). Detection of displacement of the visual world during saccades. Paper read at the Association for Research in Vision and Ophthalmology, Annual Meeting, April.

Bridgeman, B., Hendry, D. and Stark, L. (1975). Failure to detect displacment of the visual world during saccadic eye movements. *Vision Research, 15,* 719–722.

Bridgeman, B., Kirch, M. and Sperling, A. (1981). Segregation of cognitive and motor aspects of visual function using induced motion. *Perception and Psychophysics, 29,* 336–342.

Bridgeman, B., Lewis, S., Heit, G. and Nagle, M. (1979). Relationship between cognitive and motor-oriented systems of visual position perception. *Journal of Experimental Psychology: Human Perception and Performance, 5,* 692–700.

Bridgeman, B. and Stark, L. (1979). Omnidirectional increase in threshold for image shifts during saccadic eye movements. *Perception and Psychophysics, 25,* 241–243.

Bridgeman, B. and Stark, L. (1981). Efferent copy and visual direction. *Investigative Ophthalmology and Visual Science Supplement, 20,* 55.

Bridgeman, B. and Stark, L. (1991). Ocular proprioception and efference copy in perception and visually guided behavior. *Vision Research, 31,* 1903–1913.

Brindley, G. S., Goodwin, G. M., Kulikowski, J. J. and Leighton, D. (1976). Stability of vision with a paralysed eye. *Journal of Physiology, 258,* 65–66.

Brindley, G. S. and Merton, P. A. (1960). The absence of position sense in the human eye. *Journal of Physiology, 153,* 127–130.

Brune, F. and Lücking, C. H. (1969). Okulomotorik, Bewegungswahrnehmung und Raumkonstanz der Sehdinge. *Der Nervenarzt, 240,* 692–700.

Buisseret, P. and Maffei, L. (1977). Extraocular proprioceptive projections to the visual cortex. *Experimental Brain Research, 28,* 421–425.

Coren, S., Bradley, D. R., Hoenig, P. and Girgus, J. (1975). The effect of smooth tracking and saccadic eye movements on the perception of size: The shrinking circle illusion. *Vision Research, 15,* 49–55.

Craske, B., Crawshaw, M. and Heron, P. (1975). Disturbance of the oculomotor system due to lateral fixation. *Quarterly Journal of Experimental Psychology, 27,* 459–465.

Deubel, H. (1987). Adaptivity of gain and direction in oblique saccades. In J. K. O'Regan and A. Lévy-Schoen (Eds), *Eye Movements: From Physiology to Cognition* (pp. 181–190). Amsterdam: North-Holland.

Dichgans, J., Körner, F. and Voigt, K. (1969). Vergleichende Skalierung des afferenten und efferenten Bewegungssehens beim Menschen: Lineare Funktionen mit verschiedener Anstiegssteilheit. *Psychologische Forschung, 32,* 277–295.

Ditchburn, R. W. (1955). Eye movements in relation to retinal action. *Optica Acta, 1,* 171–176.

Dittler, R. (1921). Über die Raumfunktion der Netzhaut in ihrer Abhängigkeit vom Lagegefühl der Augen und vom Labyrinth. *Zeitschrift für Sinnesphysiologie, 52,* 274–310.

Donaldson, I. and Long, A. C. (1980). Interaction between extraocular proprioceptive and visual signals in the superior colliculus of the cat. *Journal of Physiology, 298,* 85–110.

Fendrich, R., Mack, A. and Pleune, J. (1977). The adaptation of position constancy during saccadic eye movements. *Investigative Ophthalmology and Visual Science Supplement* 107.

Festinger, L. and Canon, L. K. (1965). Information about spatial location based on knowledge about efference. *Psychological Review, 72*, 373–384.

Festinger, L. and Easton, A. M. (1974). Inferences about the efferent system based on a perceptual illusion produced by eye movements. *Psychological Review, 81*, 44–58.

Festinger, L., Sedgwick, H. A. and Holtzman, J. D. (1976). Visual perception during smooth pursuit eye movements. *Vision Research, 16*, 1377–1386.

Fiorentini, A. and Maffei, L. (1977). Instability of the eye in the dark and proprioception. *Nature, 269*, 330–331.

Fujii, E. (1943). Forming a figure by movements of a luminous point. *Japanese Journal of Psychology, 18*, 196–232.

Gauthier, G., Nommay, D. and Vercher, J.-L. (1990). The role of ocular muscle proprioception in visual localization of targets. *Science, 249*, 58–61.

Goodale, M. A., Meenan, J. P., Bötthoff, H. H., Nicolle, D. A., Murphy, K. S. and Racicot, C. I. (1994). Separate neural pathways for the visual analysis of object shape in perception and prehension. *Current Biology, 4*, 604–610.

Grüsser, O.-J. (1985). Possible role of efference copy signals for space and movement perception. Paper presented at the Conference on Sensorimotor Interactions in Space Perception and Action, University of Bielefeld, Germany, February.

Grüsser, O.-J. (1986a). Interaction of afferent and efferent signals in visual perception. A history of ideas and experimental paradigms. *Acta Psychologica, 63*, 3–21.

Grüsser, O.-J. (1986b). Some recent studies on the quantitative analysis of efference copy mechanisms in visual perception. *Acta Psychologica, 63*, 49–62.

Grüsser, O.-J. and Krizič, A. (1984). Time constant of pre- and postsaccadic recalibration of retinal spatial values as measured by a new afterimage method. *Investigative Ophthalmology and Visual Sciences, 25*, ARVO Suppl., 263.

Grüsser, O.-J., Krizič, A. and Weiss, L.-R. (1987). Afterimage movement during saccades in the dark. *Vision Research, 27*, 215–226.

Grüsser, O.-J., Kulikowski, J., Pause, M. and Wollensak, J. O.-J. (1981). Optokinetic nystagmus, sigma-optokinetic nystagmus and pursuit movements elicited by stimulation of an immobilized human eye. *Journal of Physiology, 320*, 210 ff.

Hallett, P. and Lightstone, A. (1974). Saccades to flashed targets. Paper read at Association for Research in Vision and Ophthalmology Annual Meeting, April.

Hallett, P. and Lightstone, A. (1976a). Saccadic eye movements towards stimuli triggered by prior saccades. *Vision Research, 16*, 99–106.

Hallett P. and Lightstone, A. (1976b). Saccadic eye movements to flashed targets. *Vision Research, 16* 107–114.

Haustein, W. and Mittelstaedt, H. (1990). Evaluation of retinal orientation and gaze direction in the perception of the vertical. *Vision Research, 30*, 255–262.

Hein, A. and Diamond, R. (1983). Contribution of eye movement to the representation of space. In A. Hein and M. Jeannerod (Eds), *Spatially Oriented Behavior* (pp. 119–133). New York: Springer.

Helmholtz, H. Von (1866/1962). *A Treatise on Physiological Optics*, vol. 3, J. P. C. Southall (Ed. and Transl.). New York: Dover, 1962. (Originally published 1866, *Handbuch der Physiologischen Optik*. Leipzig, Hamburg: Voss.)

Helmholtz, H. Von (1867/1925). *Helmholtz' Treatise on Physiological Optics* 3rd edn, J. P. C. Southall (Ed. and Transl.). Menasha, WI: Optical Society of America, 1925. (Originally published 1867.)

Hering, E. (1861/1990). *Beiträge zur Physiologie*, vol. 1. Leipzig: Engelmann. (Reissued with introduction by B. Bridgeman (1990). Berlin: Springer.)

Hering, E. (1868/1977). *Die Lehre vom binokularen Sehen*. Leipzig: Engelmann. (Translated by B. Bridgeman as *The Theory of Binocular Vision* (1977), B. Bridgeman and L. Stark (Eds). New York: Plenum Press.)

Hill, A. L. (1972). Direction constancy. *Perception and Psychophysics, 11*, 175–178.

Holtzman, J. D. and Sedgwick, H. A. (1984). The integration of motor control and visual perception. In M. S. Gazzaniga (Ed.), *Handbook of Cognitive Neuroscience* (pp. 115–133). New York: Plenum Press.

Holtzman, J. D., Sedgwick, H. A. and Festinger, L. K. (1978). Interaction of perceptually monitored and unmonitored efferent commands for smooth pursuit eye movements. *Vision Research, 18,* 1545–1555.

Honda, H. (1984). Eye-position signals in successive saccades. *Perception and Psychophysics, 36,* 15–20.

Ilg, U. J., Bridgeman, B. and Hoffmann, K. P. (1989). Influence of mechanical disturbance on oculomotor behavior. *Vision Research, 29,* 545–551.

Kashii, S., Matsui, Y., Honda, Y., Ito, J., Sasa, M. and Takaori, S. (1989). The role of extraocular proprioception in vestibulo-ocular reflex of rabbits. *Investigative Ophthalmology and Visual Science, 30,* 2258–2264.

Köllner, H. (1923). Über die Abhängigkeit der räumlichen Orientierung von den Augenbewegungen. *Klinische Wochenschrift, 2,* 482–484.

Kornmüller, A. E. (1931). Eine experimentelle Anästhesie der äußeren Augenmuskeln am Menschen und ihre Auswirkungen. *Journal für Psychologie und Neurologie, 41,* 354–366.

Ludvigh, E. (1952). Possible role of proprioception in the extraocular muscles. *Archives of Ophthalmology, 48,* 436–441.

Mach, E. (1885/1959). *Analysis of Sensations* (C. M. Williams, Ed. and Transl.). New York: Dover. (Originally published 1885.)

Mach, E. (1906). *Die Analyse der Empfindungen und das Verhältnis des Physischen zum Psychischen,* 5th edn. Jena: Fischer.

Mack, A. (1986). Perceptual aspects of motion in the frontal plane. In K. R. Boff, L. Kaufman and J. P. Thomas (Eds), *Handbook of Perception and Human Performance,* vol. I: *Sensory Processes and Perception* (pp. 17.1–17.38). New York: John Wiley.

Mack, A., Fendrich, R. and Pleune, J. (1978). Adaptation to an altered relation between retinal image displacements and saccadic eye movements. *Vision Research, 18,* 1321–1327.

Mack, A., Fendrich, R. and Sirigatti, S. (1973). A rebound illusion in visual tracking. *American Journal of Psychology, 86,* 425–433.

Mack, A. and Herman, E. (1972). The underestimation of distance during pursuit eye movements. *Perception and Psychophysics, 12,* 471–473.

MacKay, D. G. (1973). Visual stability and voluntary eye movements. In R. Jung (Ed.), *Handbook of Sensory Physiology,* vol. 7, part 3: *Central Visual Information.* New York: Springer.

Matin, L. (1972). Eye movements and perceived viaual direction. In D. Jameson and L. Hurvich (Eds), *Handbook of Sensory Physiology,* vol. 7: *Visual Psychophysics* (pp. 331–380). New York: Springer.

Matin, L. (1982). Visual localization and eye movements. In A. H. Wertheim, W. A. Wagenaar and H. W. Leibowitz (Eds), *Tutorials on Motion Perception* (pp. 101–156). New York: Plenum Press.

Matin, L. (1986). Visual localization and eye movements. In K. R. Boff, L. Kaufman and J. P. Thomas (Eds), *Handbook of Perception and Human Performance,* vol. I: *Sensory Processes and Perception* (pp. 20.1–20.45). New York: John Wiley.

Matin, L., Picoult, E., Stevens, J. K., Edwards, Jr, M. W., Young, D. and MacArthur, R. (1980). Visual context-dependent mislocalizations under curare-induced partial paralysis of the extraocular muscles. *Investigative Ophthalmology and Visual Science, Supplement, 19,* 81.

Matin, L., Picoult, F., Stevens, J. K., Edwards, Jr, M. W., Young, D. and MacArthur, R. (1982). Oculoparalytic illusion: Visual-field-dependent spatial mislocalizations by humans partially paralyzed with curare. *Science, 216,* 198–201.

Mishkin, M., Ungerleider, L. and Macko, K. (1983). Object vision and spatial vision: Two cortical pathways. *Trends in Neurosciences, 6,* 414–417.

Mittelstaedt, H. (1990). Basic solutions to the problem of head-centric visual localization. In R. Warren and A. H. Wertheim (Eds), *Perception and Control of Self-motion*. Hillsdale, NJ: Erlbaum.

Moidell, B. G. and Bedell, H. E. (1988). Changes in oculocentric visual direction induced by the recalibration of saccades. *Vision Research*, **28**, 329–336.

Morgan, C. L. (1978). Constancy of egocentric visual direction. *Perception and Psychophysics*, **23**, 61–68.

Ono, H. and Nakazimo, R. (1977). Saccadic eye movements during changes in fixation to stimuli at different distances. *Vision Research*, **17**, 233–238.

Paap, K. and Ebenholtz, S. (1976). Perceptual consequences of potentiation in the extraocular muscles: An alternative explanation for adaptation to wedge prisms. *Journal of Experimental Psychology: Human Perception and Performance*, **2**, 457–468.

Paillard, J. (1987). Cognitive versus sensorimotor encoding of spatial information. In P. Ellen and C. Thinus-Blanc (Eds), *Cognitive Processes and Spatial Orientation in Animal and Man*, vol. II (pp. 43–77). Dordrecht, Netherlands: Nijhoff.

Pola, J. and Wyatt, H. J. (1989). The perception of target motion during smooth pursuit eye movements in the open-loop condition: Characteristics of retinal and extraretinal signals. *Vision Research*, **29**, 471–483.

Post, R. B. and Leibowitz, H. W. (1982). The effect of convergence on the vestibulo-ocular reflex and implications for perceived movement. *Vision Research*, **22**, 461–465.

Post, R. B. and Leibowitz, H. W. (1985). A revised analysis of the role of efference in motion perception. *Perception*, **14**, 631–643.

Purkinje, J. E. (1825a). *Beobachtungen und Versuche zur Physiologie der Sinne*, vol. II: *Neue Beiträge zur Kenntnis des Sehens in subjectiver Hinsicht*. Berlin: Reimer.

Purkinje, J. E. (1825b). Über die Scheinbewegungen, welche im subjectiven Umfang des Gesichtssinnes vorkommen. *Bulletin der naturwissenschaftlichen Sektion der Schlesischen Gesellschaft*, **IV**, 9–10.

Roelofs, C. O. (1935). Optische Localisation. *Archiv für Augenheilkunde*, **109**, 395–415.

Sedgwick, H. A. and Festinger, L. K. (1976). Eye movements, efference and visual perception. In R. A. Monty and J. W. Senders (Eds), *Eye Movements and Psychological Processes* (pp. 221–230). Hillsdale, NJ: Erlbaum.

Shebilske, W. (1977). Visuomotor coordination in visual direction and position constances. In W. Epstein (Ed.), *Stability and Constancy in Visual Perception* (pp. 23–69). New York: John Wiley.

Shebilske, W. (1981). Visual direction illusions in everyday situations: Implications for sensorimotor and ecological theories. In D. Fisher, R. Monty and J. Senders (Eds), *Eye Movements: Cognition and Visual Perception*. Hillsdale, NJ: Erlbaum.

Shebilske, W. (1986). Baseball batters support an ecological efference mediation theory of natural event perception. *Acta Psychologica*, **63**, 117–131.

Sherrington, C. S. (1898). Further note on the sensory nerves of the eye muscles. *Proceedings of the Royal Society*, **64**, 120–121.

Sherrington, C. S. (1918). Observations on the sensual role of the proprioceptive nerve supply of the extrinsic ocular muscles. *Brain*, **41**, 332–343.

Siebeck, R. (1954). Wahrnehmungsstörung und Störungswahrnehmung bei Augenmuskellähmungen. *Von Graefes Archiv für Opthalmologie*, **155**, 26–34.

Skavenski, A. A., Haddad, G. and Steinman, R. M. (1972). The extraretinal signal for the visual perception of direction. *Perception and Psychophysics*, **11**, 287–290.

Sperry, R. W. (1950). Neural basis of the spontaneous optokinetic response produced by visual inversion. *Journal of Comparative Psychology and Physiology*, **43**, 482–489.

Stark, L. and Bridgeman, B. (1983). Role of corollary discharge in space constancy. *Perception and Psychophysics*, **34**, 371–380.

Stark, L., Kong, R., Schwartz, S., Hendry, D. and Bridgeman, B. (1976). Saccadic suppression of image displacement. *Vision Research*, **16**, 1185–1187.

Steinbach, M. J. (1987). Proprioceptive knowledge of eye position. *Vision Research*, **10**, 1737–1744.

Steinbach, M. J. and Smith, D. R. (1981). Spatial localization after strabismus surgery: Evidence for inflow. *Science*, **213**, 1407–1409.

Stevens, J. K., Emerson, R. C., Gerstein, G. L., Kallos, T., Neufeld, G. R., Nichols, C. W. and Rosenquist, A. C. (1976). Paralysis of the awake human: Visual perceptions. *Vision Research*, **16**, 93–98.

Stoper, A. E. and Cohen, M. M. (1986). Judgements of eye level in light and in darkness. *Perception and Psychophysics*, **37**, 311–316.

Teuber, H.-L. (1960). Perception. In J. Field and H. W. Magoun (Eds), *Handbook of Physiology*, sect. 1: *Neurophysiology*, vol. 3 (pp. 1595–1668). Washington, DC: American Physiological Society.

Van Essen, D. C., Newsome, W. T. and Bixby, J. L. (1982). The pattern of interhemispheric connections and its relationship to extrastriate visual areas in the macaque monkey. *Journal of Neuroscience*, **2**, 265–283.

von Holst, F. and Mittelstaedt, H. (1950). Das Reafferenzprinzip. Wechselwirkungen zwischen Zentralnervensystem und Peripherie. *Naturwissenschaften*, **37**, 464–476. [English translation in *The Behavioral Physiology of Animals and Man*. London: Methuen (1973), pp. 139–173].

von Uexküll, J. (1920). *Theoretische Biologie*. Berlin: Patel.

von Uexküll, J. (1928). *Theoretische Biologie*, 2nd edn. Berlin: Springer.

Wallach, H. and Lewis, C. (1966). The effect of abnormal displacement of the retinal image during eye movements. *Perception and Psychophysics*, **1**, 25–29.

Wolf, W., Deubel, H. and Hauske, G. (1984). Properties of parametric adjustment in the saccadic system. In A. G. Gale and F. Johnson (Eds), *Theoretical and Applied Aspects of Eye Movement Research* (pp. 79–86). Amsterdam: North-Holland.

Wong, F. and Mack, A. (1981). Saccadic programming and perceived location. *Acta Psychologica*, **48**, 123–131.

Part II

Perception of Objects, Events and Actions

Chapter 7

Perceptual Constancies: Analysis and Synthesis

Wayne L. Shebilske and Aaron L. Peters
Texas A&M University

1 INTRODUCTION

Perceptual constancies are tendencies for the appearances of objects to remain unaltered as their sensory correlates vary. Day and McKenzie (1977, p. 291) distinguish two kinds: (1) egocentric constancies, which 'refer to constancy of an object's apparent position in space in relation to the observer as the sensory representation of that position varies'; and (2) object constancies, which 'refer mainly to constancy of object properties as their sensory images vary'. Woodworth (1938, p. 595) described visual constancies as follows:

> '... the retinal image continually changes without much changing the appearance of objects. The apparent size of a person does not change as he moves away from you. A ring turned at various angles to the line of sight, and therefore projected as a varying ellipse on the retina, continues to appear circular. Part of a wall, standing in shadow, is seen as the same color as the well-lighted portion. Still more radical are the changes in the retinal image that occur when we move about a room and examine its contents from various angles. In spite of the visual flux the objects seem to remain in the same place.'

Similar constancies exist in other sensory modalities, such as constancies for loudness as a function of distance (Mershon *et al.*, 1981) and odor (we tend to perceive the same olfactory intensity whether we take a shallow or deep sniff, despite changes of the amount of stimulus reaching the olfactory receptors (Teghtsoonian *et al.*, 1978)).

Most constancy research, however, has been done on visual constancies, such as constancies of distance (Hill, 1972; Purdy and Gibson, 1955), color (Graham, 1965), position and direction (Shebilske, 1977) and motion (Richards, 1977). Much of that research was inspired by Koffka's (1935) provocative analysis of 'why things look as they do'. Excellent comprehensive reviews of that literature (Epstein, 1977) suggest that it perpetuated not only Koffka's interest in vision, but also his emphasis on appearance as opposed to performance. Despite this narrow focus, however, there was substantial divergence of theories, methods and constructs. The present chapter will analyze the divergence and provide a framework aimed toward a synthesis.

Handbook of Perception and Action: Volume 1
ISBN 0-12-516161-1

Table 7.1. *A Taxonomy of constancy theories*

	Theories	
Analysis	Unconscious inference	Relational
Psychophysical	1	2
Biopsychological	3	4

2   A TAXONOMY OF CONSTANCY THEORIES

Constancy theories can be categorized according to a simple 2 × 2 taxonomy as shown in Table 7.1. The columns contrast unconscious inference theories (Epstein, 1963; Rock, 1977) and relational theories (Gibson, 1950, 1966, 1979; Wallach, 1948) The rows contrast psychophysical versus psychobiological levels of analysis.

According to unconscious inference theory (cells 1 and 3), veridical apparent location and properties are determined by their simplest sensory correlates plus impercipient inductive reasoning, which takes into account the many factors that influence the sensory correlates. On this account, apparent size is determined by retinal image size plus unconscious inferences about the effect of distance on image

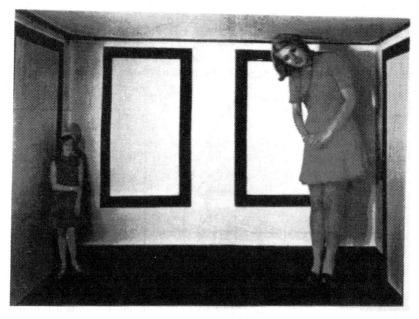

Figure 7.1. *The Ames room distorts the apparent size of the people standing in the corners.* *[Photograph courtesy of R. Berger/Science Digest; © Hearst Corporation.]*

size, so that we see size accurately when we have unerring information about retinal image size and distance. Conversely, we see size inaccurately when we have misleading information. For example, Figure 7.1 shows an Ames room (Ittelson, 1952/1968), which is designed to provide misleading information about distance. The room's left corner is actually much farther away than its right corner, yet the two corners appear equidistant. The room produces a dramatic illusion. People standing in the far corner look like dwarves, while those in the close corner look like giants. According to the unconscious inference theory, we see the distorted sizes *because* we see distorted distances. We unconsciously reason that the woman on the left is smaller because she has a small retinal image size and she appears to be the same distance away.

According to relational theories (cells 2 and 4), in contrast, constant perceptions are determined by constant aspects of the sensory stimulus, which are higher-order invariant relationships that directly convey veridical location and properties without the need for additional inductive reasoning processes. Hence, constant size perception is attributed to some aspect of the visual scene that remains unchanged when distance changes. Rock and Ebenholtz (1959) noted, for example, that an object's size remains in a constant ratio to surrounding objects as an observer changes her distance from the object. For instance, as you approach a person who is standing in a door frame, the ratio of the person's size to the door frame size remains constant. In a natural environment, such relationships should yield accurate perceptions. In a distorted environment, however, they should yield false perceptions. On this account, the Ames room misleads us by distorting stimulus relationships that are critical for constancy, such as the size of the people with respect to the size of the windows.

Unconscious inference theories and relational theories also offer opposing accounts of other constancies. Visual direction constancy is an example. It is the tendency for the apparent egocentric direction of objects to remain relatively constant, despite eye movements that change the location of the object's retinal image. According to unconscious inference theory, this constancy is a result of unconsciously applying an algorithm that takes eye position into account. Figure 7.2 presents assumptions that simplify this algorithm by making perceived visual location a simple linear function of eye position and retinal position. The algorithm yields visual direction constancy for A in the right-hand drawing and A' in the left-hand drawing, even though eye position and retinal location are different in the two drawings. The unconscious application of this algorithm could provide a general explanation for visual direction constancy. In principle, however, relational theories could also explain visual direction constancy. For instance, a straight-ahead object projects images in the two eyes that are symmetrically displaced from the nose image, regardless of eye position (Bower, 1974), and the point of maximum rate of expansion in an optic array represents the point of contact on an approaching surface, regardless of eye position (Regan and Beverley, 1982).

Lightness constancy provides another example of opposing accounts. Apparent lightness ranges from white to black through shades of grey. Lightness constancy is the tendency of apparent lightness to remain relatively constant despite changes in illumination which alters the amount of light reaching the eye. We see the ink on this page as black and the paper as white, for instance, in dim or bright light. The ink reflects about 5% of the light that strikes it and the paper reflects about

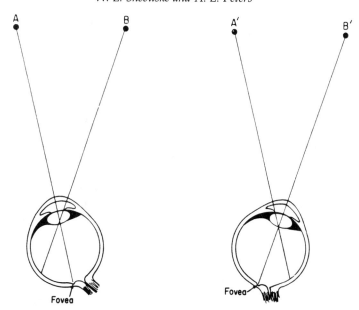

Figure 7.2. *Simplifying assumptions of an algorithm for perceiving visual direction. The assumptions are: (1) Visual location of target (VL(T)): A and A' are defined as targets located at a spatial location of 0°, B and B' as targets located 30° to the right of A and A'. (2) Retinal location (RL): The fovea is defined as a retinal location of zero. Deviations from the fovea are measured in degrees of visual angle. Target deviations to the right and left produce plus and minus changes in retinal location respectively. (3) Extraretinal eye position information (EEPI): the direction of gaze toward A and A' is defined as zero. For other targets, EEPI is defined in terms of the visual angle between the targets and A or A' (right = plus; left = minus). The algorithm is VL(T) = RL + EEPI. The algorithm specifies the locations of the targets in the figure as follows: VL(A) = 0 + 0 = 0, VL(B) = 30 + 0 = 30, VL(A') = −30 + 30 = 0, VL(B') = 0 + 30 = 30. [From Shebilske, 1987a, p. 197. © 1987 Lawrence Erlbaum Associates; reprinted with kind permission.]*

80%. Thus, when 100 units of light strike the page, the ink reflects about 5 units and the paper reflects about 80 units. When 10 000 units of light strike the page, the ink reflects about 500 units and the paper reflects about 8000 units. How do the two theories explain that 80 units of light look white in dim light, while 500 units look black in bright light? According to unconscious inference theory, we have this constancy because an unconscious reasoning process takes into account differences in lighting. In contrast, according to relational theories, this constancy stems from an invariant ratio between the brightness of an object and its surround (Wallach, 1948). This ratio is the same on this page in dim light: 5/80 = 0.0625, and in bright light: 500/8000 = 0.0625.

Both unconscious inference theories and relational theories have been analyzed at psychophysical and psychobiological levels. Psychophysical analyses (Table 7.1, cells 1 and 2) study the relationship between physical stimuli and experiences. Psychobiological analyses (cells 3 and 4) study the biological underpinnings of behavior and experience. Let us consider some applications of these analyses to the constancies.

Psychophysical experiments have supported the algorithm postulated by the unconscious inference account of visual direction constancy. Many of these were done by Leonard Matin and his colleagues (Matin, 1972, 1976, 1982). In a typical experiment, subjects judge the relative positions of briefly flashed lights in darkness. One light flashes, an eye movement occurs, and a second light flashes during or after the eye movement. The results of such experiments are usually consistent with the algorithm in Figure 7.2. Psychobiological experiments also support the algorithm and go beyond it in suggesting the source of eye position information. In one experiment, Collins (1974a, b) showed that specific efferent innervation patterns are required to hold the eyes in specific positions and to move the eyes from one position to another. Efferent innervations could therefore be a source of eye position.

Psychophysical studies have also tested relational theories of visual direction constancies. On the one hand, tests of apparent straight ahead with and without the nose visible fail to support the importance of invariant relationships with respect to the nose (Shebilske and Nice, 1976); on the other hand, experiments have supported the functional significance of the point of maximum rate of expansion in judging the contact point of an approaching surface (Regan and Beverley, 1982). Biopsychological experiments have not yet provided additional support for relational theories of visual direction constancy.

The situation is reversed for brightness constancy. Relational theories are supported by both psychophysical and biopsychological evidence. Unconscious inference theories are only supported by psychophysical evidence at this time. Psychophysical experiments by Burkhardt *et al.* (1984) have shown that perceived lightness responses to fixed brightness ratios remain constant over a broad range of background illumination, and this constancy holds when a dark object is viewed against a light background (e.g. black letters on a white page) or when light objects are viewed against a dark background (e.g. car headlights at night).

Psychobiological experiments have found that retinal ganglion cells respond in a way that could account for constant lightness responses over fixed brightness ratios. These cells have receptive fields that are antagonistic concentric circular areas, which have either an 'on'-center and 'off'-surround or an 'off'- center and an 'on'-surround. Light stimulating on-areas increases the cell's response, and light stimulating off-areas decreases the cell's response. Figure 7.3 illustrates hypothetical data from a retinal ganglion cell with an on-center. The ordinate shows the cell's firing rate; the abscissa shows the amount of light stimulating the on-center; and the three parallel, laterally displaced curves represent three levels of illumination stimulating the off-surround (low on the left; medium in the middle; and high on the right). The lines A, B and C show that three different levels of light stimulating the on-center yield the same firing rate because proportionally more light on the center is needed to yield the same response as the light increases on the surround. The simple assumption that lightness perception is based on the firing rate of retinal ganglion cells could therefore explain Burkhardt *et al.*'s (1984) data on lightness constancy. The on-center cells would explain responses for light stimuli on a darker background; off-center cells would account for perception with dark stimuli against a lighter background.

Unconscious inference theory does not have a similar tidy package of corresponding psychophysical and psychobiological results, but it does explain psychophysical results that cannot be explained by relational theory. For example, Hochberg and Beck (1954) found that an object's apparent lightness depended upon the apparent direction of illumination relative to the object, even when the ratio of

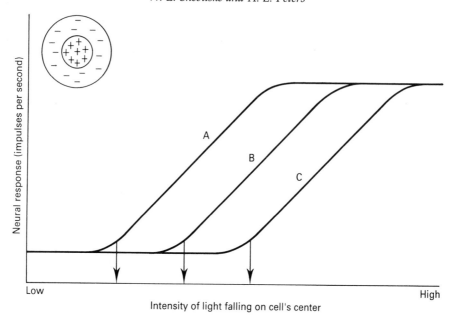

Figure 7.3. *Idealized firing rate data from an on-center retinal ganglion cell as a function of the amount of light falling on the on-center and as a function of three levels of light (A, B, C) falling on the off-surround. [From Sekuler and Blake, 1990, Figure 3.14, p. 76. © 1990 Glencoe/Macmillan/ McGraw-Hill, Mission Hills, CA; reprinted with kind permission.]*

light falling on the object and its surround were held constant. Figure 7.4 shows their display. Subjects viewed a table top containing an upright trapezoid and several small blocks, all of which were illuminated from directly above. Subjects viewed this scene through an aperture that required monocular viewing and minimized motion parallax. Under these conditions, the trapezoid tended to look like a square lying flat on the table. The observer saw the trapezoid flip up to its actual shape and position, however, when a rod was waved behind it. The apparent flipping changed neither the absolute amount of light nor the ratio of light on the trapezoid and its surround, but it did change the apparent lightness from a darker square to a lighter trapezoid. It was as if subjects unconsciously reasoned as follows: the square and the trapezoid reflect the same amount of light into my eye even though the square is directly illuminated, while the trapezoid is indirectly illuminated; therefore, the trapezoid must reflect a greater proportion of light, that is, it must be lighter.

You can see a similar effect for yourself by doing a demonstration first described by Ernst Mach (see Attneave, 1971). Fold a 7 × 14 cm white card in half along its long axis. Place the long edges on a table, so that the folded edge runs parallel to the table. It should look like a small book with the open pages down and the binding up. Sit at the table with your head directly above the table's edge and place the card 30 cm away from the edge with the long folded axis pointing directly at your nose. Illuminate the card from the right side and view it monocularly. Eventually the card will appear to flip and to look like a book standing on edge

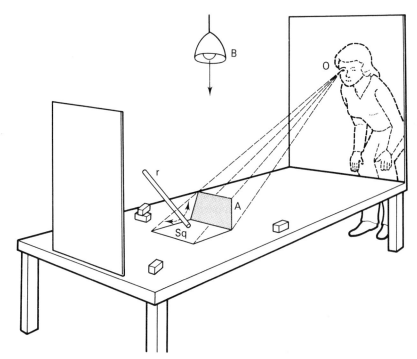

Figure 7.4. *A display used to demonstrate that apparent lightness depends on the perceived angle of illumination relative to an object. The trapezoid appears darker when it is seen as a square lying flat on the table. [From Hochberg and Beck, 1954, p. 264, modified. © 1954 The American Psychological Association; reprinted with kind permission.]*

with its open pages toward you. This apparent flip changes the apparent level of illumination on the right side without changing the actual illumination or the ratio of light from the card and its surround. Before the apparent flip, the right side appears to be an outer surface facing the light. After the apparent flip, the right side appears to be an inner surface facing away from the light and it appears much lighter as if you unconsciously reason as follows: the surface facing away from the light reflects as much light into my eye, so it must reflect a greater proportion, that is, it must be lighter.

Such demonstrations suggest that unconscious inferences might play a role in lightness constancy even though their biological underpinnings are not determined (Gilchrist, 1977).

3   ANALYSIS OF DIVERGING METHODS AND CONSTRUCTS

In addition to these main theoretical categories, the constancy literature is laden with numerous diverging methods and constructs. Some of these stem from early debates between Gestalt psychologists and introspectionists. Others emerged from later research. This section will analyze some of these.

3.1 Analytic Introspection Versus the Gestalt-Phenomenological Method

Constancy research was at the heart of the divergence between introspectionism and Gestalt psychology. Epstein (1977, pp. 1–2) described the controversy as follows:

> 'Analysis of the constancies served several objectives of Gestalt theory. Among the objectives was the Gestalt polemic against the analytic introspectionism advocated by the Leipzig–Cornell axis of Wundt and Titchener. According to Köhler (1929, Chapter 3), the introspectionist distorted the data of psychology ... The introspective method yielded data that were compatible with the core-context theory, chiefly because it was designed to yield no other. ... Gestalt psychologists were determined to redirect attention from artificially isolated sense data to immediate spontaneous perceptions. ... Whereas the introspectionist tried to strip away the constancies so that the genuine sensory core could be observed, the Gestalt psychologist considered the constancies in perception to be the primary data.'

Ironically, after criticizing the structuralists for using a method of observation that was designed to slant data in favor of a specific theory, the Gestalt psychologists limited their experiments to a single method of observation. Epstein (1977, p. 19) describes their rationale as follows:

> 'Gestalt psychologists ... insisted that the proper concern of a psychology of perception is to examine and explain perceptual reports. For this purpose the phenomenological method was advocated. The observer was urged to report how the world looked to naïve immediate observation. Careful instructions to induce the phenomenal attitude of viewing became critical to sound experimentation.'

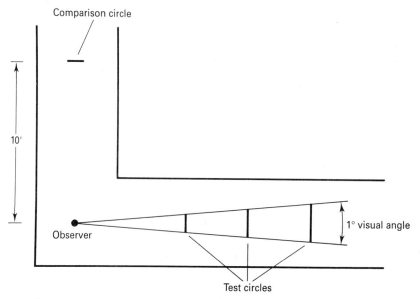

Figure 7.5. *The Holway–Boring experimental set-up used to study size constancy. [From Holway and Boring, 1941, p. 34, © 1941 University of Illinois Press; reprinted with kind permission.]*

As noted earlier, this phenomenological emphasis persisted in constancy research, which has focused on appearance as opposed to performance. An example is a study of size constancy by Holway and Boring (1941). They devised a paradigm which has since become the prototype for many constancy experiments. In their classic experiment, observers were seated at the junction of two long corridors, one being somewhat longer than the other. They then viewed illuminated disks of different physical sizes placed at different physical distances. Observers were to adjust the size of a variable disk in one corridor to be perceptually equal to a standard disk positioned in the other. The standard disks were presented at different distances from the observer, yet all disks subtended one degree of visual angle (Figure 7.5). Observers performed this size-matching task under four different viewing conditions. In descending order from the most depth information present to the least depth information present, these conditions were: (1) binocular vision; (2) monocular vision; (3) monocular vision with artificial pupil produced by looking through a pinhole in a piece of paper; and (4), an iteration of (3) with the addition of a long, black reduction tube which produced total darkness.

Results of the Holway–Boring (1941) experiment implied that human size perception involves principles of both the law of visual angle (perceived size is determined by the retinal image size of an object) and the law of size constancy (perceived size is determined by an interaction of retinal size information and perceptual processes involved in resolving the perceived distance of a target), depending on the specific environmental condition (Figure 7.6). Further research in this area has employed various nuances of the Holway–Boring paradigm to study variable effects on size constancy, such as instructions (Carlson, 1960, 1962; Epstein, 1963; Gilinsky, 1955; Leibowitz and Harvey, 1967, 1969), reduction conditions, that is, in an environment void of distance information (Epstein and Landauer, 1969;

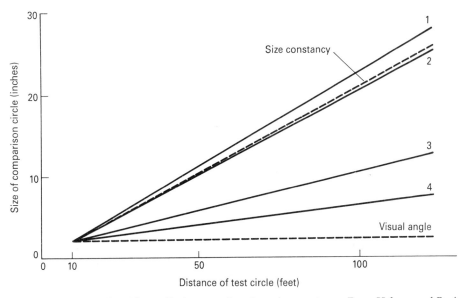

Figure 7.6. *Data from the Holway–Boring experiment on size constancy. From Holway and Boring, 1941, p. 23, modified.* © *1941 University of Illinois Press; reprinted with kind permission.]*

Hastorf and Way, 1952; Rock and Kaufman, 1962), and even cross-cultural effects (Leibowitz and Pick, 1972). All of these experiments and most other constancy experiments preserve the Gestalt phenomenological emphasis by focusing on the question of why size looks the way it does.

3.2 Perceptual and Judgmental Modes

The Gestalt psychologists also insisted upon a distinction between perceptual and judgmental modes of observation, which had been made earlier by Helmholtz (1890) and Hering (1879). According to this distinction, constancies correspond to immediate perceptions. The lack of constancy is reported when cognitive or judgmental processes intrude. This distinction was highlighted again when Gibson (1950, 1952) and Boring (1952) debated the relationship between what Gibson called the 'visual field' and the 'visual world'. In the visual field, appearances change as sensory correlates vary (i.e. no constancy); in the visual world, they do not (i.e. constancy). Observers can experience one or the other or both of these alternatives. Boring argued that the visual field is the immediate, or direct, perceptual product and that the visual world is the product of additional mental operations. Gibson aligned himself with the Gestalt psychologists in defending the view that the visual world is the direct product of perception and that the visual field represented the intrusion of judgmental operations.

In contrast to each of these traditional views, modern researchers have proposed an alternative view according to which both the visual field and the visual world correspond to immediate perceptual representations that are functionally significant in responding to stimuli (cf. Benedetti, 1988; Humphreys and Riddoch, 1984; Jameson and Hurvich, 1989; McKee and Welch, 1989). For example, Gilinsky (1986) demonstrated that we can have size constancy but not velocity constancy for the same stimulus. That is, we see the visual world with respect to size and the visual field with respect to velocity. She argued that both of these perceptions are functional. The visual world gives us a veridical representation of objects in our environment; the visual field enables us to track objects with our eyes and limbs. Representation of the proximal information, the visual field, she maintains, gives the observer the information needed to follow moving objects. Which is immediate and which is derived? Gilinsky argues that both the visual field and the visual world are immediate and both serve different functions.

3.3 Apparent, Proximal and Objective Instructions

Given the initial Gestalt versus introspectionist controversy over instructions, it is not surprising that the manipulation of instructions is a potent source of variance in constancy experiments. This variance can be attributed to the information given or implied by a particular set of instructions. In fact, Leibowitz and Harvey (1969) called this instructional information the most effective experimental variable in size-constancy experiments. Carlson (1977, p. 218) stated that:

> '... the size-constancy experiment consists essentially of asking the subject to vary the size of a test-object presented at a near distance so that it is the same size as a test-object

presented at a greater distance. ... In order for instructions to be as effective as they are, however, they must communicate with some attitude of the observer in a way that has a particular implication for how he should respond in the experimental situation.'

In an attempt to quantify size-matching behavior that is particularly sensitive to instructions, Leibowitz and Harvey (1969) employed three distinct types of instructions: 'objective', 'retinal' (proximal) and 'apparent'. They stated that objective instructions correspond most closely to the theoretical concepts implied by Gibson's (1950) 'visual world' and tend to emphasize the permanent quantities of objects. Such instructions imply that a subject should match linear sizes of two objects as if they were being measured by a ruler. Kaufman (1974) adds that objective instructions imply a match of the objects' distal sizes.

Leibowitz and Harvey noted that retinal instructions, on the other hand, are introspective in nature and stress visual angle relationships. These instructions suggest a proportional relationship between the two test-objects and are often referred to as projective instructions. Size matching, in this case, occurs as the size of one object is projected to the distance of the other. Kaufman (1974) states that successful accomplishment of such instructions would 'be equivalent to giving matches that varied with variations in the proximal distance' (p. 337).

Apparent instructions served as the third type of instructions employed by Leibowitz and Harvey. Used to evoke responses based on immediate visual impressions, these instructions, it is said, correspond most closely to the phenomenological approach of the Gestalt psychologists. This type of instruction enjoins the subject 'to set the size of a near object so that it "looks" [or appears] equal in size to the far object and he is not to be concerned about achieving equality of size in any other sense' (Carlson, 1977, p. 221).

In general, Leibowitz and Harvey found that when combined with variables, such as familiarity of a test-object and variability of depth-cue-rich environments, the influence of instructions was of greater magnitude than any other variable. Additionally, they found that the magnitude of size matches decreased with distance (underconstancy) under apparent and retinal instructions, yet remained the same (constancy) under objective instructions. Further, objective instructions tended to produce larger size matches than retinal instructions while apparent instructions produced intermediate matches. They concluded that instructions play a significant role in all size matching behavior and argued that multiple instructions should be used in any such study (size-constancy experiments), regardless of theoretical perspective.

Although their study served as a compelling impetus for further research concerning the effect of instructions on size constancy, a review of subsequent research in this area (Carlson, 1977) points to results which generally differ quite significantly from those found by Leibowitz and Harvey. Carlson's review explores size-matching responses ranging from extreme overconstancy to extreme underconstancy. A general pattern which Carlson found throughout a majority of the data consisted of a tendency to get increasing size responses with distance (overconstancy), when subjects were given objective-size instructions, and decreasing size responses with distance (underconstancy), when subjects were given retinal- or projective-size instructions. When apparent-size instructions were used, size estimates of the two test-objects remained the same, indicating that size constancy had been achieved. Carlson noted that such instructions have similar effects on other constancies, for example, brightness (Landauer and Rodger, 1964; Lindauer and Baust, 1970) and orientation (Ebenholtz and Shebilske, 1973; Wade, 1970). He further offered several possible explanations for the difference in results between the Leibowitz–Harvey study and those which followed.

In summary, Carlson suggests that it is what seems appropriate to the subject within the perceptual constraints of the particular stimulus situation, the particular instructions given by the experimenter, and the way the subject understands those instructions which govern individual response bias. He agreed with the Gestalt psychologists and Gibson that constancies are the product of perceptual processes, and he argued that instructions affect judgmental as opposed to perceptual processes. He concluded, however, that 'in order to understand what is perceived in a given situation it is necessary to understand how the subject's attitude interacts with the particular stimulus conditions'. He believed, as did Leibowitz and Harvey, that 'if the interpretation of an experimental result is to have generality, it is as important to vary instructions systematically as it is to vary the stimulus conditions' (Carlson, 1977, p. 248).

3.4   Children Versus Adults

The importance of a subject's viewing attitude was demonstrated in comparisons of children and adults. Circumspect of empirical suggestions that size constancy develops as a function of age and the concomitant assumption that it is acquired through a learned usage of distance information, Shallo and Rock (1988) tested an alternative argument. They proposed that what had continually been referred to as an incomplete size constancy in children may actually be a propensity for children to respond more readily to the proximal mode of size perception than do adults. They stated that 'the proximal mode refers to perceptual experience that reflects the absolute features of the proximal stimulus' (p. 803). They distinguished this mode from the constancy mode of perception which reflects objective properties of a distal stimulus and is based on the integration of all sensory information.

To test their hypothesis that children have accurate size perception at far and near distances and that their 'incomplete' size constancy is a result of their spontaneous accessing of proximal mode information, Shallo and Rock (1988) ran a series of experiments beginning with one conducted earlier by Brislin and Leibowitz (1970). Using children (age range 7.7–9.7 years) and adults (17.0–21.0 years) as subjects, standard objects consisting of five white cardboard disks 7.6, 9.1, 15.2, 30.5 and 61.0 cm in diameter were viewed at specific distances (7.6, 9.1, 15.2, 30.5 and 61.0 m) from the observer, so that the visual angle remained a constant of 0.53°. After viewing the standard, subjects turned 90° to view a comparison series consisting of 37 white disks ranging in size from 1.3 to 76.2 cm in diameter, at a distance of 7.6 m away. Unlike the Holway–Boring paradigm which used a method of adjustments, a method of limits was used to present the comparison stimuli. Observers were to state whether the comparison disk was 'bigger', 'smaller' or 'the same size' as the presented standard. Results from this first experiment were identical to the Brislin–Leibowitz findings which showed that size-constancy matches made by children were generally less accurate than those made by adults for farther observation distances.

In a subsequent experiment, Shallo and Rock tested their notion that in the absence of proximal mode information children – like adults – would exhibit size constancy. In this experiment only one standard disk was used, 61.0 cm in diameter at 61.0 m away. In order to 'neutralize' proximal mode information, nine comparison disks (15.2–76.2 cm in diameter) were simultaneously displayed at different distances so as to subtend the same visual angle of 9.46°. No comparison disk subtended the same visual angle as the standard, and only one of the comparison disks was the constancy match of the standard. Observers were to indicate which comparison disk was 'the same size' as the standard. Results showed that children were able to make this match with a significant degree of accuracy and tended to maintain size constancy rather than depart from it. The conclusive results of the Shallo–Rock study challenge the notion that children must acquire size-constancy capabilities through experience of using distance information because, as they showed, children do exhibit size constancy in the absence of proximal mode information. A third experiment indicated that methodological differences between the first two experiments (which were both empirical variants of Holway and Boring's (1941) classic paradigm) were not enough to account for differences in the resulting data.

3.5 Registered Versus Perceived Values

An example of a diverging construct is the distinction between 'registered' and 'perceived' values of spatial variables. Registered values are those that are assumed to be taken into account by constancy mechanisms without having a phenomenal correlate. Perceived values, of course, correspond to the apparent representation. A famous example of this distinction was made by Rock and Kaufman (1962) in their explanation of the moon illusion: the fact that the horizon moon appears larger and closer than the zenith moon, although the actual size (1342 kilometers in diameter), distance (148 447 kilometers from the earth) and retinal image (1/6 mm) of the moon remain the same. To study this phenomenon, Rock and Kaufman employed an apparatus which permitted observers to view an artificial moon on the sky (Figures 7.7 and 7.8). With instructions to adjust the moon size, observers used two such devices to compare a standard moon in one position (i.e. at the zenith) to a moon in another position (i.e. at the horizon). The size projected by the observer in relation to the standard served to measure the magnitude of the illusion.

By manipulating selected variables, Rock and Kaufman (1962) found that this illusion could be explained in terms of the context in which the moon was viewed. More specifically, they found that the moon's apparent size existed as a function of the presence or absence of distance cues provided by the horizon's terrain. What would normally be described as the large horizon moon became relatively small and more distant when viewed through a small aperture which occluded depth cues. Without the distance cues provided by the horizon, the appearance of the horizon moon was seen to be equivalent in size to the zenith moon. As expected, Rock and Kaufman successfully demonstrated a reversal of the illusion (large zenith) by 'giving the zenith moon a terrain' (1962, p. 1023).

Rock and Kaufman argued that the terrain was responsible for the illusion because of a registered distance of the horizon moon. They proposed that the

W. L. Shebilske and A. L. Peters

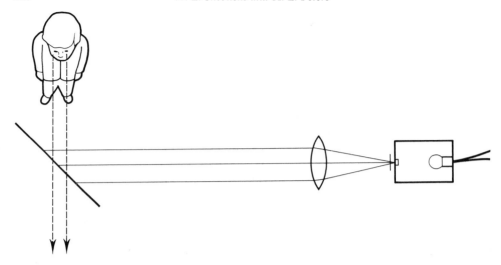

Figure 7.7. *The Rock and Kaufman experimental set-up employed to study the moon illusion. [From Kaufman, 1974, p. 326, Fig. 12.2A. © 1979 Oxford University Press; reprinted with kind permission.]*

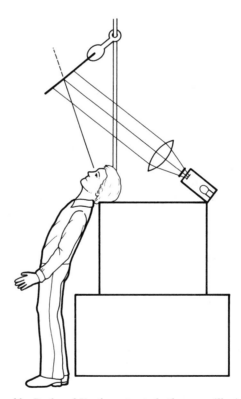

Figure 7.8. *Apparatus used by Rock and Kaufman to study the moon illusion. [From Kaufman, 1974, p. 326, Fig. 12.2B. © 1979 Oxford University Press; reprinted with kind permission.]*

crucial element was not distance as judged but distance as registered by the nervous system on the basis of certain stimuli. These stimuli, they argued, were not physical properties but rather configural properties, relationships within the stimulus pattern, such as perspective and interposition. Thus, the cues responsible for the perceived size of the horizon moon are those unconsciously registered sources of information that have no phenomenological correlates. They further state that physiological correlates cease to be important at greater distances.

3.6 Correlational Versus Causal Relationships

Rock and Kaufman's arguments raise the more general question of causal relationships in the perceptual constancies. Oyama (1977) addressed this question by using partial correlations to make causal inferences. To discriminate between direct and indirect causal relationships among three or more perceptual variables, Oyama analyzed data from various size, shape and lightness-constancy experiments using the Simon–Blalock method of causal inference by partial correlation.

Partial correlation is defined as being a net correlation between two variables (perceptual properties), when the influence of one or more additional variable(s) has been eliminated. Obtained patterns of partial correlations yielding net values close to zero suggest causal relationships among perceptual properties. In lay terms, when no correlation exists between two 'normally associated' percepts (i.e. perceived size and perceived distance) while one or more perceptual property (i.e. depth cues) is held constant, there is reason to suggest that a causal relationship exists between one (or both) of the 'normally associated' percepts and that which has been held constant. As different variables are held constant, causal relationships among variables (if any) become more clearly defined.

Analytical results of individual data led Oyama (1977) to conclude that more often than not, two perceptual properties are independently determined by stimulus variables. Further, no direct causal relationship exists between them. This conclusion rests on the assumption that the measured properties were in fact perceptual rather than judgmental.

On the other hand, Oyama found that there are times when causal relationships do exist between perceptual properties. Further, evidence shows that these percept–percept causalities can work in either direction. For example, changes in perceived size can cause changes in perceived distance as hypothesized in the Rock–Kaufman explanation of the moon illusion. Inversely, changes in perceived distance can cause changes in perceived size as is expressed by Emmert's law (1881) which states that the perceived size of an afterimage is proportional to its apparent distance (i.e. an afterimage seen on a nearby surface will be perceived as small in relation to the perception of the same afterimage projected on a more distant surface).

These percept–percept causalities imply sequential processing. However, Oyama suggests that these sequences are not fixed. Depending on observer and situation, any percept may be registered earlier than that of an associate as suggested by the results of causal inference.

3.7   Converging and Diverging Operations

The lack of causal relationships is also hinted at by the lack of agreement that is often observed between measurements that should converge if percepts were causally related. Many of these incongruities have been observed in tests of the size–distance invariance hypothesis, according to which visual angle determines a unique ratio between perceived size and perceived distance (Epstein, Park and Casey, 1961). Top-down influences have been proposed to explain failures to observe the predicted ratio. For example, Gogel (1977) attributes these failures to intrusions of cognitive factors in reports of distance. That is, objects can be cognitively judged to be in a different location than they appear, and performance can reflect these cognitive judgments. For instance, if subjects know a room is only 3 meters long, their judgments of a target's distance might be constrained to a maximum of 3 meters, even when the target looks farther away than that. Bottom-up influences have also been proposed. In one study of constancies during lateral head movement, Shebilske and Proffitt (1983) suggested that separate input modules could explain inconsistencies in the obtained constancy measurements as well, or better than, top-down processes. They argued that one module might use principles of motion organization to determine apparent motions without reference to apparent distance. Another module might simultaneously provide input for pointing responses based on distance information from one set of sources. A third module might determine apparent distance based on a different set of distance information. A fourth module might determine apparent size based on yet another set of distance information. The next section expands this modularity proposal into a framework for integrating the diverse theories, constructs and methods in the constancy literature.

4   A FRAMEWORK FOR SYNTHESIS

Most constancy research has been guided by linear models according to which information processing follows a single path of progression. An example is shown in Figure 7.9, which is taken from a textbook that uses the figure to capture prevalent views about perception (Sekuler and Blake, 1990). The figure illustrates a sequential process in which the perception of a cat guides the motor responses of picking up the cat. The process begins with sensory transduction which converts physical information into neural activity. Further neural processing results in perception which then guides action. Implicit in the figure is the assumption that the same linear process would be used to hit a baseball or to do any sensory-guided action. Many diverse philosophies and scientific theories make the assumption that sensory-guided performance is based on perception (cf. Goodale, 1988). Advocates of linear models would not deny that perception with action requires different processes than perception without action. But they would insist on the assumption that the separate sensorimotor modules diverge, after perceptual constancy mechanisms yield the stable representations needed for skilled performance. They have to insist on this assumption because it is a necessary consequence of a model in which action is based on perceptual representations. From this point of view, it makes sense to understand the early perceptual processes before considering

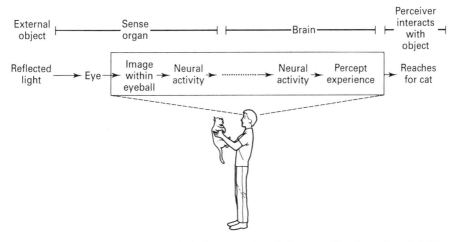

Figure 7.9. *A linear process model in which the perception of the cat guides the action of picking up the cat. [From Sekuler and Blake, 1990, p. 2, Fig. 1.1. © 1990 Glencoe/Macmillan/McGraw-Hill, Mission Hills, CA; reprinted with kind permission.]*

control processes. This rationale could account for the emphasis on appearance as opposed to performance in the constancy literature.

The preceding analysis of diverging theories and constructs suggests, however, that trying to fit constancy data into a linear model is like trying to fit five pounds of beans into a one-pound bag. You only get a sense of progress if you ignore the ones falling on the floor.

Multilinear models with multiple representations of spatial layout provide more appropriate frameworks for synthesis. The next two sections briefly consider the historical backdrop against which such models are emerging.

4.1 Multilinear Models Without Multiple Representations of Space

Multilinear models include 'New look' top-down processing models according to which knowledge and beliefs influence perception. From this point of view, separate representations of space need not be postulated to explain paradoxical relationships, such as percept–percept (the closer and larger appearance of the horizon moon) or perception–action (seeing a target in one place and reaching for it in another). Such discordance could, in principle, be accounted for by the intrusion of judgemental or higher-order, top-down processes. The 'New look' approach provides a coherent heuristic framework for studying such top-down effects.

This heuristic does not provide a useful framework, however, for interpreting the growing evidence for separate bottom-up processes (cf. Bridgeman, 1990; Goodale, 1988; Shebilske, 1990). As a result, Fodor (1983) in his book, *The Modularity of Mind*, challenged the 'New look' emphasis on top-down processing. He argues that input operations are insulated from other information and beliefs that an observer has about the environment. They are also insulated from each other and operate as independent and parallel 'smart systems' (Pylyshyn, 1984). Such modular models characterize most computational approaches to vision, including the pioneering work of Marr (1982). Many cognitive scientists, however, remain committed to the old tradition of identifying vision with visual perception. That is, these modular models are multilinear between perception and action, but they remain linear between sensory stimulation and perception.

4.2   Multilinear Models with Multiple Representations of Space

In contrast, Goodale (1988) cites evidence of independent visuomotor modules that are separate from retinal projections right through to motor nuclei (Ingle, 1982). For example, Goodale (1988, p. 263) argues that:

> '... vision evolved in vertebrates and other organisms to control movements. ... In "designing" these control systems, natural selection appears to have favored the development of a visual system that consists of a network of relatively independent sensorimotor channels, each of which supports a particular kind of visually guided behavior. ... In a now classic series of studies of vision in the frog, *Rana pipiens*, David Ingle (1973, 1982) was able to show that visually elicited feeding, visually elicited escape, and visually guided avoidance of barriers are mediated by entirely separate pathways from the retina to the motor nuclei.'

Similarly, Bridgeman (1990) cited evidence that the visual world is represented by several topographic maps in the cortex (Van Essen, Newsome and Bixby, 1982). In other words, these multiple modes of visual representation models postulate separate hard-wired visual modules.

At the same time, it is recognized that such modules alone cannot account for the integration and coordination of action in a stimulus-rich environment. Goodale (1988), for instance, calls upon researchers to work out ways that visuomotor modules are integrated in behaving animals.

Shebilske (1991) brought his ecological efference mediation theory to bear on this issue of ontological influences on modularity. He proposed that the acquisition of high-performance skills changes perception–action relationships by modifying modular input operations that produce multiple spatial representations. All of the representations are stable, but only one is consciously perceived. Unconscious representations are generated to guide specific high-skill actions.

The ecological efference mediation theory, like other ecological theories, holds that perception–action relationships are shaped by the interaction of an organism with its environment and that operations for encoding sensory information approach optimal efficiency in the environment in which a species evolved (cf. Gibson, 1979; Shebilske and Fisher, 1984; Shebilske, Proffitt and Fisher, 1984; Turvey, 1979; Turvey and Solomon, 1984). The dominant ecological theories have adhered to a direct perception approach, which assumes a one-to-one correspondence between stimulus information, perception and action (e.g., Gibson, 1979; Turvey and Solomon, 1984). These direct theories allow no room for multiple visual representations. In contrast, Shebilske (1984, 1987a, b) proposed an ecological efference mediation theory stating that: (1) efference-based information (e.g. from the oculomotor system) interacts with higher order light-based information (e.g. from optical flow patterns) to determine performance during natural events, and that: (2)

fallibility in both visual and efference-based information functions synergistically to shape both the phylogeny and ontogeny of the visual system (Shebilske, Proffitt and Fisher, 1984). Assigning a central role to efference-based information in an ecological analysis paves the way for proposing multiple representations that emerge as a result of interactions between an organism and its environment.

Shebilske (1991) hypothesized that expert performance is not based solely on input processes that determine perception. Instead, skilled performers employ unconscious representations formed by input processes that operate in parallel with those that yield conscious perceptions. The parallel processes are specialized for specific skills by utilizing content addressable, distributed information that is acquired during training. These *parallel distributed processes* (PDP) have their own equivalency mechanisms that transform varying sensory information into stable unconscious representations that are established according to different operations than those that determine perceptual impressions. For example, the PDP input modules might use (1) separate selective attention mechanisms that pick up different potential sources of information; (2) different parsing routines that result in sampling units of different spatial sizes and/or different temporal durations; (3) different weights for various sources of information; and (4) different rules (e.g. rigidity assumption) and/or different principles of processing (e.g. minimum principle). Accordingly, the stable representations that guide expert performance become available at different times and take on different values than the perceptual constancies. The PDP input modules for performance and perception diverge and become integrated as trainees interact with their environment during the acquisition of a high-performance skill. That is, high-skill performance employs unique unconscious representations that are based on *ecologically integrated event input operations* (EIEIOs).

At first, this hypothesis seems to be without the benefit of Occam's razor. But this first impression changes to one of parsimony when human adaptability is considered within the wide range of conditions in which perception and action systems operate. On the one hand, perception guides behavior day and night in highly structured environments such as forests, and in relatively low structured environments such as snow-covered fields. On the other hand, specific skills are often performed within a narrow range of this total variability. Our prehistoric ancestors navigated ocean vessels by the stars in low-information environments and piloted fresh-water vessels through raging rapids in high-information environments. Our modern-day pilots and athletes also perform skills in narrow bands of environmental variability. Night-landing on an aircraft carrier includes only the low-information end, for instance, and gymnastics usually includes only the high-information end. Adaptability would be optimized, therefore, by the development of separate representations for visual perception and visuomotor coordination in specific skills.

Whereas input operations corresponding to conscious representations must be maximally efficient over the entire range of contextual variability in which an organism perceives, EIEIOs must only be maximally efficient in a narrower variability range within which a particular skill is performed. This narrower contextual range enables the EIEIO mechanisms to take parsimonious short-cuts in establishing stable sensory representations that work best for a specific skill performed in a specific environment. These short-cuts are not feasible for the perceptual mechanisms, since they must operate over a broader contextual range.

In other words, it is proposed that EIEIOs are efficient because they take advantage of the fact that specific skills tend to be performed in specific environments.

The EIEIO heuristic affords the explanatory power of recent PDP models (Feldman and Ballard, 1982; Hinton and Anderson, 1981; Pew, 1986; Pribram, 1988; Rumelhart and McClelland, 1986; Smolensky, 1988). These models explain how practice can affect the earliest stages of sensory processing before constancy mechanisms operate. Pribram (1988), for example, proposed that memorial representations established through practice affect the structure of dendritic networks throughout the visual pathways. Each synapse is a processing unit and networks of synapses enable us to extract spatiotemporal relationships from our environment. Past experience can modify the structure of dendritic networks and thereby modify the way that they extract information from the environment (Kandel and Schwartz, 1982). Pribram argues that such distributed memory representations can affect the earliest stages of sensory information processing.

In contrast to most constancy studies, which begin with an analysis of the stimulus information and end with the appearance of objects in space, the *ecological efference mediation theory* provides a framework for investigating processes that go beyond appearance to performance. The analysis begins with stimulus information and continues on to some skilled performance that requires stable representations of space. For example, baseball pitchers throw strikes to a fixed position, despite considerable visual flux created by eye and head movements during the windup and delivery. Is this response, which seems to require some stabilized representation of the strike zone, based on perceptual impressions that are stabilized by processes of egocentric constancies? Consider also the performance of an ornithologist. When birds are on the move, ornithologists check the silhouettes to help place a bird within a recognized group. For example, the wing length to body length ratio is much greater in albatrosses than in gulls. The barest glimpse enables a skilled observer to use this information to identify species, even though projected silhouettes vary as a function of viewing angle. Is this performance based upon perceptual impressions that are stabilized by processes of object constancy? The answer for both the pitcher and the ornithologist is assumed to be 'yes' according to linear models. The answer awaits empirical investigations according to multilinear models.

The ecological efference mediation theory provides a framework for such investigations. It suggests further that the answer will depend upon the level of practice. Both the baseball and ornithology examples illustrate high-performance skills, which are defined by the following characteristics: (1) more than 100 h are required to reach proficiency; (2) more than 20% of highly motivated trainees fail to reach proficiency; and (3) substantial qualitative differences in performance exist between a novice and an expert (Schneider, 1985). The ecological efference mediation theory suggests that some of the qualitative differences stem from changes in the relationship between perceptual constancies and performance. Accordingly, the performance of a novice baseball pitcher and an ornithologist depends upon perceptual impressions that are stabilized by processes of perceptual constancies. But performance of expert pitchers and ornithologists does not. These high-performance skills depend, instead, on unconscious representations that are stabilized by processes that are different from the mechanisms that determine perceptual constancies.

The EIEIO heuristic also provides a framework for integrating other diverse consequences of extensive practice. Schmidt (1987) reviewed the history of thought on practice effects, starting with William James' observation (1890) that practice of skills seems to lead to more automatic, less mentally taxing behavior. Subsequent research suggested three separate process level changes that seem to contribute to this practice effect:

(1) tasks that are slow and guided shift from dependence on exproprioceptive information to dependence on proprioceptive information (Adams and Goetz, 1973);

(2) tasks that have predictable parameters – such as predictable target locations in pointing tasks – shift to open-loop control (Schmidt and McCabe, 1976); and

(3) tasks that have unpredictable parameters shift to fast, automatic and parallel processing of the information needed to make decisions (Schneider and Shiffrin, 1977).

We propose that all three of these effects manifest EIEIO modules, one that specializes in proprioception, one that incorporates open-loop control and one that employs parallel decision processes.

At this early stage in its development, the ecological efference mediation theory provides only a loose packaging for data. Our five pounds of beans, which cannot be captured by linear models, are easily contained; but now they are rattling around in a 100 pound container. The data are consistent with a single theory, however, which does provide a heuristic framework for investigations aimed toward a synthesis of the diverging theories and constructs in the constancy literature. For example, the theory embraces PDP models, which provide formal processing structures for those who argue that the visual world and the visual field are both primary and are both serving different functions. Data on attitude of viewing as well as registered versus perceived spatial values are also consistent with multiple representations, several of which are potentially available to consciousness. Perceptions that develop along multiple paths also account for the many patterns of causality found in percept–percept relationships and for the failure for experimental measurements to converge the way they should according to linear models.

Finally, the ecological efference mediation theory suggests that progress toward synthesis will be made when unilinear approaches that ask either–or questions about perception are replaced with a multilinear approach that investigates multiple spatial representations for perception and performance in specific integrated sensorimotor modules. For example, according to the EIEIO heuristic, unconscious inference and relational hypotheses need not be mutually exclusive. The diverse mechanisms postulated by these hypotheses might operate simultaneously in parallel modules. Accordingly, the goal of an EIEIO approach is to articulate the integration and coordination of these diverse mechanisms by specifying the boundary conditions for the operation of specific multiple representations.

5   SUMMARY AND CONCLUSION

Constancy research has been focused on perception as opposed to performance in part because the research has been guided by linear models of perception–action relationships, according to which all sensory guided action is based on perception. However, diverging theories, constructs and operations suggest that linear models cannot account for constancy data. We suggest, therefore, that a synthesis should be sought in the ecological efference mediation theory, a multilinear model with multiple representations of spatial layout.

REFERENCES

Adams, A. and Goetz, E. T. (1973). Feedback and practice of variables in error detection and correction. *Journal of Motor Behavior*, **5**, 217–224.

Attneave, F. (1971). Multistability in perception. *Scientific American*, **225**, 62–71.

Benedetti, F. (1988). Localization of tactile stimuli and body parts in space: Two dissociated perceptual experiences revealed by a lack of constancy in the presence of position sense and motor activity. *Journal of Experimental Psychology: Human Perception and Performance*, **14**, 69–76.

Boring, E. G. (1952). Visual perception as invariance. *Psychological Review*, **59**, 141–148.

Bower, T. G. R. (1974). *Development in Infancy*. San Francisco: Freeman.

Bridgeman, B. (1990). Separate visual representations for perception and for visually guided behavior. In S. R. Ellis and M. K. Kaiser (Eds), *Spatial Displays and Spatial Instruments*. Hillsdale, NJ: Erlbaum.

Brislin, R. W. and Leibowitz, H. W. (1970). The effect of separation between test and comparison objects on size constancy at various age levels. *American Journal of Psychology*, **83**, 372–376.

Burkhardt, D. A., Gottesmann, J., Kersten, S. and Legge, G. E. (1984). Symmetry and constancy in the perception of negative and positive luminance contrast. *Journal of the Optical Society of America*, **1**, 309–316.

Carlson, V. R. (1960). Overestimation in size-constancy judgments. *American Journal of Psychology*, **73**, 199–213.

Carlson, V. R. (1962). Size-constancy judgments and perceptual compromise. *Journal of Experimental Psychology*, **63**, 68–73.

Carlson, V. R. (1977). Instructions and perceptual constancy judgments. In W. Epstein (Ed.), *Stability and Constancy in Visual Perception: Mechanisms and Processes* (pp. 217–254). New York: John Wiley.

Collins, W. E. (1974a). Arousal and vestibular habituation. In H. H. Kornhuber (Ed.), *Handbook of Sensory Physiology*, vol. VI/2. New York: Springer.

Collins, W. E. (1974b). Habituation of vestibular responses with and without visual stimulation. In H. H. Kornhuber (Ed.), *Handbook of Sensory Physiology*, vol. VI/2. New York: Springer.

Day, R. H. and McKenzie, B. E. (1977). Constancies in the perceptual world of infants. In W. Epstein (Ed.), *Stability and Constancy in Visual Perception: Mechanisms and Processes* (pp. 285–320). New York: John Wiley.

Ebenholtz, S. M. and Shebilske, W. L. (1973). Differential effects of instructions on A and E phenomena in judgments of the vertical. *American Journal of Psychology*, **86**, 601–612.

Emmert, E. (1881). Größenverhältnisse der Nachbilder. *Klinische Monatsblätter der Augenheilkunde*, **19**, 443–450.

Epstein, W. (1963). Attitudes of judgment and the size–distance invariance hypothesis. *Journal of Experimental Psychology*, **66**, 78–83.

Epstein, W. (1977). Historical introduction to the constancies. In W. Epstein (Ed.), *Stability and Constancy in Visual Perception: Mechanisms and Processes* (pp. 1–22). New York: John Wiley.

Epstein, W., and Landauer, A. A. (1969). Size and distance judgments under reduced conditions of viewing. *Perception and Psychophysics*, **6**, 269–272.

Epstein, W. E., Park, J. and Casey, A. (1961). The current status of the size–distance hypothesis. *Psychological Bulletin*, **58**, 491–514.

Feldman, J. A., and Ballard, D. H. (1982). Connectionist models and their properties. *Cognitive Science*, **6**, 205–254.

Fodor, J. (1983). *The Modularity of Mind*. Cambridge, MA: MIT Press.

Gibson, J. J. (1950). *The Perception of the Visual World*. Boston: Houghton Mifflin.

Gibson, J. J. (1952). The visual field and the visual world: A reply to Prof. Boring. *Psychological Review*, **59**, 149–151.

Gibson, J. J. (1966). *The Senses Considered as Perceptual Systems*. Boston: Houghton Mifflin.

Gibson, J. J. (1979). *The Ecological Approach to Visual Perception*. Boston: Houghton Mifflin.

Gilchrist, A. L (1977). Perceived lightness depends on perceived spatial arrangement. *Science*, **195**, 185–187.

Gilinsky, A. S. (1955). The effect of attitude upon the perception of size. *American Journal of Psychology*, **68**, 173–192.

Gilinsky, A. S. (1986). How the brain recognizes meaningful objects. *Bulletin of the Psychonomic Society*, **24**, 138–140.

Gogel, W. C. (1977). The metric of visual space. In W. Epstein (Ed.), *Stability and Constancy in Visual Perception: Mechanisms and Processes* (pp. 129–182). New York: John Wiley.

Goodale, M. A. (1988). Modularity in visuomotor control: From input to output. In Z. W. Pylyshyn (Ed.), *Computational Processes in Human Vision: An Interdisciplinary Perspective* (pp. 262–286). Norwood, NJ: Ablex.

Graham, C. H. (Ed.). (1965). *Vision and Visual Perception*. New York: John Wiley.

Hastorf, A. H. and Way, K. S. (1952). Apparent size with and without distance cues. *Journal of General Psychology*, **47**, 181–188.

Helmholtz, H. von (1890/1962). A treatise on physiological optics, vol. 3. (J. P. C. Southhall, Ed. and Transl.). New York: Dover, 1962.

Hering, E. (1879). *Beiträge zur Physiologie*. Leipzig: Engelmann.

Hill, A. L. (1972). Direction constancy. *Perception and Psychophysics*, **11**, 175–178.

Hinton, G. E. and Anderson, J. A. (1981). *Parallel Models of Associative Memory*. Hillsdale, NJ: Erlbaum.

Hochberg, J. and Beck, J. (1954). Apparent spatial arrangement and perceived brightness. *Journal of Experimental Psychology*, **47**, 263–266.

Holway, A. H. and Boring, E. G. (1941). Determinants of apparent visual size with distance variant. *American Journal of Psychology*, **54**, 21–37.

Humphreys, G. W. and Riddoch, M. J. (1984). Routes to object constancy: Implications from neurological impairments of object constancy. *The Quarterly Journal of Experimental Psychology*, **36A**, 385–415.

Ingle, D. J. (1973). Two visual systems in the frog. *Science*, **181**, 1053–1055.

Ingle, D. J. (1982). Organization of visuomotor behaviors in vertebrates. In D. J. Ingle, M. A. Goodale, and R. J. W. Mansfield (Eds), *Analysis of Visual Behavior*. Cambridge, MA: MIT Press.

Ittelson, W. H. (1952/1968). *The Ames Demonstrations in Perception*. New York: Hafner.

James, W. (1890). *The Principles of Psychology*. New York: Holt.

Jameson, D. and Hurvich, L. (1989). Essay concerning color constancy. *Annual Review of Psychology*, **40**, 1–22.

Kandel, E. R. and Schwartz, J. H. (1982). Molecular biology of learning: Modulation of transmitter release. *Science*, **218**, 433–443.

Kaufman, L. (1974). *Sight and mind: An introduction to visual perception*. New York: Oxford University Press.

Köhler, W. (1929). *Gestalt Psychology*. New York: Liveright.

Koffka, K. (1935). *Principles of Gestalt Psychology*. New York: Harcourt Brace.

Landauer, A. A. and Rodger, R. S. (1964). Effect of 'apparent' instructions on brightness judgments. *Journal of Experimental Psychology*, **68**, 80–84.

Leibowitz, H. W. and Harvey, L. O., Jr (1967). Size matching as a function of instructions in a natural environment. *Journal of Experimental Psychology*, **74**, 378–382.

Leibowitz, H. W. and Harvey, L. O., Jr (1969). Size matching as a function of instructions in a natural environment. *Journal of Experimental Psychology*, **81**, 36–43.

Leibowitz, H. W. and Pick, H. (1972). Cross-cultural and educational aspects of the Ponzo illusion. *Perception and Psychophysics*, **12**, 430–432.

Lindauer, M. S. and Baust, R. F. (1970). Instructions and knowledge of situation in brightness perception. *American Journal of Psychology*, **83**, 130–135.

Marr, D. (1982). *Vision*. San Francisco: W. H. Freeman.

Matin, L. (1972). Eye movements and perceived visual direction. In D. Jameson and L. M. Hurvich (Eds), *Handbook of Sensory Physiology*, vol. 7/4: *Visual Psychophysics*. Berlin, New York: Springer.

Matin, L. (1976). Saccades and the extraretinal signal for visual direction. In R. Monty and J. Senders (Eds), *Eye Movements and Psychological Processes*, ch. 4. Hillsdale, NJ: Erlbaum.

Matin, L. (1982). Visual localization and eye movements. In A. H. Wertheim, W. A. Wagenaar and H. W. Leibowitz (Eds), *Tutorials on Motion Perception* (pp. 101–156). New York: Plenum.

McKee, S. P. and Welch, L. (1989). Is there a constancy for velocity? *Vision Research*, **29(5)**, 553–561.

Mershon, D. H., Desaulniers, D. H., Kiefer, S. A., Amerson, T. L., Jr and Mills, J. T. (1981). Perceived loudness and visually determined auditory distance. *Perception*, **10**, 531–543.

Oyama, T. (1977). Analysis of causal relations in the perceptual constancies. In W. Epstein (Ed.), *Stability and Constancy in Visual Perception: Mechanisms and Processes* (pp. 183–216). New York: John Wiley.

Park, K. and Shebilske, W. L. (1991). Phoria, Hering's laws and monocular perception of egocentric direction and Hering's laws of visual direction. *Journal of Experimental Psychology: Perception and Performance*, **17**, 219–231.

Pew, R. W. (1986). Human performance issues in the design of future Air Force systems. *Aviation, Space, and Environmental Medicine*, **57**, 78–82.

Pribram, K. H. (1988). *A Holonomic Brain Theory: Cooperativity and Reciprocity in Processing the Configural and Cognitive Aspects of Perception*. Hillsdale, NJ: Erlbaum.

Purdy, J. and Gibson, E. J. (1955). Distance judgment by the method of fractionation. *Journal of Experimental Psychology*, **50**, 374–380.

Pylyshyn, Z. W. (1984). *Cognition and Computation: Toward a Foundation for Cognitive Science*. Cambridge, MA: MIT Press.

Regan, D. M. and Beverley, K. I. (1982). How do we avoid confounding the direction we are looking and the direction we are moving? *Science*, **215**, 194–196.

Richards, W. (1977). Selective stereoblindness. In H. Spekreijae and L.H. van der Tweel (Eds), *Spatial Contrast: Report of a Workshop* (pp. 109–115). Amsterdam: North-Holland.

Rock, I. (1977). In defense of unconscious inference. In W. Epstein (Ed.), *Stability and Constancy in Visual Perception: Mechanisms and Processes* (pp. 321–373). New York: John Wiley.

Rock, I. and Ebenholtz, S. M. (1959). The relational determination of perceived size. *Psychological Review*, **66**, 387–401.

Rock, I. and Kaufman, L. (1962). The moon illusion, II. *Science*, **136**, 1023–1031.

Rumelhart, D. E. and McClelland, J. L. (Eds) (1986). *Parallel-distributed Processing I and II*. Cambridge, MA: MIT Press.

Schmidt, R. A. (1987). The acquisition of skill: Some modifications to the perception–action relationship through practice. In H. Heuer and A. F. Sanders (Eds), *Perspectives on Perception and Action* (pp. 77–103). Hillsdale, NJ: Erlbaum.

Schmidt, R. A. and McCabe, J. F. (1976). Motor program utilization over extended practice. *Journal of Human Movement Studies*, **2**, 239–247.

Schneider, W. (1985). Training high performance skills: Fallacies and guidelines. Special issue: Training. *Human Factors*, **27**, 205–300.

Schneider, W. and Shiffrin, R. M. (1977). Controlled and automatic human information processing: I. Detection, search, and attention. *Psychological Review*, **84**, 1–66.

Sekuler, R. and Blake, R. (1990). *Perception,* 2nd edn. New York: McGraw-Hill.

Shallo, J. and Rock, I. (1988). Size constancy in children: A new interpretation. *Perception,* **17,** 803–813.

Shebilske, W. L. (1977). Visuomotor coordination in visual direction and position constancies. In W. Epstein (Ed.), *Stability and Constancy in Visual Perception: Mechanisms and Processes* (pp. 23–69). New York: John Wiley.

Shebilske, W. L. (1984). Context effects and efferent factors in perception and cognition. In W. Prinz and A. F. Sanders (Eds), *Cognition and Motor Processes* (pp. 99–119). Berlin, New York: Springer.

Shebilske, W. L. (1987a). An ecological efference mediation theory of natural event perception. In H. Heuer and A. F. Sanders (Eds), *Perspectives on Perception and Action* (pp. 195–213). Hillsdale, NJ: Erlbaum.

Shebilske, W. L. (1987b). Baseball batters support an ecological efference mediation theory of natural event perception. In D. G. Bouwhuis, B. Bridgeman, D. A. Owens, W. L. Shebilske, and P. Wolff (Eds), *Sensorimotor Interactions in Space Perception and Action.* Amsterdam: North-Holland.

Shebilske, W. L. (1990). Visuomotor modularity, ontogeny, and training high-performance skills with spatial display instruments. In S. R. Ellis and M. K. Kaiser (Eds), *Spatial Displays and Spatial Instruments.* Hillsdale, NJ: Erlbaum.

Shebilske, W. L. (1991). Visuomotor modularity, ontogeny, and training high-performance skills with spatial instruments. In S. R. Ellis (Ed.), *Pictorial Communication in Virtual and Real Environments.* London: Taylor and Francis.

Shebilske, W. L. and Fisher, S. K. (1984). Ubiquity of efferent factors in space perception. In J. L. Semmlow and W. Welkowitz (Eds), *Frontiers of Engineering and Computing in Health Care 1984.* New York: IEEE Publishing.

Shebilske, W. L. and Nice, R. S. (1976). Optical insignificance of the nose and the Pinocchio effect in free-scan visual straight-ahead judgments. *Perception and Psychophysics,* **20,** 17–20.

Shebilske, W. L. and Proffitt, D. R. (1983). Paradoxical retinal motion during head movements: Apparent motion without equivalent apparent displacement. *Perception and Psychophysics,* **34,** 467–481.

Shebilske, W. L., Proffitt, D. R. and Fisher, S. K. (1984). Efferent factors in natural event perception can be rationalized and verified: A reply to Turvey and Solomon. *Journal of Experimental Psychology: Human Perception and Performance,* **10,** 455–460.

Smolensky, P. (1988). On the proper treatment of connectionism. *Behavioral and Brain Science,* **11,** 1–74.

Teghtsoonian, R., Teghtsoonian, M., Berglund, B. and Berglund, U. (1978). Invariance of odor strength with sniff vigor: An olfactory analogue to size constancy. *Journal of Experimental Psychology: Human Perception and Performance,* **4,** 144–152.

Turvey, M. T. (1979). The thesis of the efference-mediation of vision cannot be rationalized. *Behavioral and Brain Sciences,* **2,** 59–94.

Turvey, M. T. and Solomon J. (1984). Visually perceiving distance: A comment on Shebilske, Karmiohl and Proffitt (1983). *Journal of Experimental Psychology: Human Perception and Performance,* **10,** 449–454.

Van Essen, D. C., Newsome, W. T. and Bixhby, J. L. (1982). The pattern of interhemispheric connections and its relationship to extrastriate visual areas in the macaque monkey. *Journal of Neuroscience,* **2,** 265–283.

Wade, N. J. (1970). Effect of instructions on visual orientation. *Journal of Experimental Psychology,* **83,** 331–332.

Wallach, H. (1948). Brightness constancy and the nature of achromatic colours. *Journal of Experimental Psychology,* **38,** 310–324.

Woodworth, R. (1938). *Experimental Psychology,* London: Methuen; New York: Holt.

Chapter 8

The Perception of Auditory Patterns

Diana Deutsch

University of California, San Diego

1 INTRODUCTION

Over the last half-century a considerable body of knowledge has accumulated concerning visual shape perception, based on findings in experimental psychology, neurophysiology, artificial intelligence and related fields. These developments have not, however, been paralleled by analogous developments in audition. It is interesting, therefore, that the foundations of pattern perception were laid by scientists who were as much concerned with auditory and musical phenomena as they were with visual ones. Wertheimer (1924/1938) described the beginnings of Gestalt theory thus:

'Historically, the most important impulse came from von Ehrenfels who raised the following problem. Psychology has said that experience is a compound of elements; we hear a melody and then, upon hearing it again, memory enables us to recognize it. But what is it that enables us to recognize the melody when it is played in a new key? The sum of its elements is different, yet the melody is the same; indeed, one is often not even aware that a transposition has been made.' (p. 4)

In another paper in which he proposed the Gestalt principles of perceptual organization, Wertheimer (1923/1955) frequently presented musical illustrations along with visual ones. For example, in order to illustrate that 'more or less dissimilarity operates to determine experienced arrangement' he wrote: 'With tones, for example, C, C♯, E, F, G♯, A, C, C♯ ... will be heard in the grouping ab/cd...; and C, C♯, D, E, F, F♯, G♯, A, A♯, C, C♯, D ... in the grouping abc/def' (1923/1955, p. 76). Figure 8.1 shows visual arrays such as presented by Wertheimer as analogous to these musical ones.

In contrast to work on visual perception, the development of psychoacoustics around the middle of this century was characterized by a strong focus on highly restricted perceptual phenomena: namely, those that could be produced by very simple stimuli and which lent themselves to interpretations based on the workings of the peripheral hearing apparatus. Issues explored in detail included absolute and differential thresholds for pitch and loudness, lateralization of sine waves and noise bands, and various masking functions.

The reluctance over the past few decades to consider higher-level processing in audition can be attributed to a number of factors (Deutsch and Pierce, 1992). First,

Handbook of Perception and Action: Volume 1
ISBN 0-12-516161-1

(a)

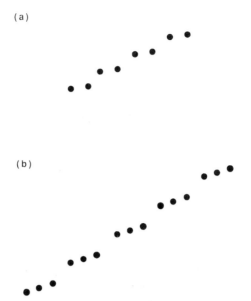

(b)

Figure 8.1 *Visual analogs of two pitch series, to illustrate perceptual grouping in the two modalities. Pattern (a) corresponds to the series C, C♯, E, F, G♯, A, C, C♯, and pattern (b) to the series C, C♯, D, E, F, F♯, G♯, A, A♯, C, C♯, D. [From Wertheimer, 1923/1955. © 1923 Springer; reprinted with kind permission of the publisher.]*

it was very difficult until recently to generate complex auditory stimuli with sufficient precision to address higher-level issues in the laboratory. A second factor was the lack of awareness of musical phenomena on the part of many researchers in the field. In the case of vision, it is evident from everyday experience that we recognize shapes as equivalent when these differ in size, in orientation and location in the visual field. Analogous perceptual equivalences in hearing are not evident from consideration of extramusical phenomena; however, music provides us with a number of convincing examples. We recognize musical passages when these are transposed to different keys; we treat as harmonically equivalent tones that are related by octaves; we perceive patterns of duration as equivalent when these are presented at different tempi, and so on. We are at present experiencing a renewed interest in mechanisms of auditory shape perception, and it appears as no surprise that this is accompanied by a resurgence of interest in music.

2   PERCEPTUAL GROUPING PRINCIPLES

Before embarking on a consideration of auditory phenomena, we first review two approaches to the issue of how elements of perceptual arrays are grouped together. The first approach, expounded by the Gestalt psychologists, assumes that the perceptual system forms groupings on the basis of a number of primitive organizational principles (Wertheimer, 1923/1955). One principle is termed *proximity* and states that perceptual connections are formed between elements that are close together, in preference to those that are further apart. Figure 8.2a presents an

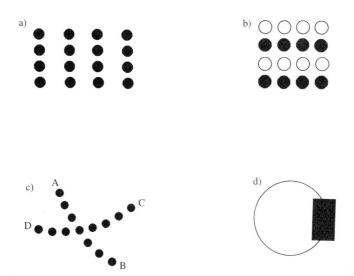

Figure 8.2. *Illustrations of several principles of perceptual organization enunciated by the Gestalt psychologists: (a) proximity; (b) similarity; (c) good continuation; (d) closure.*

example of this principle in vision. An array of dots is here displayed, which are closer along the vertical axis than along the horizontal one. These dots are perceptually connected on the basis of spatial proximity, so that columns rather than rows are perceived. A second principle, termed *similarity*, states that connections are formed between elements that are similar rather than between those that are dissimilar. Figure 8.2b presents an example from vision. Here, the open and closed circles form separate groupings, so that, in this case, rows rather than columns are perceived. A third principle, termed *good continuation*, states that connections are formed between elements that continue in the same direction. As a visual example, the dots in Figure 8.2c are perceived as forming the continuous lines AB and CD. A fourth principle, termed *closure*, states that we tend to perceive arrays as self-enclosed units. Thus, the pattern in Figure 8.2d is perceived as a circle that is partially occluded by a rectangle. A fifth principle, termed *common fate*, states that elements that move synchronously in the same direction are perceptually connected together. For example, two rows of dots moving in opposite directions are seen as belonging to two distinctly different sources.

Another approach to perceptual organization, expounded by Helmholtz (1862/ 1954), argues that the observer employs perceptual principles that give rise to the most effective interpretation of the environment. This line of reasoning could explain why the Gestalt grouping principles operate in perception. In making sense of our visual environment, it is useful to group together elements that are in spatial proximity or that are similar to each other, since these elements are more likely to belong to the same object. Analogously, sounds that are proximal in frequency or that are similar in timbre are likely to be emanating from the same source.

We now turn to the application of these organizational principles to sound perception, with an emphasis on music, and we also consider the relative contributions of pitch, timbre, spatial location and time as bases for such organization.

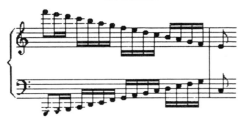

Figure 8.3. *A measure from Beethoven's* Waldstein Sonata. *The visual representation provided by the score mirrors the converging pitch lines heard in the passage.*

The most prominent characteristics of music consist of arrangements of pitches in time. As a result, the conventions of musical scores have evolved primarily to emphasize such arrangements. Generally speaking, in a written score, pitch and time are mapped respectively into the vertical and horizontal dimensions of visual space. An illustration of such a mapping is given in Figure 8.3, which reproduces a measure from Beethoven's *Waldstein Sonata*. Here, the converging lines in the score provide a good visual analog of the converging pitch movements that are heard in the passage. As we shall see, several principles of perceptual organization in music are evident in visual analogs provided by scores, although there are also important exceptions.

2.1 Pitch Proximity in the Grouping of Sound Patterns

Proximity is a powerful organizational principle in the perception of pitch structures. This is particularly manifest for series of tones which are presented in rapid succession. When such tones are drawn from different pitch ranges, the listener hears two melodic lines in parallel: one corresponding to the higher tones and the other to the lower tones. This perceptual phenomenon has frequently been exploited by composers. Figure 8.4 provides, as an example, a passage from Tarrega's *Recuerdos de la Alhambra*. The musical score is here given together with a representation in which pitch (or log frequency) and time are mapped into two dimensions of visual space. The two separate pitch lines are clearly reflected in the visual representation.

There are a number of interesting consequences to this tendency to group rapid series of tones on the basis of pitch proximity. One concerns the perception of temporal relationships. These are well perceived between tones that are in the same pitch range, but poorly perceived between tones that are in different pitch ranges (Bregman, 1990; Bregman and Campbell, 1971; Dannenbring and Bregman, 1976; Fitzgibbon, Pollatsek and Thomas, 1974; van Noorden, 1975). As an example, Figure 8.5 shows the just noticeable temporal displacement of a tone in a continuous series of alternating tones, plotted as a function of the pitch separation between the alternating tones. As can be seen, there is a gradual breakdown of temporal resolution with an increase in the pitch separation between the alternating tones.

Another interesting consequence of grouping by pitch range was demonstrated by Dowling (1973). He generated two well-known melodies such that the tones from each melody occurred in rapid alternation. When the pitch ranges of the melodies overlapped heavily, listeners perceived a single line which corresponded

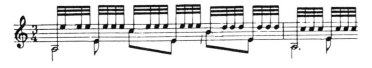

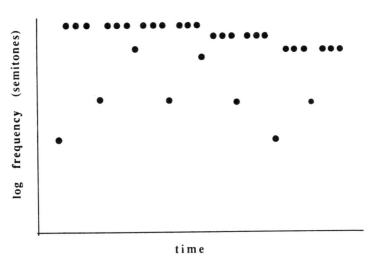

Figure 8.4. *The beginning of Tarrega's* Recuerdos de la Alhambra. *The tones are presented one at a time, but two parallel melodic lines are heard, organized in accordance with pitch proximity.*

to neither melody alone. However, when the alternating melodies were instead presented in different pitch ranges, listeners were then able to separate them perceptually.[1]

When two streams of tones arise simultaneously from different regions of space, pitch proximity can again have a substantial influence on perception. A perceptual reorganization often occurs, so that two melodic lines are heard – one corresponding to the higher tones and the other to the lower tones. Further, tones in one pitch range appear to be coming from one region of space, and tones in another pitch range from a different region, this being true regardless of where each tone is indeed coming from.

Deutsch (1975a,b) first demonstrated this phenomenon with the use of stereo headphones, employing the basic pattern shown in Figure 8.6. This pattern consists of a major scale, with successive tones alternating from ear to ear. The scale is presented simultaneously in both ascending and descending form, so that when a tone from the ascending scale is in one ear, a tone from the descending scale is in the other ear. This basic pattern is repeatedly presented without pause. This pattern, together with its properties, is known as the *scale illusion*.

---

[1]This effect need not necessarily occur, however, and depends on other characteristics of the tones and the relationship between them (see later).

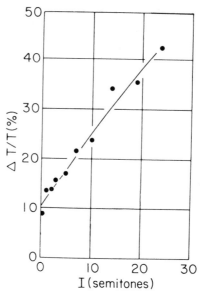

Figure 8.5. *Just noticeable temporal displacement of a tone in a continuous series of alternating tones, as a function of the pitch separation between the alternating tones. The larger the pitch separation, the poorer the ability to detect temporal displacement. [Adapted from van Noorden, 1975.]*

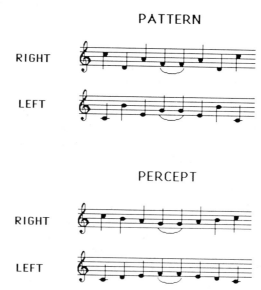

Figure 8.6. *The pattern giving rise to the scale illusion, and the percept most commonly obtained. When the pattern is presented through stereo headphones, most listeners obtain the illusion of two melodic lines that move in contrary motion. The higher tones appear to be coming from one earphone and the lower tones from the other, regardless of where the tones are indeed coming from. [From Deutsch, 1975a. © 1975. The American Institute of Physics, New York; reprinted with kind permission.]*

PATTERN

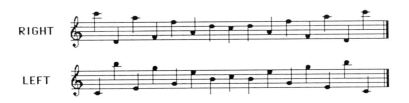

PERCEPT

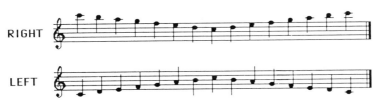

Figure 8.7. *Variant of the scale illusion using a two-octave major scale. The visual representation in the score depicting the percept mirrors the perceptual reorganization of the tones in accordance with pitch proximity.*

Interestingly, listeners very rarely perceive the pattern correctly. Instead, most listeners obtain the illusory percept also shown in Figure 8.6. This consists of two melodic lines that move in contrary motion. Furthermore, tones comprising the higher line all appear to be coming from one earphone and those comprising the lower line from the other. When the earphone positions are reversed, for most listeners the apparent locations of the higher and lower tones remain fixed. So it seems as though the earphone that had been producing the higher tones is now producing the lower tones, and that the earphone that had been producing the lower tones is now producing the higher tones!

As a further unexpected finding, the apparent locations of the higher and the lower tones vary in correlation with the handedness of the listener: most right-handers hear the higher tones on the right and the lower tones on the left; however, left-handers as a group do not show this tendency.

Variants of the scale illusion can readily be produced. Figure 8.7 presents a two-octave major scale, which switches from ear to ear in the same fashion. When the two channels are played together in stereo, most listeners hear a higher scale that moves down an octave and then back, and they simultaneously hear a lower scale that moves up an octave and back, with the two meeting in the middle. However, when each channel is played separately, the tones are heard correctly as jumping around in pitch. In this illustration, the smoothing out of the visual representation in the score depicting the percept reflects well the way that the sounds are perceptually reorganized (see also Butler, 1979a).

Although the scale illusion was originally discovered with the use of stereo headphones, it was later found to occur also with tones presented through spatially

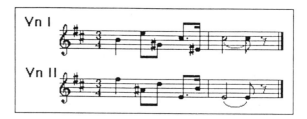

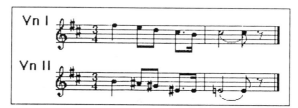

Figure 8.8. *Part of a passage from the final movement of Tchaikovsky's* Sixth Symphony (The Pathétique). *The upper box shows the pattern as it is played, the lower box shows the pattern as it tends to be perceived.*

separated loudspeakers. Indeed, analogous phenomena can even be found in listening to live music in concert halls. Figure 8.8 shows part of a passage from the last movement of Tchaikovsky's *Sixth Symphony (The Pathétique)*. Here, the theme is formed of notes which alternate between the first and second violin parts, and a second voice alternates in converse fashion. Yet the passage is not perceived this way; instead, one violin part appears to be playing the theme and the other violin part the accompaniment. Whether Tchaikovsky intended to produce an illusion here, or whether he assumed that audiences would hear the passage as in the written score, will probably remain a mystery (Butler, 1979b)

Another example occurs in the second movement of Rachmaninoff's *Second Suite for Two Pianos*. At the end of this movement there is a passage in which the first and second pianos play the two patterns shown in Figure 8.9. Yet it appears to the listener that one piano is consistently producing the higher tone, and that the other piano is consistently producing the lower tone (Sloboda, 1985).

We may ask why such illusions should occur, and here the following line of reasoning can be advanced: because of the complexity of our auditory environment, we cannot rely on first-order localization cues alone (e.g. differences in amplitude or time of arrival between the ears) to determine where each of two simultaneous sounds is coming from. Other cues must therefore be taken into account determining the sources of simultaneously presented sounds. One such cue is similarity of frequency spectrum: it is probable that similar sounds are coming from the same source and that dissimilar sounds are coming from different sources. So with patterns such as described here, it makes sense for the auditory system to assume that tones in one frequency range are coming from one source, and that tones in a different frequency range are coming from a different source. The tones are therefore reorganized perceptually in accordance with this interpretation.

So far we have been considering patterns in which sounds presented through the two earphones or loudspeakers are simultaneous. This leads us to enquire what

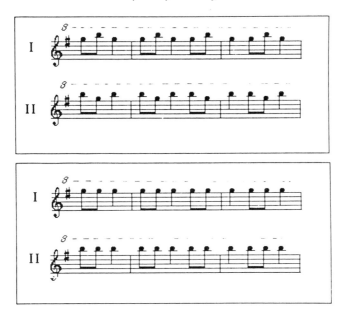

Figure 8.9. *Part of a passage from the second movement of Rachmaninoff's* Second Suite for Two Pianos. *The upper box shows the pattern as it is played, the lower box shows the pattern as it is often perceived.*

happens when the factor of simultaneity is removed. Two experiments were performed to examine this issue (Deutsch, 1979). In each experiment, two repeating melodic patterns were presented and listeners were asked to identify on each trial which one they had heard. The two patterns are displayed in Figure 8.10.

The experiment consisted of four conditions. In all conditions, the patterns were presented through stereo headphones. The different conditions, together with their associated error rates, are illustrated in Figure 8.11. In the first condition, the patterns were delivered to both ears simultaneously, and it can be seen that here identification levels were very high. In the second condition, the tones were switched haphazardly between the ears. As can be seen, the switching procedure made the task much more difficult. The third condition was exactly as the second, except that the melody was accompanied by a drone. Whenever a tone from the melody was delivered to the right ear, the drone was delivered to the left ear and vice versa. Thus, the tones were again delivered to both ears simultaneously, even though the melody was switching from ear to ear, exactly as in the second condition. As can be seen, the contralateral drone caused the melody to emerge perceptually, with the result that identification performance was again very high. In the fourth condition, a drone again accompanied the melody, but now it was delivered to the same ear as the melody component. In this condition, therefore, input was again to one ear at a time. As can be seen, identification performance was here again very low; indeed, it was slightly below chance.

This experiment, taken together with the findings from the scale illusion, demonstrates that with tones which emanate from different spatial locations, temporal relationships between them are important in determining how they are perceptually grouped together. When the tones arriving at the two ears are

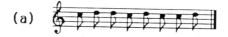

(a)

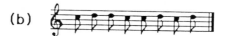

(b)

Figure 8.10. *The two patterns employed in the experiment to investigate the effect on melody identification of switching input between the ears. See text for details. [From Deutsch, 1979. © 1979 The Psychonomic Society, Inc.; reprinted with kind permission.]*

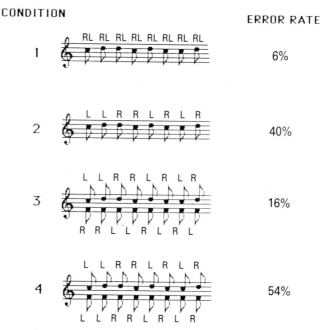

Figure 8.11. *Different conditions employed in the experiment to investigate the effect on melody identification of switching input between the ears, together with associated error rates. See text for details. [From Deutsch, 1979. © 1979 The Psychonomic Society, Inc.; reprinted with kind permission.]*

simultaneous, organization on the basis of pitch proximity occurs, so that patterns composed of such tones are readily integrated. On the other hand, when the tones arriving at the two ears are clearly separated in time, grouping by spatial location is so powerful as to virtually obliterate the listener's ability to integrate them into a single coherent pattern.

We may then ask what happens in the intermediate condition, that is, where the tones arriving at the two ears are not strictly simultaneous but overlap in time. This situation is much more like that found in normal listening to music. In the second experiment this intermediate case was found to produce intermediate results: when the tones from the melody and the contralateral drone were asynchronous, identification performance was at a lower level than when they were strictly synchronous, but at a higher level than when there was no temporal overlap between the tones.

This leads us to enquire why such results should have been obtained, and here the following line of reasoning may be advanced. Temporal relationships between sounds are important indicators of whether they are coming from the same source or from different sources. Thus, the more clearly the signals arriving at the two ears are separated in time, the greater should be the tendency to treat them as coming from separate sources, and so the greater should be the tendency to group them by spatial location. When such grouping is sufficiently strong, it should prevent us from forming perceptual connections between tones that arise from different sources.

2.2 Illusory Conjunctions in Hearing

A doctrine stemming from the British empiricists of the seventeenth and eighteenth centuries is that objects are perceived as bundles of attribute values. For example, it is assumed that when we see an object, we separately apprehend its shape, its color, its location and so on. It is further assumed that the different values of these attributes are later combined by the perceptual system, so that an integrated percept results. Similarly, when we hear a sound, it is assumed that we separately apprehend its pitch, its location, its loudness and so on, and that these attribute values are later combined so as to form a unitary percept.

The view that different attributes of a stimulus are analyzed at some stage separately by the perceptual system accommodates the processing of single stimuli without difficulty. However, a problem arises when we consider the case where more than one stimulus is presented at a time. For example, suppose that a red square and a green circle are simultaneously presented. The color-analyzing mechanism produces the two outputs 'red' and 'green' and the shape-analyzing mechanism produces the two outputs 'square' and 'circle'. The question then arises of how we know which output of the color-analyzing mechanism to combine with which output of the shape-analyzing mechanism. In other words, how do we know that it is the square that is red and the circle that is green, rather than the other way round? Analogously, suppose that a 1000 Hz signal is presented to the right and a 300 Hz signal to the left. The pitch-analyzing mechanism produces two outputs: one corresponding to the high tone and the other to the low tone. The localization mechanism also produces two outputs: one signalling 'right' and the other 'left'. But how do we then know that it is the high tone that is to the right and the low tone to the left, rather than the other way round?

We have seen that in the scale illusion, when two series of tones are simultaneously presented, the process of recombination of attribute values does indeed go wildly wrong, so that illusory conjunctions occur. Another sound pattern that produces illusory conjunctions is known as the *octave illusion* (Deutsch, 1974, 1975b). This is produced by the pattern depicted in Figure 8.12. As can be seen, it consists of two tones that are spaced an octave apart and are repeatedly presented in alternation. The identical series of alternating tones is presented to both ears simultaneously but out of step with each other; thus, when one ear receives the high tone, the other ear receives the low tone, and vice versa.

D. Deutsch

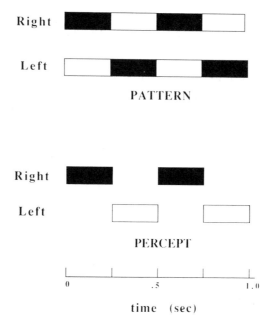

Figure 8.12. *Pattern giving rise to the octave illusion, and percept most commonly obtained. Filled boxes represent tones of 800 Hz and unfilled boxes tones of 400 Hz. This basic pattern is repeatedly presented without pause. Most listeners obtain the illusion of a pattern consisting of a high tone alternating with silence in the right ear, and a low tone alternating with silence in the left ear. This percept is obtained regardless of positioning of the earphones.*

Interestingly, it is extremely rare for anyone to hear this pattern correctly. The illusion most commonly obtained is also shown in Figure 8.12. This consists of a single tone that switches from ear to ear and, as it switches, its pitch simultaneously shifts back and forth between high and low. In other words, the listener hears a repeating high tone in one ear which alternates with a repeating low tone in the other ear.

There is clearly no simple way to explain this illusion. The perception of alternating pitches can be explained by assuming that the listenener processes the input to one ear and ignores the other. But on this hypothesis both of the alternating pitches should appear localized in the same ear. Similarly, the perception of a tone that alternates from ear to ear can be explained by assuming that the listener suppresses the input to each ear in turn. But on this hypothesis the pitch of the tone should not appear to change with the change in its apparent location. The illusion of a single tone that alternates both in pitch and in location appears as a paradox.

A further surprise occurs when the listener's headphones are placed in reverse position. Now most people hear exactly the same thing: the tone that had appeared in the right ear still appears in the right ear, and the tone that had appeared in the left ear still appears in the left ear. So it seems to the listener that the earphone that had been producing the high tone is now producing the low tone, and that the earphone that had been producing the low tone is now producing the high tone!

There is clearly no simple way to explain this illusion. However, if we suppose that two separate decision mechanisms exist, one to determine *what* pitch we hear, the other to determine *where* the tone is coming from, we are in a position to advance an explanation. The model proposed by Deutsch (1975b) is depicted in Figure 8.13. To determine the perceived pitch, the information arriving at one ear is followed and the information arriving at the other ear is suppressed. However, to determine the perceived location, each tone is localized at the ear receiving the higher tone, regardless of whether the higher or the lower tone is in fact perceived.

Let us take the case of a listener who follows the pitches presented to his right ear. When the high tone is presented to his right and the low tone to his left, this listener hears a high tone, since this is presented to his right ear, and he localizes the tone in his right ear, since this ear is receiving the higher tone. However, when the low tone is presented to his right ear and the high tone to his left, this listener now hears a low tone, since this is the tone presented to his right ear, but he localizes the tone in his left ear instead, since this ear is receiving the higher tone. So the entire pattern is heard as a high tone to the right ear alternating with a low tone to the left.

We can see that on this model, reversing the position of the earphones would not alter the basic percept. However, if we take the case of a listener who follows the pitches presented to his left ear instead, holding the localization rule constant, the entire pattern is now heard as a high tone to the left alternating with a low tone to the right.

A further test of this model employed the following pattern: one ear received three high tones followed by two low tones, while simultaneously the other ear received three low tones followed by two high tones. This basic pattern was presented ten times without pause. Subjects were asked to report separately the pattern of pitches and also the pattern of locations that they heard (Deutsch and Roll, 1976). It was found that, in confirmation of the model, most subjects reported hearing either three high tones alternating with two low tones, or two high tones alternating with three low tones. Further, also in confirmation of the model, each tone was localized in the ear receiving the higher tone, regardless of whether the higher or the lower tone was in fact perceived. So, as with the original octave illusion, when a low tone was heard, it appeared to be coming, not from the earphone which was indeed delivering it, but from the opposite earphone.

Another interesting characteristic of the octave illusion is that the way it is perceived varies in correlation with the handedness of the listener. Right-handers tend to hear the high tone on the right and the low tone on the left; however, left-handers do not show this tendency (Deutsch, 1974). Indeed, regardless of the handedness of the listener, the tendency to hear the high tone on the right and the low tone on the left is higher among those without left-handed parents or siblings than among those with a left-handed parent or sibling (Deutsch, 1983). These findings indicate that the way the octave illusion is perceived might serve as a reliable indicator of the direction of cerebral dominance.

At all events, experiments on the octave illusion provide strong evidence for the view that the mechanism deciding *what* pitch we hear and the mechanism deciding *where* a sound is located are at some stage separate in the auditory system, and that at this stage they operate according to independent, and in some cases even contradictory, criteria. As a result, for certain stimulus configurations, we end up perceiving a sound that does not exist; that is, with its pitch taken from one source and its location from another.

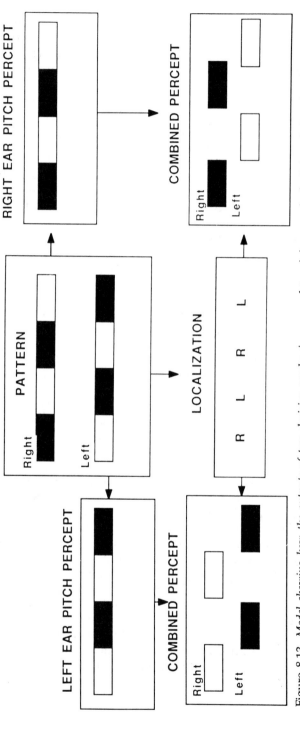

Figure 8.13. Model showing how the outputs of two decision mechanisms, one determining perceived pitch and the other determining perceived location, can combine to produce the octave illusion. Filled boxes represent tones of 800 Hz and unfilled boxes tones of 400 Hz. See text for details.

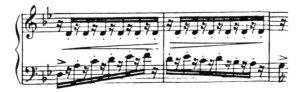

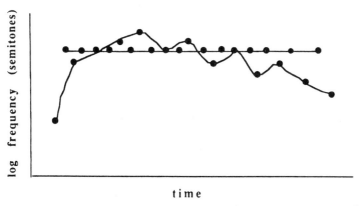

Figure 8.14. *Two measures from Albinez's* Leyenda. *The listener hears two distinct melodic streams; one formed of the repeating pitch and the other is composed of the moving pitch line, even though the pitch ranges of the streams overlap. This illustrates perceptual grouping by good continuation.*

2.3 Good Continuation in the Grouping of Pitch Patterns

When a series of tones is presented in rapid succession, the listener may organize these on the basis of good continuation. One situation in which this occurs is where a repeating pitch alternates with a moving pitch line. The continuity provided by the single repeating pitch enables the other pitches to be separated out perceptually. Figure 8.14 depicts a passage from Albinez's *Leyenda* which exploits this phenomenon.

There are a few laboratory findings related to other aspects of good continuation. Bregman and Dannenbring (1973) showed that when a series of tones is presented at a rapid tempo and the pitches of these tones alternate between high and low, the series appears more coherent when the tones are related by pitch glides. Several other investigators have reported that when subjects are asked to identify the order of occurrence of tones in a rapid series, performance levels are higher when the tones form a unidirectional pitch change than when they do not do so (Divenyi and Hirsh, 1974; Warren and Byrnes, 1975).

violin

piano

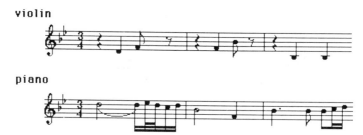

Figure 8.15. *Part of a passage from the beginning of the second movement of Beethoven's* Spring Sonata *for violin and piano. Although the tones played by the two instruments overlap in pitch, the listener perceives two parallel melodic lines, which correspond to those played by each instrument. This illustrates perceptual grouping by similarity.*

2.4   Grouping of Sounds by Similarity or by Sound Quality

When different types of instrument perform in parallel, the sounds are often grouped on the basis of timbre. Figure 8.15 is taken from the beginning of the second movement of Beethoven's *Spring Sonata* for violin and piano. Here, the pitch ranges of the two instruments overlap, and yet the listener perceives two parallel melodic lines which correspond to those played by each instrument.

Warren *et al.* (1969) produced a striking demonstration of the influence of sound quality on the perception of rapidly presented sounds. A series of four unrelated sounds was generated, and this was repeatedly presented without pause. The sounds were a high tone, a low tone, a hiss and a buzz. When each sound was 200 ms in duration, listeners were unable to identify the order in which they occurred. However, when the presentation rate was slowed down, so that each sound was 500 ms in duration, listeners were able to order the sounds correctly.

Another consequence of grouping by timbre was demonstrated by Wessel (1979). He generated a repeating three-tone ascending line by means of two alternating timbres. When the difference between the timbres was small, listeners perceived the three-tone ascending line and so followed the pitch contour of the pattern. However, when this difference was large, listeners instead perceived two interwoven descending lines which were defined on the basis of timbre.

2.5   The Principle of Closure

The perceptual organization of sound patterns is also influenced by the principle of closure. For example, when two sounds of differing amplitude are presented in alternation, the softer sound may appear to continue through the louder one (Miller and Licklider, 1950; Thurlow, 1957; Vicario, 1960). As another example, when a gliding tone is presented, and a portion of the glide is removed and replaced by a noise burst, the listener obtains the impression of an uninterrupted glide that continues through the noise (Dannenbring, 1976).

2.6   Grouping of Sounds by Common Fate

The principle of common fate has been shown to influence grouping in music. Chowning (1980) demonstrated that, in synthesizing a singing voice, the superposition of a small amount of vibrato on all the harmonic components, so that they fluctuated in synchrony with each other, enabled these components to fuse together so as to produce a unitary percept. He further demonstrated that the superposition of different patterns of vibrato on different components of a tone complex led to these components being heard as perceptually distinct from each other. A related finding was obtained by Rasch (1978). He found that the superposition of a frequency modulation on one component of a two-tone chord led to enhanced perceptual separation between the components of this chord.

3   MUSICAL SHAPE ANALYSIS

We may consider musical shape analysis as occurring at several levels of abstraction. We first enquire into the types of abstraction that give rise to the perception of local features, such as intervals, chords and pitch classes (Deutsch, 1969). Features such as these are analogous to visual features such as line orientation and angle size. Global features are also abstracted at this primitive level. These include contour (the sequence of rises and falls in pitch), general pitch range, approximate sizes of melodic and of harmonic intervals, and so on. At the next level of abstraction, low-level features are combined so as to form more elaborate features. At yet higher levels, abstract encodings are created.

The present approach to musical shape analysis does not assume that processing always occurs from lower levels to higher ones. Indeed, it will be shown that the opposite is sometimes the case. As will be shown below, the testing of hypotheses by the listener based on previously acquired information, can be important in determining how sound patterns are perceived.

3.1   Low-level Features

3.1.1   Pitch Class

Tones whose fundamental frequencies stand in the ratio of $2:1$ are described as in octave relation. Such tones have a certain perceptual equivalence and so are described by music theorists as being in the same *pitch class*. In Western musical notation, a tone is represented first by a letter name (C, C♯, D, etc.) which designates its pitch class, and then by a number which designates the octave in which the tone occurs. For example, the symbols E_3, E_4 and E_5 refer to tones that are in the same pitch class but in successively higher octaves. Conversely, the symbols E_3, A_3 and G♯ $_3$, refer to tones that are in different pitch classes but in the same octave. It should be observed that octave equivalence is not confined to Western tonal music but is built into most musical systems (Burns and Ward, 1982).

As a consequence of perceptual equivalence based on the octave, listeners with absolute pitch sometimes make octave errors in naming notes (Bachem, 1954; Baird,

1917; Ward and Burns, 1982). Further, generalization of response to tones that stand in octave relation occurs both in humans (Demany and Armand, 1984; Humphreys, 1939) and in animals (Blackwell and Schlosberg, 1942). As yet further evidence for octave equivalence, interference effects in short-term memory for pitch generalize across octaves (Deutsch, 1973).

3.1.2 Intervals and Chords

When two tones are presented, either simultaneously or in succession, a musical *interval* is perceived, and intervals are perceived as being the same in size when the fundamental frequencies of their component tones stand in the same ratio. This principle serves as a basis of the traditional musical scale. The smallest unit of this scale is the semitone, which corresponds to a frequency ratio of roughly 18:17. Intervals that comprise the same number of semitones are given the same name. Thus, for example, the interval that comprises four semitones is termed a major third; the interval that comprises five semitones is termed a perfect fourth, and so on. Table 8.1 displays the 12 intervals within the octave, together with their names, the frequency ratios to which they correspond and the number of semitones they comprise.

When three or more tones are presented simultaneously, a *chord* is perceived. One way of characterizing a chord is in terms of its component intervals. Thus, the major triad (e.g. C, E, G) is composed of a major third, a minor third and a perfect fifth. However, we may observe that a mere listing of these intervals is not sufficient to define a chord. The minor triad (e.g. C, E♭, G) is also composed of a major third, a minor third and a perfect fifth. However, major and minor triads are perceptually quite distinct. For the major triad the major third lies below the minor third, yet for the minor triad the major third lies above the minor third (Figure 8.16). This difference in the ordering of intervals is evidently of perceptual importance (Deutsch, 1969).

3.1.3 Interval Class

Given perceptual equivalence based on pitch class and on interval, some music theorists have claimed that perceptual equivalence must also exist between intervals that are composed of tones that are in the same pitch class but in different octaves (see, for example, Babbitt, 1960, 1965; Forte, 1973). Such intervals are described as in the same *interval class*. The experimental evidence on this point, however, is complex; it appears that perceptual equivalence based on interval class occurs under certain circumstances but not others.

In considering this issue, we should first draw a distinction between harmonic and melodic intervals. For the case of harmonic intervals, evidence for perceptual equivalence based in interval class has indeed been obtained (Deutsch and Roll, 1974; Plomp, Wagenaar and Mimpen, 1973). To investigate the issue for the case of melodic intervals, the following experiment was performed (Deutsch, 1972). A well-known melody was presented which was transformed in such a way that the pitch classes were preserved but the octave placement of the tones varied randomly across three adjacent octaves. Subjects were simply asked to name the melody. The results of the experiment were unequivocal: identification performance was no better than in a control condition in which the melody was presented as a series of

Table 8.1. *The 12 intervals within the octave*

Approximate ratio	17:18	8:9	5:6	4:5	3:4	5:7	2:3	5:8	3:5	5:9	11:21	1:2
Number of semitones	1	2	3	4	5	6	7	8	9	10	11	12
Musical interval	Minor second	Major second	Minor third	Major third	Perfect fourth	Tritone	Perfect fifth	Minor sixth	Major sixth	Minor seventh	Major seventh	Octave

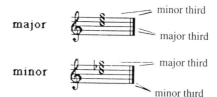

Figure 8.16. *The major and minor triads. Both are composed of a major third, a minor third, and a perfect fifth. However, in the major triad the major third lies below the minor third, whereas in the minor triad the major third lies above the minor third. This ordering of the intervals is of perceptual importance. [From Deutsch, 1969. © 1969 The American Psychological Association; reprinted with kind permission.]*

clicks, so that the rhythm was retained but the pitch information was removed entirely. It is evident, then, that the subjects were quite unable to use interval class to identify the melody.

However, when the subjects were later given the name of the melody, they were able to follow the 'octave-randomized' version with ease and so confirm that each tone was indeed in the correct pitch class. In other words, the subjects were able to identify the melody through a process of hypothesis-testing, even though they had not been able to recognize it in the absence of cues on which to base a hypothesis. The present phenomenon thus provides a striking demonstration of the role of hypothesis-testing in listening to music: when given no clues on which to base a hypothesis, listeners cannot recognize melodies that have been transformed in this fashion. However, when appropriate clues are furnished, listeners can draw on long-term memory so as to enable them to identify such melodies with ease.

In a further experiment on the issue of interval class equivalence, Deutsch and Boulanger (1984) presented novel melodic patterns to musicians and asked them to recall these in musical notation. Each pattern consisted of a random ordering of the first six notes of a major scale. In one condition, all tones were taken from a higher octave. In another condition, all tones were taken from a lower octave. In a third, 'across-octaves' condition, the tones in each pattern alternated between the higher and lower octaves. Performance in the 'across-octaves' condition was found to be markedly inferior to performance in the other two. This provides further confirmation of the view that interval class identity does not entail perceptual equivalence.

3.1.4 Global Cues

Global cues involved in music perception include overall pitch range, the distribution of interval sizes, the proportion of ascending relative to descending intervals, and contour.

3.2 Musical Shape Analysis at Higher Levels of Abstraction

We next consider how low-order features in music are combined by the perceptual system so as to give rise to perceptual equivalences and similarities. Visual shapes are recognized as equivalent when they differ in size, location, orientation, and so on. We may then ask what transformations result in analogous equivalences in music.

As described by von Ehrenfels (1890), melodies retain their perceptual identities when they are transposed to different keys, in the same way as visual shapes retain their perceptual identities when they are translated to different regions of the visual field. In transposition, the intervals formed by the tones are preserved, although these intervals are invoked with respect to different pitches.[2]

This leads us to enquire what other types of transformation leave the perceptual identities of musical shapes intact. Schönberg (1951) employed an intermodal analogy in which pitch and time are translated into two dimensions of visual space and argued that transformations analogous to reflection and rotation in vision give rise to perceptual equivalences in music also:

'THE TWO-OR-MORE-DIMENSIONAL SPACE IN WHICH MUSICAL IDEAS ARE PRESENTED IS A UNIT.... The elements of a musical idea are partly incorporated in the horizontal plane as successive sounds, and partly in the vertical plane as simultaneous sounds.... *The unity of musical space demands an absolute and unitary perception.* In this space...there is no absolute down, no right or left, forward or backward....To the imaginative and creative faculty, relations in the material sphere are as independent from directions or planes as material objects are, in their sphere, to our perceptive faculties. Just as our mind always recognizes, for instance, a knife, a bottle or a watch, regardless of its position, and can reproduce it in the imagination in every possible position, even so a musical creator's mind can operate subconsciously with a row of tones, regardless of their direction, regardless of the way in which a mirror might show the mutual relations, which remain a given quantity.' (pp. 220, 223; italics as in original work)

Based on this intermodal analogy, Schönberg argued that series of tones would be perceived as equivalent when the tones are played backwards (retrogression), when the directions of the melodic intervals are reversed (inversion) and when they are transformed by both these operations (retrograde-inversion). Schönberg's theory of the abstract representation of musical shapes is illustrated in Figure 8.17. As he wrote: '...The employment of these mirror forms corresponds to the principle of *the absolute and unitary perception of musical space.*' (p. 225)

It is interesting to note that Ernst Mach (1889) had argued earlier against this view. In addressing the question of 'whether there is anything similar to the symmetry of figures in the province of sounds', he wrote:

'Now, although in all the preceding examples I have transposed steps upward into equal and similar steps downward, that is, as we may justly say, have played for every movement the movement which is symmetrical to it, yet the ear notices little or nothing of symmetry. The transposition from a major to a minor key is the sole indication of symmetry remaining. The symmetry is there for the mind but is wanting for sensation. No symmetry exists for the ear, because a reversal of musical sounds conditions no repetition of sensations. If we had an ear for height and an ear for depth, just as we have an eye for the right and an eye for the left, we should also find that symmetrical sound-structures existed for our auditory organs.' (p. 103)

We can here observe an important difference between the approach taken by Mach and that taken by Schönberg. Mach (and the Gestalt psychologists after him)

---

[2]However, there can be exceptions to this rule (see later).

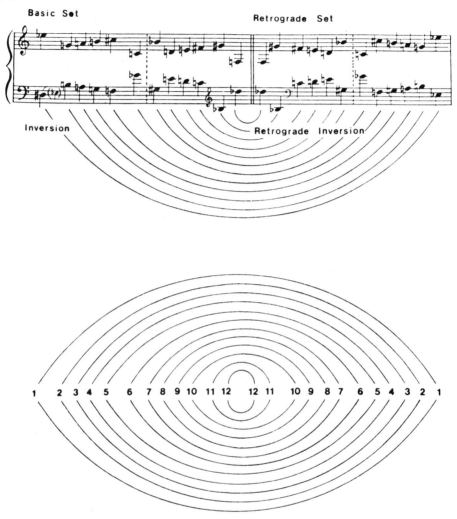

Figure 8.17. *Schönberg's concept of 'musical space'. Series of pitches are considered perceptually equivalent when these are related by inversion, retrogression or retrograde-inversion. [From Schönberg, 1951. © 1951 A & C Black; reprinted with kind permission.]*

treated theories of perceptual organization as *hypotheses* which require experimental verification or, at least, convincing demonstration by observation. In contrast, Schönberg propounded his theories by fiat and did not believe that they should be subject to empirical investigation.

A few experimental studies bearing on Schönberg's theoretical speculations have been performed. Francès (1958) carried out an experiment in which musicians (including composers of serial music[3]) were asked to discriminate between tone series which had been transformed in accordance with Schönberg's rules. Very poor

---

[3]Serial music is the name given to music composed in accordance with the principles laid down by Schönberg and his followers.

performance was obtained and Francès concluded that the transformations proposed by Schönberg did not in fact give rise to perceptual equivalences.

In a further experiment, White (1960) studied the ability of subjects to identify well-known melodies which were played in retrogression. He found that identification of such melodies was no better than for melodies in which the pitch information was removed entirely, with rhythm alone remaining. In yet another experiment, Dowling (1972) explored the ability of subjects to recognize melodies that had been transformed by retrogression, inversion and retrograde-inversion. Again, very poor performance was obtained.

General considerations also cast doubt on the view that transformations analogous to rotation and reflection in vision should result in perceptual equivalences in music. For the case of vision, clear evolutionary advantages are conferred by mechanisms that enable us to identify objects when these have been placed in different positions or orientations relative to the observer. However, there are no analogous advantages associated with the ability to recognize patterns of sound which have been presented backward in time, or in which the pitch relationships have been inverted; such perceptual tasks are never required in our natural environment.

From general considerations of tonal music, however, it appears that short melodic fragments that have been transformed by retrogression and inversion can be recognized in a short-term memory situation (Meyer, 1973). However, it also appears that such recognition occurs at a higher level of abstraction, rather than being based on melodic intervals as proposed by Schönberg. This higher level of abstraction is explored in the next section.

3.3   Hierarchical Encoding of Pitch Patterns

When observers are presented with artificial patterns which lend themselves to hierarchical encoding, they generally form encodings which reflect the structures of these patterns (Bjork, 1968; Kotovsky and Simon, 1973; Restle, 1970; Restle and Brown, 1970; Simon and Kotovsky, 1963; Vitz and Todd, 1969). This consideration has led several researchers to propose models of the cognitive representation of serial patterns in terms of hierarchies of operators (Deutsch and Feroe, 1981; Greeno and Simon, 1974; Restle, 1970; Simon, 1972; Simon and Sumner, 1968).

To document that such cognitive representations can indeed be formed, Restle (1970) and Restle and Brown (1970) employed the following paradigm: subjects were presented with arrays of lights that repeatedly turned on and off in succession. On each trial, the subjects' task was to predict which light would turn on next. The orders in which the lights were turned on were such as to form compact structural descriptions. For example, assuming an array of six lights, we may take the basic subsequence $X = (1\ 2)$. The operation T (transposition $+1$ of X) then produces the sequence $1\ 2\ 2\ 3$; the operation R (repeat of X) produces the sequence $1\ 2\ 1\ 2$; and the operation M (mirror image of X) produces the sequence $1\ 2\ 6\ 5$. It can be seen that recursive application of such operations will generate long sequences which nevertheless have compact structural descriptions. For example, the sequence $1\ 2\ 1\ 2\ 6\ 5\ 6\ 5$ can be represented as $M(R(X))$. This example corresponds to the structural tree shown in Figure 8.18.

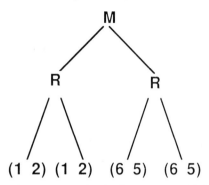

Figure 8.18. *Structural tree that corresponds to the sequence 1 2 1 2 6 5 6 5, according to the formalism of Restle (1970) . [From Restle, 1970, p. 487, Fig. 5. © 1970 The American Psychological Association; reprinted with kind permission.]*

Restle and Brown (1970) showed that for sequences that were constructed in accordance with such structural trees, the probability of error increased monotonically the higher the level of transformation along the tree. Thus, in our present example, the highest probability of error would occur at locations 1 and 5 and the next highest would occur at locations 3 and 7. Restle and Brown concluded that observers can indeed develop representations of patterns in accordance with such structural trees.

We may note, however, that the patterns used in these studies were such as to enable only a single type of parsimonious encoding. This leads us to wonder how well this model would generalize to the encoding of patterns that have not been artificially contrived to conform with these particular rules.

In this context, we may note that the organization of tonal music is hierarchical in nature (Keiler, 1983; Lerdahl and Jackendoff, 1983; Meyer, 1973, 1989; Narmour, 1977, 1983, 1990; Schenker, 1935, 1906/1973). It appears reasonable to assume that such hierarchical structure has evolved to optimize the use of our processing mechanisms. Thus, examining the structure of tonal music can generate useful hypotheses concerning the ways in which we naturally generate hierarchical representations.

Using this line of reasoning, Deutsch and Feroe (1981) proposed a model for the cognitive representation of pitch series in tonal music. This model takes the structure of tonal music into account, and also demonstrates how various characteristics of tonal music can be exploited so as to produce parsimonious representations. The model assumes that the listener encodes series of pitches as hierarchies. At each level of such a hierarchy, elements are organized as structural units in accordance with principles of figural goodness (good continuation, proximity, and so on). Elements that are present at any given level of the hierarchy are elaborated by further elements so as to form structural units at the next-lower level, until the lowest level is reached. Here follows a simplified set of rules for the system:

(1) A *structure* A, of length n, is notated as $A_0, A_1, \ldots, A_{l-1}, {}^*, A_{l+1}, \ldots, A_{n-1})$ where A_j is one of the operators n, p, s, n^i or p^i. A string of length k of an operator is here abbreviated as kA.

(2) Associated with each structure is an alphabet, α. The combination of a structure and an alphabet produces a *sequence*. A sequence, in combination with the reference element r, produces a *sequence of notes*.

(3) The effect of an operator is determined by that of the operator next to it, on the same side as *. Thus, for example, the operator n refers to traversing one step up the alphabet that is associated with the structure. The operator p refers to traversing one step down this alphabet. The operator s refers to remaining in the same position. The operators n^i and p^i refer to traversing up or down i steps along the alphabet, respectively. The values of the sequence of notes $(A_0, A_1, \ldots, A_{l-1}, *, A_{l+1}, \ldots, A_{n-1})$ α, r, are obtained by taking the value of * to be that of r.

(4) Given two sequences $A = (A_0, A_1, \ldots, A_{l-1}, *, A_{l+1}, \ldots, A_{n-1})$ α and $B = (B_0, B_1, \ldots, B_{l-1}, *, B_{l+1}, B_{m-1})$, β, the compound operator pr (prime) is defined as follows. A [pr] B; r , refers to the assignation of values to the notes produced from $(B_0, B_1, \ldots, B_{l-1}, *, B_{l+1}, \ldots, B_{m-1})$ such that the value of * is the same as the value of A_0, when the sequence A is applied to r. Next, values are assigned to the notes produced from $(B_0, B_1, \ldots, B_{l-1}, *, B_{l+1}, \ldots, B_{m-1})$ so that the value of * is the same as that of A_1, and so on. In this way, a sequence of length $n \times m$ is produced. Other compound operators such as inv (inversion) and ret (retrograde) are defined analogously.

Figure 8.19 provides an example of such a representation. This pattern can be parsimoniously represented on two hierarchical levels. At the higher level, a

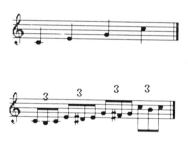

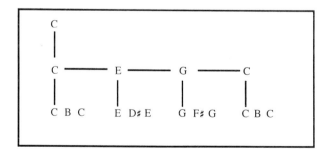

Figure 8.19. *A series of pitches represented at two hierarchical levels. At the higher level there is an arpeggiation of a major triad (C–E–G–C). At the lower level each note of the triad is elaborated by a pattern that moves one step down and then up the chromatic scale.*

series of notes moves stepwise up the alphabet of a major triad (C–E–G–C). At the lower level, each of these notes is elaborated by a further series that moves one step down and then up the chromatic scale. In this way, the full series ((C–B–C) (E–D♯–E)(G–F♯–G) (C–B–C)) is produced.

The associated encoding is as follows:

$$A = \{(*, 3n); 1\}$$
$$B = \{(n, p, *); \mathrm{Cr}\}$$
$$S = \{A \,[\mathrm{pr}]\, B; 1\}\, C$$

We may observe that, where this pattern is not encoded hierarchically, one would have to employ a considerably more cumbersome notation to represent it, for example:

$$\{\{(*, p, n, n^4, p, n, n^3, p, n, n^5, p, n); \mathrm{Cr}\}; 1\}C$$

The present hierarchical representation therefore has several cognitive advantages. First, since two alphabets are employed, it is possible to encode the pattern in terms of single steps along each alphabet, so conforming to the principle of proximity. As a second point, the present representation involves only two structures, each of which is of small chunk size. Further, since notes that are present at the higher level are also present at the lower level, these notes are redundantly represented and so are given prominence over the other notes. In this way, the higher-level notes serve to cement the lower-level notes together.

In an associated experiment to test the assumptions of the model, Deutsch (1980) presented musically trained subjects with series of tones that could be parsimoniously encoded in this hierarchical fashion. The subjects were required to recall these series in musical notation. Each such series was matched with another in which the identical set of tones were ordered haphazardly. It was found that, for the series that could be hierarchically encoded, performance levels were very high. However, for the matched series which could not be so encoded, performance levels were considerably lower. This result provides further evidence in favor of the view that we readily form encodings of this hierarchical type.

Another issue examined in the experiment of Deutsch (1980) was the role of temporal segmentation in the processing of pitch structures. The tone series described above were presented either unsegmented, or they were temporarily segmented in accordance with their pitch structure, or they were temporarily segmented in conflict with their pitch structure. It was found that, whereas segmentation in accordance with pitch structure was associated with enhanced performance, segmentation in conflict with pitch structure resulted in substantial performance decrements. We can conclude that grouping by temporal proximity can be so powerful as to virtually abolish the listener's ability to apprehend the pitch structure of a series, when this structure conflicts with temporal segmentation.

A further related experiment was performed by Oura (1991). She presented subjects with a melody which they were required to recall in musical notation. She found that notes that were situated at higher hierarchical levels were well recalled and that most errors in recall occurred for notes that were situated at lower levels. This finding is in accordance with the above model.

3.4 Pitch Class and Pitch Height

Given that tones which stand in octave relation have a strong perceptual similarity, the pitch of a tone may be held to vary along two dimensions: the rectilinear dimension of height defines its position on a continuum from low to high, and the circular dimension of pitch class defines its position within the octave (Bachem, 1948; Charbonneau and Risset, 1973; Deutsch, 1969, 1973, 1982; Meyer, 1904, 1914; Révész, 1913; Ruckmick, 1929; Shepard, 1964, 1982; Ward and Burns, 1982). The circular dimension of pitch class is depicted in Figure 8.20.

We may then enquire whether these two dimensions of pitch are orthogonal, or whether they interact in some way. Common sense would lead one to argue that surely they must be orthogonal. If one were asked: 'Which tone is higher, C or F♯?' one could reasonably answer that such a question is nonsensical, since this would depend on the octave in which each of the two tones was placed.

In an experiment designed to produce a formal demonstration of such orthogonality, Shepard (1964) generated a series of tones, each of which was clearly defined in terms of pitch class, but ambiguously defined in terms of height. Each tone consisted of a series of sinusoids which were separated exactly by octaves. The amplitudes of these sinusoidal components were scaled by a fixed, bell-shaped spectral envelope in such a way that those in the middle of the musical range were loudest, with the lowest and highest falling off below the hearing threshold. He then varied the pitch classes of the tones, while keeping the position and shape of the spectral envelope constant. He argued that since the envelope was invariant, the perceived heights of these tones should remain constant in face of variations in pitch class.

Shepard found that when a sequential pair of such tones was presented, listeners heard either an ascending or a descending pattern, depending on which was the shorter distance along the pitch class circle. For example, the series C–C♯ was always heard as ascending, since the shorter distance here was clockwise. Analogously, the series F–E was always heard as descending, since the shorter distance here was counter-clockwise.

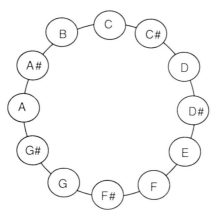

Figure 8.20. *The pitch class circle.*

Based on these findings, Shepard produced a striking demonstration. A series of tones was presented which repeatedly traversed the pitch class circle in clockwise steps. As a result, listeners perceived a series of tones that appeared to ascend endlessly in pitch: C♯ was heard as higher than C, D as higher than C♯, ..., B as higher than A♯, C as higher than B, C♯ as higher than C, and so on infinitely. Analogously, a series of tones that traversed the circle in counter-clockwise direction appeared to descend endlessly.

Perhaps an even more compelling version of this paradox was produced by Risset (1971). He generated a single gliding tone that moved around the pitch class circle in clockwise or counter-clockwise direction, so that listeners heard a single tone that appeared to glide endlessly up or down in pitch. (For related work see also Burns, 1981; Nakajima *et al.*, 1988; Pollack, 1978; Schroeder, 1986; Ueda and Ohgushi, 1987.)

These endlessly ascending and descending pitches demonstrate that under conditions of ambiguity, listeners will invoke pitch proximity in making judgments of relative height. This leads us to enquire what would happen when the opportunity to exploit the proximity principle were removed. For example, what happens when a sequential pair of tones is presented which are related by a half-octave (i.e. a tritone), so that they are separated by the same distance along the pitch class circle in either direction? Would judgments of relative height for such tones be haphazard, or would the perceptual system invoke some other principle to resolve the ambiguity?

In considering this question, it occurred to me that there is a further cue to draw on: reference could be made to the absolute positions of the tones along the pitch class circle. Supposing the listener tagged tones in one region of the circle as higher and tones in the opposite region as lower, the ambiguity would be resolved. As an analogy, let us consider the pitch class circle as a clockface with the pitch classes arranged as numbers on the clock. Assume that a listener oriented this clockface, so that C was in the 12:00 position, C♯ in, the 1:00 position, and so on. He would then tend to hear tone series such as B–F, C–F♯ and C♯–G as descending and tone series such as F–B, F♯–C and G–C♯ as ascending. Now assume, on the other hand, that a listener oriented this clockface so that F♯ was in the 12:00 position instead, with G in the 1:00 position, and so on. He would then tend to hear the tone series B–F, C–F♯ and C♯–G as ascending and the tone series F–B, F♯–C and G–C♯ as descending. Figure 8.21 illustrates this point with respect to the tone pair D–G♯.

In order to test this hypothesis, listeners were presented with just such tritone pairs (i.e. C–F♯, C♯–G, etc.), so that each pitch class served equally often as the first tone of a pair. Subjects judged for each pair whether it formed an ascending or a descending pattern. Judgments were then plotted as a function of the pitch class of the first tone of the pair (Deutsch, 1986).

The hypothesis was strikingly confirmed: the judgments of most subjects showed orderly relationships between pitch class and perceived height, so that tones situated in one region of the pitch class circle were heard as higher and tones situated in the opposite region were heard as lower. Another striking – and unexpected – finding was that the direction of the relationship between pitch class and perceived height differed radically across subjects.

As an example, Figure 8.22 shows, for two subjects, the percentages of judgments that a tone pair formed a descending pattern, as a function of the pitch class of the first tone of the pair. As can be seen, there were striking differences between these subjects in the way the pitch class circle was oriented with respect to height.

STIMULUS

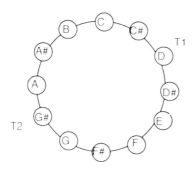

PERCEPTS

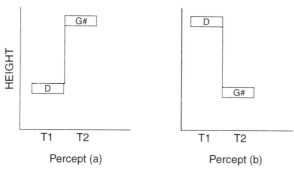

Percept (a)   Percept (b)

Figure 8.21. *Example of pattern employed to generate the tritone paradox, together with two alternative perceptual organizations. Tone D is presented at time T1, and tone G♯ at time T2. Some listeners perceive D as lower and G♯ as higher and so hear the pattern as ascending (percept (a)). However, other listeners perceive D as higher and G♯ as lower and so hear the pattern as descending (percept (b)).*

The first subject heard patterns beginning with F♯, G, G♯, A, A♯ and B as descending and patterns beginning with C♯, D, D♯ and E as ascending. Thus, if we envision the tritone pattern as successively transposed up in semitone steps, starting with C as the first tone of the pair, followed by C♯ as the first tone, and so on, the pattern was first heard ambiguously, then as ascending and then, when F♯ was reached, the pattern was heard as descending.

The other subject produced judgments that were almost the converse of the first. Patterns beginning with B, C, C♯, D, D♯ and E were heard as descending and those beginning with F♯, G, G♯ and A were heard as ascending. Thus, if we envision the tritone pattern as successively transposed up in semitone steps, it was first heard as descending, then when F♯ was reached, the pattern was heard as ascending, and finally when B was reached, it was heard as descending again.

For both subjects, then, as this pattern (the *tritone paradox*) was transposed up in semitone steps, it was heard first one way and then as upside-down. But for the

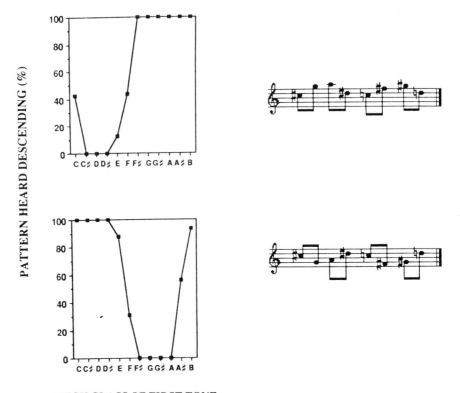

PITCH CLASS OF FIRST TONE

Figure 8.22. *Percentage of judgments that a tone pair formed a descending series, plotted as a function of the pitch class of the first tone of the pair. The graphs on the left display the data from two subjects, averaged over four spectral envelopes, which were positioned at half-octave intervals. The notations on the right show how the identical series of tone pairs was perceived by these two subjects. [Data from Deutsch, 1986 © 1986 The Regents of the University of California; reprinted with kind permission.]*

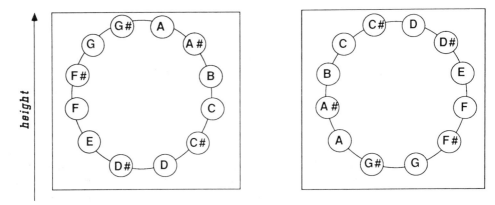

Figure 8.23. *Perceptual orientations of the pitch class circle with respect to height, derived from the judgements of the two subjects displayed in Figure 8.22. The pitch classes that define the highest position along the circle are termed* peak pitch classes.

most part when the first subject heard an ascending pattern, the second subject heard a descending one, and vice versa. In consequence, extended patterns produced by concatenating such tone pairs were heard by these two subjects as forming entirely different melodies. This is illustrated on the right-hand part of Figure 8.22.

Figure 8.23 shows the perceptual orientations of the pitch class circle with respect to height derived from the subjects' judgments shown in Figure 8.22. As can be seen, these two orientations were almost the converse of each other. For the first subject the peak pitch classes (i.e. those that defined the highest position along the pitch class circle) were G♯ and A, whereas for the second subject the peak pitch classes were C♯ and D instead.

Figure 8.24 shows the judgments of four more subjects. As can be seen, they all displayed orderly relationships between pitch class and perceived height. However, the form of this relationship varied from subject to subject.

What happens when more than one tone is presented at a time? To examine this question, I created the pattern known as the *semitone paradox*. This consisted of two

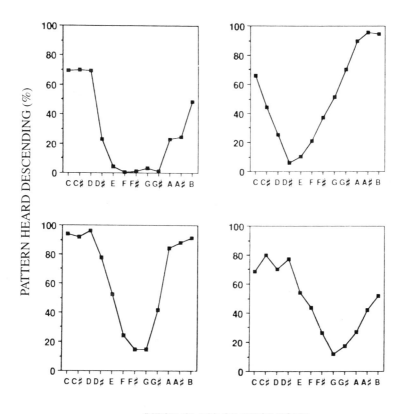

PITCH CLASS OF FIRST TONE

Figure 8.24. *Percentage of judgments that a tone pair formed a descending series, plotted as a function of the pitch class of the first tone of the pair. The data from four subjects are here displayed, averaged over 12 spectral envelopes, which were positioned at 1/4 octave intervals. [From Deutsch, 1987, p. 567, Fig. 5. © 1987 The Psychonomic Society, Inc.; reprinted with kind permission.]*

STIMULUS

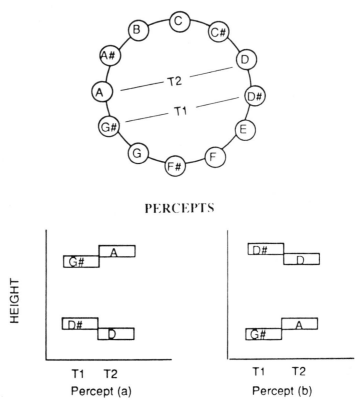

PERCEPTS

Figure 8.25. *Example of the pattern employed to generate the semitone paradox, together with two alternative perceptual organizations. Tones D♯ and G♯ are presented simultaneously at T1, tones D and A at time T2. Listeners perceive this pattern as two stepwise lines that move in contrary motion. However, some listeners hear the higher line as ascending and the lower line as descending (percept (a)), whereas others hear the higher line as descending and the lower line as ascending (percept (b)).*

sequential pairs of tones, one of which ascended by a semitone while the other descended by a semitone (Deutsch, 1988a). The tone pairs were diametrically opposed along the pitch class circle so that, again, proximity could not be invoked in making judgments of relative height. Subjects generally perceived this pattern as two stepwise lines that moved in contrary motion. However, the higher line could be heard as ascending and the lower line as descending, or alternatively the higher line could be heard as descending and the lower line as ascending. These two percepts are illustrated in Figure 8.25.

Subjects were presented with such patterns and judged for each one whether the line that was higher in pitch ascended or descended. From these judgments it was inferred which pitch classes were heard as higher and which as lower. Taking as an example the pair shown in Figure 8.25: if the subject judged the higher line to be ascending, this showed that he heard tones G♯ and A as higher and tones D♯ and D as lower (percept (a)). If, however, he judged the higher line to be

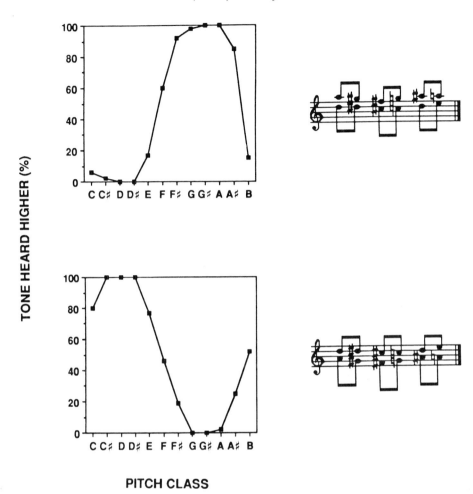

Figure 8.26. *The semitone paradox as perceived by two subjects. Graphs on left show percentages of trials in which a tone was heard as part of the higher line, plotted as a function of the pitch class of the tone. For both subjects, as the pattern was transposed, the ascending and descending lines were perceived to interchange positions. However, in general when the first subject heard the higher line as ascending the second subject heard it as descending, and vice versa. Illustration on right shows how the identical series of patterns was perceived by these two subjects.*

descending, this showed that he heard tones D♯ and D as higher and tones G♯ and A as lower (percept (b)).

Just as with the tritone paradox, judgments reflected an orderly relationship between the perceived heights of the tones and their positions along the pitch class circle. Also as with the tritone paradox, the form of this relationship varied substantially across subjects. This is exemplified by the judgments shown in Figure 8.26. For the first subject, tones F♯, G, G♯, A and A♯ were heard as higher and tones B, C, C♯, D, D♯ and E as lower. Yet for the second subject, tones C, C♯, D, D♯ and E were heard as higher and tones F♯, G, G♯, A and A♯ as lower instead!

D. Deutsch

STIMULUS

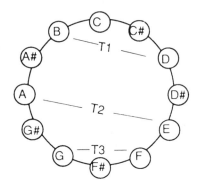

PERCEPTS

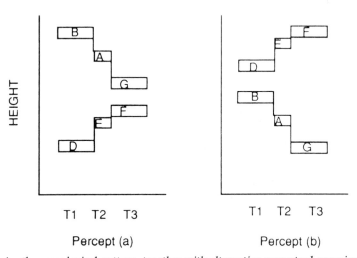

Figure 8.27. *Another paradoxical pattern, together with alternative perceptual organizations. Tones D and B are presented simultaneously at time T1, tones E and A at T2, and tones F and G at T3. Listeners in general hear this pattern as two stepwise lines that move in contrary motion. However, some listeners hear the higher line as descending and the lower line as ascending (percept (a)), whereas other listeners hear the higher line as ascending and the lower line as descending (percept (b)).*

As a result, passages produced by concatenating such patterns were heard quite differently by these two subjects. An example is given in the right-hand part of Figure 8.26.

What happens when more complex patterns are presented? This question was explored using the pattern depicted in Figure 8.27 (Deutsch, Moore and Dolson,

1986). Subjects generally heard this pattern as two simultaneous lines – a higher one and a lower one – that moved in contrary motion. However, some subjects heard the higher line as descending and the lower line as ascending (percept (a)), whereas others heard the higher line as ascending and the lower line as descending (percept (b)).

When the pattern was transposed by a half-octave, the relative heights of the pitch classes were again preserved, so that there resulted a perceived interchange of voices. Thus, subjects who had heard the higher line as descending now heard it as ascending, and subjects who had heard the higher line as ascending now heard it as descending!

In a further experiment this pattern was presented in six different keys, corresponding to six equal steps along the pitch class circle: C major, D, E, F♯, G♯ and A♯. Highly orderly effects of key were apparent in the subjects' judgments, and they also differed from each other in terms of the direction in which their judgments were influenced by key. Figure 8.28 illustrates these points for two of the subjects. Taking the first and moving from left to right, the pattern in the key of C was heard with the higher line descending. However, in the key of D it was heard with the higher line ascending instead, as also in the keys of E, F♯ and G♯. In the key of A♯ the pattern was heard with the higher line descending again. It can be seen that the second subject produced judgments that were for the most part the converse of the first. This is exemplified in the series of patterns shown in the right-hand part of Figure 8.28 (Deutsch, 1988b).

As an interesting demonstration, the pattern can be played with the keys shifting up in whole tone steps, so that the pattern is first in C major, then in D major, and so on. Most listeners hear the pattern first one way, then ambiguously, then it turns itself upside-down and finally rights itself again. Indeed, many listeners report that they perceive the pattern as rotating, analogous to the rotation of shapes in vision.

The patterns which we have been exploring provide striking counter-examples to the principle of equivalence under transposition – a perceptual principle that has generally been assumed to be universal (see above). A convincing way to demonstrate this feature is to tape-record the patterns and then play them back at different speeds. This manipulation results in rigid shifts in the spectra up or down in log frequency, so that different pitches are perceived. In the case of normal patterns, such shifts result simply in perceived transpositions, but the patterns we have been exploring are heard as having radically changed their shapes as well.

For example, we can take the tritone pattern consisting of the tone pair D–G♯, and two listeners – one who hears it as ascending and the other who hears it as descending. First we play the pattern at normal speed, then we speed the tape up so that the pitches are shifted up a half-octave, with the result that the tone pair becomes G♯–D instead. As a result solely of this manipulation, the listener who had heard the pattern as ascending now hears it as descending, and the listener who had heard the pattern as descending now hears it as ascending! One can achieve the same result by decreasing the tape speed instead, so that the pitches are shifted down a half-octave.

Analogously, we can take an example of the semitone pattern, and two listeners – one who hears it with the higher line ascending, and the other who hears it with the higher line descending. We record this example on tape and then speed the tape up, so that the pitches are shifted up a half-octave. As a result, the first listener now hears this example with the higher line descending, and the second listener

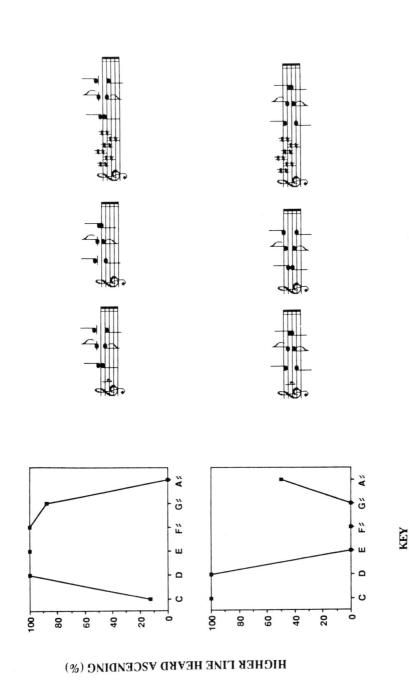

Figure 8.28. Paradoxical pattern shown in Figure 8.27 as perceived by two subjects when presented in different keys. In general, as the pattern was transposed, the ascending and descending lines were perceived to interchange positions. However, for the most part when the first subject heard the higher line as ascending the second subject heard it as descending, and vice versa. Illustration on right shows how the identical series of such patterns was perceived by the two subjects.

now hears it with the higher line ascending! So, for the semitone paradox, changing the tape speed results in an apparent interchange of voices.

A surprising theoretical conclusion from these paradoxes concerns the phenomenon of absolute pitch; that is, the ability to identify the name of a note just from hearing it. This is considered a rare faculty which is much prized by musicians. However, the paradoxes we have been exploring show that the large majority of us possess a form of absolute pitch, in that we hear tones as higher or as lower depending simply on their pitch classes or note names. Further evidence that absolute pitch is more prevalent than had been supposed was provided by Terhardt and Seewann (1983) and Terhardt and Ward (1982). These authors found that musicians were able to determine whether or not well-known passages were played in the correct key, even though most of their subjects did not have absolute pitch as conventionally defined. It appears that absolute pitch is considerably less rare than had been supposed, at least in partial form.

What are the implications of these paradoxes for everyday listening to music? In other experiments, I found that the paradoxes were not confined to octave-related complexes, but occurred also with different types of complex tones that contained ambiguities of height. For example, the phenomena persisted when each of the sinusoidal components in each tone complex was itself replaced by a complex tone which constituted a full harmonic series. The spectra of such more elaborate tone complexes are similar to those produced by a group of natural instruments when playing simultaneously in octave relation. And, for some subjects at least, the tritone paradox was found to persist when each tone complex was composed of a single harmonic series, but where the amplitudes of the odd and even harmonics differed so as to produce ambiguities of perceived height. The paradoxes also persisted when the tones were subjected to a number of time-varying manipulations, such as imposing a vibrato (rapid fluctuations in pitch), a tremolo (rapid fluctuations in loudness), or a fast decay such as to produce the impression of a plucked string. Given the variety of sounds that can produce these paradoxes, we may speculate that they may also be found in natural musical situations, although this remains to be demonstrated.

What can be the basis for these unexpected relationships between pitch class and perceived height? In one experiment, the tritone paradox was found to occur in the large majority of subjects in a sizable population, showing that it is not confined to a few selected individuals (Deutsch, Kuyper and Fisher, 1987). Within this population, no correlate with musical training was found, either in terms of the size of the effect, or its direction, or the probability of obtaining it. It would appear, therefore, that the phenomenon is extramusical in origin. Further studies have also ruled out explanations in terms of low-level characteristics of the hearing mechanism. For many subjects, the form of relationship between pitch class and perceived height was largely unaltered when the position of the spectral envelope was shifted over a three-octave range (Deutsch, 1987). In addition, such relationships were found not to correspond to patterns of relative loudness for the sinusoidal components of the tones when these were compared individually (Deutsch, in prep.).

Based on a number of informal observations, I hypothesized that perception of the tritone paradox might be related to the processing of speech sounds. More specifically, I conjectured that the listener develops a long-term representation of the pitch range of his or her speaking voice, and that included in this representation is a delimitation of the octave band in which the largest proportion of pitch values

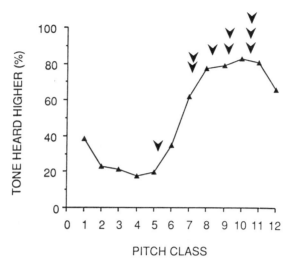

Figure 8.29. *Percentages of trials in which a tone was heard as the higher of a pair in making judgements of the tritone paradox, with the orientation of the pitch class circle normalized and averaged across subjects. Arrows show the limit of each subject's octave band for speech, in relation to the highest position along the pitch class circle. [From Deutsch, North and Ray, 1990. © 1990 The Regents of the University of California; reprinted from* Music Perception *with kind permission.]*

occurs. I also conjectured that the pitch classes delimiting this octave band for speech are taken by the listener as defining the highest position along the pitch class circle (i.e. the 12:00 position on the clockface analogy) and that this in turn determines the listener's orientation of the pitch class circle with respect to height.

A study was undertaken to examine this hypothesis (Deutsch, North and Ray, 1990). Subjects were selected who showed clear relationships between pitch class and perceived height in their judgments of the tritone paradox. A 15-minute recording of spontaneous speech was then taken from each subject, and from this recording the octave band that contained the largest number of pitch values was determined. Comparing across subjects, a significant correspondence was indeed obtained between the pitch classes delimiting this octave band for speech and those defining the highest position along the pitch class circle, as manifest in judgments of the tritone paradox (Figure 8.29).

The results of this experiment are in accordance with the conjecture that perception of the tritone paradox is based on a representation of the pitch class circle by the listener, and the orientation of this representation is related to the pitch range of his or her speaking voice. Two versions of this hypothesis may then be proposed. The first, and more restricted version does not assume that the listener's vocal range for speech is itself determined by such an acquired template. The second version assumes that such a template is acquired developmentally through exposure to speech produced by others, and that it is employed both to evaluate perceived speech and also to constrain the speech produced by the listener. One would therefore expect the characteristics of this template to vary across individuals who speak in different languages or dialects, in a fashion analogous to other speech characteristics such as vowel quality. Given this line of reasoning, the orientation of the pitch class circle with respect to height, as manifest in judgments of the tritone paradox, should be similar for individuals who speak in the same language or dialect but should vary for individuals who speak in different languages or dialects.

Evidence for the latter hypothesis was provided by the study by Deutsch, Kuyper and Fisher (1987) described earlier. An orderly distribution of peak pitch classes (Figure 8.22) was found among these subjects: C# and D occurred most frequently as peak pitch classes, and the frequency of occurrence of the other pitch classes fell off gradually on either side of these. Although no information was obtained concerning the linguistic backgrounds of these subjects, they were UCSD undergraduates, so we may assume that the majority had grown up in California and were from the same linguistic subculture.

As a further test of this hypothesis, I carried out a study to examine whether individuals who speak in the same language or dialect would tend to agree in terms of the orientation of the pitch class circle with respect to height, and whether individuals who speak in different languages or dialects would tend to disagree on this measure (Deutsch, 1991). Two groups were chosen to test this hypothesis: the first consisted of 24 individuals who had grown up in California, the second consisted of 12 individuals who had grown up in the south of England.

Figure 8.30 shows the distributions of peak pitch classes for the English and Californian groups. As can be seen, these distributions were strikingly different: for the English group, F#, G and G# occurred most often as peak pitch classes, yet for the Californian group, B, C, C#, D and D# occurred most frequently.

The results of this experiment provide strong evidence for the view that, through a developmental learning process, the individual acquires a representation of the pitch class circle which has a particular orientation with respect to height. Further, the form of this orientation is derived from exposure to speech produced by others and varies from one language or dialect to another. We can conclude from the present findings that for Californians, the agreed-upon orientation of the pitch class circle is such that the highest position occurs around C# and D. Yet, for people from the south of England, the agreed-upon orientation is such that the highest position occurs around G instead. We may further assume that such a template is employed both in our own speech production and in the interpretation of speech produced by others. We should note that a template which is based on pitch class rather than pitch has the useful feature that it can be invoked for both male and female speakers, even though they speak in different pitch ranges.

What would be the usefulness of such an acquired template? As one line of reasoning, it could be of considerable social advantage to make rapid determination of the emotional state of a speaker through the pitch of his or her voice. A template such as this could serve to provide a framework, common to a particular dialect, within which the pitch of a speaker's voice may be evaluated, so providing evidence concerning his or her emotional state. Such a template might also be employed in the communication of syntactic aspects of speech.

The suggestion that music and speech are in some way related is not new. However, the reasons for any such relationships have so far been undetermined. One may speculate, for example, that music and speech might share certain features because they are based on overlapping perceptual and cognitive structures. The present findings provide, to the author's knowledge, the first demonstration of a direct influence of the one form of communication on the other.

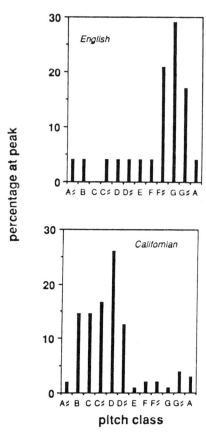

Figure 8.30. *Distributions of peak pitch classes in a group of subjects who grew up in the south of England, and also in a group who grew up in California. [From Deutsch, 1991. © 1991 The Regents of the University of California; reprinted from* Music Perception *with kind permission.]*

4 SUMMARY

In this chapter we have considered the perception of auditory and musical patterns from several points of view. The first part of the chapter explored ways in which elements of auditory arrays are perceptually grouped together. The second part was concerned with the types of shape abstractions carried out by the auditory system. Paradoxical and illusory percepts were also explored, as were individual differences in sound perception, some of which appear to be biological in origin while others appear to be culturally determined.

It is clear from the phenomena described here that auditory perception is mediated by a highly complex and sophisticated system. With recent advances in audio technology now within the reach of the individual researcher, we should expect to see considerable advances in understanding this system in the years ahead.[4]

---

[4]Sound demonstrations of the octave and scale illusions, together with an entire experiment on the tritone paradox, are available on compact disc (Deutsch, D. (1995). Musical illusions and paradoxes. Philomel Records, P.O. Box 12189, La Jolla, CA 92039-2189, USA).

REFERENCES

Babbitt, M. (1960). Twelve-tone invariants as compositional determinants. *The Musical Quarterly*, **46**, 246–259.

Babbitt, M. (1965). The structure and function of musical theory. *College Music Symposium*, **5**, 10–21.

Bachem, A. (1948). Note on Neu's review of the literature on absolute pitch. *Psychological Bulletin*, **45**, 161–162.

Bachem, A. (1954). Time factors in relative and absolute pitch: Studies in psychology *Journal of the Acoustical Society of America*, **26**, 751–753.

Baird, J. W. (1917). Memory for absolute pitch: Studies in psychology. in *Titchener Commemorative Volume*. Worcester.

Bjork, R. A. (1968). All-or-none subprocesses in the learning of complex sequences. *Journal of Mathematical Psychology*, **5**, 182–195.

Blackwell, H. R. and Schlosberg, H. (1942). Octave generalization, pitch discrimination, and loudness thresholds in the white rat. *Journal of Experimental Psychology*, **33**, 407–419.

Bregman, A. S. (1990). *Auditory scene analysis*. Cambridge: MIT Press/Bradford.

Bregman, A. S. and Campbell, J. (1971). Primary auditory stream segregation and perception of order in rapid sequence of tones. *Journal of Experimental Psychology*, **89**, 244–249.

Bregman, A. S., and Dannenbring, G. L. (1973). The effect of continuity on auditory stream segregation. *Perception and Psychophysics* **13**, 308–312.

Burns, E. M. (1981). Circularity in relative pitch judgments for inharmonic tones: The Shepard demonstration revisited again. *Perception and Psychophysics* **30**, 467–472.

Burns, E. M. and Ward, W.D. (1982). Intervals, scales, and tuning. In D. Deutsch (Ed.), *The Psychology of Music* (pp. 241–269). New York: Academic Press.

Butler, D. (1979a). A further study of melodic channeling. *Perception and Psychophysics*, **25**, 264–268.

Butler, D. (1979b). Melodic channeling in a musical environment. Research Symposium on the Psychology and Acoustics of Music, Kansas.

Charbonneau, G. and Risset, J. C. (1973). Circularité de jugements de hauteur sonore. *Comptes Rendus de l'Académie des Sciences, Serie B*, **277**, 623 ff.

Chowning, J. (1980). Computer synthesis of the singing voice. In E. Jansson and J. Sundberg (Eds), *Sound Generation in Winds, Strings, Computers*. Stockholm: Royal Swedish Academy of Music.

Dannenbring, G. L. (1976). Perceived auditory continuity with alternately rising and falling frequency transitions. *Canadian Journal of Psychology*, **30**, 99–114.

Dannenbring, G. L. and Bregman, A. S. (1976). Stream segregation and the illusion of overlap. *Journal of Experimental Psychology: Human Perception and Performance*, **2**, 544–555.

Demany, L. and Armand, F. (1984). The perceptual reality of tone chroma in early infancy. *Journal of the Acoustical Society of America*, **76**, 57–66.

Deutsch, D. (1969). Music recognition. *Psychological Review*, **76**, 300–307.

Deutsch, D. (1972). Octave generalization and tune recognition. *Perception and Psychophysics*, **11**, 411–412.

Deutsch, D. (1973). Octave generalization of specific interference effects in memory for tonal pitch. *Perception and Psychophysics*, **13**, 272–275.

Deutsch, D. (1974). An auditory illusion. *Nature*, **252**, 307–309.

Deutsch, D. (1975a). Two-channel listening to musical scales. *Journal of the Acoustical Society of America*, **57**, 1156–1160.

Deutsch, D. (1975b). Musical illusions. *Scientific American*, **233**, 91–104.

Deutsch, D. (1979). Binaural integration of melodic patterns. *Perception and Psychophysics*, **25**, 399–405.

Deutsch, D. (1980). The processing of structured and unstructured tonal sequences. *Perception and Psychophysics*, **28**, 381–389.

Deutsch, D. (1982). The processing of pitch combinations. In D. Deutsch (Ed.), *The Psychology of Music* (pp. 271–316). New York: Academic Press.

Deutsch, D. (1983). The octave illusion in relation to handedness and familial handedness background. *Neuropsychologia*, **21**, 289–293.

Deutsch, D. (1986). A musical paradox. *Music Perception*, **3**, 275–280.

Deutsch, D. (1987). The tritone paradox: Effects of spectral variables. *Perception and Psychophysics*, **42**, 563–575.

Deutsch, D. (1988a). The semitone paradox. *Music Perception*, **6**, 115–131.

Deutsch, D. (1988b). Pitch class and perceived height: Some paradoxes and their implications. In E. Narmour and R. A. Solic (Eds), *Explorations in Music, the Arts, and Ideas: Essays in Honor of Leonard B. Meyer*. Stuyvesant, NY: Pendragon Press.

Deutsch, D. (1991). The tritone paradox: An influence of language on music perception. *Music Perception*, **8**, 335–347.

Deutsch, D. (in prep.). The tritone paradox in relation to patterns of relative loudness for the components of the tones.

Deutsch, D. and Boulanger, R. C. (1984). Octave equivalence and the immediate recall of pitch sequences. *Music Perception*, **2**, 40–51.

Deutsch, D. and Feroe, J. (1981). The internal representation of pitch sequences in tonal music. *Psychological Review*, **88**, 503–522.

Deutsch, D., Kuyper, W. L. and Fisher, Y. (1987). The tritone paradox: Its presence and form of distribution in a general population. *Music Perception*, **5**, 79–92.

Deutsch, D., Moore, F. R. and Dolson, M. (1986). The perceived height of octave-related complexes. *Journal of the Acoustical Society of America*, **80**, 1346–1353.

Deutsch, D., North, T. and Ray, L. (1990). The tritone paradox: Correlate with the listener's vocal range for speech. *Music Perception*, **4**, 371–384.

Deutsch, D. and Pierce, J. R. (1992). The climate of auditory imagery and music. In D. Reisberg (Ed.), *Auditory Imagery* (pp. 237–260). Hillsdale, NJ: Erlbaum.

Deutsch, D. and Roll, P. L. (1974). Error patterns in delayed pitch comparison as a function of relational context. *Journal of Experimental Psychology*, **103**, 1027–1034.

Deutsch, D. and Roll, P. L. (1976). Separate 'what' and 'where' decision mechanisms in processing a dichotic tonal sequence. *Journal of Experimental Psychology: Human Perception and Performance*, **2**, 23–29.

Divenyi, P. L. and Hirsh, I. J. (1974). Identification of temporal order in three-tone sequences. *Journal of the Acoustical Society of America*, **56**, 144–151.

Dowling, W. J. (1972). Recognition of melodic transformations: Inversion, retrograde, and retrograde-inversion. *Perception and Psychophysics*, **12**, 417–421.

Dowling, W. J. (1973). The perception of interleaved melodies. *Cognitive Psychology*, **5**, 322–337.

Fitzgibbon, P. J., Pollatsek, A. and Thomas, I.B. (1974). Detection of temporal gaps within and between perceptual tonal groups. *Perception and Psychophysics*, **16**, 522–528.

Forte, A. (1973). *The Structure of Atonal Music*. New Haven, CT: Yale University Press.

Francès, R. (1958). *La Perception de la Musique*. Paris: Vrin.

Greeno, J. G. and Simon, H. A. (1974). Processes for sequence production. *Psychological Review*, **81**, 187–196.

Helmholtz, H. von (1862/1954). *On the Sensations of Tone as a Physiological Basis for the Theory of Music*, 2nd English edn, 1954; originally published in German 1862, 1st edn). New York: Dover.

Humphreys, L. F. (1939). Generalization as a function of method of reinforcement. *Journal of Experimental Psychology*, **25**, 361–372.

Keiler, A. (1983). On the properties of Schenker's pitch derivations. *Music Perception*, **1**, 200–228.

Kotovsky, K. and Simon, H. A. (1973). Empirical tests or a theory of human acquisition of concepts of sequential events. *Cognitive Psychology*, **4**, 399–424.

Lerdahl, F. and Jackendorff, R. (1983). *A Generative Theory of Tonal Music.* Cambridge, MA: MIT Press.

Mach, E. (1889). *Popular Scientific Lectures.* Chicago, La Salle: The Open Court.

Meyer, L. B. (1973). *Explaining Music: Essays and Explorations.* Berkeley, CA: University of California Press.

Meyer, L. B. (1989). *Style and Music: Theory, History, and Ideology.* Philadelphia: University of Pennsylvania Press.

Meyer, M. (1904). On the attributes of the sensations. *Psychological Review,* **11,** 83–103.

Meyer, M. (1914). Review of G. Révész, 'Zur Grundlegung der Tonpsychologie' (publ. 1913), *Psychological Bulletin,* **11,** 349–352.

Miller, G. A. and Licklider, J. C. R. (1950). The intelligibility of interrupted speech. *Journal of the Acoustical Society of America,* **22,** 167–173.

Nakajima, Y., Tsumura, T., Matsuura, S., Minami, H. and Teranishi, R. (1988). Dynamic pitch perception for complex tones derived from major triads. *Music Perception,* **6,** 1–20.

Narmour, E. (1977). *Beyond Schenkerism.* Chicago: University of Chicago Press.

Narmour, E. (1983). Some major theoretical problems concerning the concept of hierarchy in the analysis of tonal music. *Music Perception,* **1,** 129–199.

Narmour, E. (1990). *The Analysis and Cognition of Basic Melodic Structures: The Implication–Realization Model.* Chicago: University of Chicago Press.

Oura, Y. (1991). Constructing a representation of a melody: Transforming melodic segments into reduced pitch patterns operated on my modifiers. *Music Perception,* **2,** 251–266.

Plomp, R., Wagenaar, W. A. and Mimpen, A. M. (1973). Musical interval recognition with simultaneous tones. *Acustica,* **29,** 101–109.

Pollack, I. (1978). Decoupling of auditory pitch and stimulus frequency: The Shepard demonstration revisited. *Journal of the Acoustical Society of America,* **63,** 202–206.

Rasch, R. A. (1978). The perception of simultaneous notes such as in polyphonic music. *Acustica,* **40** 1–72.

Restle, F. (1970). Theory of serial pattern learning: Structural trees. *Psychological Review,* **77,** 481–495.

Restle, F. and Brown, E. (1970). Organization of serial pattern learning. In G. H. Bower (Ed.), *The Psychology of Learning and Motivation,* vol. 4: *Advances, Research, and Theory* (pp. 249–331). New York: Academic Press.

Révész, G. (1913). *Zur Grundlegung der Tonpsychologie.* Leipzig: Feit.

Risset, J. C. (1971). Paradoxes de hauteur: Le concept de hauteur sonore n'est pas le même pour tout le monde. 7th International Congress of Acoustics, Budapest.

Ruckmick, C. A. (1929). A new classification of tonal qualities. *Psychological Review,* **36,** 172–180.

Schenker, H. (1935). *Neue musikalische Theorien und Phantasien: III. Der Freie Satz,* 1st edn. Vienna: Universal-Edition.

Schenker, H. (1906/1973). *Harmony* (O. Jonas, Ed., E. M. Borgese, transl.) Cambridge, MA: MIT Press. (Originally published in German 1906).

Schönberg, A. (1951). *Style and Idea.* London: Williams and Norgate. Citations from: Schönberg, A. (1905). *Style and Idea – Selected Writings of Arnold Schönberg,* L. Stein (Ed.). London: Faber and Faber.

Schroeder, M. R. (1986). Auditory paradox based on fractal wave-form. *Journal of the Acoustical Society of America,* **79,** 186–188.

Shepard, R. N. (1964). Circularity in judgments of relative pitch. *Journal of the Acoustical Society of America,* **36,** 2345–2353.

Shepard, R. N. (1982). Structural representations of musical pitch. In D. Deutsch (Ed.), *The Psychology of Music* (pp. 343–390). New York: Academic Press.

Simon, H. A. (1972). Complexity and the representation of patterned sequences of symbols. *Psychological Review,* **79,** 369–382.

Simon, H. A. and Kotovsky, K. (1963). Human acquisition of concepts for sequential patterns. *Psychological Review*, **70**, 534–546.

Simon, H. A. and Sumner, R. K. (1968). Pattern in music. in B. Kleinmuntz (Ed.), *Formal Representation of Human Judgment*. New York: John Wiley.

Sloboda, J. A. (1985). *The Musical Mind*. Oxford: Clarendon Press.

Terhardt, E. and Seewann, M. (1983). Aural key identification and its relationship to absolute pitch. *Music Perception*, **1**, 63–83.

Terhardt, E. and Ward, W. D. (1982). Recognition of musical key: Exploratory study. *Journal of the Acoustical Society of America*, **72**, 26–33.

Thurlow, W. R. (1957). An auditory figure-ground effect. *American Journal of Psychology*, **70**, 653–654.

Ueda, K. and Ohgushi, K. (1980). Perceptual components of pitch: Spatial representation using a multidimension scaling technique. *Journal of the Acoustical Society of America*, **82**, 1193–1200.

van Noorden, L. P. A. S. (1975). Temporal coherence in the perception of tone sequences. Unpublished doctoral dissertation, Technische Hogeschoel, Eindhoven, The Netherlands.

Vicario, G. (1960). L'effetto tunnel acustico. *Revista di Psicologia*, **54**, 41–52.

Vitz, P. C. and Todd, T. C. (1969). A coded element model of the perceptual processing of sequential stimuli. *Psychological Review*, **76**, 433–449.

von Ehrenfels, C. (1890). Über Gestaltqualitäten. *Vierteljahresschrift für Wissenschaftliche Philosophie*, **14**, 249–292.

Ward, W. D. and Burns, E. M. (1982). Absolute pitch. In D. Deutsch (Ed.), *The Psychology of Music* (pp. 431–451). New York: Academic Press.

Warren, R. M. and Byrnes, D. L. (1975). Temporal discrimination of recycled tonal sequences: Pattern matching and naming of order by untrained listeners. *Journal of the Acoustical Society of America*, **18**, 273–280.

Warren, R. M., Obusek, C. J., Farmer, R. M. and Warren, R. P. (1969). Auditory sequence: Confusions of patterns other than speech or music. *Science*, **164**, 586.

Wertheimer, M. (1923/1955). Untersuchung zur Lehre von der Gestalt, Teil II. *Psychologische Forschung*, **4**, 301–350. (Abridged translation as Laws of organization in perceptual forms. In W. D. Ellis (Ed.) (1955), *A Source Book of Gestalt Psychology*, 2nd edn). New York: Harcourt Brace.)

Wertheimer, M. (1924/1938). *Ueber Gestalttheorie*. Lecture at the Kant Society, Berlin, December 17, 1924. (Abridged translation in W. D. Ellis (Ed.) (1938), *A Source Book of Gestalt Psychology* (pp. 1–11). New York: Harcourt Brace; complete translation in *Social Research*, **11**, 78–99 (1944).)

Wessel, D. L. (1979). Timbre space as a musical control structure. *Computer Music Journal*, **3**, 45–52.

White, B. (1960). Recognition of distorted melodies. *American Journal of Psychology*, **73**, 100–107.

Chapter 9
Visual Object Recognition

Joachim Hoffman
University of Würzburg

1 THE FUNCTION OF OBJECT RECOGNITION

1.1   The 'Units' of Perception

This chapter addresses the fact that we recognize structures in our environment without any effort, although these structures are always embedded in a variety of visual contexts. For example, when we look out of the window, we do not see lights and colors, nor a tangle of continuously varying contours or the like whose meanings have to be decoded. Rather, we directly see meaningful scenes containing objects, such as a street with houses and stores, hurrying and idle pedestrians, automobiles and trees, and the sky above. Within the complexity of stimulation, we cannot avoid this instantaneous recognition of familiar objects, such as trees and automobiles, as well as more comprehensive units like streets, stores, and so forth. Hence, in most cases, we can say that perceiving means recognizing. What would be the significance of perception if it did not enable us to recognize the objects and units in our environment? What exactly are the 'objects' and the 'units' of our environment that have to be recognized?

Visual stimuli can mostly be decomposed into many different structures. Even a simple configuration like that depicted in Figure 9.1 can be structured into two squares, eight triangles, or various irregular polygons. Yet, out of all these possible structures, we actually see only one: namely, two squares.

As in this simple example, our perception typically realizes only one of the innumerable possible structures in everyday stimulation. This raises a first fundamental problem with our topic: Which relationships determine the selection of those units that perception lets us recognize? That is, why does perception make us see two squares when we look at Figure 9.1, and people, trees, automobiles and so forth when we look out of the window instead of making other distinctions from the given stimulation? Why do we see a tree structured into its trunk and crown, or a human being structured into a trunk, arms, legs and a head, and not see them somehow differently? That is, what determines the units that visual perception lets us recognize?

Even if we could find a satisfactory answer to this question, another problem still remains: the units we see, that is, scenes, objects and their constituents, mostly offer

Handbook of Perception and Action: Volume 1
ISBN 0-12-516161-1

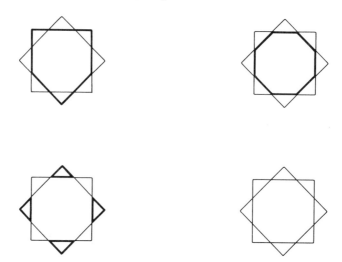

Figure 9.1. *Two rectangles, eight triangles, an octagon plus triangles, or...*

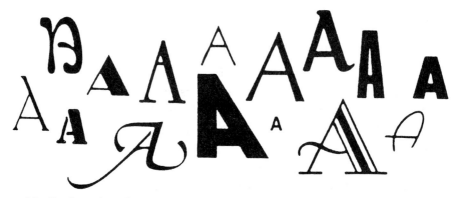

Figure 9.2. *Configurations that are all identified as the letter A. [From Bruce and Green, 1990 p. 175, Fig. 8.1. © 1990 Lawrence Erlbaum Associates Ltd; reprinted with kind permission.]*

themselves in different manifestations. For example, Figure 9.2 presents some figures that are all seen instantaneously as the letter A.

The same applies to objects in daily life. An automobile, for example, produces a wide variety of stimulations depending on the manufacturer's model and the perspective from which it is viewed. Stimulations characterizing a dog, for example, vary even more: a dog produces a great variety of different stimulus patterns depending on whether it is lying down, sitting, standing or running. Despite this enormous variability, we rarely have any difficulty in recognizing dogs, automobiles, and so forth. Hence, the ability to recognize objects and units seems to be unaffected by the variability of the mediating stimulus structures. As a result, we can speculate that perception somehow manages to abstract invariants from the great number of stimulations produced by objects and units, and uses these invariants to recognize objects confidently and directly.

If perception is to abstract invariants for the recognition of units, the class of stimuli over which invariants are to be abstracted has to be specified. For example, if perception is to find the characteristic invariants for recognizing a car or a dog, it has to recognize what kind of stimulation is produced by automobiles and what kind by dogs. However, recognizing that a stimulus structure is produced by a certain object is based – as pointed out above – on invariants abstracted from the diversity of possible stimuli produced by that object. That is, perception is in the same difficult position as, for example, a teacher in a schoolyard crowded with students who is asked to determine characteristic features of students from different grades without knowing how many grades there are and without being able to recognize to which grades the students belong. If our teacher is to be able to abstract invariants for recognizing grade membership, she must already possess the ability to recognize which grade a student belongs to. Returning to perception, we can formulate this paradox as follows: the invariants that form the basis for the recognition of objects need to be known before they can be abstracted.

The compelling consequence of this argument is that the contents of perception cannot be determined by the perceptual process itself. Hence, that which has to be perceived must be determined by criteria that lie outside of perception. For example, our teacher could solve the problem by asking each student to report his or her grade. Then, she could look for characteristic features in those students who gave the same answers. Uniformity of answers would thus become the criterion for forming the classes that have to be recognized. If uniform answers are matched to characteristic features of students, these can be abstracted as invariant features for the recognition of members of one specific grade. That is, recognition then serves to characterize a class of students who can be predicted to give the same answer when asked to name their school grade.

It can be assumed that the perceptual processes underlying object recognition use similar relationships to solve the above-mentioned paradox as those applied by our imaginary teacher: the teacher's questions are replaced by actions on the environment and, instead of answers, we now have the consequences arising from these actions. Relationships between the given stimuli and those occurring as a consequence of actions are registered, and invariants are sought for classes of stimuli when actions lead to uniform consequences. If such invariants are found, they are abstracted, and these, in turn, determine the contents of perception in terms of visual features that can be used to recognize classes of stimuli for which a comparable consequence of a certain action can be anticipated. In this view, perceptions that underlie recognition serve to anticipate behavioral consequences. They should be understood as instruments for predicting alterations of reality induced by one's own behavior, and they consequently serve as a means of controlling the outcome of behavior.

1.2 Perception and Anticipation

Ideas on the functional relationship between perception and behavior have a long tradition in psychology (Neumann and Prinz, 1990a). If we look at some of these ideas, we soon see that we are not the first to speculate that perception serves to predict the consequences of actions. William James (1890/1981, p. 1104) has written: 'At the moment when we consciously will a certain act, a mental conception made up of memory images of the sensations, defining which special act it is, must be there.' The same holds for Dewey (1896, p. 368) when he wrote, 'We must have an anticipatory sensation, an image, of the movements that may occur, together with their respective values, before attention will go to the seeing...'. Both quotes express the notion that a volitional act is related to anticipations of its sensory consequences. Within the same context, Ach (1905, 1935) has discussed a 'deter-minierende Tendenz' (a determining tendency) that controls behavior. He has used this concept to describe, 'the strange aftereffect that particularly originates in the *imagining of the goal*... that results in a realization of the occurrence in terms of this imagining of the goal' (Ach, 1935, p. 143, translated).

Anticipation of the perceptions that accompany the performance of a behavior is the core of the reafference principle (Anochin, 1967; von Holst and Mittelstaedt, 1950):

'We no longer look for the relation between a given afference and the efference it produces, that is, for the reflex. On the contrary, we start from the efference and ask: "What happens in the central nervous system to the afference caused by this efference over effectors and receptors, which we wish to label reafference?"' (von Holst and Mittelstaedt, 1950, p. 464, translated)

In the 'Gestaltkreis' approach, von Weizsäcker and his students have added an intentional component to the reafference principle. In this concept, the reafferences to be expected when executing an efference depend not only on the motor command but also on the underlying intention. Efference and afference, motion and perception, are not only interrelated but also form an inseparable unit: 'Perception does not simply contain self-movement as a factor that produces it, it is self-movement (von Weizsäcker, 1950, p. 21, translated).

Gibson (1979) has worked out that the relationship between motion and percep-tion is probably mediated by the abstraction of invariants in the ambient light accompanying motion. Invariants can determine the respective type of motion so unequivocally that its execution can be controlled by determining whether the respective invariants have been produced. For example, 'To start, make the array flow. To stop, cancel the flow.... To approach is to magnify a patch in the array' (Gibson, 1979, p. 233). Neisser (1976, 1978) has also emphasized the function of anticipations in perception: with reference to Bartlett (1932), he has assumed that anticipations are realized by constantly changing schemata: 'The schema accepts information as it becomes available at sensory surfaces and is changed by that in-formation; it directs movements and exploratory activities that make more informa-tion available, by which it is further modified' (Neisser, 1976, p. 54).

In a comprehensive analysis of the interactions between perception and action control, Prinz (1983) has additionally assumed that behavioral acts are related to exteroceptive execution criteria that are 'tagged' in the case of a corresponding behavioral readiness: 'The strength of the tag determines the probability that the attribute will influence behavior if activated, that is, that it will be used to control the behavior of the observer' (Prinz, 1983, p. 338, translated). Hence, it is assumed that the readiness for a specific behavior is accompanied by expectations regarding not only its consequences but also those stimuli that are a necessary precondition for its successful execution. Dörner *et al.* (1988) have also assumed that action programs are linked to sensory schemata through which they become activated.

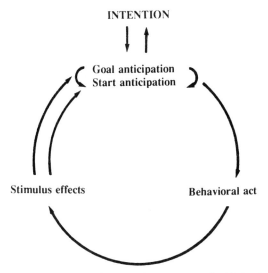

INTENTION

Goal anticipation
Start anticipation

Stimulus effects

Behavioral act

Figure 9.3. *The assumed structure of an anticipatory control of behavior.*

Furthermore, they assume that:

> '... an action program "points" in turn to one or more new sensory schemas that represent the anticipated effect of the execution of the operation and it preactivates them. This permits a very simple and effective control of the execution of motor action programs.' (pp. 220–221, translated)

It should now be evident that the conceptions mentioned here as examples commonly assume that anticipations of the stimulation accompanying successful behavior may be the basic mechanism that integrates perception and behavior into one entity. This assumption is illustrated in Figure 9.3.

An intentional behavioral act is triggered by at least two types of anticipation: (1) an anticipation of features of a goal state that has to be achieved or produced; and (2) an anticipation of those features of an initial state that experience has shown to be necessary in order to transpose the initial state into the goal state through active behavior. Actual stimulation is compared with expectation: If there is sufficient correspondence to anticipated starting conditions, the one intended behavioral act will be executed that experience has shown to be capable of producing the goal state by applying it to the present one. Changes in stimulation produced by this behavior are compared with the goal anticipations. Using these comparisons, both anticipations and executed behavior can be adapted continuously to the conditions that actually exist (Hoffmann, 1990, 1992).

1.3 Functional Equivalence and the Abstraction of Invariants

I started this discussion by asking which relationships determine the units that perception lets us recognize. Taking into account the interweaving of perception and action by anticipations of behaviorally induced stimulus changes sketched in

Figure 9.3, it can be assumed that the units we perceive are formed as classes of stimulus structures that can be changed in a predictable way through behavioral acts. Invariant features of these classes are sought that then become starting conditions for the successful realization of the behavioral act that achieves the anticipated goal. Hence, these speculations imply that what we perceive is determined by functional equivalence of stimulus structures in the context of behavioral acts. However, *how* something is perceived is determined by the mechanisms underlying the abstraction of invariants. Thus, object recognition has to serve action control. By recognizing objects or other units, perception acquires the necessary information for a successful execution of behavior – essentially the information that enables the prediction of the consequences of potential behavioral acts under the given circumstances.

   These considerations favor a position that – as mentioned above – has often been maintained in psychology. It tries to understand the phenomena of perception by placing them in a functional relationship to action control (Neumann and Prinz 1990b). The next five sections discuss the following phenomena:

(1) the dominance of global features in visual recognition;
(2) the preference for recognizing objects at a certain level of conceptual generality;
(3) the recognition of parts in visual structures;
(4) contextual influences on object recognition; and
(5) the dependence of object recognition on the spatial orientation of objects.

This discussion will be limited to studies of visual object recognition. Studies of recognition in special domains such as the recognition of letters, words or faces, as well as nonvisual recognition are not included. in addition to discussing current approaches, I will try to link experimental findings on each topic to the functional view outlined above.

2   THE DOMINANCE OF GLOBAL FEATURES

2.1   Global Dominance in Visual Perception

Everyday experience already demonstrates that global form usually dominates local detail in visual perception. For this reason, the difference between a saw and a lime tree, for example, is more 'obvious' than the difference between a lime tree and a plane tree, which only differ in details. Beyond everyday experience, several experiments have demonstrated the dominance of global visual stimulation. Pomerantz, Sager and Stoever (1977) asked subjects to discriminate between an arrow and a triangle and between a positively and negatively slanted diagonal (Figure 9.4a).

   Arrows and triangles were discriminated much more quickly than diagonals even though the only actual difference lies in the position of the diagonal. Hence, a difference in detail becomes effective more rapidly when it leads to a change in the global form of a configuration than when it is perceived in isolation (Pomerantz, 1983; Wandmacher and Arend, 1985).

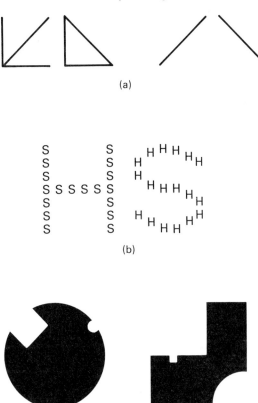

Figure 9.4. *Figures containing global and local features as used in: (a) Pomerantz, Sager and Stoever (1977) [© 1977 The American Psychological Association]; (b) Navon (1977) [p. 360, Fig. 2, modified; © 1977 Academic Press]; (c) Hoffman and Zießler (1986) [p. 69, Fig. 1; © 1986 Springer. All figures reprinted with kind permission of the publishers.]*

Navon (1977, 1981a) has used the stimuli illustrated in Figure 9.4b. These so-called global letters are composed of a corresponding arrangement of local letters. The advantage of such stimuli is that both global and local components are structurally identical. Therefore, differences in their processing cannot be traced back to structural differences (Kinchla, 1974). Navon has demonstrated that recognition of global letters is not influenced by the identity of the local letters from which they are constructed. However, recognition of local letters is influenced by the identity of the global letter that they form. Hence, it seems possible to recognize a global letter without taking into account the local ones, while local letters cannot be recognized without recognizing the global one.

Finally, Figure 9.4c presents materials that have been used by Hoffmann and Zießler (1986). These are globally different outlines in which local details are cuts of different size and shape. Once more, differences in global form are registered more quickly than differences in the cuts, just as subjects react faster to the global form than to the shape of one of the cuts (Hoffmann and Zießler, 1986; Zießler, and Hoffmann, 1987).

Despite the different relationships between local and global features in the three sets of stimuli (see Pomerantz, 1981, for a systematization of these relationships), the dominance of global features can be demonstrated unanimously. This phenomenon has been accounted for by assuming that: (1) stimuli exert distinctive influences on the visual system that are specific for their global and their local features; and (2) that global features exert their influence more quickly, and hence are also available more quickly for decision-making than local details (Hughes *et al.*, 1984; Navon, 1977, 1981a, b). According to this perspective, the dominance of global features is based on their faster availability during the course of visual processing.

Navon's studies (1977, 1981a), in particular, have stimulated critical examinations demonstrating that the dominance of global over local letters can be modified by several factors: the effect disappears when global letters only contain a few local letters (Martin, 1979); it inverts when the visual angle of the global letters exceeds 7 degrees (Kinchla and Wolfe, 1979); it depends on how well the letters can be discriminated on the global and local level (Hoffman, 1980); compared to a fixed presentation, it is strengthened by varying the presentation positions (Pomerantz, 1983); and, finally, it is influenced by attentional factors (Kinchla, Solis-Macias, and Hoffman, 1983; Miller, 1981a; Ward, 1982).

2.2 Explanations of Global Dominance

The impact of these factors permits several assumptions about the causes underlying the faster availability of global letters: it is assumed to be because they are simply larger, only easier to discriminate, visually more dominant, or can be localized more quickly than local letters (Navon, 1981a).

The difficulties in determining the causes of global dominance reflect the currently unsatisfactory theoretical differentiation of global and local features. At present, there are three accounts:

(1) A visual structure can be described as consisting of basic components that combine to form units depending on the relationships between the components. These units can, in turn, recombine to form higher-order units; and this procedure can continue until the entire stimulus structure is grasped (Biederman, 1987; Palmer, 1975; Winston, 1975). From this perspective, a visual structure can be viewed as a hierarchically structured entity that integrates increasingly larger sections of the stimulus structure from the bottom up. Global and local features are determined relatively in this case: structures on a certain descriptive level are global in relation to lower-level components, and they are local in relation to the higher level of which they, in turn, form a component.

(2) A visual structure can also be described as consisting of an outline figure in which visual features are embedded at certain (relative) locations (Bouma, 1971; Kosslyn and Schwartz, 1978). In this case, global features are provided by the form of the outlines and local details by the fine-grained structures within the outline.

(3) Finally, any visual stimulus can be segmented into spatial frequencies. It can be assumed that the visual system possesses selective sensitivity to spatial frequen-

cies of different bandwidth (De Valois and De Valois, 1980; Ginsburg, 1986). It has also been demonstrated that recognition data sometimes covary more closely with their 'spatial frequency content' than with other descriptions of the patterns to be recognized (Harvey, 1986; Harvey, Roberts and Gervais, 1983). In terms of spatial frequency, low frequencies represent global features and high frequencies represent local features.

If these conceptions are to explain global dominance, they need to be supplemented by respective process assumptions; that is, it would have to be assumed that the hierarchical structure of a configuration is built up from the top, perceptual processing starts by analyzing the outline of a configuration, or that the visual system responds more quickly to low spatial frequencies than to high ones (Breitmeyer and Ganz, 1977; Wilson and Bergen, 1979). At present, it is difficult to decide which of these assumptions accounts most appropriately for the dynamics of visual perception.

The impact of attention mentioned above suggests yet another approach. Miller (1981a, b), for example, has shown – in contrast to the studies of Navon (1977, 1981a) – that recognition of global letters is influenced by the identity of local letters if subjects do not have to attend to either global letters alone or local letters alone but to both simultaneously (see also Ward, 1982). He has concluded that information about the identity of local letters must already be available when decisions are reached on the identity of global letters. Boer and Keuss (1982) have reached the same conclusion on the basis of speed–accuracy analyses. They have shown that the impact of local letters on the recognition of global letters does not change as a function of recognition time. This also supports the idea that local details exert their influence at the same time as global ones (Wandmacher and Arend, 1985). According to these ideas, global features do not receive preferential processing because they are available more rapidly but because they preferentially attract attention (Boer and Keuss, 1982; Miller, 1981a, b; Wandmacher and Arend, 1985; however, see also Hughes *et al.*, 1984).

The distinction between availability and usability of visual information formed the basis of a study by Kämpf and Hoffmann (1990). Subjects had to classify geometrical figures similar to those in Figure 9.4c according to an algorithm that required features to be used in a sequence from either global to local or local to global. That is, the sequence was either congruent or incongruent with the assumed sequence of the feature's availability. The study showed: (1) increased classification times as a function of the number of features to be considered; (2) faster classification when global features had to be considered first; and, above all, (3) interactions between both factors. These interactions indicate that the sequence in which information about global and local features becomes available and the sequence in which these features have to be used when making decisions are not independent but can be coordinated with each other.

The same conclusion is suggested by observations reported by Paquet and Merikle (1988): Reactions to a global letter were influenced only by the global identity of a second letter that was presented but had to be ignored. However, reactions to local letters were influenced solely by the local identity of the letter to be ignored. That is, only that aspect (global or local) of the letter to be ignored has an impact that determines the reaction to the letter that is attended to. Hence, it would seem that visual processing is not an encapsulated modular process in which global aspects always become available before local ones. Instead, findings indicate that the visual dominance of features is also determined by their respective behavioral relevance – by their functional dominance.

2.3   Functional Advantages of Global Dominance

Considering function increases the significance of another aspect of global dominance that has not yet received much attention: while recognition of a local detail typically requires fixation, global features can be grasped mostly without specific fixation, at first glance. This independence from fixation makes global features ideal starting conditions for locating details. This is particularly true when details are located systematically at certain positions in a global structure. Under this condition, recognition of the global structure permits the anticipation of details at certain locations, and hence their 'generation' through respective eye movements to these locations. In this approach, global dominance is less a result of a fixed sequence in the availability or usability of global and local features but more a necessary precondition for an aimed generation of visual information through eye movements.

3   BASIC CONCEPTS

3.1   Basic Levels in Taxonomies

Objects can be recognized at different levels of generality. For example, we can recognize the configuration in Figure 9.5 as a titmouse, a bird, or an animal; each with the same degree of accuracy.

However, these different recognitions are not equivalent: most objects can be recognized more easily at an intermediate level than at either a more specific or a more general one. The titmouse is easier to recognize as a bird than as a titmouse or as an animal, and an oak tree is easier to recognize as a tree than as an oak or a

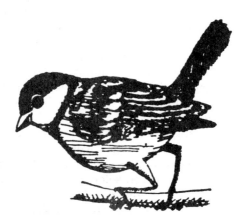

Figure 9.5. *A titmouse, a bird, and an animal.*

plant. The concepts of intermediate generality that are favored in object recognition have been labeled 'basic concepts' (Rosch, 1977).

Object recognition is required in three distinct behavioral contexts:

(1) if an object unexpectedly requires a reaction (what is this?)
(2) when a decision has to be made on whether an object belongs to a certain category (is it this?); and
(3) when a search is made for an object (where is it?).

A preference for basic concepts has been confirmed in all three contexts: for example, if subjects are asked to name objects as quickly as possible (what is this?), the names selected are almost exclusively basic concepts. Furthermore, basic names are generally reported more quickly than the less frequent specific names and the even rarer general ones (Hoffmann and Kämpf, 1985; Jolicoeur, Gluck and Kosslyn, 1984; Rosch *et al.*, 1976; Seguí and Fraisse, 1968). Language acquisition also reveals that children first use basic concepts before mastering more specific differentiations and more general abstractions (Anglin, 1977; Brown, 1958; Mervis and Crisafi, 1982; Mervis and Rosch, 1981).

If subjects are asked to verify that an object is a member of a given concept as quickly as possible (is it this?), they are once more able to do this more quickly for basic concepts than for more specific or more general ones (Hoffmann, 1982; Hoffmann, Zießler *et al.*, 1985; Rosch *et al.*, 1976; Zimmer, 1983). Finally, if subjects are asked to search for an object (where is it?), it is detected more quickly when it is sought as an object belonging to a basic concept than when sought as an object belonging to a more specific or more general concept (Hoffmann and Grosser, 1985, 1986). All these results (exceptions will be dealt with below) indicate a preference for recognizing objects at the level of basic concepts.

The preference for basic concepts is considered to be due mainly to the particularities of their features. For example, Rosch and Mervis (1975) have argued that basic-level concepts are distinguished by a particularly high 'family resemblance' (Wittgenstein, 1953). Objects that belong to them possess many features in common that they do not share with objects in adjacent categories. They are the concepts at the level of generality on which similarity within categories and dissimilarity between categories are equally maximized (Mervis and Rosch, 1981; Murphy and Brownell, 1985; but see also Medin, Wattenmaker and Hampson, 1987). Rosch *et al.* (1976, p. 435) have defined basic concepts as: '... the most general classes at which attributes are predictable, objects of the class are used in the same way, objects can be readily recognized by shape, and at which classes can be imaged'. Jones (1983) has defined basic categories as those concepts in which the features can be inferred reliably from category membership, and category membership can be inferred reliably from the features of an object. Hoffmann and Zießler (1982) have emphasized the distinction between features related to perceivable characteristics of objects and those related to nonperceivable ones. Accordingly, basic concepts seem to be the ones with the highest generality that are still characterized mainly by perceivable features. Tversky and Hemenway (1984) have stated that basic concepts are characterized by a particularly large number of constituent features (an automobile has wheels, a tree has leaves, a chair has a back, etc.), and that these are less frequent in feature associations to both higher- and lower-level concepts (see also Hoffmann, 1986a, 1986b).

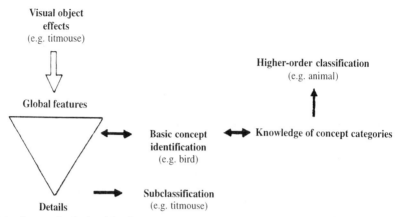

Figure 9.6. *Assumed relationships between visual processing and conceptual recognition of objects. [From Hoffmann, 1986. © 1986 Psychologie-Verlags-Union, Weinheim; reprinted with kind permission.]*

3.2   Basic Concepts and Global Dominance

To understand the preference for recognizing objects at the basic level, it is necessary to supplement assumptions on the structure of basic concepts with process assumptions. Of particular significance here are the observations that characterize basic concepts as the most general categories with perceivable features (Hoffmann and Zießler, 1982) that particularly share the same form (Rosch *et al.*, 1976) and the same configuration of parts (Tversky and Hemenway, 1984). Hence, basic concepts are distinguished by common global features. Relating this to the phenomenon of global dominance discussed in the previous section suggests the following explanation of the preference for basic concepts (Hoffmann, 1982, 1986a; Hoffmann, Zießler and Grosser, 1984):

> Visual recognition of an object is a process during which the object's visual effects are used continuously to specify its conceptual identity (Figure 9.6).

The early availability of global features of an object (e.g. the titmouse in Figure 9.5) allows it to be identified initially as belonging to only one category that (if it exists) is characterized by global features, that is, the basic concept (bird). Recognition at a more specific level (as a titmouse) requires the processing of additional visual features such as the specific form of a local detail at a specific location within the global form of the object (e.g. the shape of the beak or the special coloring of head feathers. In contrast, classifying an object as belonging to a higher-level concept (animal) does not depend on the processing of further visual features but on appropriate knowledge about the recognized basic concept's conceptual membership in higher-order categories. In this perspective, the preference for recognizing objects at the basic level is due mainly to the dominance of global features in visual perception.

The model in Figure 9.6 has been tested in various ways. If an object is displayed briefly with a tachistoscope, and subjects are asked, first, to classify it to a basic or higher-level concept, and then to specify the object they have seen providing their classification was correct (e.g. 'Yes, that was a tree/animal. Can you also say what kind of tree/animal it was?'), specifications of higher-level concepts (animal) are almost always independent of presentation time. However, correct specifications of basic concepts (tree) increase as a function of presentation time (Hoffmann, 1982). This result supports the assumption that recognition of an object at the lower level is only a precondition for classification to a higher-level concept and not to a basic one.

In another experiment, subjects again had to classify tachistoscopically presented objects to concepts of varying generality. Classifications to specific lower-level concepts (titmouse) were impaired much more by shortening the presentation time than classifications to basic and higher-level concepts (bird/animal), while classifications to basic and higher-level concepts did not differ (Hoffman, Zießler and Grosser, 1984). This confirms that recognitions of lower-level concepts depend on visual details that become available later during the perception process, and that classification to higher concepts always functions just as well as classification to basic concepts. It could also be demonstrated that verbal training in atypical memberships (e.g. a cypress is a tree, a fungus is a plant) accelerated classification to higher concepts only (plant) but not to basic ones (tree). This finding supports the assumption that explicit knowledge about conceptual membership is involved in classifying objects to higher-level concepts only (Hoffmann, Zießler and Grosser, 1984)

Studies using artificial conceptual hierarchies of geometric figures (Hoffmann and Grosser, 1986; Hoffmann and Zießler, 1983, 1986) have shown additionally that it is only necessary to characterize a class of figures by global features in order to observe 'basic concept' phenomena. Hence, they cannot be attributed to other factors (e.g. shorter namings at the basic concept level, higher frequencies of basic names; see also Murphy and Smith, 1982). One of these studies also demonstrated that the phenomena of basic concepts occur only when the respective object class is characterized by a global feature but not when it is characterized by a local feature under otherwise identical conditions (Hoffmann and Grosser, 1986; Hoffmann, Grosser and Klein, 1987; cf. also Zimmer and Biegelmann, 1990).

In all, the results support:

(1) the significance of global features for the generation and stabilization of basic concepts;
(2) the assumption that a more specific object recognition requires a greater perceptual effort than a basic one; and
(3) the assumption that the relative increase in effort necessary for a more general recognition is not determined by perceptual processes.

From this point of view, phenomena of basic recognition are based on a narrow interplay between a visual analysis proceeding from global to local features and an object identification proceeding from more basic classifications to more specific ones. Presumably, the ability to identify global features independently from fixation permits rapid classification to a basic concept. At the same time – as discussed in the previous section – this permits directed focusing in order to recognize anticipated details that lead to a further conceptual specification of the object.

3.3   Basic Concepts and Functional Equivalence

Nonetheless, basic concepts are not generated for all classes of objects that possess common global features. For example, there is no common basic concept for tennis balls, oranges and dumplings; or for pencils, chopsticks and macaroni, which are at least as similar to each other as the oaks, pines and birches lumped together in the basic concept *tree*. Even such simple examples demonstrate that common global features are not sufficient to integrate objects into a basic concept. It seems that global features have to be used in a common functional context in order to form a basic concept. According to this argument, basic concepts are prominent not only because of their global features but also because they discriminate between objects that we usually have to differentiate in everyday life. In most cases it is sufficient to treat, for example, an oak tree as a tree, a titmouse as a bird, or a carp as a fish; more specific differentiations are rarely required. Hence, basic concepts are determined primarily by their functional appropriateness and only secondarily by their features.

One of the facts that clearly reveals the decisive influence of 'functional fit' on the formation of basic concepts is the existence of 'basic concepts' within the set of objects assigned to a basic concept. In naming experiments, Hoffmann and Kämpf (1985) have found that more specific names are sometimes preferred instead of basic concept names. Examples are *chicken* and *rose*. The concepts at the basic level are *bird* and *flower*. However, pictures of chickens and roses are called exclusively *chicken* or *rose* with reaction times that are comparable to those for basic concepts (see also Jolicoeur, Gluck and Kosslyn, 1984; Murphy and Brownell, 1985). Subcategories like *chicken* and *rose* seem to have acquired a similar status to their higher-ordered basic concepts. Intuitively, both examples are subcategories that differ sufficiently from other subcategories of the same basic concept not only in appearance but also in function (i.e. chickens compared to other birds, roses compared to other flowers) as to have specific behavior references.

Zimmer (1984) has reported comparable findings. In his experiments, novices and florists had to recognize flowers. While novices recognized the same basic level (flower) more quickly than the subcategory level (carnation, lily, crocus, tulip, etc.), florists classified flowers just as quickly at both levels. Their familiarity with flowers and their professional need to distinguish them continuously seems to make it possible for subcategories assigned to one basic concept to themselves acquire the status of a basic concept.

These observations suggest that the phenomenon of basic concepts is not bound to concepts of the same generality. No level has been distinguished within taxonomic hierarchies at which basic concepts are to be found exclusively. Instead, basic concepts seem to be categories of objects whose functional equivalence has been experienced with sufficient frequency, and whose visual qualities provide suitable preconditions for the abstraction of common invariants that are as global as possible. With reference to my introductory speculations, basic concepts could be viewed as representing classes of stimulation that are characterized by invariant global features and that serve as starting conditions for intentional behavior. Hence, basic concepts are an outcome of the conjunction of mutually facilitating functional and perceptual properties that can hold for classes of very different generality and are not restricted to a specific level (Hoffmann, 1986a).

4 THE PERCEPTION OF WHOLES AND PARTS

4.1 The Origin of Partial Structures in Perception

Typically, the objects we deal with are made up of parts. A knife consists of a handle and a blade; a teapot of a body, a handle, a spout and a lid; a chair of a seat, legs, and an arm rest; and so forth. In more complex entities, parts themselves are again composed of parts: a part of the human body is the head, a part of the head is the face, a part of the face is the eye, and a part of the eye is the pupil. Here, parts and wholes are related hierarchically and form so-called partonomies (Tversky and Hemenway, 1984). In recognizing an object, we generally perceive its parts just as self-evidently as we perceive objects in a scene. Even when looking at an unknown object like that in Figure 9.7, we see a container with superstructures, a kind of handle, a kind of wheel and a somewhat strange appendage.

Even though we do not know the object, we directly see the parts it seems to consist of. Perception is probably organized in such a way as to provide a description in which some of the stimuli seem to belong more closely together than others, so that the entire configuration is seen mostly as a whole consisting of parts. The rules governing this are to a large extent unknown and one of the fundamental problems of object recognition.

It was particularly the proponents of Gestalt theory who systematized such phenomena of perceptual organization and described them with 'Gestalt laws' (Koffka, 1935; Köhler, 1929; Metzger, 1975; Wertheimer, 1923; see also Boring, 1942). For example, the law of proximity maintains that stimuli lying close together are more likely to be seen as belonging to each other than stimuli that are further apart. The law of good continuation maintains that lines at intersections are preferably seen as continuing the previous line. The law of similarity states that similar stimuli are experienced as belonging more to each other than dissimilar ones; and the law of closure refers to the tendency to see closed lines as structural units (Figure 9.8).

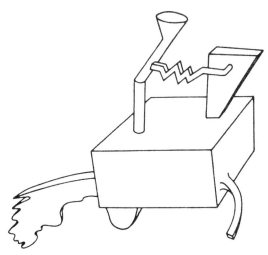

Figure 9.7. *An unknown object.* [*From Biederman, 1987, p. 116, Fig. 1. © 1987 Academic Press; reprinted with kind permission.*]

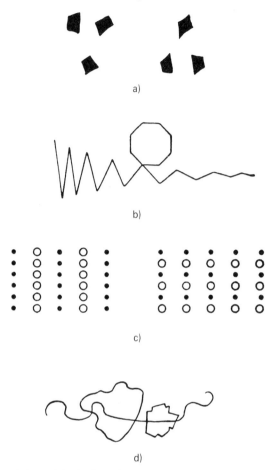

Figure 9.8. *Some Gestalt laws. (a) The law of proximity: two groups of figures are seen. (b) The law of good continuation: an octagon and a zigzag line are seen. (c) The law of similarity: identical figures are seen as columns or lines, respectively. (d) The law of closure: two figures and one line are seen so that the hidden number 4 is not recognized.*

Palmer (1977) has tried to assess the impact on perception of some of these Gestalt factors experimentally. He employed figures generated by choosing 6 out of a total of 16 basic lines or segments. Analyzing perceptual organizations in such a microworld offers three advantages: (1) the basic perceptual units can be assumed to be given by the individual segments used to form all the figures; (2) properties of these basic units are easy to determine as they only vary in length, position and orientation; and (3) relationships between them can be defined precisely. Drawing on Gestalt theory, Palmer has investigated the relationships of proximity, closure, good continuation, and similarity in length and orientation. For any subset of segments of a figure, it is possible to determine the relationships between them within the subset in comparison to relationships to segments lying outside the subset. The more strongly the elements of a subset are interrelated and the more weakly they are related to outside elements, the more the subset forms a good part of the figure.

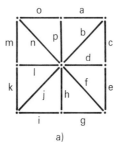

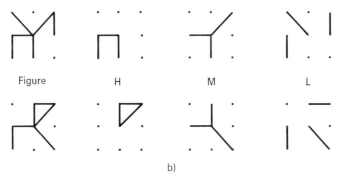

Figure 9.9. *Examples of figures used by Palmer: (a) the basic lines from which the figures are composed; (b) two figures with examples of parts with high (H), medium (M) and low (L) goodness. [From Palmer, 1977, p. 445, Fig. 2. © 1977 Academic Press; reprinted with kind permission.]*

Figure 9.9 depicts the entire set of 16 segments, two figures each made up of six segments, as well as parts of these figures of three segments each that are regarded as parts with high (H), medium (M) or low (L) goodness. Palmer asked his subjects to decompose given figures into their 'natural parts', to rate the goodness of parts within figures, to determine as quickly as possible whether a part is contained in a presented figure, and finally to combine two separately presented and mutually exclusive parts to an imaginary figure. It was demonstrated that subjects' performance depended on the 'goodness' of the respective parts on all these tasks: they decomposed figures almost exclusively into good (high goodness) parts; ratings corresponded to the calculated goodness; good parts were detected much faster than bad (low goodness) parts; and they were also integrated much faster in imagination. Bower and Glass (1976) have shown additionally that subjects were much better at reproducing configurations out of memory when they were cued by good parts than when they were cued by bad parts.

Results confirm the fundamental insight of Gestalt theory that visual configurations are perceived as holistic entities consisting of related parts, which are determined by their inner coherence and their relation to the whole. Furthermore, they confirm the influence of proximity, closure, good continuation and similarity on visual structures, although without providing an explanation of why it is exactly these relationships that permit a prediction of visual organization. As Palmer has noted explicitly, these considerations are an approach to the assessment of perceptual structures and not a description of the processes leading to them.

Goodness of parts was predicted so convincingly because the elements on which the perception of the figures was probably based (the segments) could be assessed exactly. However, as soon as we leave Palmer's microworld, we are once more confronted with the three problems: (1) What are the basic units of visual perception under natural conditions? (2) What properties does perception use to differentiate between these elements? (3) What relationships between them determine their integration into wholes? In the following section a few selected approaches to these issues will be discussed.

4.2   The Gestalt Approach

According to Gestalt theory (Koffka, 1935; Köhler, 1924, 1929; Wertheimer, 1925), visual stimuli lead to activations in the central nervous system that are subject to self-organization. For example, Köhler (1924, pp. 189–190) has maintained that the physical entities whose states correspond to the optical-phenomenal fields make up a connected system in which psychophysical processes adopt qualities of physical 'Raumgestalten'. The most important qualities in the present context are that: (1) time-independent states ('psychophysische Gestalten') are generated that are maintained for the system as a whole; (2) psychophysical processes are always dependent on the entire retinal stimulus configuration; and (3) 'psychophysische Gestalten' adopt that structure that, 'under the retinal and other conditions of the respective processes, yields the smallest possible structural energy in the whole' (Köhler, 1924, p. 253, translated). In this approach, perceptual structures evolve as a result of the self-organization of activations elicited that strive toward a state of minimum energy expenditure.

Gestalt laws are considered to result from this self-organization. Consequently, visual elements whose interrelationships would determine the perceptual structure are not discriminated. The effects of stimulation are always holistic: '... instead of reacting to local stimuli by local and mutually independent events, the organism reacts to an actual *constellation* of stimuli by a total process which, as a functional whole, is its response to the whole situation' (Köhler, 1929, p. 106; italics as in original work).

4.3   Structural Information Theory

The proponents of structural information theory (SIT) (Buffart and Leeuwenberg, 1983; Buffart, Leeuwenberg and Restle, 1981; Hochberg and McAlister, 1953; Leeuwenberg, 1969, 1971; Leeuwenberg and Buffart, 1983) also assume that perceptual organization strives toward a minimum expenditure of effort (Hatfield and Epstein, 1985). However, in contrast to Gestalt theory, they propose a formal description of configurations that allows the specification of the structure with the lowest 'information load' from the set of all possible structures. The procedure can be depicted as follows. A stimulus pattern is described as a sequence of basic units that are stringed together starting from one point on the pattern and proceeding in one direction. A coding of the pattern arises as a string of basic coding elements. This string is called the primitive code. Further processing is directed toward detecting regularities in the primitive code in order to reduce its length by describing the pattern as a structured string of subsequences.

For example, the string *ababababab* (the letters correspond to any kind of basic coding element) repeats the pair *ab* four times. Hence, the string can also be described by applying a repetition operator, R4(*ab*). A string such as *abccba* can be described by applying a symmetry operator SYM(*abc*). A string *cabdabeabfabg* contains the *ab* subsequence several times at different positions. This can be described with a distribution operator DIST(*ab*) [(*c*) (*d*) (*e*) (*f*) (*g*)], and so forth. That is, applying such 'redundancy operators' reduces the length of the primitive code and thus permits a reduction in the effort required to describe the pattern.

The procedure implies that primitive codes can be reduced in several ways. For example, if symmetry is stressed in a string like *aabccbaabc*, structures like SYM(*aabc*) (*bc*) arise. However, instead of symmetry, repetition of elements or the distribution of subsequences can also be emphasized. This would lead to structures such as R2(*a*) (*b*) R2(*c*) b R2(*a*) (*bc*) or DIST(*aa*) [(*bccb*) (*bc*)]. If symmetry and repetition are considered jointly, a structure like R2(*a*) SYM(*bc*) R2(*a*) (*bc*) would result. Each such 'endcode' decomposes the pattern into different substructures, that is, in each case, the whole seems to be composed of different parts. It is assumed that from the set of all possible interpretations, preference is given to perceiving the one that corresponds to the shortest endcode. This coding is called the 'minimal code'. By determining the minimal codes of configurations, it should be possible to predict which organization will be preferably perceived.

Corresponding studies have been able to demonstrate a fair degree of agreement with theoretical predictions in: (1) judgements on visual complexity; (2) interpretations of complex patterns; (3) complementing incomplete patterns; (4) the strength of subjective contours; and (5) the origin of ambiguous patterns (Buffart, Leeuwenberg and Restle, 1981; Leeuwenberg, 1971; Leeuwenberg and Buffart, 1983).

The main contribution of SIT is its proposal regarding a formal definition of what is called 'simplest structure' or 'Prägnanz'. The minimal code enables us not only to observe 'natural' structures of visual configurations but also to derive them from a formalized theory. Of course, this does not provide an explanation as to how perception generates these structures: 'It is important to emphasize that structural information theory is not a theory about the perceptual process' (Leeuwenberg and Buffart, 1983, p. 44). However, the assumptions regarding the shortening of primitive codes suggest processes that are particularly sensitive to repetitions of identical units and that mainly search for regularities in their distribution (redundancy is based exclusively on repetition, continuation or distribution of identities).

Any application of SIT requires the compilation of an alphabet of basic units that can be considered to compose the patterns to be perceived. For geometrical figures, the most frequently defined units have been length and angle: 'Every length or angle that differs from another in a shape corresponds to an information unit' (Leeuwenberg, 1971). Such a definition is based on the experimenter's knowledge about the total number of differentiations that have to be made. However, for a perceptual system, such knowledge is not given *a priori*. It would seem to be a hopeless task to derive a necessary and sufficient number of basic units to cover the diverse structures we have to discriminate under natural conditions (see also Pomerantz and Kubovy, 1986). Hence, this approach is also unable to answer the question on the units from which perception constructs its structures.

4.4   Recognition by Components

Biederman (1987) made an attempt to define the basic units that underlie the recognition of natural objects and their parts. He started with the idea that the visual system takes certain qualities of two-dimensional contours as evidence that the represented objects have these same qualities in the three-dimensional world (Witkin and Tenenbaum, 1983). Thus, straight lines infer straight edges and bent lines infer bent edges. Symmetries in a contour refer to a symmetrical object. Parallel lines infer parallel edges, and lines that end together at the same point refer to converging edges. Furthermore, concave discontinuities in the contour infer that two parts of an object are joined together at this position (Hoffman and Richards, 1984).

These features have been termed 'nonaccidental' insofar as they would be produced only very infrequently by accidental alignments of perspective and object properties and, consequently, are generally unaffected by variations in perspective. Biederman (1987) refers to studies demonstrating that nonaccidental features of contours such as straightness versus bendedness, symmetry versus asymmetry, parallelism versus nonparallelism, or different forms of line concurrence (T-, Y-, L- or arrow-formed) can be discriminated with extraordinary rapidity and are therefore possible candidates for basic units of perception. A corresponding combination of features, Biederman (1987) assumes, leads to a perception of the one respective body that would project the given contour. Hence, the number of possible feature combinations determines the number of bodies that are possible to differentiate. Such volumetric primitives are called 'geons' (for geometrical ions). Biederman (1987) has derived the existence of 36 geons from combinations of nonaccidental features and argues that it is possible to derive the seemingly uncountable diversity of perceivable structures and figures from combinations of even such a small number of geons.

In this conception, recognizing objects is based on the perceivable edges of an object as given in a line drawing. The totality of edge configurations is decomposed into partial configurations that are perceived as geons. Which object is seen is determined consecutively by the relationships between geons. Biederman (1987) considers four of these: (1) their relative sizes; (2) their arrangement (vertical versus horizontal); (3) how they are linked together; and (4) the relative location of this linkage. Again, only nonaccidentally projected relationships are taken into consideration. The identity of an object finally discloses itself to the perceiver by matching the perceived structure of the geons to stored structures for thousands of (basic) concepts (Figure 9.10).

Biederman (1987) has reported a series of experimental observations to support his 'recognition-by-components' theory. For example, it can be demonstrated that objects are still recognized rapidly when some detail components are eliminated. This supports the hypothesis that object recognition is based on the perception of only some main components in a 'correct' relationship (Figure 9.11a).

Other experiments have degraded the contours of objects that had to be recognized. Although the same amount of contour was always deleted, in one case, it was taken from regions that were intended to ensure the identification of nonaccidental features, while in other cases these features remained intact (Figure 9.11b). A drastic impairment of recognition is only found in the first case. This supports the assumption that object recognition builds upon the nonaccidental

Stages in Object Perception

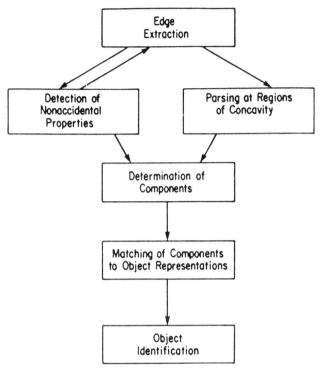

Figure 9.10. *Stages in object perception. [From Biederman, 1987, p. 118. © 1987 Academic Press; reprinted with kind permission.]*

features of the contour. Furthermore, presenting objects as line drawings or colored photographs does not change their recognizability in any systematic way (Biederman and Ju, 1988; Hoffmann *et al.*, 1985). Color information does not seem to play a decisive role in object recognition (but see Zimmer, 1984, on the role of color in the classification of flowers by florists). This supports the claim that it is the contour that provides the main visual components for object recognition.

According to the 'recognition-by-components' theory, a visual configuration is structured into parts because elementary visual features cause perception of those volumetric primitives (geons) that have probably (nonaccidentally) projected the given stimuli; that is, perception is directed basically toward the recognition of the three-dimensional world. From this point of view, Gestalt factors do not result from an autonomous striving of perception toward the least complicated description but from its orientation toward (nonaccidental) features in order to recognize geons (Biederman, 1987). Nonetheless, this approach fails to specify several points: no concrete statements are given on the process of parsing a given contour; ideas on the relationships between geons need to be extended; and there are only vague ideas on how the matching of the structures of geons with object representations in memory is organized.

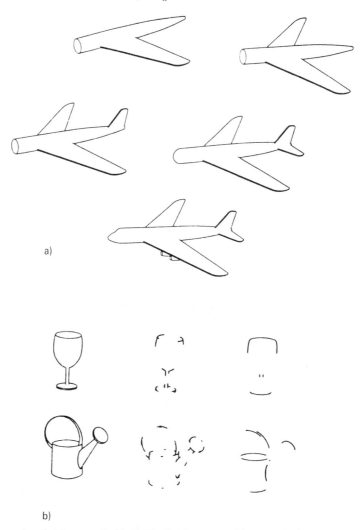

a)

b)

Figure 9.11. *Examples of: (a) removal of individual object parts; (b) removal of contour elements that scarcely (in the middle) and greatly (on the right) impair recognition. [From Biederman, 1987, Fig. 13, p. 132. © 1987 Academic Press; reprinted with kind permission.]*

In particular, there is a need to specify ideas about the relationships among parts against the background of the wholes to be recognized. Relationships between contour elements (concerning parallelism, symmetry, etc.) have to be defined with respect to the geon whose recognition they permit, and relationships among geons concern the object whose recognition they are a part of. In other words, recognizing relationships between the 'right' parts requires the determination of which parts constitute the whole that has to be recognized. We are once more faced with the problem that the units of perception have to be determined in advance in order to abstract features from the given stimulation that can identify these units.

4.5   The Functional Determination of Parts

One crucial element in recognition-by-components theory is the assumption that objects are inferred from the stimulations that are most likely to have elicited them. This assumption is based on the 'likelihood principle' that can be traced back to Helmholtz (1910), who spoke about 'unconscious inferences' in the process of perception (see also Brunswik, 1956; Gregory, 1974; Hochberg, 1978, 1981; Klix, 1962). One critical nonaccidental feature for recognizing parts might well be what Hoffman and Richards (1984) have called 'transversality'. These authors have shown that the outer contour of an object composed of parts always has concave discontinuities (cusps that point into the object and not into the background) at the locations at which the parts meet. They assume that this regularity permits the decomposition of contours into parts at concave discontinuities. Hence, concave discontinuities represent an invariant that is abstracted across object contours and permits inferences on their partitions.

However, why should a perceptual system abstract such an invariant and assign it the status of a feature at which configurations are parsed into parts? The abstraction of an invariant for the demarcation of parts should only result when perception particularly needs to recognize parts, and why should this be so? In addition, the invariant can be abstracted only when the classes of stimuli for which the invariants have to be found are determined by criteria that lie beyond perception. How else could it be possible to find an invariant for otherwise nondeterminable entities? In my opinion, there is an obvious answer to these questions: behavior directed toward and with objects has to be oriented toward parts in order to be successful.

Typically, parts of objects determine the way in which we deal with them. To start the computer, we have to press a switch; to drink from a cup, we have to grasp it by the handle; to open a door, turn the door knob; and so forth. The manipulatory use of objects, their incorporation into the most diverse activities, indeed, practically every use of them, requires the recognition of those substructures at which our actions have to be applied, and whose characteristics have to be taken into account if actions are to succeed. It is these behavioral constraints that not only define what has to be considered as a part but also force perception to search for possible ways of reliably recognizing them. Hence, perception does not – from this point of view – 'infer' the existence of parts of an object from existing concave discontinuities. Rather, it abstracts from the diversity of stimulations those invariants that are necessary for orienting behavior toward parts. Of course, these can only control behavior successfully if they reliably represent the respective parts of an object.

If the parts of an object are given, the relationships between them determine its identity. A handle, a spout, a body and a lid do not make a teapot if they are not structured in the characteristic way for a teapot. It can be assumed that object-specific structures are determined mainly by the relative locations of their parts: handle and spout generally lie at opposite sides of the dominating body of the teapot; and the lid is on the long side that is marked as 'top' by the spout. This relatively stable configuration of parts is an essential aid in handling objects. If we want to pick up a teapot, we have to determine the position of its handle. If the handle's relative position within the appearance of the teapot is largely stable, the 'search' for the handle is facilitated decisively as it can be reduced to the 'search' for the teapot. Once the teapot is located, the location of the handle can be anticipated with high certainty. In more general terms, handling objects requires not only the recognition of behaviorally relevant parts but also their egocentric location. This is facilitated by regularities in the relative location of the parts within the object's appearance or contour. Therefore, relatively stable locations of parts within the context of their global configurations are appropriate invariants to be abstracted for an efficient handling of objects as well as being invariants for their recognition.

These speculations on a functional determination of parts through the need to determine their location have been supported by observations showing that: (1) the recognition and location of objects and parts are performed by apparently different processes (Pollatsek, Rayner and Henderson, 1990; Ungerleider, 1985); and (2) there may additionally be separate mechanisms that register relative locations (Kosslyn et. al., 1989). However, I do not know of any empirical tests of the consequences of these ideas for the learning-dependent formation of perceptual structures. It is necessary to study, for example, how strongly the variability of the relative locations of parts influences the recognition of the respective objects, or to what extent covariations in relative locations of parts of an object influence their 'seen' unity.

However, two studies conducted in another context have already confirmed that visual perception actually does react very sensitively to regular relative locations of stimuli (Lambert, 1987; Lambert and Hockey, 1986; Miller, 1988). These studies presented different stimulus categories above chance at certain positions. The results reveal that stimuli from the different categories were each detected and classified more quickly at those positions at which they had been seen more frequently. Such a sensitivity for specific stimuli at specific (relative) locations agrees with the above considerations (see also Hoffmann, 1990, 1992). However, further studies will be needed to determine the influence of this sensitivity on visual organization.

The assumption that perceptual structures are based on the abstraction of behaviorally related invariants necessarily implies learning processes. Phylogenetic and ontogenetic learning (Brunswik, 1956; Gregory, 1974; Pomerantz and Kubovy, 1986) are to be distinguished. It can be argued that phylogenetic learning has already led to a genetic determination of perceptual processes that inevitably delivers behaviorally relevant structures. Accordingly, the previously mentioned use of concave discontinuities for visual parsing could be attributed to the idea that perceptual systems that use concave discontinuities for parsing have been selected during phylogenesis because of behavioral advantages. Further mechanisms may have been selected in the same way that now form a set of elementary features that determine human perception.

Nonetheless, it is scarcely possible to confirm such an assumption in preference to other approaches. For example, it is difficult to decide empirically whether Gestalt factors should be interpreted as phylogenetically selected elementary features, as a result of dynamic self-organization, or as a by-product of minimal coding (Leeuwenberg and Boselie, 1988). This argument has to rest mainly on demonstrations of developmental or experimentally induced change in visual organization. The studies carried out by Gottschaldt (1926) are often cited in this context. He has demonstrated that even if we perceive a certain figure hundreds of times, this does not facilitate its recognition if it is embedded as a hidden part into a more comprehensive configuration. This is evidence that visual organization is scarcely changed by experience. It is argued that it is always the totality of stimulations that determines visual organization and not the familiarity of single parts. Indeed, as far as I know, there is still no convincing empirical evidence that visual structures depend on experiences such as the experience of covariations between global and local features mentioned above. On the other hand, numerous contextual influences on visual object recognition confirm that acquired knowledge about structural relationships can in fact exert an enduring influence.

5 CONTEXTUAL INFLUENCES

5.1 Behavior Sequences and Surroundings as Context

Under natural conditions, most object recognition is embedded in two contexts: (1) actions; and (2) visual surroundings. If, for example, I want to write a letter, such objects as my desk, notepaper, pen, envelope, postage stamp, and so forth have to be recognized where they are needed in order to perform the respective action. At the same time, the objects are embedded in the surroundings of, say, my study, that is, in a familiar visual structure. Performing the behavioral sequence can lead to expectations concerning the specific object that is needed to continue, and the visual surroundings can provide a more or less familiar framework for its recognition and location.

5.2 Priming

Initially, I shall consider the influence of expectations on object recognition. Experimentally, expectations of an 'object' generally are not operationalized by requiring subjects to perform an object-specific action but through an experimental paradigm called 'priming'. In priming experiments, subjects have to react to a sequence of two stimuli: the first called the prime, and the second, the target. For some of these stimulus pairs, there is a relationship between prime and target; other pairs are unrelated. Such studies investigate the impact of the prime on target processing as a function of the relationship between prime and target. This section is particularly interested in experiments in which the target is a picture of an object. For example, if a picture of a dog has to be recognized after reading the word dog (word–picture) or after recognizing a picture of a cat (picture–picture), there are similarities between the two tasks that can facilitate recognition of the dog compared to neutral conditions. Such facilitation effects, like faster target recognition, are called priming effects and are interpreted as resulting from preparation of target recognition through the processing of the preceding prime.

An inspection of studies in which subjects have had to recognize two objects in succession permits the following generalized observations. If the two objects belong to the same category, for example, two birds, two musical instruments, or two vehicles, the second object is always recognized more quickly or more confidently compared with conditions in which the first object does not belong to the same category (Carr et al., 1982; Guenther, Klatzky and Putnam, 1980; Huttenlocher and Kubicek, 1983; Irwin and Lupker, 1983; Kroll and Potter, 1984). Conversely, object recognition is impaired when an object of the same category is presented shortly before as a stimulus to be ignored (Tipper, 1985; Tipper and Driver, 1988). In addition, the strength of priming effects depends on the visual similarity of the two objects: the strongest effects are observed when the second picture is identical to the first one (repetition priming, e.g. Jacoby, Baker and Brooks, 1989; Warren and Morton, 1982). Repetition priming is still effective after an interval of six weeks (Mitchell and Brown, 1988). Strong priming effects are also observed when objects belong to the same basic category (two birds, two trees, etc.) and thus share a common global form. In comparison, objects that only have a similar form without belonging to the same category (e.g. a tennis racquet and a banjo) show weaker priming effects, while the smallest effects are observed when objects are chosen from a common abstract category (e.g. clothes, furniture; see Flores d'Arcais and Schreuder, 1987; Pollatsek, Rayner and Collins, 1984). Priming effects can also be observed if category names are used as primes instead of pictures of objects. However, these effects are usually weaker than corresponding picture–picture conditions (Carr et al., 1982; Irwin and Lupker, 1983; McEvoy, 1988; Sperber et al., 1979; Warren and Morton, 1982; however, see also Guenther, Klatzky and Putnam, 1980; Lupker, 1988).

In summary, the observations permit the following conclusions. At least three factors are involved in the priming of object recognition:

(1) A priming of the conceptual meaning of the target. This can be held responsible for the effects of conceptual identity.
(2) A priming of visual processing that is considered to be responsible for effects of visual similarity.
(3) Finally, a priming of the required reaction to the objects in cases in which both prime and target call for the same reaction (see also Farah, 1989).

5.3 Perceptual Effects of Priming

Most of the experiments cited above studied the representation of word- and picture-specific information in memory, which will not be dealt with any further (see Carr et al., 1982; Glaser, 1992; Hoffmann and Klimesch, 1984; Kroll and Potter, 1984; Rosch, 1975; Theios and Amrhein, 1989). However, little research has dealt explicitly with the priming of visual processing. Sperber et al. (1979) have analyzed priming effects in naming two object pictures in succession belonging to either the same (cat–horse) or different categories (trumpet–horse). They also varied stimulus quality by presenting focused and defocused photographs of the targets. Priming effects for defocused photographs were about twice as high as those for focused photographs (122 ms versus 51 ms). This interaction supports the assumption that priming effects are due partly to influences on visual processing. It is assumed that recognizing an object from a certain category facilitates the processing of visual features that also trigger the recognition of other objects of the same category. This facilitation becomes increasingly apparent when visual conditions become more difficult (Becker and Killion, 1977; Seymor, 1973; but see also Lupker, 1988, for a different interpretation)

These ideas on the facilitation of visual processing have been elaborated even further by Reinitz, Wright and Loftus (1989). They displayed object pictures for between 30 and 90 ms under masking conditions. Before each presentation, subjects were shown either a neutral prime, the object name, or the name of another object. Compared with the other two conditions, the object name enhances the probability of correct object recognition. After initial enhancement, the effect remains constant with increasing presentation time. That is, interactions between priming and presentation time seem to be restricted to early phases of visual processing. This indicates that the name prime mainly facilitates processing of global visual features that are available relatively quickly and that determine the conceptual identity of the object. However, further visual processing in order to determine the object's individuality is scarcely influenced by the prime: '...knowledge of a picture's category increases the rate at which visual information is encoded, and once a picture's category is known, subsequent processing is independent of the means by which the category was recognized' (Reinitz, Wright and Loftus, 1989, p. 1989, p. 292; see also Loftus and Hogden 1988; Loftus, Nelson and Kallman, 1983). Hence, the prime is only effective up until an object has been recognized as belonging to its (basic) category. This is in agreement with the above-mentioned observations that priming effects are particularly strong when both prime and target belong to a common basic concept (Hoffmann and Klimesch, 1984; Warren and Morton, 1982).

This section started with the assumption that object expectations are aroused by intended actions, particularly in that those objects that have to be included next in the action are anticipated. The reported priming effects confirm the possibility that object recognition can be facilitated by prior processing. Thus, they show that it is principally possible to facilitate recognition of an object by means of its expectation. However, whether the same effects are engendered by behaviorally induced expectations as those induced by the consecutive processing of prime and target will require further research.

5.4 Priming by Surroundings

The second class of context effects is those due to objects being embedded in familiar surroundings. Just like the above-mentioned categorical priming, prior information about a context in which an object is frequently embedded can facilitate its recognition. If subjects are informed that they will have to identify, for example, kitchen objects, context-congruent objects like bread or toaster are recognized more quickly and confidently than when either no or a misleading contextual cue is given (Gerling, 1979; Hoffmann and Klein, 1988; Palmer, 1975). Similar effects can be observed when the objects to be recognized are not presented individually but as elements of complex pictures (Antes, Penland and Metzger, 1981; Biederman, 1972; Biederman, Glass and Stacy, 1973; Boyce, Pollatsek and Rayner, 1989; Hoffmann and Klein, 1988). Compared with being embedded in an incongruent context (a toaster in a ticket booth) or in a random collection of objects, recognition is facilitated by a congruent context (toaster in a kitchen) On average, effects are comparable to those obtained for prior explicit contextual information (Hoffmann and Klein, 1988, Exp. 1). Furthermore, how much an object profits from congruent embedding depends on its degree of congruence and its relative size. Highly congruent objects that are particularly typical for a specific context (e.g. cooking pot for kitchen) profit more than less typical ones (e.g. dustpan for kitchen). Likewise, context has a much stronger influence on the recognition of small objects than large ones (Hoffmann and Klein, 1988, Exp. 2 and 3).

Objects given in a natural context frequently belong to the same category. A kitchen contains other cooking utensils alongside cooking pots; a living room, all kinds of furniture; and an orchestra, a whole range of different musical instruments. Hence, pictures displaying natural contexts mostly contain various objects from the same categories (Murphy and Wisniewski, 1989). Against this background, the observed context effects may possibly be due to categorical priming (Friedman, 1979; Henderson, Pollatsek and Rayner, 1987).

If several objects are to form a natural context, certain relationships have to be maintained: objects have to be arranged so that they all make contact with a surface on which they stand. Overlapping objects must cover each other, they must be presented in their natural relative sizes, and their spatial arrangement also has to correspond to natural conditions (Biederman, Mezanotte and Rabinowitz, 1982). If these context-forming relationships between objects are violated so that the same objects are shown without creating the impression of a natural setting, context effects disappear (Antes, Penland and Metzger, 1981; Biederman, 1972; Biederman, Glass and Stacy, 1973; Biederman et al., 1988; Boyce, Pollatsek and Rayner, 1989). Biederman, Mezanotte and Rabinowitz (1982) have even shown that recognition performance on a single object deteriorates the more it violates such context-forming relationships, while Boyce, Pollatsek and Rayner (1989) have shown that removing a few lines from a picture is sufficient to eliminate context effects if these lines suggest a background (such as a street) that links the objects together. Hence, context effects are not due to categorically related objects alone, but are above all due to the specific arrangement of these objects that conveys the impression of a familiar scene.

Presumably, natural scenes will be recognized just as directly as the identity of single objects. Presentation times of 20 ms are already sufficient to observe scene-specific context effects (Biederman, Glass and Stacy, 1973). When presentation time is gradually increased, it is not so much individual objects but above all context-forming sections of a picture of a scene that are recognized up to a presentation time of 150 ms (Metzger and Antes, 1983). Compared with an unorganized presentation of objects, context effects increase as a function of lengthening presentation time up to about 100 ms and then decline again (Biederman et al., 1974). Furthermore, context effects are not influenced by manipulations rendering it more difficult to identify single objects within a scene (Klatzky, 1983).

All these observations support the assumption that when viewing a complex picture, the recognition of a scene is not based primarily on the recognition of scene-specific objects. Instead, it seems that global features of the picture first determine its perception. These features are determined by the arrangement of objects as well as the background stimuli. It can be assumed further that although these global features enable recognition of a scene, they do not yet enable recognition of single objects. This assumption has been supported by studies conducted by Antes and Mann (1984): recognition of scenes and objects was brought into conflict by having to recognize objects in congruent and incongruent scenes, and scenes with congruent and incongruent objects. Scene recognition only dominated object recognition when the scene could be viewed at one glance (about 6 degrees of visual angle). However, in a condition in which the same pictures were greatly enlarged (16 degrees), object recognition dominated scene recognition. Initial recognition seems to be determined by the global stimulus structures that are effective at first glance (i.e. independent of fixation): a scene will be recognized if the global impression corresponds sufficiently to a familiar surrounding; and an object, if it corresponds sufficiently to a basic category.

If these suppositions are correct, recognition of an object that is congruent with its scene is facilitated mainly by a recognition of the scene as a whole that precedes object recognition. Recognizing the scene creates a framework that facilitates the recognition of objects that are congruent with it, just like recognizing an object at its basic level creates a framework that facilitates the recognition of its details. In analogy to basic concepts, we can speak of scenes in the sense of basic categories that differentiate natural scenarios according to common global features (Hoffmann, 1986a, Klix, 1984; Tversky and Hemenway, 1983).

One important function of basic scene categories is probably to facilitate the location of objects. This assumes that congruent objects will be detected more quickly in pictures of scenes than incongruent ones (Hoffmann and Klein, 1988; Meyers and Rhoades, 1978; Reinert, 1985): that is, given a picture of a kitchen containing a cooking pot and a safety helmet, the pot is detected faster than the helmet. If a congruent object is located in an unusual place, however, the advantage of congruence is more than lost. The search for the object takes even longer than in an incongruent scene, and, additionally, it is more often overlooked (Hoffmann and Klein, 1988; Meyers and Rhoades, 1978)

In summary, observations have shown that embedding an object into a familiar visual context facilitates both recognition and location. The dynamics of context effects suggest that familiar scenes can be recognized as wholes on the basis of global stimulations even before single objects are recognized. Global scene structures can be related to expectations about objects at certain places, and these can be tested by a fixation of these places. Expectations prime object recognitions, and the fact that they are tied to certain places in the global reference framework results in the phenomena of visual search. Presumably, congruent parts are fixated only briefly for the same reasons: they merely confirm corresponding expectations, giving the observer more time to inspect incongruent and therefore unexpected parts of the picture (Friedman, 1979; Loftus, 1976; Loftus and Mackworth, 1978). This is probably also why only few scene-congruent details are stored in memory (Mandler and Johnson, 1976; Mandler and Parker, 1976; Mandler and Ritchey, 1977; Pezdek *et al.*, 1988, 1989).

5.5 Contexts as a Prerequisite of Intended Actions

If the present discussion is related to the introductory considerations on the relationship between visual recognition and behavior control, then global features of natural scenes seem to be the starting conditions for scene-specific acts. These also include eye movements to specific locations with the expectation of perceiving certain objects there. In other words, global scene features seem to be starting conditions for intentionally generating anticipated stimulations so that the recognition of scenes and objects within them arises from the confirmation of such anticipations (Wolff, 1985, 1986)

Such speculations imply that the impressive directness of object recognition is based to a large extent on expectations, in particular, on expecting to generate details through fixation on specific locations in global frameworks. The available data do not contradict such an interpretation. However, further experiments are needed to test it more precisely. In particular, it would be necessary to systematically vary covariations between global and local stimulations in order to elucidate their influence on visual recognition. Previously mentioned studies carried out by Lambert (1987), Lambert and Hockey (1986) and Miller (1988) are already pursuing this – my view, promising – approach.

6 PERCEPTUAL PERSPECTIVE AND ORIENTATION

6.1 Three-dimensional Models and Canonical Representations

The objects that have to be recognized can elicit very different stimulations depending on the perspective from which they are viewed. Usually, this diversity of stimulation does not impair the directness with which we recognize objects. For example, we recognize an automobile instantaneously, regardless of whether we are seeing it from the front, the side, or the top. The differences, and even, to a certain extent, the incomparability of the resulting stimulations, hardly seems to influence recognizability.

This apparent independence of recognition from the angle at which an object is perceived suggests that the representation that is derived from the given stimulation during the course of visual processing is independent of visual angle. Marr and Nishihara (1978) have proposed a series of processing steps that should render such a transformation of a perspective-dependent stimulus structure into an independent representation (see also Marr, 1982). After early contour processing, a coordinate system is set up, which is centered on the as yet unrecognized object. Elongations and symmetries of the given stimulus distribution are used to determine main axes, first, for the configuration as a whole; and then, in increasing detail, for individual parts. The relative positions of the axes form a structural description of an object in terms of the arrangement of its parts. Thus, an object-centered, three-dimensional (3-D) model is derived from the given, subject-centered stimulus structure. The identity of this 3-D model description is then determined by comparing it with corresponding object models represented in memory. Hence, object identification is independent from visual angle insofar as visual processing always leads to the same 3-D model; and it is dependent on visual angle insofar as different views can require different effort to derive the model.

An alternative conception assumes that objects are not represented in 3-D models but by one (or more) prototypical (canonical) two-dimensional stimulus structure(s) (Palmer, Rosch, and Chase, 1981; Reed, 1978; Rock, 1973). Furthermore, it is assumed that stimuli proceeding from an object can be mentally transformed in a way that corresponds to the effects of changing its orientation in space. Such transformations are conceived as mental rotation. Object recognition is based accordingly on comparing given with represented canonical stimulations that either correspond directly or can be made congruent by mental rotation. This concept replaces the effort required to derive a 3-D model with the effort of performing mental rotations.

6.2 Mental Rotation

Most support for the notion of mental rotation has come from studies in which subjects had to discriminate between standard versions and mirror images of two- and three-dimensional figures presented in different orientations (Cooper and Shepard, 1973; Metzler and Shepard, 1974; Shepard and Metzler, 1971). The crucial finding is that decision time monotonously increases as a function of the distance of orientations from the standard orientation and/or as a function of the distance between the orientations of the two figures to be compared. This has been confirmed for orientations in the two-dimensional plane and in three-dimensional space (Metzler and Shepard, 1974; Shepard and Metzler, 1971, 1988; but see also Rock and DiVita, 1987; Rock, DiVita and Barbeito, 1981). It has additionally been shown that subjects are able to imagine a figure in any orientation in order to compare it directly with a second figure presented in that orientation (Cooper and Shepard, 1973; but see also Rock, Wheeler and Tudor, 1989).

These results are interpreted as indicating a genuine mental process that alters representations of a given stimulus in a way that is analogous to changes that would arise from rotating a figure in space. There is a controversial discussion on whether this mental rotation should be understood as a holistic rotation of an image, a step-wise transformation of relational information, or as a reorientation of an egocentric reference system (Bethell-Fox and Shepard, 1988; Carpenter and Just, 1978; Cooper and Podgorny, 1976; Just and Carpenter, 1976; Robertson, Palmer and Gomez, 1987; Rock, Wheeler and Tudor, 1989; Shepard and Cooper, 1982). Rather than taking up this discussion, I shall address the issue of how far mental rotation plays a role in object recognition.

In some investigations, subjects simply have to recognize two-dimensional figures presented in different orientations without having to discriminate them from their mirror images. Recognition time does not depend on orientation here (Corballis and Nagourney, 1978; Corballis *et al.*, 1978; Eley, 1982; Shepard and Cooper, 1982; White, 1980). However, Palmer, Rosch and Chase (1981) have shown that there certainly exists a preferred orientation for the recognition of three-dimensional drawings of objects (i.e. objects drawn in perspective). Recognition time increases continuously as a function of the degree of deviation from this 'canonical' perspective. Dependence of recognition on orientation has also been reported for two-dimensional drawings of objects (Jolicoeur, 1985; Maki, 1986), alphanumeric symbols (Jolicoeur and Landau, 1984; Kolers and Perkins, 1969a, b), or symbols resembling letters (Tarr and Pinker, 1989). Hence, findings are contra- dictory.

6.3 Familiarity and Dependence on Orientation

The familiarity of figures may well be a factor that modifies the strength of the dependence of recognition on orientation (Koriat and Norman, 1985). It could be supposed that orientation effects will only be found when subjects have little experience with the figures. This assumption is supported by Jolicoeur's (1985) finding that the dependence of recognition on orientation dropped clearly as a function of increasing test experience. However, training effects were restricted to the object drawings that were actually experienced during the course of the experiment. That is, if new drawings are presented following extensive training with a fixed set of object drawings, the orientation dependence of recognizing these new objects corresponds closely to that for the trained objects at the beginning of the experiment (Jolicoeur, 1985, Exp. 3). Subjects do not acquire a general ability to perform orientation-independent recognition but merely one for objects that have been perceived repeatedly under different orientations. Furthermore, if an object is perceived repeatedly in an upright orientation only, the dependence of its recognition on orientation is not reduced (Jolicoeur and Milliken, 1989, Exp. 1). However, repeated perception of an object in an upright position can improve its recognition in other orientations when experienced in the context of other objects whose orientations change continuously (Jolicoeur and Milliken, 1989, Exp. 2).

These observations show that an object has to be perceived (or at least expected) repeatedly in several orientations before the recognition mechanisms for this object, and only this object, can become less dependent on its orientation. They suggest a learning-dependent abstraction of features that remains invariant across all perceived (or expected) orientations of an object, so that recognition can rely increasingly on these invariants. Then after training, the object is no longer recognized through the derivation of a 3-D model, nor through mental rotation, but through the use of object-specific invariants (Selfridge and Neisser, 1960).

Findings reported by Tarr and Pinker (1989, Exp. 2) suggest an alternative explanation. Subjects had to name letter-like figures as quickly as possible. During learning trials, the figures were each presented in three or four selected orientations. Training these orientations makes recognition time independent of orientation. However, if figures are presented in additional orientations that have not been trained previously, recognition of these unaccustomed orientations once more proves to be orientation-dependent: recognition time increases as a function of the distance between these new orientations and the previously trained ones. The authors interpreted this result as indicating that a specific representation was acquired for each trained orientation. They concluded that the reduction of orientation dependence is not based on orientation-independent features but rather on several orientation-bound representations with which actual perceptions are compared either directly or following mental rotation.

Against the background of the above-mentioned training effects, familiar stimuli such as letters or digits should be recognized independently from orientation because of our extensive perceptual experience with them. In contrast, recognizing unfamiliar figures should remain dependent on their orientation as long as such experience has not been made. However, even this reasoning cannot account for all the findings. While, in some studies, recognition of letters and digits has proved to be orientation-dependent (Jolicoeur and Landau, 1984; Kolers and Perkins, 1969a,b), Eley (1982) has shown that recognition of artificial figures is orientation-independent even if subjects are only slightly familiar with them. The interaction between familiarity and orientation seems to be influenced by further factors.

6.4 Orientation-free and Orientation-bound Features

How far it is possible to achieve orientation-independent recognition also depends on the differences between the figures that have to be recognized. If global differences permit a confident recognition, then orientation independence is more likely than when details of the figure determine its identity. Whether a figure portrays, for example, a face can be decided immediately from all orientations, while making gender distinctions or recognizing individuals increases in difficulty the more the face deviates from the upright orientation (Rock, 1973; Sergent and Corballis, 1989). Likewise, a configuration can be recognized as a hand independent of orientation, while distinguishing between a right and a left hand is orientation-dependent (Cooper and Shepard, 1975; Parsons, 1987). Some alphanumeric symbols change identity with orientation: rotation turns a *6* into a *9*, a *b* into a *q*, and an *M* into a *W*, while a mirror image of a *b* is a *d*. If these symbols have to be distinguished, their recognition requires the ascertainment of the relative position of details in each case. However, if the task is only to distinguish between letters and digits, one can ignore the relative position of details, and recognition proves to be independent from orientation (Corballis and Nagourney, 1978).

On the basis of such considerations, Takano (1989) has proposed a discrimination between orientation-free and orientation-bound features. He has argued that the orientation dependence of recognition should depend on the kinds of feature on which it is based: recognition should be orientation-independent if the figures can be distinguished through orientation-free features. This was certainly the case in the above-mentioned studies of Corballis and Nagourney (1978), Corballis *et al.* (1978), and Eley (1982) that reported orientation-independent recognition performance. On the other hand, orientation-dependent recognition should always be observed when distinctions are based on spatial relationships between parts, that is, on orientation-bound features.

Why this should be so can be illustrated by the following example. In many typefaces, the letters *b*, *q*, *d* and *p* can be described as being composed of a straight line and a semicircle. They differ according to whether the semicircle is located on top or at the bottom and on the left- or right-hand side of the line. These relationships – *top*, *bottom*, *left-hand* and *right-hand* – are, indeed, relations between the parts of the figure, and they are thus object-centered in the sense of Marr (1982). However, their recognition requires relating the figure to a coordinate system that is anchored in the observer. Just as describing whether a person walks up or down a street or turns left or right depends on one's perspective, the definition of spatial relationships between parts of a figure depends on the perspective of the observer. Hence, if the figures to be recognized differ only with regard to the spatial relations of their parts, recognition requires the orientation of the figures to be related to spatial directions determined by the observer. As a consequence, this leads to an orientation dependence of recognition.

This notion agrees with the fact that orientation dependence has always been found for the recognition of mirror images, because mirror images differ in nothing other than the left–right orientation of their parts. The letter-like figures employed by Tarr and Pinker (1989) also differed mainly in the left–right arrangement of their elements (unlike those used by Eley, 1982), and they also produced an orientation dependence of recognition. Hence both observations confirm the notion that the orientation dependence of recognition is based on the need to determine the relative position of parts of a figure in order to identify it.

Takano (1989) has reported experiments in which the figures to be recognized differed in orientation-free or orientation-bound features. Figures that permit different codings are of particular interest. The shapes in Figure 9.12 differ in the relative orientation of the upper hook: one points to the left, the other to the right. This is an orientation-bound feature (left–right). However, the figures also differ in

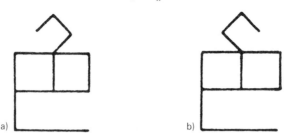

Figure 9.12. *Figures with orientation-bound and orientation-free differences. [From Takano, 1989, p. 36, Fig. 6, top. © 1989 Academic Press; reprinted with kind permission.]*

that in one figure, the lower opening and the point of the hook point in the same direction; in the other, they point in opposite directions. This is an orientation-free feature. Takano (1989) has been able to show that recognition is either orientation-dependent or orientation-independent depending on whether subjects encode the figure by the orientation-bound or the orientation-free feature, respectively.

This result offers an explanation of the training effects reported earlier (Jolicoeur, 1985; Jolicoeur and Milliken, 1989; Tarr and Pinker, 1989). If figures that are normally perceived in an upright orientation, such as letters, digits and most of the objects surrounding us, suddenly have to be recognized again and again in the most varied orientations, it can be assumed that the way these figures are encoded changes so that orientation-bound features lose and orientation-free features gain in impact. Hence, with increasing training, figure recognition becomes more independent of orientation. However, if the figures do not differ in such orientation-free features, no training – no matter how long it may last – can lead to their abstraction. In such cases, an alternative possibility is to store several orientation-specific representations of the figures, as Tarr and Pinker's (1989) results suggest.

6.5   Orientation-free Invariants and Concept Formation

This section started by asking which mechanisms enable reliable identification of objects despite differences in stimulation due to different perspectives. The majority of the studies cited do not concern the recognition of three-dimensional objects but focus on two-dimensional drawings. Varying the visual angle from which a three-dimensional object is viewed and varying the orientation of a two-dimensional drawing certainly lead to very different changes in stimulation. While the internal structure of a two-dimensional pattern remains constant, views of three-dimensional objects can arise in which substantial parts are hidden so that stimulation undergoes fundamental changes. This is in line with the difficulties subjects have in imagining different views of unfamiliar three-dimensional wire objects compared to the ease of mentally rotating two-dimensional figures (Rock and DiVita, 1987; Rock, Wheeler and Tudor, 1989). Hence, the mechanisms underlying orientation-independent recognition of two-dimensional object drawings may not be assumed to be the same mechanisms that ensure the recognition of three-dimensional objects from different perspectives. Despite these limitations in generalizability, the reported results permit some conclusions whose validity may be assumed to extend to object recognition in three-dimensional space.

Our discussion suggests that the orientation independence of recognition is not based upon one mechanism alone. Instead, there are at least two possible ways of compensating for orientation-dependent stimulation. Apart from recognition based on orientation-free invariants, recognition can also be based on a comparison of given stimulations with orientation-bound prototypes that each represent one 'typical' orientation.

Orientation dependence changes with the required level of recognition and with the specificity of the distinctions that have to be made. If only a rough classification of objects at the level of basic concepts is required, orientation independence is more probable than when objects have to be recognized more specifically. If it is agreed that the identity of basic concepts is determined mainly by global features and the identity of subconcepts by additional local features at specific relative locations (see Section 3), recognition may be expected to be orientation-dependent if it calls for the consideration of details (Corballis, 1988). However, if global features are sufficient to recognize an object's identity, recognition may be expected to be independent of orientation as long as the global features are not orientation-bound.

The orientation independence of recognition depends on corresponding experience. It is finally obtained through the repeated recognition of objects under different orientations. Mechanisms can be assumed that abstract 'orientation-free' invariants from the variety of experienced stimulations. Presumably, these are the same mechanisms as those that underlie concept formation, that is, mechanisms for representing functionally equivalent 'configurations' by visual invariants. Since the functional value of an object usually does not change as a function of its spatial orientation, conceptual invariants have to be orientation-independent in order to represent functional equivalence. That is, invariants have to be invariant over not only the range of functionally equivalent objects but also the range of experienced orientations of these objects. It follows that to indicate conceptual (functional) identity, it is preferable to abstract those invariants that are orientation-free, and these are mainly global features with a preference for representing basic concepts. Therefore, it is probably more appropriate not to say that recognition of basic concepts is orientation-independent because it is based on global features, but to say that basic concepts are based on global features because, in general, only these are orientation-free.

The invariants on which a specific recognition is based depends on the variability of orientations under which the respective recognition has been experienced, and then the orientation independence only holds for this range of experienced variability. Accordingly, we find it difficult to recognize, for example, an automobile from underneath, or a coffee machine from a bird's-eye view (Biederman, 1987). This experience dependence of the invariants underlying object recognitions certainly does not exclude the possibility of general invariants also being effective, particularly those that covary with depth (binocular and monocular criteria) or those that indicate volumetric characteristics (nonaccidental features, Biederman, 1987; Hoffman and Richards, 1984; Marr, 1982). However, from the perspective presented in this chapter, such invariants do not serve to reconstruct a three-dimensional model from a two-dimensional stimulus. Rather, they serve a structuring of two-dimensional stimuli that corresponds broadly to its three-dimensional origins, thus facilitating the abstraction of orientation-free invariants (Lowe, 1987).

The usual experimental task, in which subjects have to recognize an object that appears suddenly in an unpredictable orientation, occurs very rarely under natural conditions. Typically, changes in perspective are generated by one's own behavior, so that the resulting stimulations do not confront us unexpectedly but in a predictable way. These controllable voluntary changes in stimulation contain information about the identity of objects as well, which is presumably also used (Gibson, 1979; Turvey and Carello, 1986). At times, we fall into the routine of gaining further information by varying the visual angle, even when looking at pictures–for example, when we look at a puzzling picture in a newspaper from different perspectives. This active form of gaining information about an object's identity through an aimed generation of stimulations from different perspectives is still an unelaborated research topic (see, for example, Turvey, Solomon and Burton, 1989, for current studies on gaining information through handling objects).

7 CONCLUSIONS

7.1 Functional Equivalence in Perception

In my introduction, I tried to justify the idea that the 'organization' of visual stimulation into units corresponding to objects, to their arrangements in scenes, and to their parts and features cannot be based on characteristics of the perceptual process itself if we wish to avoid the assumption that these correspond *a priori* to environmental structure. The preceding discussions have revealed the importance of this problem whenever proposed mechanisms of object recognition presupposed the performances they have to account for in order to achieve them. Determining the minimal code of a configuration, from which its decomposition into parts should result, presupposes, for example, the determination of its primitive code, that is, its decomposition into elementary parts. Likewise, the employment of nonaccidental features for parsing a whole into parts presumes that the parts have already been determined, so that the visual system can ascertain which features covary nonaccidentally with them. Or mentally rotating a configuration into its 'standard orientation' in order to recognize it presupposes its recognition, because otherwise, how can a decision be reached on what should be regarded as the 'standard orientation?' Perhaps I can generalize by saying that if the structures we perceive have to be derived from the identity of the units from which they originate, the identity of the units cannot be derived from the structures we perceive.

I shall briefly return to the notions discussed in the introduction: the units to be perceived are determined by functional equivalences, that is, by the fact that behavioral acts lead to the same predictable consequences when applied to different stimulus configurations. It is above all these similar changes engendered by one behavioral act that determine the functional equivalence of stimulus configurations. Visual object recognition, one can speculate, is based on the visual system's ability to learn to distinguish between stimulus configurations that differ in their functional equivalence. For configurations with the same functional equivalence, it is assumed that the visual system 'searches' for invariants that differentiate them from configurations with another functional equivalence.

The functional equivalence of stimulus conditions is determined in two ways: first by the behavioral act for which the equivalence holds, and second by the features of the source of stimulation on which the equivalence is based. Both determinants are integrated by coding functional equivalence in perceptual invariants. This permits a perception based on these invariants to mediate between object features and object manipulation, between environment and behavior (see also Prinz, 1984, 1990).

The functional equivalences of objects usually do not change either with viewing perspective or with different fixations. Hence, the invariants underlying object recognition have to be determined not only for different, functionally equivalent objects but also for the stimulations arising from different visual angles and fixations of each object. The stimulus structures that are invariant to these diverse variations are mostly global features such as the specific form of an outline or the like. The phenomena of global dominance suggest that the visual system is adapted to these relationships insofar as it is particularly able to perform a rapid discrimination between global features of stimuli.

From this point of view, two stimulus configurations are functionally equivalent if a behavioral act has the same consequence when applied to either of them. Hence, equivalence should be recognizable for perception in that configurations can be changed by some behavioral act in a comparable and thus predictable manner. Anticipations about the ways in which stimulus structures can be changed by varying visual angle or fixation should therefore play an important role in object recognition.

According to this assumption, an object is recognized according to a stepwise and expectation-bound differentiation of visual information in which each given state defines the starting conditions for the generation of further information. Such a speculation is in line with findings on the dominance of scene identification, the dominance of object recognition at the basic level, and the priming and context effects related to these dominances.

These speculations suggest that the visual structures underlying object recognition may be described as expectations of certain stimulations at certain locations in a still unstructured global stimulus distribution. The most basic features for object recognition are accordingly the global (fixation-independent) features. They 'define' expectations of stimulations that can be produced mainly by eye movements or changes in perspective. Hence, the identity of scenes, contexts, persons, objects, and so forth will be deduced by producing the expected stimulation, that is, in the repetition of past perceptual experiences.

The prevailing conceptions about the processes of object recognition differ fundamentally. It is assumed that the identity of a stimulus structure is determined by comparing the outcome of its visual processing with conceptual entities stored in memory; that is, visual processing and identification through comparison are viewed as being separated. According to Marr (1982), for example, visual processing leads to a three-dimensional model that is then compared with object models stored in memory. Biederman (1987) has proposed that the components of a stimulus structure acquired through perception are matched with memorized object representations (see Figure 9.10). Prinz (1983) has assumed that early visual processes generate features that are able to activate respective feature tags in knowledge memory. Other authors have assumed that stimulations are compared with conceptual prototypes (Bransford and Franks, 1971; Rosch, 1975, 1977) after having been 'normalized' by, for example, mental rotation.

My premise that object recognition is based on the repetition of past perceptual experiences transcends the distinction between visual processes and comparison processes. According to my view, visual processing is a process aimed toward the generation of stimulations: a stimulus structure is recognized to the degree that it evokes anticipations about how it could be altered, and its identity is realized to the degree that these anticipations are confirmed. Thus, the visual features of objects are not represented independently from the mechanisms of their processing but, in contrast, as 'instructions' for purposefully changing a stimulus structure. Those stimulus structures, conditions or situations in which instructions can be executed successfully correspond to the extensional meaning of the objects; and their successful execution corresponds to their recognition.

7.2   Current Issues and Future Directions

The present speculations are derived from the idea that the units that perception permits us to recognize must be determined by the distinctions necessary for a successful execution of behavior. In the individual sections of this chapter, I have tried to show that the framework resulting from this speculation allows us to understand a variety of phenomena of visual object perception in a functionally coherent way. This should encourage the use of this traditional psychological perspective in future research (see Heuer and Sanders, 1987; Neumann and Prinz, 1990b). I shall conclude by at least outlining some of the most important issues that need to be studied.

An essential element of the speculations presented here is the assumption of the visual system's ability to grasp global features of a stimulation independently of and preferably before local details. However, what are global features? I have already discussed the difficulty of defining them. Under the assumption that global features have to be abstracted as invariants in order to be visually effective, it would seem to be worth testing the constraints of the human visual system for abstracting and processing them (Hoffmann and Grosser, 1986). If the adaptivity of visual processing is explored systematically with differently defined (global and local) invariants, further insights into the distinctions between elementary and composed as well as local and global features can be expected.

There is also insufficient specification of the learning processes that lead to the formation of the assumed visual invariants. Assuming that these invariants are based on the experience of regular transformations leads to the speculation that a 'need' to anticipate behaviorally bound transformations drives the underlying learning processes. Following up this speculation will require studies that analyze the impact of the reciprocal predictability of visual features on perception.

Finally, some observations have indicated that the behavioral effects of visual stimulations can be dissociated from the features of their conscious recognition. The perceived distance between two points, for example, does not always correspond to the size of the saccade between them (Hajos and Fey, 1982), and the perceived position of a point does not always correspond to the point indicated with the hand (Bridgeman, 1989). Further, the perceived curvature of a line does not always correspond to the eye movements when it is visually scanned (Miller and Festinger, 1977), and stimuli can influence behavior without being identified consciously (Neumann and Prinz, 1987). Such findings draw attention to the fact that the features (invariants) that underlie the successful control of a certain behavior (e.g. eye movements) do not necessarily determine the phenomenal structure of the stimulus (Bridgeman, this volume; Neumann, 1989). Once more, we must await future research in order to understand the relationships between the mechanisms of visual behavior control and those used for the conscious recognition of visual structures.

ACKNOWLEDGEMENTS

This chapter was written while the author was a guest at the Max Planck Institute for Psychological Research, Munich. I wish to thank both my colleagues at the Institute and the Max Planck Society for their support and W. Prinz and B. Bridgeman for their comments on an earlier version of this manuscript. Special thanks are due to Jonathan Harrow for his translation.

REFERENCES

Ach, N. (1905). *Über die Willenstätigkeit und das Denken*. Göttingen: Vandenhoeck und Ruprecht.

Ach, N. (1935). *Analyse des Willens*. Berlin, Wien: Urban und Schwarzenberg.

Anglin, J. M. (1977). *Word, Object, and Conceptual Development*. New York: Norton.

Anochin, P. K. (1967). *Das funktionelle System als Grundlage der physiologischen Architektur des Verhaltens*. Jena: Fischer.

Antes, J. R. and Mann, S. W. (1984). Global–local precedence in picture processing. *Psychological Research*, **46**, 247–259.

Antes, J. R., Penland, J. G. and Metzger, R. L. (1981). Processing global information in briefly presented pictures. *Psychological Research*, **43**, 277–292.

Bartlett, F. C. (1932). *Remembering, a Study in Experimental and Social Psychology*. Cambridge: Cambridge University Press.

Becker, C. A. and Killion, T. H. (1977). Interaction of visual and cognitive effects in word recognition. *Journal of Experimental Psychology: Human Perception and Performance*, **3**, 389–401.

Bethell-Fox, C. E. and Shepard, R. N. (1988). Mental rotation: Effects of stimulus complexity and familiarity. *Journal of Experimental Psychology: Human Perception and Performance*, **14**, 12–23.

Biederman, I. (1972). Perceiving real-world scenes. *Science*, **177**, 77–80.

Biederman, I. (1987). Recognition-by-components: A theory of human image understanding. *Psychological Review*, **94**, 115–147.

Biederman, I., Blickle, T. W., Teitelbaum, R. C. and Klatsky, G. J. (1988). Object search in nonscene displays. *Journal of Experimental Psychology: Learning, Memory, and Cognition*, **14**, 456–467.

Biederman, I., Glass, A. L. and Stacy, E. W. (1973). Scanning for objects in real world scenes. *Journal of Experimental Psychology*, **97**, 22–27.

Biederman, I. and Ju, G. (1988). Surface versus edge-based determinants of visual recognition. *Cognitive Psychology*, **20**, 38–64.

Biederman, I., Mezanotte, R. J. and Rabinowitz, J. C. (1982). Scene perception: Detecting and judging objects undergoing relational violations. *Cognitive Psychology*, **14**, 143–177.

Biederman, I., Rabinowitz, J. L., Glass, A. L. and Stacy, E. W. (1974). On the information extracted from a glance at a scene. *Journal of Experimental Psychology*, **103**, 596–600.

Boer, L. C. and Keuss, P. J. G. (1982). Global precedence as a postperceptual effect: An analysis of speed-accuracy trade-off functions. *Perception and Psychophysics*, **31**, 358–366.

Boring, E. G. (1942). *Sensation and Perception in the History of Experimental Psychology*. New York: Appleton-Century-Crofts.

Bouma, H. (1971). Visual recognition of isolated lower-case letters. *Vision Research*, **11**, 459–474.

Bower, G. H. and Glass, A. L. (1976). Structural units and the redintegrative power of picture fragments. *Journal of Experimental Psychology: Human Learning and Memory*, **2**, 456–466.

Boyce, S. J., Pollatsek, A. and Rayner, K. (1989). Effect of background information on object identification. *Journal of Experimental Psychology: Human Perception and Performance*, **15**, 556–566.

Bransford, J. D. and Franks, J. J. (1971). The abstraction of linguistic ideas. *Cognitive Psychology*, **2**, 331–350.

Breitmeyer, B. G. and Ganz, L. (1977). Temporal studies with flashed gratings: Inferences about transient and sustained systems. *Vision Research*, **17**, 861–865.

Bridgeman, B. (1989). Separate visual representations for perception and for visually guided behavior. In S. R. Ellis and M. K. Kaiser (Eds), *Spatial Displays and Spatial Instruments*. Moffett Field, CA: NASA (14.1–14.15).

Brown, R. (1958). How shall a thing be called? *Psychological Review*, **65**, 14–21.

Bruce, V. and Green, P. R. (1990). *Visual Perception: Physiology, Psychology and Ecology*. Hillsdale, NJ: Erlbaum.

Brunswik, E. (1956). *Perception and the Representative Design of Psychological Experiments*. Berkeley, CA: University of California Press

Buffart, H. F. J. and Leeuwenberg, E. L. J. (1983). Structural information theory. In H.G. Geissler, H. F. J. Buffart, E. L. J. Leeuwenberg, and V. Sarris (Eds), *Modern Issues in Perception* (pp. 48–74). Amsterdam: North-Holland.

Buffart, H. F. J., Leeuwenberg, E. L. J. and Restle, F. (1981). Coding theory of visual pattern completion. *Journal of Experimental Psychology: Human Perception and Performance*, **7**, 241–274.

Carpenter, P. A. and Just, M. A. (1978). Eye fixations during mental rotation. In J. W. Senders, D. F. Fisher and R. A. Monty (Eds), *Eye Movements and Higher Psychological Functions*, vol. 2 (pp. 115–133). Hillsdale, NJ: Erlbaum.

Carr, T. H., McCauley, C., Sperber, R. D. and Parmelee, C. M. (1982). Words, pictures, and priming: On semantic activation, conscious identification, and the automaticity of information processing. *Journal of Experimental Psychology: Human Perception and Performance*, **8**, 757–777.

Cooper, L. A. and Podgorny, P. (1976). Mental transformations and visual comparison processes: Effects of complexity and similarity. *Journal of Experimental Psychology: Human Perception and Performance*, **2**, 503–514.

Cooper, L. A. and Shepard, R. N. (1973). Chronometric studies of the rotation of mental images. In W. G. Chase (Ed.), *Visual Information Processing* (pp. 75–176). New York, London: Academic Press.

Cooper, L. A. and Shepard, R. N. (1975). Mental transformation in the identification of left and right hands. *Journal of Experimental Psychology: Human Perception and Performance*, **1**, 48–56.

Corballis, M. C. (1988). Recognition of disoriented shapes. *Psychological Review*, **95**, 115–123.

Corballis, M. C. and Nagourney, B. A. (1978). Latency to categorize disoriented characters as letters or digits. *Canadian Journal of Psychology*, **32**, 186–188.

Corballis, M. C., Zbrodoff, J., Shetzer, L. I. and Butler, P. B. (1978). Decisions about identity and orientation of rotated letters and digits. *Memory and Cognition*, **6**, 98–107.

De Valois, R. L. and De Valois, K. K. (1980). Spatial vision. *Annual Review of Psychology*, **31**, 309–341.

Dewey, J. (1896). The reflex arc concept in psychology. *Psychological Review*, **3**, 357–370.

Dörner, D., Schaub, H., Stäudel, Th. and Strohschneider, S. (1988). Ein System zur Handlungsregulation oder – Die Interaktion von Emotion, Kognition und Motivation. *Sprache und Kognition*, **7**, 217–232.

Eley, M. G. (1982). Identifying rotated letter-like symbols. *Memory and Cognition*, **10**, 25–32.

Farah, M. J. (1989). Semantic and perceptual priming: How similar are the underlying mechanisms? *Journal of Experimental Psychology: Human Perception and Performance*, **15**, 188–194.

Flores d'Arcais, G. B. and Schreuder, R. (1987). Semantic activation during object naming. *Psychological Research*, **49**, 153–159.

Friedman, A. (1979). Framing pictures: The role of knowledge in automatized encoding and memory for gist. *Journal of Experimental Psychology: General*, **108**, 316–355.

Gerling, M. (1979). Kontexteffekte beim Identifizieren von Bildern: Kongruenz vs. Inkongruenz. *Zeitschrift für experimentelle und angewandte Psychologie*, **26**, 541–560.

Gibson, J. J. (1979). *The Ecological Approach to Visual Perception*. Boston: Houghton.

Ginsburg, A. P. (1986). Spatial filtering and visual form perception. In K. R. Boff, L. Kaufman, and J. P. Thomas (Eds), *Handbook of Perception and Human Performance*, vol. 2: *Cognitive Processes and Performance* (pp. 34.1–34.41). New York: John Wiley.

Glaser, W. R. (1992). Picture naming. *Cognition*, **42**, 51–105.

Gottschaldt, K. (1926). Über den Einfluß der Erfahrung auf die Wahrnehmung von Figuren. *Psychologische Forschung*, **8**, 261–317.

Gregory, R. L. (1974). Choosing a paradigm for perception. In E. C. Carterette and M. P. Friedman (Eds), *Handbook of Perception*, vol. 1.1: *Historical and Philosophical Roots of Perception* (pp. 255–283). New York: Academic Press.

Guenther, R. K., Klatzky, R. L. and Putnam, W. (1980). Commonalities and differences in semantic decisions about pictures and words. *Journal of Verbal Learning and Verbal Behavior*, **19**, 54–74.

Hajos, A. and Fey, D. A. (1982). Lernprozesse des okulomotorischen Systems. *Psychologische Beiträge*, **24**, 135–158.

Harvey, L. D. Jr (1986). Visual memory: What is remembered. In F. Klix and H. Hagendorf (Eds), *Human Memory and Cognitive Capabilities: Mechanisms and Performances* (pp. 173–187). Amsterdam: North-Holland.

Harvey, L. D. Jr, Roberts, J. O. and Gervais, M. J. (1983). The spatial frequency basis of internal representations. In H. G. Geissler, H. F. J. M. Buffart, E. L. J. Leeuwenberg and V. Sarris (Eds), *Modern Issues in Perception* (pp. 217–226). Amsterdam: North-Holland.

Hatfield, G. and Epstein, W. (1985). The status of the minimum principle in the theoretical analysis of visual perception. *Psychological Bulletin*, **97**, 155–186.

Helmholtz, H. von (1910/1962). *Handbuch der physiologischen Optik*, vol. 3. Hamburg, Leipzig: Voss. (J. P. C. Southall, Ed. and Transl., *A Treatise on Physiological Optics*. New York: Dover, 1962.)

Henderson, J. M., Pollatsek, A. and Rayner, K. (1987). The effects of foveal priming and extrafoveal preview on object identification. *Journal of Experimental Psychology: Human Perception and Performance*, **3**, 449–463.

Heuer, H. and Sanders, A. F. (Eds) (1987). *Perspectives on Perception and Action*. Hillsdale, NJ: Erlbaum.

Hochberg, J. (1978). *Perception*, 2nd edn. Englewood Cliffs, NJ: Prentice-Hall.

Hochberg, J. (1981). Levels of perceptual organization. In M. Kubovy and J. R. Pomerantz (Eds), *Perceptual Organization* (pp. 255–278). Hillsdale, NJ: Erlbaum.

Hochberg, J. and McAlister, E. A. (1953). A quantitative approach to figural 'goodness'. *Journal of Experimental Psychology*, **46**, 361–364.

Hoffman, D. D. and Richards, W. A. (1984). Parts of recognition. *Cognition*, **18**, 65–96.

Hoffman, J. E. (1980). Interaction between global and local levels of a form. *Journal of Experimental Psychology: Human Perception and Performance*, **6**, 222–234.

Hoffmann, J. (1982). Representation of concepts and the classification of objects. In F. Klix, J. Hoffmann and E. van der Meer (Eds), *Cognitive Research in Psychology* (pp. 72–89). Amsterdam: North-Holland.

Hoffmann, J. (1986a). *Die Welt der Begriffe*. Weinheim: Psychologie Verlags-Union.

Hoffmann, J. (1986b). A simulation approach to conceptual identification processes. In I. Kurcz, G. W. Shugar, and J. H. Danks (Eds), *Knowledge and Language* (pp. 49–68). Amsterdam: North-Holland.

Hoffmann, J. (1987). Semantic control of selective attention. *Psychological Research*, **49**, 123–129.

Hoffmann, J. (1990). Über die Integration von Wissen in die Verhaltenssteuerung. *Schweizerische Zeitschrift für Psychologie*, **49**, 250–265.

Hoffmann, J. (1992). Konzentration durch Antizipation. In J. Beckmann, H. Strang, and E. Hahn (Eds), *Konzentration und Leistung*, vol. 2. Göttingen: Hogrefe.

Hoffmann, J. and Grosser, U. (1985). Automatismen bei der begrifflichen Klassifikation. *Spache und Kognition*, **4**, 28–48.

Hoffmann, J. and Grosser, U. (1986). Die lernabhängige Automatisierung begrifflicher Identifikation. *Sprache und Kognition*, **5**, 27–41.

Hoffmann, J., Grosser, U. and Klein, R. (1987). The influence of knowledge on visual search. In E. van der Meer and J. Hoffmann (Eds), *Knowledge-aided Information Processing* (pp. 81–100). Amsterdam: North-Holland.

Hoffmann, J. and Kämpf, U. (1985). Mechanismen der Objektbenennung – Parallele Verarbeitungssakkaden. *Sprache und Kogition*, **4**, 217–230.

Hoffmann, J. and Klein, R. (1988). Kontexteffekte bei der Benennung und Entdeckung von Objekten. *Sprache und Kognition*, **7**, 25–39.

Hoffmann, J. and Klimesch, W. (1984). Die semantische Codierung von Wörtern und Bildern. *Sprache und Kognition*, **3**, 1–25.

Hoffmann, J. and Zießler, M. (1982). Begriffe und ihre Merkmale. *Zeitschrift für Psychologie*, **190**, 46–77.

Hoffmann, J. and Zießler, C. (1983). Objektidentifikation in künstlichen Begriffshierarchien. *Zeitschrift für Psychologie*, **191**, 135–167.

Hoffmann, J. and Zießler, M. (1986). The integration of visual and functional classifications in concept formation. *Psychological Research*, **48**, 69–78.

Hoffmann, J., Zießler, M. and Grosser, U. (1984). Psychologische Gesetzmäßigkeiten der begrifflichen Klassifikation von Objekten. In F. Klix (Ed.), *Gedächtnis, Wissen, Wissensnutzung* (pp. 74–107). Berlin: Verlag der Wissenschaften.

Hoffmann, J., Zießler, M., Grosser, U. and Kämpf, U. (1985). Struktur- und Prozeßkomponenten in begrifflichen Identifikationsleistungen. *Zeitschrift für Psychologie*, **193**, 51–70.

Hughes, H. C., Layton, W. M., Baird, J. C. and Lester, L. S. (1984). Global precedence in visual pattern recognition. *Perception and Psychophysics*, **35**, 361–371.

Huttenlocher, J. and Kubicek, L. F. (1983). The source of relatedness effects on naming latency. *Journal of Experimental Psychology: Learning, Memory, and Cognition*, **9**, 486–496.

Irwin, D. I. and Lupker, S. J. (1983). Semantic priming of pictures and words: A levels-of-processing approach. *Journal of Verbal Learning and Verbal Behavior*, **22**, 45–60.

Jacoby, L. L., Baker, J. G. and Brooks, L. R. (1989). Episodic effects on picture identification: Implications for theories of concept learning and theories of memory. *Journal of Experimental Psychology: Learning, Memory, and Cognition*, **15**, 275–281.

James, W. (1890/1981). *The Principles of Pschology*, vol. 2. Cambridge, MA: Harvard University Press (original work published 1890).

Jolicoeur, P. (1985). The time to name disoriented natural objects. *Memory and Cognition*, **13**, 289–303.

Jolicoeur, P., Gluck, M. and Kosslyn, S. (1984). Pictures and names: Making the connection. *Cognitive Psychology*, **16**, 243–275.

Jolicoeur, P. and Landau, M. J. (1984). Effects of orientation on the identification of simple visual patterns. *Canadian Journal of Psychology*, **38**, 80–93.

Jolicoeur, P. and Milliken, B. (1989). Identification of disoriented objects: Effects of context-prior presentation. *Journal of Experimental Psychology: Learning, Memory, and Cognition*, **15**, 200–210.

Jones, G. V. (1983). Identifying basic categories. *Psychological Bulletin*, **94**, 423–428.

Just, M. A. and Carpenter, P. A. (1976). Eye fixations and cognitive processes. *Cognitive Psychology*, **8**, 441–480.

Kämpf U. and Hoffmann, J. (1990). The latency course of feature encoding interfaced with a logorithm-based figure classification. In H. G. Geissler (Ed), *Psychophysical Explorations of Mental Structures* (pp. 456–468). Goettingen: Hogrefe.

Kinchla, R. A. (1974). Detecting target elements in multi-element arrays: A confusability model. *Perception and Psychophysics*, **15**, 149–158.

Kinchla, R. A., Solis-Macias, V. and Hoffman, J. E. (1983). Attending to different levels of structure in a visual image. *Perception and Psychophysics*, **33**, 1–10.

Kinchla, R. A. and Wolfe, J. (1979). The order of visual processing: 'Top down', 'bottom up', or 'middle out'. *Perception and Psychophysics*, **25**, 225–231.

Klatzky, G. J. (1983). Getting to the top: On the access routes to scene schemata. Unpublished doctoral dissertation, State University of New York at Buffalo.

Klix, F. (1962). *Elementaranalysen zur Psychophysik der Raumwahrnehmung*. Berlin: Verlag der Wissenschaften.

Klix, F. (1984). Über Erkennungsprozesse im menschlichen Gedächtnis. *Zeitschrift für Psychologie*, **192**, 18–46.

Koffka, K. (1935). *Principles of Gestalt Psychology*. New York: Harcourt Brace.

Köhler, W. (1924). *Die physischen Gestalten in Ruhe und im stationären Zustand*. Erlangen: Verlag der Philosophischen Akademie.

Kolers, P. A. and Perkins, D. N. (1969a). Orientation of letters and errors in their recognition. *Perception and Psychophysics*, **5**, 265–269.

Kolers, P. A. and Perkins, D. N. (1969b). Orientation of letters and their speed of recognition. *Perception and Psychophysics*, **5**, 275–280.

Koriat, A. and Norman, J. (1985). Mental rotation and visual familiarity. *Perception and Psychophysics*, **37**, 429–439.

Kosslyn, S. M., Koenig, O., Barrett, A., Cave, C. B., Tang, J. and Gabrieli, J. D. E. (1989). Evidence for two types of spatial representations: Hemispheric specialization for categorical and coordinate relations. *Journal of Experimental Psychology: Human Perception and Performance*, **15**, 723–735.

Kosslyn, S. M. and Schwartz, S. P. (1978). Visual images as spatial representations in active memory. *Computer Vision Systems*, **5**, 223–241.

Kroll, J. K. and Potter, M. C. (1984). Recognizing words, pictures, and concepts: A comparison of lexical, object, and reality decisions. *Journal of Verbal Learning and Verbal Behavior*, **23**, 39–66.

Lambert, A. J. (1987). Expecting different categories at different locations and spatial selective attention. *The Quarterly Journal of Experimental Psychology*, **39A**, 61–76.

Lambert, A. J. and Hockey, R. (1986). Selective attention and performance with a multidimensional visual display. *Journal of Experimental Psychology: Human Perception and Performance*, **12**, 484–495.

Leeuwenberg, E. L. J. (1969). Quantitative specification of information in sequential patterns. *Psychological Review*, **76**, 216–220.

Leeuwenberg, E. L. J. (1971). A perceptual coding language for visual and auditory patterns. *American Journal of Psychology*, **84**, 307–349.

Leeuwenberg, E. L. J. and Boselie, F. (1988). Against the likelihood principle in visual form perception. *Psychological Review*, **95**, 485–491.

Leeuwenberg, E. L. J. and Buffart, H. F. J. (1983). An outline of coding theory, summary of some related experiments. In H. G. Geissler, H. F. J. Buffart, E. L. J. Leeuwenberg and V. Sarris (Eds), *Modern Issues in Perception* (pp. 25–47). Amsterdam: North-Holland.

Loftus, G. R. (1976). A framework for a theory of picture recognition. In R. A. Monty and J. W. Senders (Eds), *Eye Movements and Psychological Processes*. Hillsdale, NJ: Erlbaum.

Loftus, G. R. and Hogden, J. (1988). Extraction of information from complex visual stimuli: Memory performance and phenomenological appearance. In G. H. Bower (Ed.), *The Psychology of Learning and Motivation* (vol. 22, pp. 139-191). New York: Academic Press.

Loftus, G. R. and Mackworth, H. M. (1978). Cognitive determinants of fixation location during picture viewing. *Journal of Experimental Psychology: Human Perception and Performance, 4,* 565–572.

Loftus, G. R., Nelson, W. W. and Kallman, H. J. (1983). Differential acquisition rates for different types of information from pictures. *Quarterly Journal of Experimental Psychology,* **35A,** 187–198.

Lowe, D. G. (1987). Three-dimensional object recognition from single two-dimensional images. *Artificial Intelligence,* **31,** 355–395.

Lupker, S. J. (1988). Picture naming: An investigation of the nature of categorical priming. *Journal of Experimental Psychology: Learning, Memory, and Cognition,* **14,** 444–455.

Maki, R. H. (1986). Naming and locating the tops of rotated pictures. *Canadian Journal of Psychology,* **40,** 368–387.

Mandler, J. M. and Johnson, N. S. (1976). Some of the thousand words a picture is worth. *Journal of Experimental Psychology: Human Learning and Memory,* **2,** 256–263.

Mandler, J. M. and Parker, R. E. (1976). Memory for descriptive and spatial information in complex pictures. *Journal of Experimental Psychology: Human Learning and Memory,* **2,** 38–48.

Mandler, J. M. and Ritchey, G. H. (1977). Long-term memory for pictures. *Journal of Experimental Psychology: Human Learning and Memory,* **3,** 386–396.

Marr, D. (1982). *Vision.* San Francisco: Freeman.

Marr, D. and Nishihara, H. K. (1978). Representation and recognition of the spatial organization of three-dimensional shapes. *Proceedings of the Royal Society of London (series B),* **200,** 269–294.

Martin, M. (1979). Local and global processing: The role of sparsity. *Memory and Cognition,* **7,** 476–484.

McClelland, J. L. and Rumelhart, D. E. (1981). An interactive activation model of context effects in letter perception: Part 1. An account of basic findings. *Psychological Review,* **88,** 375–407.

McEvoy, C. L. (1988). Automatic and strategic processes in picture naming. *Journal of Experimental Psychology: Learning, Memory, and Cognition,* **14,** 618–626.

Medin, D. L., Wattenmaker, W. D. and Hampson, S. E. (1987). Family resemblance, conceptual cohesiveness, and category construction. *Cognitive Psychology,* **19,** 242–279.

Mervis, C. B. and Crisafi, M. A. (1982). Order of acquisition of subordinate-, basic-, and superordinate-level categories. *Child Development,* **53,** 258–266.

Mervis, C. B. and Rosch, E. (1981). Categorization of natural objects. *Annual Review of Psychology,* **32,** 89–115.

Metzger, R. L. and Antes, J. R. (1983). The nature of processing early in picture perception. *Psychological Research,* **45,** 267–274.

Metzger, W. (1975). *Die Gesetze des Sehens,* 3rd edn. Frankfurt: Kramer.

Metzler, J. and Shepard, R. N. (1974). Transformational studies of the internal representation of three-dimensional objects. In R. L. Solso (Ed.), *Theories in Cognitive Psychology: The Loyola Symposium* (pp. 147–201). San Francisco: Freeman.

Meyers, L. S. and Rhoades, R. W. (1978). Visual search of common scenes. *Quarterly Journal of Experimental Psychology,* **30,** 297–310.

Miller, J. (1981a). Global precedence in attention and decision. *Journal of Experimental Psychology: Human Perception and Performance,* **7,** 1161–1174.

Miller, J. (1981b). Global precedence: Information availability or use? Reply to Navon. *Journal of Experimental Psychology: Human Perception and Performance,* **7,** 1183–1185.

Miller, J. (1988). Components of the location probability effect in visual search tasks. *Journal of Experimental Psychology: Human Perception and Performance,* **14,** 453–471.

Miller, J. and Festinger, L. (1977). Impact of oculomotor retraining on the visual perception of curvature. *Journal of Experimental Psychology: Human Perception and Performance,* **3,** 187–200.

Mitchell, D. B. and Brown, A. S. (1988). Persistent repetition priming in picture naming and its dissociation from recognition memory. *Journal of Experimental Psychology: Learning, Memory, and Cognition,* **14,** 213–222.

Murphy, G. L. and Brownell, H. H. (1985). Category differentiation in object recognition: Typicality constraints on the basic category advantage. *Journal of Experimental Psychology: Learning, Memory, and Cognition,* **11,** 70–84.

Murphy, G. L. and Smith, E. E. (1982). Basic level superiority in picture categorization. *Journal of Verbal Learning and Verbal Behavior,* **21,** 1–20.

Murphy, G. L. and Wisniewski, E. J. (1989). Categorizing objects in isolation and in scenes: What a superordinate is good for. *Journal of Experimental Psychology: Learning, Memory, and Cognition,* **15,** 572–586.

Navon, D. (1977). Forest before trees: The precedence of global features in visual perception. *Cognitive Psychology,* **9,** 353–383.

Navon, D. (1981a). Do attention and decision follow perception? Comment on Miller. *Journal of Experimental Psychology: Human Perception and Performance,* **7,** 1175–1182.

Navon, D. (1981b). The forest revisited: More on global precedence. *Psychological Research,* **43,** 1–32.

Neisser, U. (1967). *Cognitive Psychology.* New York: Appleton-Century-Crofts.

Neisser, U. (1976). *Cognition and Reality.* San Francisco: Freeman.

Neisser, U. (1978). Anticipations, images, and introspection. *Cognition,* **6,** 169–174.

Neumann, O. (1989). Kognitive Vermittlung und direkte Parameterspezifikation. Zum Problem mentaler Repräsentation in der Wahrnehmung. *Sprache und Kognition,* **8,** 32–49.

Neumann, O. and Prinz, W. (1987). Kognitive Antezedenzien von Willkürhandlungen. In H. Heckhausen, P. M. Gollwitzer, and F. E. Weinert (Eds), *Jenseits des Rubikon: Der Wille in den Humanwissenschaften* (pp. 195–215). Berin: Springer.

Neumann, O. and Prinz, W. (1990a). Prologue: Historical approaches to perception and action. In O. Neumann and W. Prinz (Eds), *Relationships between Perception and Action* (pp. 5–19). Berlin, New York: Springer.

Neumann, O. and Prinz, W. (Eds) (1990b). *Relationships between Perception and Action.* Berlin, New York: Springer.

Palmer, S. (1975). The effects of contextual scenes on the identification of objects. *Memory and Cognition,* **3,** 519–526.

Palmer, S. (1977). Hierarchical structure in perceptual representation. *Cognitive Psychology,* **9,** 441–474.

Palmer, S., Rosch, E. and Chase, P. (1981). Canonical perspective and the perception of objects. In J. Long and A. Baddeley (Eds), *Attention and Performance,* vol. 9 (pp. 135–151). Hillsdale, NJ: Erlbaum.

Paquet, L. and Merikle, P. M. (1988). Global precedence in attended and nonattended objects. *Journal of Experimental Psychology: Human Perception and Performance,* **14,** 89–100.

Parsons, L. M. (1987). Imagined spatial transformations of one's hands and feet. *Cognitive Psychology,* **19,** 178–241.

Pezdek, K., Maki, R., Valencia-Laver, D., Whetstone, T. Stoeckert, J. and Dougherty, T. (1988). Picture memory: Recognizing added and deleted details. *Journal of Experimental Psychology: Learning, Memory, and Cognition,* **14,** 468–476.

Pezdek, K., Whetstone, T., Reynolds, K., Askari, N. and Dougherty, T. (1989). Memory for real-world scenes: The role of consistency with schema expectation. *Journal of Experimental Psychology: Learning, Memory, and Cognition,* **15,** 587–595.

Pollatsek, A., Rayner, K. and Collins, W. E. (1984). Integrating pictorial information across eye movements. *Journal of Experimental Psychology: General,* **113,** 426–442.

Pollatsek, A., Rayner, K. and Henderson, J. M. (1990). Role of spatial location in integration of pictorial information across saccades. *Journal of Experimental Psychology: Human Perception and Performance,* **16,** 199–210.

Pomerantz, J. R. (1981). Perceptual organization in information processing. In M. Kubovy and J. R. Pomerantz (Eds), *Perceptual Organization* (pp. 141–180). Hillsdale, NJ: Erlbaum.

Pomerantz, J. R. (1983). Global and local precedence: Selective attention in form and motion perception. *Journal of Experimental Psychology: General,* **112,** 516–540.

Pomerantz, J. R. and Kubovy, M. (1986). Theoretical approaches to perceptual organization: Simplicity and likelihood principles. In K. R. Boff, L. Kaufman and J. P. Thomas (Eds), *Handbook of Perception and Human Performance,* vol. 2 (pp. 36.1–36.46). New York: John Wiley.

Pomerantz, J. R., Sager, L. G. and Stoever, R. J. (1977). Perception of wholes and of their component parts: Some configural superiority effects. *Journal of Experimental Psychology: Human Perception and Performance,* **3,** 422–435.

Prinz, W. (1983). *Wahrnehmung und Tätigkeitssteuerung.* Berlin: Springer.

Prinz, W. (1984). Modes of linkage between perception and action. In W. Prinz and A. F. Sanders (Eds), *Cognition and Motor Processes* (pp. 185–194). Berlin, New York: Springer.

Prinz, W. (1990). A common-coding approach to perception and action. In O. Neumann and W. Prinz (Eds), *Relationships between Perception and Action* (pp. 5–19). Berlin, New York: Springer.

Reed, S. K. (1978). Schemes and theories of pattern recognition. In E. C. Carterette and M. P. Friedman (Eds), *Handbook of Perception,* vol. 9: *Perceptual Processing* (pp. 137–162). New York: Academic Press.

Reinert, G. (1985). Schemata als Grundlage der Steuerung von Blickbewegungen bei der Bildverarbeitung. In O. Neumann (Ed.), *Perspektiven der Kognitionspsychologie* (pp. 113–146). Berlin: Springer.

Reinitz, M. T., Wright, E. and Loftus, G. R. (1989). Effects of semantic priming on visual encoding of pictures. *Journal of Experimental Psychology: General,* **118,** 280–297.

Robertson L. C., Palmer, S. E. and Gomez, L. M. (1987). Reference frames in mental rotation. *Journal of Experimental Psychology: Learning, Memory, and Cognition,* **13,** 368–379.

Rock, I. (1973). *Orientation and Form.* New York: Academic Press.

Rock, I. and DiVita, J. (1987). A case of viewer-centered object perception. *Cognitive Psychology,* **19,** 280–293.

Rock, I., DiVita, J. and Barbeito, R. (1981). The effect on form perception of change of orientation in the third dimension. *Journal of Experimental Psychology: Human Perception and Performance,* **7,** 719–732.

Rock, I., Wheeler, D. and Tudor, L. (1989). Can we imagine how objects look from other viewpoints? *Cognitive Psychology,* **21,** 185–210.

Rosch, E. (1975). Cognitive representations of semantic categories. *Journal of Experimental Psychology: General,* **104,** 192–233.

Rosch, E. (1977). Human categorization. In N. Warren (Ed.), *Studies in Crosscultural Psychology,* vol. 1 (pp. 3–49). London: Academic Press.

Rosch, E. and Mervis, C. B. (1975). Family resemblances: Studies in the internal structure of categories. *Cognitive Psychology,* **7,** 573–605.

Rosch, E. Mervis, C. B., Gray, W. D., Johnson, D. M. and Boyes-Braem, P. (1976). Basic objects in natural categories. *Cognitive Psychology,* **8,** 382–439.

Rumelhart, D. E. and McClelland, J. L. (1982). An interactive activation model of context effects in letter perception. Part 2: The contextual enhancement effect and some tests and extensions of the model. *Psychological Review,* **89,** 60–94.

Seguí, J. and Fraisse, P. (1968). Le temps de réaction verbale. iii. Réponses spécifiques et réponses catégorielles à des stimulus objets. *Année Psychologigue,* **68,** 69–82.

Selfridge, O. G. and Neisser, U. (1960). Pattern recognition by machine. *Scientific American,* **203,** 60–68.

Sergent, J. and Corballis, M. C. (1989). Categorization of disoriented faces in the cerebral hemispheres of normal and commissurotomized subjects. *Journal of Experimental Psychology: Human Perception and Performance*, **15**, 701–710.

Seymor, P. H. K. (1973). A model for reading, naming, and comparison. *British Journal of Psychology*, **64**, 35–49.

Shepard, R. N. and Cooper, L. A. (1982). *Mental Images and their Transformation*. Cambridge, MA: Bradford Books/MIT, Press.

Shepard, R. N. and Metzler, J. (1971). Mental rotation of three-dimensional objects. *Science*, **171**, 701–705.

Shepard, S. and Metzler, D. (1988). Mental rotation: Effects of dimensionality of objects and type of task. *Journal of Experimental Psychology: Human Perception and Performance*, **14**, 3–11.

Sperber, R. D., McCauley, C., Ragain, R. D. and Weil, C. M. (1979). Semantic priming effects on picture and word processing. *Memory and Cognition*, **7**, 339–345.

Takano, Y. (1989). Perception of rotated forms: A theory of information types. *Cognitive Psychology*, **21**, 1–59.

Tarr, M. J. and Pinker, S. (1989). Mental rotation and orientation-dependence in shape recognition. *Cognitive Psychology*, **21**, 233–282.

Theios, J. and Amrhein, P. C. (1989). Theoretical analysis of the cognitive processing of lexical and pictorial stimuli: Reading, naming, and visual and conceptual comparisons. *Psychological Review*, **96**, 5–24.

Tipper, S. P. (1985). The negative priming effect: Inhibitory priming by ignored objects. *Memory and Cognition*, **7**, 339–345.

Tipper, S. P. and Driver, J. (1988). Negative priming between pictures and words in a selective attention task: Evidence for semantic processing of ignored stimuli. *Memory and Cognition*, **16**, 64–70.

Turvey, M. T. and Carello, C. (1986). The ecological approach to perceiving–acting: A pictorial essay. *Acta Psychologica*, **63**, 133–155.

Turvey, M. T., Solomon, H. Y. and Burton, G. (1989). An ecological analysis of knowing by wielding. *Journal of the Experimental Analysis of Behavior*, **52**, 387–407.

Tversky, B. and Hemenway, K. (1983). Categories of environmental scenes. *Cognitive Psychology*, **15**, 121–149.

Tversky, B. and Hemenway, K. (1984). Objects, parts, and categories. *Journal of Experimental Psychology: General*, **113**, 169–193.

Ungerleider, L. G. (1985). The corticocortical pathways for object recognition and spatial perception. In C. G. Chagas, R. Gattass, and C. Gross (Eds), *Pattern Recognition Mechanisms*. Rome: Pontificiae Academiae Scientiarum Scripta Varia.

von Holst, E. and Mittelstaedt, H. (1950). Das Reafferenzprinzip. Wechselwirkungen zwischen ZNS und Peripherie. *Naturwissenschaften*, **37**, 464–476.

von Weizsäcker, V. (1950). *Der Gestaltkreis – Theorie der Einheit von Wahrnehmen und Bewegen*, 4th edn. Stuttgart: Georg Thieme.

Wandmacher, J. and Arend, U. (1985). Superiority of global features in classification and matching. *Psychological Research*, **47**, 143–157.

Ward, L. M. (1982). Determinants of attention to local and global features of visual forms. *Journal of Experimental Psychology: Human Perception and Performance*, **8**, 562–581.

Warren, C. and Morton, J. (1982). The effects of priming on picture recognition. *British Journal of Psychology*, **73**, 117–129.

Wertheimer, M. (1923). Untersuchungen zur Lehre von der Gestalt. *Psychologische Forschung*, **4**, 301–350.

Wertheimer, M. (1925). *Drei Abhandlungen zur Gestaltpsychologie*. Erlangen: Palm und Enke.

White, M. J. (1980). Naming and categorization of tilted alphanumeric characters do not require mental rotation. *Bulletin of the Psychonomic Society*, **15**, 153–156.

Wilson, H. R. and Bergen, J. R. (1979). A four-mechanism model of spatial vision. *Vision Research*, **19**, 19–32.

Winston, P. H. (1975). Learning structural descriptions from examples. In P. H. Winston (Ed.), *The Psychology of Computer Vision* (pp. 157–209). New York: McGraw-Hill.

Witkin, A. P. and Tenenbaum, M. (1983). On the role of structure in vision. In A. Rosenfeld, B. Hope, and J. Beck (Eds), *Human and Machine Vision* (pp. 481–543). New York: Academic Press.

Wittgenstein, L. (1953). *Philosophical Investigations*. New York: Macmillan.

Wolff, P. (1985). Wahrnehmungslernen durch Blickbewegungen. In O. Neumann (Ed.), *Perspektiven der Kognitionspsychologie* (pp. 63–111). Berlin: Springer.

Wolff, P. (1986). Saccadic exploration and perceptual motor learning. *Acta Psychologica*, **63**, 263–280.

Zießler, M. and Hoffmann, J. (1987). Die Verarbeitung visueller Reize und die Steuerung motorischen Verhaltens: Zwei sich wechselseitig beeinflussende Prozesse. *Psychologische Beiträge*, **29**, 524–557.

Zimmer, H. D. (1983). *Sprache und Bildwahrnehmung*. Frankfurt: Haag und Herchen.

Zimmer, H. D. (1984). Blume oder Rose? Unterschiede in der visuellen Informationsverarbeitung bei Experten und Laien. *Archiv für Psychologie*, **136**, 343–361.

Zimmer, H. D. and Biegelmann, U. E. (1990). Klassifikation globaler und lokaler Basisbegriffe bei Variation des Merkmal-Onset. *Arbeiten der Fachrichtung Psychologie*, **152**. Saarbrücken, Germany: University of the Saarland.

Chapter 10
Dimensions of Event Perception

Robert E. Shaw*, Oded M. Flascher* and William M. Mace[†]

*University of Connecticut and [†]Trinity College, Connecticut

'The essence of rhythm is the fusion of sameness and novelty; so that the whole never loses the essential unity of the pattern, while the parts exhibit the contrast arising from the novelty of detail. A mere recurrence kills rhythm as surely does a mere confusion of differences. A crystal lacks rhythm from excessive pattern, while a fog is unrhythmic in that it exhibits a patternless confusion of detail.' (Alfred North Whitehead, 1919, *Principles of Natural Knowledge*)

'We should begin thinking of events as the primary realities and of time as an abstraction from them... It is the same with space as with time.... There is always some degree of recurrence and some degree of nonrecurrence in the flow of ecological events.' (James J. Gibson, 1979, *The Ecological Approach to Visual Perception*)

1 INTRODUCTION: ISSUES, PROBLEMS AND ATTITUDES

What makes stimulation informative? Although there is not an abundance of research on this topic, no field of perceptual psychology other than event perception addresses the issue of how we perceive change. Since the topic is essentially new, having but a few pioneers such as Michotte, Gibson and Johansson, no general terminology, principles or methodology is shared by researchers in the area. Hence, reports pertaining to event perception are often more difficult to recognize than they should be. Rarely do we find a clear statement by authors as to what they take the problem of event perception to be. Relevant reports typically must be selected by *prima facie* evidence alone.

A report may seem relevant on the surface because it purports to describe the information specifying some kind of change, such as the detection of motion, or simply because it uses the term 'event'. Such usage is rarely technically precise. We found that such *prima facie* evidence often led nowhere and sometimes was even misleading.

On too many occasions when a report seemed of obvious interest, the discussion of results would leave unanswered what conclusions the authors wished to draw about event perception. Consequently, it was left to us not only to explain the relevance and to supply such conclusions but also to fashion a framework in which relevance might be ascertained and conclusions drawn. In doing so, it was inevitable that we should have to draw on our own perspectives to do so. This, of

Handbook of Perception and Action: Volume 1
ISBN 0-12-516161-1

course, made it impossible to keep this 'review' theoretically neutral. The reader is, therefore, forewarned.

A persistent problem encountered is that studies offering models for the detection of event-related properties typically fail to distinguish between description and explanation. Too often the only explanation given for how the event in question was perceived was to describe some hypothetical mechanism which undergoes a given state transition whenever the event undergoes a correlated transition. Clearly, nothing is gained if a theory introduces as an explanation of how some x occurs, an indicator that some y occurs (where x and y refer to different acts, experiences or processes). Such descriptive mechanisms, even if true, are not explanations but are themselves to be explained.

Clearly, nothing is gained if one attempts to explain the perception of x by describing the detection of something that is not x itself. For then we must face the conundrum of how the occurrence of one kind of thing (say, an event in the central nervous system CNS) can be taken as detection of another kind of thing (say, the causally contributing environmental event). The two may be *coextensive* (i.e. occur together) and yet not be *cointensive* (i.e. mean the same thing). Why are some state transitions informative about other state transitions? Why do they point beyond themselves rather than merely at themselves? And even if they point beyond themselves (what philosophers call their *intentionality*), of what consequence is this pointing? And for whom? The author of the model? Or the perceiver being modelled? Not only is this patently unclear, but the ambiguity goes essentially unacknowledged in the literature.

Hence, the fundamental problem for perceptual psychology is to explain how the coextensive can somehow be equivalent to the cointensive. A solution to this problem calls for a theory of perceptual information and an understanding of the nature of its specificity to the underlying environmental referents. The details of such a theory have yet to be given. Consequently, we must proceed without such help.

A related problem is recognizing that having a model for a mechanism that detects stimulation (not information) from some referent x is not equivalent to having an explanation of the perception of x, that is, how stimulation is made informative by the act of detection. It does not obviously resolve the puzzle of how a change in state of some internal mechanism, even if truly triggered by a specific change in environmental state (i.e. even if coextensive), can be informative (i.e. cointensive) about the associated environmental event. For a surrogate (e.g. a representation, a specification) to be useful, it must already be known to be a surrogate of something – to have intentionality – otherwise it is merely itself. Thus, the problem of the specificational import of information is the problem of how properties in the medium that are coextensive with the properties of the object of perception can be taken as cointensive with them. Coextensionality, say even as perfect correlation, does not logically guarantee cointensionality – having the same meaning – even if the specification is unique.

Often psychologists, following Helmholtz, will suggest that meaning accrues from stimulation by some kind of unconscious inference process. This contrasts with the view championed by those psychologists following Gibson, who claim that the relationship between the two is fundamentally noninferential – a view they call specificational. Neither of these approaches is adequate as it stands but demands clarification of its relevance to the intentionality problem. An attempt is made later to elucidate these contrasting views (see Section 1.3).

At this time, in the early development of the embryonic field of event perception, there seems to be no lucid discussion of this intentionality problem among those who evoke information or cue detection models. Coextensionality of predicates with properties referred to is addressed but their cointensionality is ignored. Smoke may be coextensive with fire but does not mean fire. Smoke is dark and billowy while fire is bright and licking. Similarly, certain cues (e.g. height in the picture plane, interposition) may accompany (be coextensive with) certain perceptual experiences of three-dimensional layout, but they are not the content of (cointensive with) the phenomenological experience of 'depth'. For instance, height in the picture plane is not 'depth'. For two objects may have different heights while being at the same distance from the observer, while two objects at different distances may have the same height. The fundamental question is: under what circumstances do physical features take on cue functions or information functions?

Attempts by Gestaltists (their principle of psychophysical isomorphism), by Wittgenstein, Russell, by Gibson and Gibsonians, and by Fodor and other contemporary correspondence theorists provide no notable help on this problem. For some of us, the coextensional aspects of stimulation with event or object properties is all that science should realistically be expected to address – leaving the cointensive aspects of information for the semanticists or philosophers. If so, then the concept of information collapses onto the concept of stimulation to which it is specific and cointension collapses onto coextension. This is like the message collapsing onto the signal in communication theory. Such reductionism makes the problem of perception a mystery rather than just a difficult problem. Gibson (1979) was quite aware of these dangers in that he emphasized the distinction between the type of change in the world (e.g. translation of one object in front of another), as the physicist might describe it, and the kind of disturbances in the optic array (e.g. certain accretion and deletion disturbances of texture) that embody the information about such changes, in the sense of being specific to them, without need of inferential enhancement.

Consequently, since this important issue is not adequately covered in the perception literature, the reader should not expect it to be laid to rest here. Instead, ecological psychologists believe the field is better served by directing its efforts toward discovering and describing the useful dimensions of stimulation for the control of action, while traditional theorists believe that perception is the having of an experience in the theater of the mind and the making of judgments thereof. The challenge of the intentionality problem is still worthy of pondering by both kinds of theorists since neither camp has a lock on the issue.

Even if there is no known solution to the recalcitrant intentionality problem, it still makes sense to ask what makes some information more informative than other stimulation. This means that in addition to showing that an event is causally responsible for a state transition in a model, one has to show how the state transition is informative – how the result not only entails the causally antecedent conditions that give rise to it but also how it does so for the agent for whom the model is intended. The key difficulty with this form of reasoning is that it is *post hoc ergo ante hoc* – meaning 'that which comes after entails that which goes before' – and is not causal since its entailment inverts the usual (chronological) order of antecedents and consequents required for them to represent a cause and effect sequence. Perceptual theory cannot avoid nor justify, under current theories of logical inference, this form of reasoning. (But see Rosen, 1991, for an interesting discussion of finality and entailment.)

Of course, perceptual psychologists are not the only theorists who have failed to resolve this thorny logical problem. But perhaps we are most guilty of ignoring it. By failure to acknowledge this problem of acausal specification (backward entailment), we imply that the perception of x might be explained by the mere existence of a putative mechanism that responds uniquely to the occurrence of x. In doing so, we are not only guilty of tolerating faulty reasoning but egregiously so. Until the hypothesized mechanisms incorporate a general theory of specificational information (i.e. includes an explanation of the backward entailment required of intentionality), then any solution to the problem of how x is detected leaves an unbridgeable gap to explaining how x is perceived.

When the general field of perception is ill-defined, it makes it difficult to delimit the scope of inquiry into a subfield. Lacking a consensus, it is nevertheless necessary to impose questions to set the bounds on the review. Consequently, we have tried to formulate these questions in such a way as to provide a generic framework to guide the selection and discussion of research on event perception. The fact that we are ecological psychologists, we hope, did not reduce our appreciation of the efforts of our colleagues of a different ilk, but no doubt has put a spin on the discussion that will not be to everyone's liking. A true review, perhaps, must be left to some later time, when sufficient consensus has been reached on the problem of intentionality and perceptual entailment to fashion a field with shared empirical and theoretical foundations. We hope the directions and dimensions of event perception discerned here help in this regard.

1.1   Stretching the Boundaries of Event Perception

More than a decade has passed since the last major review of the event perception literature (Johansson, von Hofsten and Jansson, 1980). In opening their review the authors say: '...We have broadened the term "event perception" in an important respect. The review will not be limited to perception of object motion in a passive perceiver, but will pay attention also to recent studies dealing with motion and movement perception in an active perceiver, thus motion and space perception in connection with action...' (p. 28). Johansson *et al.* point out that most traditional research had focused on static displays and emphasized the role of spatial information, such as position, shape and configuration. With the aid of certain technological advances, the field first broadened to include strobotic or cinematic sampling of motion and other forms of change. Later, by the time of their review, the field had broadened again to include real motion displays, where the change was continuously presented rather than merely discretely sampled. They were clearly justified in this extension of the topic, for it has been established that, other things being equal, the range of temporal factors for the perception of apparent motion and real motion events are quite different (Braddick, 1974); and that, in general, they have both different causes and different effects (Kolers, 1972; see below).

In the current review we should like to broaden once again the terrain to be covered. We should like to pay attention not only to motion and space perception in connection with action but to replace the traditional treatment of time as but an additional spatial dimension – a geometric view of time – (with a true appreciation that event perception has its referents in *space–time*. The nineteenth-century view that change is but a sequence of static displacements in a structureless space must give way to the twentieth-century insight that change is itself a real process that acts to deform the structure of space–time (Capek, 1961). Here events replace objects and change replaces displacements. Until we psychologists master this more demanding concept of space–time and replace the less adequate and inaccurate space and time geometry, the true basis of perceptual information will no doubt continue to be elusive. This chapter is organized so as to present graded steps to this end. The reader is first introduced to space and time geometries of events and then is moved toward an appreciation of the space–time geometries of events. If the reader bears this in mind, then the motivation for the various event descriptions will be apparent.

In addition to broadening the topic from space and time to space–time, we shall introduce some refinements to help focus the field, most notably as pertains to the description of events and the information by which they are perceived. We make no pretense to offering a full review of the existing literature (but see Johansson, von Hofsten and Jansson, 1980; Warren and Shaw, 1985); rather, our main goal will be to clarify certain fundamental problems and issues that lie at the foundations of the field.

1.2 Approaches to Event Perception

It seems an incontrovertible fact that animals and humans have the general perceptual capability not only to distinguish between change and nonchange but also to classify styles of change as well as the objects that undergo change. Event perception, then, can be defined as: *the detection of information about a style of change that a structure undergoes over some determinate region of space–time.* Two fundamental aspects of event perception must be accounted for: first, how one perceives change at all; and, second, how one perceives particular styles of change as such. Pittenger and Shaw (1975a, b) introduced the terms *transformational invariant* (TI) and *structural invariant* (SI) as denoting the style of change that is perceived and that which undergoes the style of change, respectively.

Using these terms, an event (E) is said to be perceptually specified when both of these terms of invariant information (i.e. TI and SI) are available to be detected – that is, when the two-variable function E(TI, SI) can be evaluated. For instance, an event involving a bouncing ball might be denoted as E(TI = bouncing, SI = ball) = bouncing ball. A major aim of this chapter is to show how such event functions might be conveniently diagrammed and their separable space–time component functions studied.

A third corollary problem has to do with the distinction between extracting information specific to a style of change from a background of complex change, as opposed simply to detecting a style of change in an isolated context. We might ask what makes a given style of change more visibly salient, say at one scale, when other styles of change might, in principle, be informationally specified at other scales of description? To extract such information calls for some additional constraint over and beyond specification, what we might call *objectification* of the information in question. More will be said about this later.

Finally, a fourth important question that will not be considered in much detail concerns how one perceives object properties (e.g. rigidity) or properties of the layout of objects (e.g. distance, depth) under conditions of change that are not perceived under static conditions. The detection of information for structurally invariant properties (i.e. SIs) under various styles of change (i.e. given TIs) is an important related problem for event perception research without actually *being* event perception as such. For in focusing primarily on the perception of SI properties involved in an event, the TI properties play but an ancillary role. The importance of this question for event perception proper would be more assured if TIs were perceptually classified in terms of SIs, rather than the other way around which seems to be the case.

This is not, however, to overlook the fact that information for change and information for structures involved in the change often do interact. Clearly, objects must be detectable or there would be no informational support for the perception of change. Consequently, some discussion of the role that object properties (SIs) play in setting the necessary boundary conditions on event perception is unavoidable (Mark, Shapiro and Shaw, 1986).

The study of the detection (as opposed to the extraction) of information for the TI component of events can be broken down into two fundamental issues. The first issue concerns the nature of information for change (variants) as opposed to nonchange (invariants). Here, the majority of the research has addressed the distinction between real and apparent motion events. The second fundamental issue has received much less study. This issue concerns the information by which different styles of change, or categories of TIs, are perceptually recognized. Here, how one chooses to describe events (e.g. motion) is of the utmost importance.

Three event geometries are logically possible: the first approach attempts to reduce change to nonchange so that events might be spatialized. Differences in positional or configurational information are deemed sufficient to express change, with the implication that events may be captured in Euclidean space by the use of time tags. A second approach uses spatiotemporal descriptions but without restrictions on the range of values the temporal dimension might assume relative to the spatial dimension. We call this the orthogonal *space and time* geometry of events and identify it with the Galilean (space plus time) frame of classical physics. It is still Euclidean but with time treated as but another spatial dimension.

Finally, there is the possibility of a Minkowski-like space–time (event) geometry derived from special relativity which treats the two dimensions of time and space nonorthogonally and, therefore, as capable of interacting. Here, in order to keep our intuitions intact, the Minkowski space–time continuum, for convenience, is treated as embedded in Euclidean geometry (although more properly it might be treated as a separate geometry that is intrinsically hyperbolic; for a helpful introduction, see Caelli, 1981, and Caelli, Hoffman and Lindman, 1978). Over the past decade or so, there has been a growing interest in variants of such space–time descriptions of events for describing both perceptual information and action control (Adelson and Bergen, 1985; Brown, 1931; Caelli, 1981; Caelli, Hoffman and Lindman, 1978; Kugler *et al.*, 1985; Shaw and Kinsella-Shaw, 1988).

1.3   Attitudes Toward Event Information

There are three basic attitudes that one might hold regarding the origin and nature of perceptual information for change.

1.3.1 Change Inferred from Structure

The first attitude follows a Helmholtzian-like assumption that information from structural differences detected over time provides the premises, or deductive basis, by which change over time might be unconsciously inferred. It assumes that information about change involves inferences from a successively ordered sequence of samples (e.g. glimpses) of continuous motion (see Haber, 1983, for a review). Many contemporary views of cognitive science assume that change perception consists of mental representations of the successive samples that are related by computations (Fodor and Pylyshyn, 1981, 1986). Although computations, formally speaking, are not inferences, they provide a means by which the inferences are represented. Both the inferential and computational views treat such discrete perceptual samples as if they were cinematic frames. Here, change is thought to be derived from an act of cognitively comparing positional differences over successive frames while ignoring the in-between blackout interval. Perceptual persistence is typically argued to be responsible for our inability to see the blackout interval. Hence, there is no information for change as such, rather change is treated as an inferential construction. Evidence for this view is often taken from picture perception, stroboscopic and cinematic motion perception. It contrasts sharply with the noncognitive views – to be discussed next – that information for change is somehow made available by events themselves through direct (noninferential) specification.

The inferring-of-change-from-structure hypothesis suffers from three problems: first, the paradox of how change might somehow be derived from nonchange; second, how perceiving might be interpreted as inferring; and third, the need to have an internal observer that glimpses what is cinematically projected and then carries out the 'perceptual' (unconscious) inference. Since the inner observer might be the first but not necessarily the last internal observer required, the cinematic metaphor can lead to an infinite regress if not terminated by some principled final state. No one has suggested a terminating principle that is consensually accepted. Thus, the potential regress is typically ignored or, if not ignored, then terminated arbitrarily, say, by a final step that treats the static differences in position as being inferentially equivalent to the phenomenological content and ushers the experiences of change into the theater of the mind.

How this last inferential step from information to experience is made, no one knows. More is known about the first step where environmental energy from events is transduced into information events in the nervous system. Consequently, incommensurability of environmental energy distributions, physiological processes and psychological experiences is generally recognized as a serious problem for any causal chain model of perception. By using the word 'inference' to bridge the gaps, the incommensurability problem is not resolved but is compounded for two reasons.

First, and a point usually ignored that deserves careful attention, is that since computational steps may represent either valid or invalid inferences equally well, then valid inference cannot be identified with computation (e.g. as Hochberg, 1964; Rock, 1975; Ullman, 1980, do). Inferences are syntactical and truth-functional, while computations are merely syntactical. Second, it is generally agreed that to make an inference requires that the inferrer intend an inference, in the sense of recognizing the truth of the premises, following the train of reasoning, and 'seeing' that the conclusion follows. If so, then how can an inference be unconscious and intended at the same time? An unconscious inference is an oxymoron, for either it is conscious or not an inference. (For instance, the full-blown hypothesis asserts that unconscious conclusions from unnoticed sensations can be used to explain perceptual achievements; Hochberg, 1964, p. 55.)

Our point is not that no sense might be made of this hypothesis but that no sense has been made of it in the literature that uses the hypothesis or entails it. The hypothesis has often been asserted but the problem of rationalizing it has been chiefly ignored by psychologists (although Fodor and Pylyshyn's, 1986, attack on connectionism brings a variant of this issue to the forefront). Given these problems, why, then, is this a perennially favorite view?

The presumed strength of this view is that apparent motion effects and other *virtual* events can be treated as examples of *real* event perception. Given the putative role of inference or 'computation', nothing essential is assumed to be lost by studying the perception of strobotically or cinematically produced events in lieu of the more difficult-to-study real world events. If, however, real events produced in the world kinetically and virtual events produced strobotically or cinematically (and here we must also include video and computer graphics) are not essentially the same information sources, for the reasons pointed out earlier, then we have two phenomena to study that require two theories. Under the change-inferred-from-structure view both empirical research and theory construction seem to be made simpler. This feature may account for the perennial popularity of this view. Unfortunately, the difficulty of making clear, how perceiving, inferring and computing may be the same process in all relevant ways, makes this virtue more apparent than real.

1.3.2 Change Extracted from Structure

A second view, in contrast with the first view, eschews the inferential hypothesis and argues from information detection alone. This view assumes that information about change does exist and is specific to the properties of an object left invariant while undergoing a given style of change. (Recall that information about change may be conveyed by stimulation from change but is functionally and logically distinct from it.) Invariant properties are those that do not change *relative to other properties* under a given style of change. This is the inverse of the *structure-extracted-from-change* view (Cutting, 1986; Ullman, 1979), where the term extraction is used advisedly. (Here, it refers to the process by which a given property is detected among the background of other properties.)

For instance, an object whose shape does not change while undergoing a rotation or translation is said to be a rigid object and the change a rigid transformation. Hence, rotation and translation are both rigid transformations. These transformations may then be distinguished from other nonrigid styles of change like compression, stretching, bending and breaking that alter the shape of the object. This approach treats information for a TI as being reducible to information for some SI.

But what invariant structural property, SI, distinguishes rotation from translation? There simply is none. For with respect to structural invariants like shape, rotating an object is no different from translating it. No change in any object property is introduced by either. Reorientation by rotation or relocation by translation involve no object properties but rather involve properties of the object's relationship to the spatiotemporal frame in which it is reoriented or relocated. Such context-dependent properties are functionally defined, like axis points or closed circular traces (as opposed to rectilinear traces); these do indeed serve to distinguish rotation from translation. But these are not object properties (SIs): they are transformationally defined invariants (TIs). They are dynamical, existing only over time – disappearing whenever rotation stops. These properties are visible as blur streaklines when the rates of rotation or translation become too fast for the visual system to process (where rate is measured in arc units of visual angle per unit time) or when a long time-exposure photographic record is made.

Finally, the change-extracted-from-structure approach also suffers from the obvious defect that it explains the source of information for structure (e.g. rigidity) but not the source of the information for change itself (rolling versus spinning). Therefore, to argue that structural invariants extracted from the persistence of certain object properties somehow specifies change encounters the same conundrum as the change-inferred-from-structure view; namely: *how can types of spatial persistence specify types of temporal nonpersistence*? (See Ullman, 1979, for a discussion of how the extraction processes in both of these views might operate; but see Todd, 1981, for a telling criticism of Ullman's account.)

Under this extraction view the notion of specification is open to two different interpretations: a style of change can either be uniquely specified by a structurally invariant property determined under that style of change or it might be multiply specified by more than one structural property. If one invariant property can be specific to the change that revealed it, why cannot another? And if another, why not another and another and another and so forth? One would need a proof that only a single SI was associated with a given TI for uniqueness to hold. We underscore this problem but do not attempt to resolve it (see Pittenger, 1989, 1990; Stoffregen, 1990, for a relevant debate).

1.3.3   Only Change Specifies Change

Finally, there is a third alternative which might be called the *extraction-of-change-from-change* view. Under this approach events are defined in terms of invariants that are stationary over spatiotemporal dimensions. The detection of these invariants over the continuants (e.g. streamlines) of the change constitutes the direct perception of the style of change by which the event can be classified (Shaw and Pittenger, 1978). Assuming this view can be made coherent, it is very attractive. For under this view the most troublesome issues encountered under the first two views do not even arise. However, this view is less familiar than the other two; thus, we pause to place it in perspective. We do so in the next two sections.

1.4   Transformational Invariant as a Persistence Over Change

The first view considered holds that information for change can be inferred from information derived from structure. Thus, under this view change as such (i.e. a TI) is not perceived at all but is derived inferentially from positional or configurational information (i.e. from SIs). The second view is related; it holds that structural properties are informationally specified rather than inferred and, therefore, directly perceived. However, it also assumes that styles of change (TIs) do not stand on their own but are derived from structural information (SIs).

Different events may involve the same objects while the same event may involve different objects. For instance, a ball may bounce or it may spin or roll. These are not the same events simply because they involve the same object; nor are they the same events because the (elastically restored) shape of the ball is shared as a structural invariant. Rather, bouncing, spinning and rolling are three different events because they involve three different transformations, or styles of change, each characterized by its own distinct TI.

Conversely, a ball may roll smoothly down an inclined plane or a rock may roll erratically down a bumpy hill. In both cases, the verb tells us what *kind* of event it is – that the general style of change is rolling, while the adverbial modifier tells us what particular *manner* of that style of change is involved – that the manner of rolling is smooth or bumpy. There is no difficulty in speaking of variants of the same transformational invariant, nor is this to change the accepted mathematical meaning of the terms *transformation* and *invariant* as has been claimed (Cutting, 1986). Transformations may undergo a change in parameters without the change destroying the dynamical invariants that specify their identity. For example, let x be an object, R a rotational transformation applied to x, and k the number of rotations applied, then kRx expresses the rotation of the object x k times (say, in radians). It is clear that k is a parameter whose value might change without changing the definition of the style of change, R. This important point is further elucidated below.

Under the first two views a recalcitrant puzzle is encountered if we assume that information for change comes from the persistence of structural properties *under* the same styles of change. But now we see no such puzzle is encountered if we assume that information for change comes from the persistence of dynamical properties *over* different manners of the same style of change. If object-specific information corresponds to invariants extracted from structural properties that persist *under* a transformation, then change-specific information must correspond to invariants extracted from dynamical properties that persist *over* different transformations. The *under* and *over* relationships are important here, logically carrying the sense of being an SI or a TI, respectively. In another context, we have spoken of this as 'change constancy' and offered it in counterpoint to 'object constancy' (Mark, Todd and Shaw, 1981). This argument has implications for resolving the so-called *multiple specification controversy* (Bruno and Cutting, 1988; Cutting and Bruno, 1988; Massaro, 1988; Pittenger, 1989), but we shall not pursue this issue further.

1.5   Is the Concept of Transformational Invariant an Oxymoron?

Does the only-change-specifies-change view also have shortcomings? At least one leading psychologist thinks so, for he argues that the notion of a transformational invariant is self-contradictory – an oxymoron (Cutting, 1983, 1986). Presumably, the complaint is that transformation is synonymous with change and invariant with nonchange. Therefore, under this interpretation, a transformational invariant would refer to a *changing nonchange*, which is indeed an oxymoron. But this objection rests on a misunderstanding – on confusing the notion of something being relatively invariant with that of it being absolutely changeless.

As defined earlier, invariant means relatively unchanging with respect to other things *which change in the same way*, not absolutely unchanging with respect to things that do not change at all. To determine that two things change in the same way already presupposes that there is information for distinguishing one style of change from another. Thus, to be invariant does not necessarily mean to be static; rather, it means to be stationary in the sense of relatively unchanging. Mathematics is explicit on this issue.

Stationarity is the property of a function (or functional) that equals a constant for some values in its domain. It is not required that it do so for all values. Nor is the constant required to be zero – so long as it can always be rescaled to zero. More explicitly, a differentiable function is said to be stationary if its first derivative is zero and, correspondingly, an integrable function if its first variation is zero. A curve plotting a function (or a transformation) is stationary if it does not move in the space in which it is plotted under a change in parameter evaluation. Whether such functions are plotted over time, over space or over space–time dimensions the definition still holds. Under our usage, *transformational invariants are functions or functionals that are stationary over time while structural invariants are those stationary over space*. Thus, mathematically they have equal status although they are not intersubstitutable.

For instance, two or more things might be comoving and therefore be stationary relative to each other. This shows up in their relative plotting if the origin of the coordinate system is initialized with respect to either one. Consider the relative stationarity of individual geese in a migrating flock (defined by placing the origin of the coordinate system on one of the birds in the flock in question). The flock may be moving, or nonstationary, with respect to another flock of geese floating below it on a pond. However, assuming their behaviors are perfectly coordinated, a velocity function for each bird in the same flock will have first derivatives equal to zero since they share the same velocity vectors. The space–time path integrals (i.e worldlines) of each bird likewise have first variations that are equal to zero since they covary. Here, the structural invariants are the same – geese are geese – but the transformational invariants between flocks are different – for flying is not floating. The Gestalt 'law' of common fate expresses what it means for more than one object to share the same transformational invariant. In waltzing, the couple must share the same TI or they would not stay together on the dance floor.

The notion of covariant functions (e.g. her waltzing versus his waltzing) can be made explicit under various mathematical descriptions. For two or more objects to share the same TI means their covariant derivatives are symmetrical (differential geometry; Burke, 1987) or that their Lie brackets equal zero (continuous group theory; Belinfante and Kolman, 1972), thereby expressing the fact that no linear deficiency exists in their shared forms of relative change. Using these latter descriptions, it is important to note that departures from symmetry by their covariant derivatives, like departures from zero for their Lie bracket commutators, can be measured (Arnold, 1978). Hence, the degree that transformations share a transformational invariant may be measured.

Consider the Lie bracket commutator for the operator description of two styles of change, where Tx and Ty represent the quantitative descriptions of the space–time path followed by each style of change (e.g. the man waltzing and the woman waltzing). Their bracket product is written as $[Tx, Ty] = (TxTy - TyTx) = k$, where k is a measure of the linear deficiency of the two styles of change – that is, their degree of asymmetry (arising from the dancing couple being out of step). If $k = 0$, then the two styles of change share the identical TI (and the couple is in step). On the other hand, if $k \neq 0$, then they do not share the same TI but differ by the amount designated by the number k. Event descriptions, then, are not restricted to ideal invariances but may approximate them within some tolerance measure $\alpha_1 < k < \alpha_2$, where α_1 and α_2 specify the lower and upper 'threshhold' limits, respectively (say, as given by the resolution of the perceptual system) (Shaw, Kugler and Kinsella-Shaw, 1990). Imperceptible differences are sufficiently small differences, namely, those differences that are less than a *jnd* (a 'just noticeable difference'). A difference in k greater than a jnd between two TIs would allow them to be perceptually discriminated.

Take another example: in classical mechanics the concept of the total energy of a conservative system, the so-called *Hamiltonian action function*, is stationary over time. The components of total energy, the potential and kinetic energy of the system, are not, in general, stationary functions. The Hamiltonian is said to be a motion invariant or a dynamical invariant. Likewise, any quantity that covaries with it (i.e. defined by a Poisson bracket, used analogously to a Lie bracket) is also said to be a dynamical invariant (Goldstein, 1980). Hence, there is nothing unusual in talking about transformational invariants if by that one means dynamical invariants. Under this view a TI is definitely not an oxymoron. Notice also that because we may in general be talking about energy or information flows, no reference need be made to structural invariants at all.

The Gestaltists recognized that symmetry of motions ('common fate') may be as important to perceptual theory as symmetry of forms ('good form'). We would be wise to do likewise. We turn next to the important question of how symmetry theory might be used to describe both structural and transformational invariants.

2 SYMMETRY THEORY OF EVENT INFORMATION

In this section we attempt to formulate an event perception hypothesis whose ramifications will be pursued throughout the chapter. A decision is made to view events as physical objects in their own right, rather than as cognitively constructed fictions. This working hypothesis has enormous implications for perceptual theory, for it suggests that what might require a complicated and yet undiscovered mechanism of cognitive mediation might be more simply handled by an information detection mechanism. Philosophically, this will be recognized as a move from a cognition-based phenomenalism (an indirect theory of perception) to a perception-based realism (a direct theory of perception). (For a defense of the former, see Fodor and Pylyshyn, 1981; and for a defense of the latter, Turvey *et al.*, 1981.)

2.1 The Event Perception Hypothesis: Generative Specification

The notion of invariant is synonymous with the concept of symmetry. As argued earlier, events involve two kinds of symmetry: successive symmetry expressed by the transformational invariant and adjacent symmetry expressed by the structural invariant. Events are not unextended instantaneous points in a space–time but occupy a 'window' which extends beyond the *here and now* continuously, both backward and forward to the *there and then*. Events, therefore, are sources of retrospective, perspective and prospective information because the 'current' state of an event is spatiotemporally extended from the past through the present to the future. There is no cutting edge to time that is the specious moment so that perception takes place instantaneously (Gibson, 1975). Consider: a redwood forest grows for centuries; it rained all day over the whole state; the tennis game lasted for four hours; the ball bounced fifty feet in thirty seconds; the lightning flashed from the cloud to the flagpole in a fraction of a second; the particle track indicated a half-life of only a few billionths of a second.

Real events must be thought of as being both spatially and temporally extended while at the same time being limited in their extent. They cover places and have durations. Hence, they occupy a 'window' in space–time. Perception is the process that connects information samples that fill the window. The window expands or contracts depending on the nature of the event. Under this view, since perception shades off into cognition, it cannot be mediated by cognition – for this would be to be mediated by itself.

Because information is symmetry based, it is abstract. Thus, it matters not one whit whether the event is fast or slow so long as the detection mechanism is capable of somehow regenerating the event's symmetry structure (Shaw and Pittenger, 1978; Shaw and Wilson, 1976). Gestaltists recognized the need for this redintegrative process in the application of their so-called 'laws' (e.g. continuity, completion, good form) to patterns or events transposed or fragmented over space and time. Feature theories, on the other hand, fail to acknowledge this requirement for perception because of their strong locality assumption. The mere fact that we can recognize transposed events attests to the need for an abstract basis to event information that treats events as objects of perception *per se* with differentiable features (e.g. symmetries) rather than as featural differences over static spatial compositions.

After a century of fruitless scientific debate, perhaps, it is not imprudent to suggest that the proponents of these opposing views are philosophically incorrigible in the sense that no argument is likely to dissuade them from their position or to move them closer together. Believing this to be so, further polemics will be eschewed in this chapter in favor of a positive statement of the event perception hypothesis. (For the polemics one might see, for instance, Carello *et al.*, 1984; Fodor and Pylyshyn, 1981, 1986; Gibson, 1979; Hochberg, 1986; Shaw and Turvey, 1981; Shaw, Turvey and Mace, 1982; Turvey and Shaw 1979; Turvey *et al.*, 1981).

If we accept this view of event information as specifying a restricted spatio-temporal continuant (i.e. a spatially 'fat' temporal trace of limited duration), then a hypothesis is required to explain how the present information about an event can also entail information about its past and future. From an information sample of an event over the extended present, we perceive where something most likely came from and where it is most likely going. Perhaps, event perception involves a mechanism of generative specification (Shaw and Wilson, 1976) – a recursive application of a rule or operator to a base structure.

Generative specification requires two things: a set of connectable elements and a generator that can connect them. More precisely, a generator is one of the set of elements of an algebraic structure, such as a group, ring or module, which determines all other elements belonging to that structure when all admissible operations are performed upon them. Assume that an event continuant is an algebraic structure and that current information for the event continuant is an element of that structure. Further assume that the operation of detecting the perspective information acts as a generator of the whole structure – that is, as a specification of how the perspective portion of the event connects its retrospective and prospective portions. For instance, an expert batter can anticipate where the pitched ball is going to be so as to start swinging the bat early, in time to connect. Drivers in traffic repeatedly use *time-to-contact* information to brake their cars to avoid the prospects of colliding with another car. One has a natural tendency to look in the direction from which a snowball was thrown to detect the culprit. Numerous studies have been directed at determining the visual information for time-to-contact (Lee, 1976, 1980). Consequently, one can likewise imagine a complementary set of studies to determine the retrospective optical or acoustic information for the source of an event.

The set of graded examples presented below are designed to illustrate the use of the symmetry properties of algebraic structures to describe how event information (TIs and SIs) might be generatively specified. From a mathematical point of view, symmetry theory provides the most natural expression of invariant event information (Shaw and McIntyre, 1974; Shaw, McIntyre and Mace, 1974). However the perceptual mechanism is designed, a minimal requirement is that it be able to detect such symmetries. Let us consider a few simple examples of such symmetries that underlie TIs and SIs.

A light on a disk rotating in the dark when viewed edgewise will project a harmonic motion whose spatiotemporal continuant is a sinusoidal trace (Figure 10.1). The amplitude of the sine wave generated by the rotation will be the diameter of the disk and the period of one cycle of the sine wave is equivalent to the length of the disk's circumference stretched out over time. A double rotation of the disk determines two cycles of the sine wave, a triple rotation, three cycles, and so forth. These cycles are *isometries,* that is, segments of the trace that exhibit recurrent self-similarity (e.g. self-congruence). In real events these isometric periods are not perfectly recurring but do so only within some tolerance range. Structural properties that belong to the object generating the trace, such as size and shape, may also exhibit isometries over spatially adjacent relationships rather than over temporally successive relationships.

Intuitively, such orthogonal isometries comprise the SI and TI of an event. Hence, to change size or shape is to change a parameter on the SI of the event trace, while to change period or wavelength is to change a parameter on the TI of the

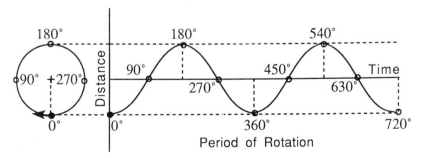

Figure 10.1. *The sinusoidal trace of a rotation event.*

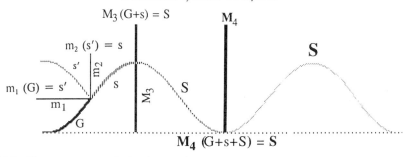

Figure 10.2. *The symmetry analysis of a rotation event trace.*

event trace. Since these SI and TI event components are based on isometries, they intrinsically scale the size of the spatiotemporal window within which perception operates.

The generator for this harmonic motion is a sequence of reflections of element G over the mirrors $[m_1, m_2, M_3, M_4]$ (Figure 10.2). This reflective sequence defines the successive symmetry, or TI, of any rotation event. Clearly, the generating element G could be chosen from any elemental portion of the symmetric spatiotemporal trace. For instance in Figure 10.1, if G were the trace element selected over the period $[0–90°]$, then *prospective* generation forward in time would specify the completion of the trace over $[90–360°]$ via the successive reflective symmetry. Likewise, if G were the trace element selected over the period $[360–270°]$, then *retrospective* generation backward in time would specify the completion of the trace over $[270–0°]$ via the successive reflective symmetry. Finally, given a middle portion of an event as a generator, say $G = [180–270°]$, then *perspective* generation would specify the impletion of the trace in both the forward and backward temporal directions via the successive reflective symmetry.

For an asymmetric event trace the only generator, of course, would be the whole trace itself. But in all those cases where the event has nontrivial symmetry, then the perceptual sample that acts as a generator is necessarily some portion of the event smaller than the window.

While a rotation viewed edgewise (a linear event) can be depicted in two dimensions – one of space and one of time – a rotation viewed perpendicularly in the frontal plane requires three dimensions – two of space and one of time. Here, instead of a harmonic motion trace, there would be a helical trace wrapped around the rectilinear trace of its fixed axial point (like a coil spring surrounding a thin stiff rod).

It is important to note that the successive symmetry underlying the TI of any event trace is abstract in the sense of being independent of the object involved in the event. All points on any rotating object would trace out the same helical successive symmetry in three-dimensional space–time when viewed frontally, or the same sinusoidal successive symmetry in two-dimensional space–time when viewed edgewise. The successive symmetry achieved by application of an event generator is the basis of generative specification and provides an abstract informational basis for detecting events and classifying them according to their distinctive TIs. In Gestalt terms, however, we recognize that the TI is not only transposable over time (retrospective, perspective and prospective) but transposable over space as well (i.e. over different adjacent structures that are involved in the same event type) This is the basis of the Gestalt law of 'common fate'.

If the sample detected is a generator, then the whole event is redintegrated to fill the window's symmetry-specified dimensions. A repeating event defines a sequence of such windows. Under this view, whether the event is slow (like growth or the motion of the hour-hand) or fast (like locomotion or the motion of the second-hand) does not matter so long as the generator information for the event can be detected (Shaw and Pittenger, 1978). The generative specification approach to event perception depends on the logically prior noticeability, or perceptual saliency, of the generator samples as opposed to the perceptually inert samples. If the generator samples are not more likely to be attended to than other inert samples – in the sense of standing out like figure against ground – then there would be no way to get the act of event perception started.

The hypothesis for event perception start-up rests on the assumption that *the more invariant the property in the stimulation, then the more available it is to be noticed* – hence its greater perceptual salience (its *attensity*; Shaw and McIntyre, 1974). Many studies show that subjects tend to become selectively attuned to systems of invariant properties even when these properties are nested among noninvariant ones. Invariance seems to carry its own built-in noticeability quotient. After reviewing a variety of such studies investigating event perception, Johansson (1985) concluded that 'what the visual system evidently records are not absolute measures but instead hierarchies of certain spatial relations which stay invariant under change' (p. 51).

Objects with different shapes generate distinct spatial complexes of successive symmetries that intertwine over time in ways specific to their respective shapes. The abstract basis for structurally invariant information specifying the objects that undergo change can therefore be found in the phase relationships (i.e. adjacent symmetries) that hold under the successive symmetries. This can be seen by studying the phase relationships among the successive symmetry complexes peculiar to objects of different shapes (as shown in Figures 10.3–10.5).

For simplicity of graphical presentation, the shape of an object can be represented by certain selected points of high information. For polygons, vertices are useful choices. In Figures 10.3 and 10.4 we see the event traces for a rotating equilateral triangle and a square. The sinusoidal shape of each point trace specifies that these

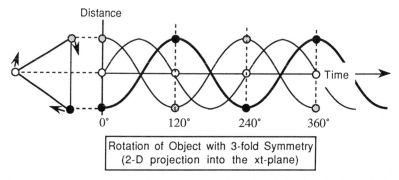

Figure 10.3. *The 3-fold symmetry of the trace of a rotating triangle (2-D projection into the* xt *plane).*

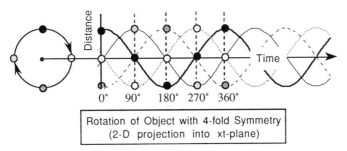

Rotation of Object with 4-fold Symmetry
(2-D projection into xt-plane)

Figure 10.4. *The 4-fold symmetry of the trace of a rotating squares (2-D projection into the* xt *plane).*

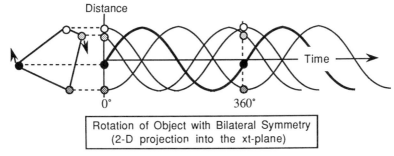

Rotation of Object with Bilateral Symmetry
(2-D projection into the xt-plane)

Figure 10.5. *The 2-fold symmetry of the trace of a rotating trapezoid (2-D projection into the* xt *plane).*

points, regardless of the overall shape of the object, are involved in events that share the same TI characteristic of its harmonic motion. The degree of regularity of the phase angles apparent among the individual point-generated sinusoidal traces specifies the symmetry, SI, of the object to which the common TI is applied. It is this information that specifies that the rotary object is an equilateral, isosceles or scalene triangle, or a square or trapezoid.

The beauty of event diagrams is that they can disambiguate over time those objects whose static perspective forms are spatially indistinguishable. For example, at an appropriately selected distance, a static square viewed from an oblique perspective may be indistinguishable from a selected trapezoid viewed in a frontal perspective. Yet, as we can readily see from comparing the event traces depicted in Figures 10.4 and 10.5, dynamical information for rotating square objects is quite different from that made available by rotating trapezoidal objects. The event approach rids us of the troublesome ambiguity allowed by the classic projective geometry of static retinal image samples.

Thus, the SI information for distinctly shaped objects is itself distinct, namely, the phase angles between sinusoidal traces determine different spacing and the periods of their successive isometries are also different. One merely has to see the rotation of the different objects to break the perspective symmetry. No taxation need be placed on memory or cognition to achieve a feature-by-feature image comparison of each object. If events are themselves objects of perception, then period and phase can be considered complex features (i.e. event information). For the properly designed and attuned perceptual mechanism (e.g. a Grossberg-type neural network; see Marshall, 1990), such global patterns of information can be assumed to be picked up as directly as any local feature.

To summarize the argument so far: a transformational approach can be used to express the successive symmetry exhibited by an event. A transformational description of this symmetry is synonymous with the concept of transformational invariant and expresses mathematically the intuitive content of the phrase 'style of change'. The detectable optical disturbances that emanate from the event source and that express the relevant TI comprise the perceptual information for the *event-type*. Likewise, the same optical disturbances convey information for size and shape and other structural properties. Information samples that are generators, in the technical sense, generatively specify the event. The spatiotemporal windows for such events are intrinsically scaled by their SI and TI isometries. The dimensions of phasing, amplitude and number of traces generated by feature singularities (e.g. vertices for polygons) express the relevant SI and comprise the perceptual (generative) information for the *object-type* to which the TI is applied. The specific values of manner parameters on the TI (e.g. its rate, number of iterations on its period, smoothness in its application) comprise the perceptual information for the *event-token*.

The hypothesis that event perception has a generative basis as explained by symmetry theory suggests an alternative to the cognitive hypothesis that events are constructed rather than perceived: consider the following line of argument. Traditionally, animal gaits have been given symmetry analyses (Gambaryan, 1974; Hildebrand, 1965). Recently, the hypothesis of cognitive programs that mediate locomotive pattern generation has been theoretically challenged by the assumption of central pattern generators. These pattern generators are treated as CNS-based oscillators that are coupled by information rather than being neurologically 'hard-wired' (Cohen, Rossignol and Grillner, 1988; Schöner, Jiang and Kelso, 1990). Here, recurrent gait isometries of animals are not cognitively mediated in the traditional sense of motor programs nor cognitive rules but are governed by natural law (Kugler and Turvey, 1987).

Analogously, we might assume a noncognitive perceptual mechanism that generatively specifies the impletion or completion of events according to their intrinsic isometries. If, on the other hand, we choose to think of visual information as 'cognitive' by definition (which broadly speaking it must be), then the coupling of elemental pattern generators by information in action theory (Schmidt, Carello and Turvey, 1990), and a similar coupling of central pattern generators by information in perceptual theory is not so strange a cognitive assumption.

Finally, under this event perception hypothesis, we need not know the details of the functional architecture of the CNS-based perceptual mechanism before we determine the informational basis of an event and, thereby, describe the functional requirements of the job that the stipulated mechanism must perform. It will be useful to examine the event perception hypothesis in the context of a well-known example. We do so next.

2.2   Perceiving a Rolling Wheel Event: An example

When a distinguished point on the rim of a wheel is rotated around a fixed axis point, it generates a highly symmetrical trace in the xy-plane: a circle (Figure 10.6). By plotting the circular motion over time, some of the symmetry is broken and more structure of the event is revealed. Recall that in the three-dimensional

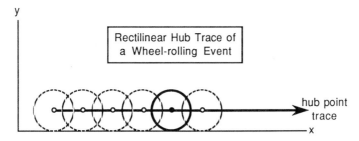

Figure 10.6. *Trace of the hub point of a rolling wheel.*

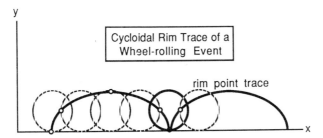

Figure 10.7 *Trace of the rim point of a rolling wheel.*

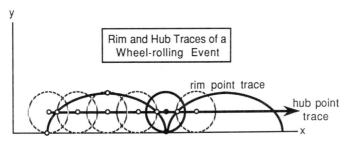

Figure 10.8. *Hub point and rim point traces of a rolling wheel.*

space–time we would see a helical trace coiled around a line of axial points – like a spring coiled around a straight wire. However, when we view the projection of this dynamical three-dimensional trace in the *xt*-plane, we see a sinuoidal shadow of the event trace indicative of a rotational TI – its harmonic motion. Rolling events have a related but more complex space–time structure.

If a wheel with a hub light is rolled over a flat surface in the dark, we see a rectilinear trace that maintains a constant radial distance from the surface. However, if – as Duncker (1929) showed – we view the rolling wheel with only a rim light, then we see a more complex trace in the frontal plane known as a cycloid (Figure 10.7). Apparently, an event TI can have more than one trace. How many?

Following Johansson (1975, 1985), one might hypothesize that the number of isolatable distinct traces should correspond to the number of component vectors associated with the event's resultant TI vector. Two component trace vectors are shown together in Figure 10.8. This depicts a wheel rolled as before but this time with a hub light and a rim light. Both a cycloidal and a rectilinear trace vector are generated simultaneously. Surprisingly, what is seen is neither of these isolatable trace vectors but rather a composite event vector that is quite different from either.

What is seen is a rotating object undergoing rectilinear translation. The invariant center of rotation perceptually anchors the event information because it maintains a constant radial distance from the horizontal surface over which the wheel rolls. Consequently, the most stationary motion trace is generated by the hub light. The next simplest motion trace is the circular orbit of the rim light which maintains a constant radial distance from the moving hub light. The least stationary motion trace is the rim light which follows a complicated nonlinear trace as defined relative to the surface of support. Hence, if we assume that the decomposition of the resultant event proceeds from the most invariant to the least invariant (a principle of minimal change), then there is no real surprise that we see the event as being organized as we do (Cutting and Proffitt, 1982; Proffitt and Cutting, 1980; Shaw and Verbrugge, 1975). This fact provides important support of the event perception hypothesis, for the event is seen as consisting of a rotation TI (i.e. motion around a center) and a translation TI (i.e. the rectilinear motion of that centered motion). How does the TI of the cycloidal trace relate to the TI of the rotation trace and the translation TIs?

Figure 10.9 shows how a perceptually persistent (spatially stationary) cycloidal trace is smoothly related to a rotation-only sinusoidal trace. The sequence of sinu-cycloidal traces represents rotating systems that have various degrees of translatory velocity, indicated by the slope of the hub trace in the xt-plane. These dynamic traces define a *homotopic* (topologically smooth) sequence (i.e. a coordinate transformation) that is interpolated between the pure adjacent symmetries (projection of the event's SI into the xy-plane) and the pure successive symmetries (projection of the event's TI into the yt-plane). Before, we argued that perception, construed formally as generative specification, operates to complete (or implete) a whole event (one that fills the space–time window) from smaller samples (that do not fill the window). Now we extend the argument to a higher level of generative specification.

Recognizing an event-token as belonging to an event-type (i.e. a class) is tantamount to perception involving a mechanism for extrapolating (or interpolating) homotopically from one token to another token, say, from a cycloidal trace to a sinusoidal trace. This homotopic relation can be seen in the event-token sequence (the sinu-cycloidal traces) that connects the SI boundary condition to the TI boundary condition. Moreover, slow events may be homotopically (transformationally) related to fast events (i.e. $dx/dt = 0$ may be related to $dx/dt = \infty$ by $dx/dt > 0$, as shown in Figure 10.9), because they lie on the same manifold whose local structure generatively specifies more remote structures. Thus, by assuming that event perception is generative, the Gestaltist's transposition problem receives a reformulation that implies a potential solution (Boring, 1942; Köhler, 1917).

The transposition problem is reformulated as the problem of explaining how one recognizes the common structure shared by event-tokens that have been transposed to different locations on their event-type manifold (e.g. like a melody played on different but related instruments). The solution is to recognize that this problem is now synonymous with discovering a manifold on which the event-tokens can be defined. This manifold must possess an information function that specifies a generative (homotopic) connection among the event-tokens corresponding to how they are perceived. Under this view, information as specification might be

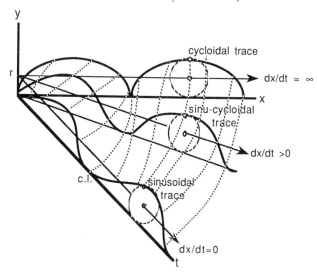

Figure 10.9. *Dynamical traces of a wheel rolling event. Here, r is the radius of rotation and c.l. is the circumferential length. The information specifying the TIs for such events clearly has an intrinsic scale.*

given a precise interpretation (Kugler and Turvey, 1987; Turvey, 1990; Turvey *et al.*, 1981).

In general, for event perception to be generative requires that there be the detection of event information intrinsic to a space–time geometry (e.g. window) for which the neural architecture that underlies detection is appropriately attuned. Specifically, it must be attuned to the homotopic sequences that dynamically relate an adjacent symmetry boundary (SI) condition to a successive symmetry boundary condition (TI). Again how such event traces are set up in the CNS, of course, needs to be explained, but the job putatively performed by such mechanisms can be made quite clear at an abstract level of description.

Consequently, this interpretation of Duncker's (1929) results supports the event perception hypotheses that the successive symmetry exhibited by an event is synonymous with the concept of transformational invariant. It also suggests a way that information for event-types may, indeed, be a form of generative specification in the sense discussed above. Adoption of the event perception hypothesis requires justification for believing that perceptual information exhibits spatiotemporal dependencies and that TIs and SIs are orthogonal dimensions of event space. These issues are addressed in due course.

2.3 Do Transformational Invariants Depend on Structural Invariants?

The evidence for the relative independence of TI from SI is mixed. Wertheimer's (1912) experiments on phi movement suggest independence, while Wallach's (1976) research on viewing motion through a rectangular window suggests dependence. These contrasting cases are considered next.

Wertheimer (1912) discovered a form of objectless motion that he called *phi movement*. As the interstimulus interval (ISI) is increased beyond that required for optimal motion, a ghostly motion is seen to pass between the two successively illuminated stimuli (see Figure 10.14 below). Wertheimer took the phi motion effect to be evidence that motion information is detected as such without any admixture of object information. G. H. Schneider (1878; cited in Boring, 1942) found that a shadow, too faint to be perceived at rest, becomes noticeable when it moves. Similarly, an object that is invisible in peripheral vision becomes visible when it moves.

Reversal of motion after-effects, like the so-called *waterfall illusion* or the *spiral illusion*, provide evidence that motion (TI) and spatial structure (SI) are independent. Stationary objects are seen as moving in a direction opposite to the direction of apparent (spiral after-effect) or real motion (waterfall illusion) of previously viewed objects (Boring, 1942). Phenomenological reports typically include a rather startling experience. During the after-effect the apparent counter-motion of a target object seems to become dissociated from that object's position. Such objects are sometimes claimed to be moving or changing size, even though they keep their place or size relative to other objects. This is a paradox unless one regards motion information (TI) and position information (SI) as having some independence (Gregory, 1966). Like Wertheimer's (1912) phi motion, this odd motion also seems objectless (see below).

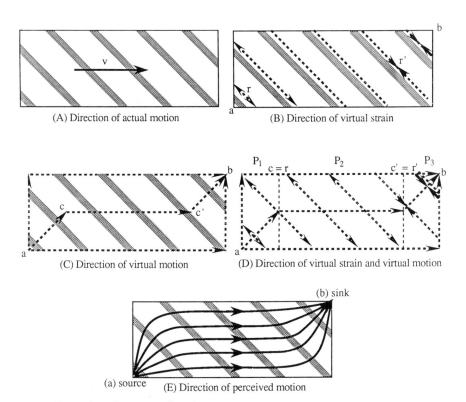

Figure 10.10. *Perception of apparent direction.*

Wallach (1935) developed a set of displays where subjects viewed stripes that moved behind a window in a direction specific to the interaction of the slant of the pattern to the window's shape (e.g. rectangular) (see Figure 10.10A–E). For example, the perceived motion, as depicted in (E), undergoes three directional phases: in phase 1 the motion is directed diagonally, in phase 2 horizontally, and in phase 3 diagonally again. Each stripe undergoes a positive (virtual) strain in phase 1, no strain in phase 2, and negative strain in phase 3. This phenomenon poses a significant problem for any local property approach to perception, whether it be an ecological approach aimed at describing the information made available by such events or a cognitive science approach aimed at modelling the mechanism by which such information is detected.

In Figure 10.10 the following holds: in (A), velocity vector v specifies left-to-right horizontal direction of real motion of the striped pattern. Figure (B) depicts the striped pattern emerging from a source-point singularity at a (lower left corner) and disappearing at a sink-point singularity at b (upper right corner). These dynamically specified initial and final conditions along with the spatial boundaries determine the perceived direction motion. As the stripes emerge and disappear, they undergo a positive and negative strain, respectively, which specifies a *relatively fixed-point property* (r.f.p.p.) on each stripe, represented by r and r'. Figure (C) shows the analytically defined motion vectors: on the one hand, the shearing of the stripes on the spatial boundary condition (perimeter motion vectors) defines the direction of motion as a function of edge-rate while, on the other hand, the connected flow of r.f.p.s defines a central motion vector with critical points (point-nonlinearities) at c and c'. Figure (D) combines the lateral strains with the edge rates due to the actual motion vector. Figure (E) shows the smooth continuous motion that is actually perceived. How do we explain the disappearance of the nonlinearities (e.g. critical points) generated under the vectorial description?

The perceptual information for aperture shape-directed motion events cannot be explained by local properties of neural networks or by information specific to local properties of the display that stimulates such networks (Marshall, 1990). The receptor network must be sensitive to both the changing local boundary conditions (the ends of each stripe) and the fixed nonlocal boundary condition (the aperture's overall shape). Each local boundary condition adjusts to satisfy the fixed nonlocal boundary condition, that is, the stripes increase or decrease continuously in length to fill the aperture's shape while moving continuously over the aperture's length. The relationship of the angled stripes to the shape of the window cannot be encoded into independent receptors but require global distributed attunement over the distributed receptor array (Marshall, 1990).

How does the shape of the window determine the trajectory of the motion event? It is one thing to explain how the information for such events is detected as a proximal stimulus but another to explain how that information is determined as a distal stimulus. Clearly, the design of the perceptual mechanism must conform to the TI for the event perceived. Let us consider how the TI for these events might be formally described.

A mapping from one set of points to another that leaves at least one point fixed is said to have a *fixed-point property* (f.p.p.). One-dimensional strains that operate in opposite directions on the ends of the stripes leave a point fixed at the center of the stripe. Since the direction of strain reverses in the neighborhood of such fixed-point properties, they may be called *reversal points*. Examples of reversal points are denoted by r and r' as shown in Figure 10.10B, D. But because these reversal points translate with the stripes, they are only relatively fixed-point properties (r.f.p.p.)

The r.f.p.p. of a given stripe is determined by the contravalent strains that act on the stripes toward the beginning (phase 1) and the end (phase 3) of the window. A reversal point is mathematically determined at the midpoint of each stripe as a function of the counter-directional strains at the end-points. The motion trajectory follows a direction mathematically defined as a path integral over the spatio-temporal interval from the initial condition a to the final condition b. The direction of the motion path is defined successively from the reversal point of one stripe to another. But what defines the motion path in the middle of the window (phase 2) where there are no contravalent strains, and hence no reversal points?

Another problem that must be resolved is why the TI for the event is smooth rather than jerky at the nonanalytic critical points, denoted by c and c', where the direction of motion abruptly changes. Is there some way to temper the stringency of the mathematics? The nonlinear abruptness arises mathematically because the path of motion is not integrable in the region of these singular (nonanalytic) points – that is, the vertices of the flow vectors at the phase transition boundaries. If these critical points are identified with the last reversal point in phase 1 and the first reversal point in phase 3, then a line of moving points is defined from $r = c$ to $c' = r'$. In this way the continuity of rectilinear flow across phase 2 is specified and our first problem is resolved.

In formal models of the CNS (e.g. neural networks or connection machine models), perceptual integration of contours and trajectories is likened to mathematical integration. Hence, we must take seriously the mathematical problems that arise in representing formally the process of integration. For instance, singular points that are not integrable by mathematical techniques cannot be blithely assumed to be integrable by perceptual techniques inherent in the CNS. Under either view, vertices of angles pose a problem. They act as critical points that are nonintegrable because they interrupt the continuity of a curve or the smoothness of a trajectory of flow. One can integrate up to but not including a vertex point. Such points constitute jump discontinuities and therefore are only piecewise integrable. Furthermore, the singularities at the vertices, through vectorial superposition effects, convolve to create the critical points (c and c') inherited by the flow in the middle of the window as well. On the other hand, if vertices can be slightly rounded off by perception, the trajectory of flow passing through their neighborhood could then be made smoothly integrable.

One way to smooth over nonlinear kinks in curves or trajectories is to reduce the precision of the mathematical description of the vertex singularity. Let the length of a chord be the minimum length that can be perceptually resolved. We do not care what the length is but only that it be realistically finite rather than ideally infinitesimal. Next, assume that the distribution of these short chords of equal length subtend the two sides of the angle in question. This distribution then defines an envelope of tangents to a curve generated by rolling a circle with a radius of $1/4R$ inside a circle with radius R. Figure 10.11 shows this curve stretching from T1 to T2 at a distance of $2R$ from the vertex point of the angle.

'The only thing that distinguishes one potential flow from another is the shape of the boundaries' (Gerhart and Gross, 1985, p. 590) . Because flowlines of a medial trajectory deform continuously onto the boundary of the flow (e.g. the aperture window), this guarantees that the smoothness of medial flow must be preserved in

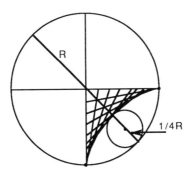

Figure 10.11. *A chord distribution geometry. An integral geometry based on chord-sets rather than point-sets provides one way of smoothing out discontinuities (Moore, 1971, 1972) (see text for details).*

the boundary flow, and vice versa. Likewise, vertex singularities that create non-linear flow on the boundaries would promulgate as nonlinearities into the medial flow and be perceived. But they are not. Consequently, smoothness on the boundary is both a necessary mathematical and perceptual assumption of the Wallach aperture viewing situation.

Perhaps, then, boundary flow around sharp corners is perceptually abraded because the space of perception is based on a set of minimally discriminable lengths (e.g. chords) rather than on real points (Shaw and Cutting, 1980). Perhaps, also, the curve is smoothed by considering c and c' perceptually to be fuzzy set distributions (Kaufmann, 1975) of flow vectors that satisfy some tolerance limit (e.g. a perception of length threshold) rather than as topological neighborhoods of single points. The perceived flowfield characteristics would then be the result of the TI of the motion being the mean free path through these regions of fuzzy set distributions.

The Wallach aperture viewing case raises several questions regarding the relationship of apparent motion events to real motion events. Are they information-ally equivalent or disequivalent? We turn next to the so-called *equivalence thesis* which asserts that since real motion and apparent motion have equivalent perceptual effects, then they must have equivalent underlying information and/or mechanisms. Both the antecedent and the consequent of this proposition have been challenged.

2.4   Is the Perception of Apparent Motion Equivalent to the Perception of Real Motion?

Is it a fallacy to assume that real motion and apparent motion are the same in some or most essential ways? A surprising number of first-rate thinkers have strongly disagreed on this question. Some have begun with the affirmative opinion and later switched to the negative one as evidence accrued. Others have staunchly maintained their respective attitudes toward this issue despite evidence to the contrary. Perhaps the most persuasive evidence that the equivalence thesis must be weakened comes from the important discovery that distinctions exist between apparent and real motion events (Kolers, 1974).

The equivalence hypothesis is a logically tenuous claim at best. For even if apparent and real motion events appeared identical under all parametric conditions (which of course they do not), it would still be fallacious to argue from the presumed equivalence of two effects that the underlying mechanisms were necessarily the same. This would be to commit the well-known fallacy of affirming the consequent. Let x be the premise that similar mechanisms produce similar effects, and let y be the observed equivalence of the phenomenal attributes of real and apparent motion. The equivalence thesis has the form: *if x, then y. Given y. Therefore x.* The only way that the equivalence thesis could be valid is if mechanisms had unique effects, that is, if a given mechanism were the only possible cause for explaining the occurrence of the observed effects. Consequently, we should not be surprised to find that distinctions exist between apparent and real motion events. But do these differences make a perceptual difference?

Among the most important of these distinctions is that between 'short-range' and 'long-range' information detection. Braddick (1974) presented evidence for the existence of two kinds of information in apparent events: low-level information for a *short-range process* that detects information over relatively short durations and short distances and a higher-level information for a *long-range process* that detects information over relatively long durations and long distances. Given this evidence, it now seems unwarranted to hold to the strong form of the equivalence thesis, although expert opinion in the field is still mixed. Let us consider examples of the most polarized opinion on this issue.

Some of the most notable psychologists who have maintained that apparent motion events are equivalent in essential ways to real motion are Gibson (1968), Gregory (1966), Hochberg (1987) and Wertheimer (1912). For instance, Gregory has likened their equivalence to a loosely fitting lock and key; Gibson once remarked that it was unfortunate that a distinction had ever been drawn between veridical and illusory motion – a sentiment he later recanted (see below). The most notable exceptions to the equivalence hypothesis have been taken by Gibson (1979), Haber (1983), Johansson (1975) and Kolers (1964). After nearly a decade of research on the topic, Kolers (1964) summarized his findings as follows:

'In sum, what our experiments reveal, in addition to several behavioral criteria that distinguish real and apparent movement, is that the "mechanism" for illusory movement has more in common with the "mechanism" controlling the formation of simple visual figures than it has with real movement. What one sees "moving" in an illusion is the result of an impletion, but the impletion occurs only at rates of stimulation associated with forming the perception of simple visual figures. The more difficult problem remaining is to elaborate the rules that govern impletion.... Experiments of this kind also support a hypothesis that has been advanced tentatively in the past few years. It is that perceptions are constructed by means of a number of different operations occurring at different times and places in the nervous system.' (p. 323)

Johansson (1975) voiced his dissent from the equivalence thesis as follows:

'The eye is often compared to the camera, but there is one enormous difference between the two. In all ordinary cameras a shutter "freezes" the image; even in a television camera, which has no shutter, the scanning raster of an electron beam serves the same purpose. In all animals, however, the eye operates without a shutter. Why, then, is the world we see through our eyes not a complete blur?... Whether we are standing still or moving

through space the eye effortlessly sorts moving objects from stationary ones and transforms the optic flow into a perfectly structured world of objects, all without the benefit of
a shutter.... Thus, the eye is basically an instrument for analyzing changes in light flux
over time rather than an instrument for recording static pattern.' (p. 67)

A decade after Kolers' monograph seemed to have established the counter-thesis,
Haber (1983) thought it still worthwhile to argue against the equivalence thesis. In
arguing for a 'natural ecology of vision', he summarizes his remarks as follows:

'I described the most typical instances of how we perceive in terms of our movements
and the movements of objects in the scene. I argued that all such combinations of
perception could easily be explained if the stimulus for vision is conceived of as dynamic
change. Conversely, if the stimulus is conceived of as an initial static picture, explaining
perception is inordinately difficult, implausible, and often impossible.' (pp. 49–50)

The only context in which perception might be legitimately treated as static
persisting glimpses is, perhaps, when brief flashes of lightning during a stormy
night are the only sources of illumination, or when searching a dark room one uses
brief intermittent illuminations by a flash-light. However, it is worth noting that out
of the nearly three dozen leading psychologists who offered peer commentaries on
Haber's arguments, only three saw fit to agree with his view that perceptual
information is a dynamical abstraction from stimulation whose source is change
itself – a change whose information we have sought to construe formally as
generative specification.

Still more recently, as notable of a figure in perceptual psychology as Hochberg
(1987) still gamely expressed support for the equivalence thesis, although certain
notable differences were duly recognized (Hochberg and Brooks, 1978):

'Some of these mechanisms and processes must also be engaged when we build up a
continuous percept of our physical environment by taking successive discrete and
discontinuous glances at it.' (Hochberg, 1987, p. 604) '... Research in this area has barely
begun. The cognitive skills by which the information from successive glances is integrated – skills that are of the utmost importance to perceptual theory that aspires to apply
beyond the momentary glance – are open to study through the medium of motion picture
cutting.' (p. 608)

Thus, despite mitigating evidence the equivalence thesis seems atavistically
healthy.

The cognitive approach to event perception opposes the direct pick-up of
information for change and treats change as a representation constructed by
inference. This view is exemplified by Oatley (1978). He asserts that the problem of
perception is to understand:

'... the processes that von Helmholtz (1866) called unconscious inference that allow us to
create in our minds a representation which we experience of what it is like out there,
given a fragmentary, changing two dimensional set of receptor excitations.' (p. 167)

The constructive view requires memory so that the positional and configurational information that act as 'premises' might persist long enough for the
inferences to 'change' to be drawn, presumably, as mental computations. If one is
willing to allow 'unconscious inference' mechanisms to construct more elaborate

perceptions than given in the stimulus information, then why not begin with static snapshots of events? Consequently, it is often (although not always) the case that those who accept the Helmholtzian thesis also have no qualms in accepting the strongest form of the equivalence thesis.

On the other hand, if generative information for change is available in the stimulation, then neither of these theses are required. Thus, the counter-Helmholtzian thesis asserts that the problem of event perception is to understand how we perceive events from the information for change *per se* without need of cognitive elaboration. Is there any evidence to favor this counter-thesis?

In a recent, thorough review of evidence for mechanisms proposed to explain visual processing of real and apparent motion, Nakayama (1985) evaluates the thesis that motion perception requires memory or persistence of position information over time (Dimmick and Karl, 1930; Kinchla and Allan, 1969):

> 'It is likely that the appreciation of motion as a fundamental sense was retarded by these alternative interpretations. Mounting evidence, accumulated over the past century and especially of late, however, leaves no doubt that motion is indeed a fundamental visual dimension.' (Nakayama, 1985, p. 626)

After reading Hochberg and Brooks (1978), what he called the only serious account of motion picture perception, Gibson (1979) expressed the ecological psychology thesis that runs counter to both the Helmholtzian and the equivalence thesis as follows:

> 'The artificially produced *glimpse* is an abnormal kind of vision, not the simplest kind on which normal vision is based.... If perception of the environment is truly based on glimpses, it *has* to be a process of construction. If the data are insufficient, the observer must go beyond the data. How? Some of the greatest minds in history have undertaken to answer this question without success.' (p. 304)

He goes on to say that explanations of perception based on discrete sensory inputs fail because they all come down to this:

> 'In order to perceive the world, one must already have ideas about it. Knowledge of the world is explained by assuming that the knowledge of the world exists. Whether the ideas are learned or innate makes no difference; the fallacy lies in the circular reasoning.
>
> But if, on the other hand, perception of the environment is not based on a sequence of snapshots but on invariant-extraction from a flux, one does not need to have ideas about the environment in order to perceive it.' (p. 304)

These represent the primary opinions of the field toward perception in general and event perception in particular. Event perception is either a cognitive construction from impoverished stimulation or it is the detection of information that generatively specifies exactly what is seen. If the observer perceives by going beyond the data, then perception is a constructive process that adds something to the event data that was not there. But if, as the event perception hypothesis purports, the observer perceives by extracting invariants from the event data, then perception is an extraction and generative completion (or impletion) process that adds nothing to the event data that was not already there. If so, then this is the basis for a realism rather than a phenomenalism regarding perception.

So far our concern has focused primarily on linear descriptions of event information. However, there are important nonlinear issues to which we now turn.

3 PHASES OF MOTION EVENTS

One of the most perplexing aspects of event perception is that a continuous change of an extensive parameter can lead to discontinuous intensive effects. One style of change can make an abrupt transition to another style of change so that: $f: TI_1 \rightarrow TI_2$ may be a nonlinear function even though the controlling independent variable undergoes only smooth linear change. The issue is whether such differential 'thresholds' in perception can be explained in terms of the information made available by the event or whether some cognitive construction or 'inferential' activity must be postulated. In other words, can the perception be direct in the sense of generative specification, or must it be indirect and go beyond the information given? This issue is addressed next.

3.1 Slipping, Rolling and Sliding

A real world rolling event is rarely perfect. Usually the traction of objects rolling over a surface varies as a function of changing coefficients of friction so that the object may slide or slip to some extent instead of rolling. These three event phases can be graphed in such a way that they are shown to be homotopically related and therefore lie on the same manifold. A generative specification of how these phases relate can be given by changing the value of a free parameter, called a *control parameter* (R or T as discussed below) which then determines the value of an *order parameter* (R/T). A control parameter is a variable in an equation that describes the order parameter of a dynamical system such that changing it gives rise to a successive order of distinct but related phases of a given phenomenon. An order parameter is a measure of, and determiner of, the phases of orderliness that the dynamical system moves through when the control parameter is manipulated (Bruce and Wallace, 1989; Haken, 1977; Landau and Lifschitz, 1985). Here, the order parameter is the ratio of the amount of rotation to the amount of translation, as measured in circumferential distance units of $2\pi r$. Notice in Figure 10.12 that the slip phase graph is for the case where the rotation R is greater than the relative translation T, that is, $R > T$ (as measured in circumferential units of distance); the roll phase graph depicts the case where $R = T$; and the slide phase graph the case where $R < T$. The entire event is comprised of three phases that show up as distinct segments satisfying different transformational invariants – ranging from pure slipping (where $T \rightarrow 0$) through pure rolling (where $R = T$) to pure sliding (where $R \rightarrow 0$). Hence, the complex event depicted satisfies the transformational invariant with the boundary conditions $0 \leqslant R \leqslant 2k\pi r$ and $0 \leqslant T \leqslant 2k\pi r$ – where k and r are constants specifying the number of periods through which the event cycles.

A real world event to which this complex event might correspond is a car slipping its wheels in mud as it attempts to go up a hill (slip phase), rolling with good traction on dry pavement (roll phase), and sliding across a wet pavement as the wheels lock-up under heavy braking (slide phase). These three phases comprise three different lower-order transformational invariants that belong to the same higher-order transformational invariant; namely, although they specify three distinct styles of rolling, they are all cases of rolling (except at limit). Here, the order parameter implicated is *degree of rotation/unit distance translated*. Degenerate cases of

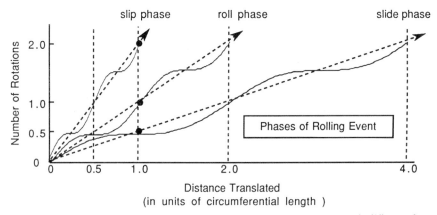

Figure 10.12. *Three phases of a rolling event arise from an object rotating with different degrees of frictional contact with a given surface. Slip phase: with some slipping the wheel rotates more than once for each circumferential length over which it translates. Roll phase: with perfect traction the wheel rotates exactly once for each circumferental length over which it translates. Slide phase: with the application of some outside pulling force the wheel rotates less than once for each circumferential length over which it translates*

these phases are *pure rotating* representing a wheel slipping without traction on a frictionless surface and *pure translating* representing a wheel sliding over a surface without any rotation whatsoever.

One might consider the existence of any object, in principle, to be mathematically describable in terms of its worldline over a variety of phases with different periods. If, as we have argued, event perception should be considered the scientific study of how people and animals detect and classify the successive symmetry of various styles of change, then a task for the field is to work toward empirical validation of a taxonomy of candidate transformational invariants.

In this regard, Figure 10.12 illustrates a key feature of phase diagrams for event information. Transformational invariants occupy temporal degrees of freedom while structural invariants occupy spatial degrees of freedom. If we assign a unit time to a rotation, then the ordinate of the graph plays the role of a temporal dimension, while the abscissa plays the role of a spatial dimension. The regularities in adjacent order that appear as constant intercept values along the spatial axes denote structurally invariant properties, while regularities in successive order that appear as constant intercept values along the temporal axis denote transformationally invariant properties.

For instance, in the roll phase the isometries comprising the SI along the abscissa are circumferential distance units that are in the ratio of $1:1$ with the isometries comprising the TI time to rotate. The breaking of the symmetry relationship between the TI and SI in the slip phase, where the ratio is $1:2$, or in the slide phase, where the ratio is $2:1$, is responsible for the transition from one event phase to another. The breaking of symmetry between TIs and SIs, therefore, can be an important way both to classify events (i.e. by phases) and to characterize the parameter over which this higher-order generative information is defined.

In the next section, we show that taxonomies of event phases can be found not only in cases of real motion but also in cases of apparent motion.

3.2 Phases of Apparent Events

Perceptual phases are found to exist for apparent motion events as well as for real motion events. Perhaps the most famous and most studied apparent motion event was created by Wertheimer (1912). By changing the relative frequency of successive events, say a pair of small flashing lights, a range of apparent movement phenomena can be created. The interstimulus interval (ISI) is the temporal period separating the off-set of one event from the on-set of another such event. Such events may contain a pair of identical, similar or highly distinct objects. Some of the other most relevant variables are distance between the lights, time between flashes, and their intensity relative to each other and the background. Assuming we hold all the other parameters constant, then as the ISI is shortened the frequency of the successive flashing increases and a range of apparent motion effects is typically experienced by a person observing these events (Figures 10.13 and 10.14).

With a sufficiently long range of ISIs the flashes are seen as two separate, successive events But as the range of the ISI is decreased, a remarkable new event is seen – a 'pure' objectless motion passes between the two lights. This is Wertheimer's famous phi phenomenon and was taken by him to be evidence that motion as such is a fundamental dimension of experience independent of sensations of successive locations (i.e. positional information). This might be taken as arguing that information for transformational invariants may be available independent of information for structural invariance.

At still shorter ISIs one no longer sees two separate events but one event: a single object moving continuously from one place to the other. This is called *optimal motion*

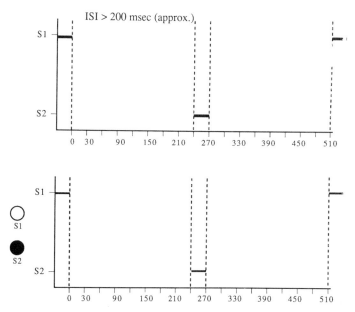

Figure 10.13. *Apparent motion (phase 1): at an ISI of approx. 200ms successive events are seen. The top diagram depicts the actual parameters of the display while the bottom one depicts what is seen. Here, there is no significant discrepancy between the two.*

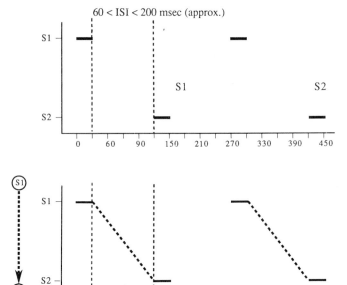

Figure 10.14. *Apparent motion (phase 2) at an ISI of approx. 60–200 ms phi (objectless) motion between the two stimuli is seen. Notice the discrepancy between what is actually presented (top diagram) and what is seen (bottom diagram). The pure objectless phi motion is shown as a dotted line.*

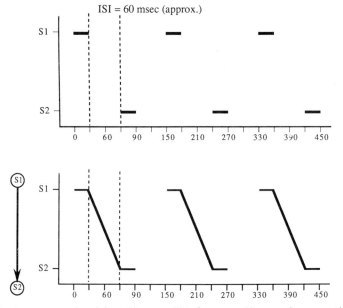

Figure 10.15. *Apparent motion (phase 3): at an ISI of approx. 60 ms optimum motion of one object is seen. The solid line connecting the events at positions S1 and S2 represent the optimal motion that is seen.*

(Figure 10.15). As the ISIs become even shorter, two partial movement events are seen (Figure 10.16). One object begins moving toward the other but then stops without making the full transit. Then the other light picks up the motion somewhat later and completes the transit to its own location. Finally, at the shortest ISI, two lights are seen in two locations at the same time (Figure 10.17).

Koffka's student Korte (1915) formulated principles that Koffka named Korte's 'laws', or as Anstis (1986) suggests are more aptly rules of thumb. These principles define the conditions for optimal apparent motion as involving three linear functions f, g and h of the variables T (ISI), S (spatial separation) and I (stimulus intensity),

(1) For T = constant: $S = f(I)$ and $I = g(S)$, i.e. the spatial separation and the intensity are directly related.
(2) For S = constant: $I = 1/h(T)$ and $T = 1/f(I)$ i.e. the intensity and the ISI are inversely related.
(3) For I = constant: $T = g(S)$ and $S = h(T)$ i.e. the ISI and spatial separation are directly related.

These first two laws are tolerant over wide ranges of values. For instance, Korte (1915) recognized that displays with fine patterns and small distances separating them required shorter ISIs than displays with coarse patterns and longer distances (see Anstis, 1986, for a summary of the tolerance ranges for Korte's laws). The third law has been characterized as being more problematic than the first two – even being in error. Neuhaus (1930) maintained that the duration of exposure rather than intensity was a determinant of apparent motion. We will return to discuss these 'laws' later.

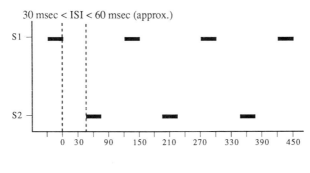

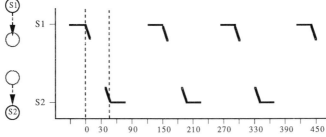

Figure 10.16. *Apparent motion (phase 4): at an ISI of approx. 30–60 ms partial motions are seen to take place near each terminus. These partial motions are shown as the short solid lines*

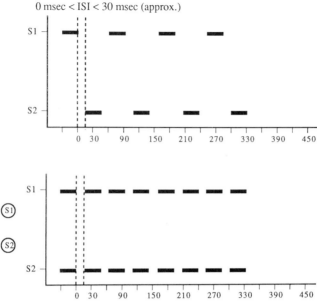

Figure 10.17. *Apparent motion (phase 5): at an ISI of less than approx. 30 ms two simultaneous events with no motion of any kind are seen.*

4   EVENT DIAGRAMS: THE RELATION OF APPARENT MOTION EVENTS TO REAL MOTION EVENTS

We now wish to examine the advantage of treating apparent and real motion phenomena as true spatiotemporal objects rather than as time-tagged, loosely ordered spatial objects. Many changes in spatial configurations look arbitrary and give rise to puzzling perceptual effects when treated as static frames edited into arbitrary temporal sequential order. By contrast, many aspects of event perception that are difficult to explain under sequencing of static samples are seen to arise as intrinsic properties of the appropriate space–time geometry. We consider next how spatial and temporal dimensions may depend on each other.

4.1   Space and Time Dependencies

There is considerable evidence that spatial and temporal dimensions of events are not processed equivalently by the visual system. In Korte's data for maintaining optimum apparent motion spatial separation, S, seems to relate to temporal separation by an approximate measure of $3:2$ (i.e. $3S = 2T$) (Koffka, 1935). As Kolers (1972) observes, the ratios are more than $3:2$ for Neuhaus' (1930) data. Judged spatial extent and measured physical distance are in close accord, while judged duration does not fit clocked duration very well at all.

In an experiment to determine the relationship of perceived spatial extent to duration, Mashhour (1964) had observers view and scale numerically a small object

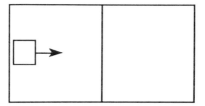

Figure 10.18. *Perceived velocity as a function of context. The perceived velocity of the small object moving in the frame is affected by the amount of background detail. The speed of the object appears faster near the end and middle lines of the frame than in between.*

moving at various speeds over various distances. The results were then plotted against the physically measured values to determine any discrepancies. He found that perceived velocity v^* related to physical velocity v by a power law estimate rather than $1:1$, i.e. $v^* = kv^p$, $0.63 \leqslant p \leqslant 0.94$. This and the fact that there are many other determinants for perceived velocity makes the relating of perceived velocity to physically measured velocity a complicated affair. In many cases of velocity detection there are significant effects of the context in which the motion takes place (Brown, 1931). Figure 10.18 shows once again how context (SI) might have an effect on the TI – similar to Wallach's aperture window, only the effect is on velocity rather than the direction of motion. Thus, if Korte's laws apply at all, they must apply nonlinearly rather than linearly.

In keeping with the idea that velocity estimates may, more likely, reflect rates of processing event information than detection of velocity as such, Caelli, Hoffman and Lindman (1978) introduced a new metric consideration. Perhaps the data from apparent and real motion experiments should be analyzed in a space other than Euclidean space plus time – what physicists call the *Galilean view of space and time*. Numerous studies have shown that the perception of spatial and temporal factors are interrelated so that 'velocity seems to be a directly perceived attribute of moving stimulation' (Lappin *et al.*, 1975, p. 393) Furthermore, form (line of dots) detection seems also to depend on total space–time distance among component dots, independent of their distance apart or their temporal separation *per se* (Falzett and Lappin, 1983).

The perceived length of objects in real motion has been shown to be different from the perceived length of the same objects when viewed stationary (Ansbacher, 1944; Bhatia and Verghese, 1964; Brown, 1931). An inverse relationship has been shown to hold between separation of events in space–time and the so-called *threshold on motion detection* (Henderson, 1973). This threshold seems to be higher when the events are far apart than when they are closer together. After reviewing the available evidence and running three studies to verify the hypothesis, Caelli (1981) concluded that perceived time, length and velocity are all interdependent so that any attempt to base a theory of velocity detection on a fixed concept of distance and time treated as independent is bound to fail.

Hence, what is needed is a geometry of events that systematically and elegantly incorporates these interdependencies of time, length and velocity. Minkowskian geometry, used to express special relativity, as opposed to Galilean space and time geometry of classical mechanics, seems to offer the appropriate method of description. We turn next to this approach to event geometry.

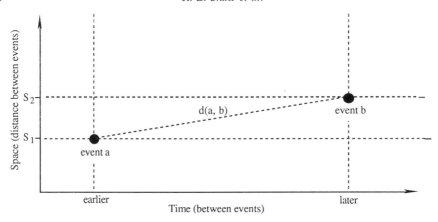

Figure 10.19. *Galilean event diagram.*

4.2   Event Descriptions

Events, by definition, have a four-dimensional spatiotemporal structure. They unfold simultaneously over space and time. Spatiotemporal structure need not, however, have a Euclidean distance metric. For instance, just as the two-dimensional Euclidean distance metric, $d = (x^2 + y^2)^{1/2}$, and the three-dimensional Euclidean distance metric, $d = (x^2 + y^2 + z^2)^{1/2}$, is a generalization of the Pythagorean theorem for two dimensions, $d^2 = x^2 + y^2$, and three dimensions, $d^2 = x^2 + y^2 + z^2$, respectively, so the four-dimensional Euclidean distance metric for space–time structures (i.e events) has the analogous form $d^2 = x^2 + y^2 + z^2 + t^2$. Or, as defined under Minkowski's hyperbolic geometry for space–time, we have the distance metric $d^2 = x^2 + y^2 + z^2 - t^2$. Let us begin with a simple Galilean event geometry as illustrated in Figure 10.19.

Newtonian physics assumes a Galilean event geometry embedded in Euclidean space with time as an added spatial dimension. Events, therefore, are objects in this space and time geometry that have both spatial and temporal coordinates. The interval separating two events, $d(a, b)$, has both a spatial separation and a temporal separation. The ratio of the spatial and temporal intervals separating the two events defines a rate or velocity. Instantaneous velocities are also possible in this coordinate system. A spatial dimension is needed to show the distances separating their sources (e.g. a pair of blinking lights) and another dimension to represent their timing (e.g. ISI).

A restriction must be imposed on Newtonian physics with its Galilean event geometry (Figure 10.19) to express our perceptual inability to discriminate very brief ISIs between two events. Even though an event is actually later in time, it can be seen as moving backwards in time to become simultaneous with an earlier event if the ISI between the two events is sufficiently brief (recall Figure 10.17). The limitation on the rate of causal action in physics is set by the extremely high but finite velocity of light. Since no physical process involving objects with a nonzero moving mass can exceed this rate, a null region in space–time exists in which such events are deemed to be effectively simultaneous – even though by an absolute Newtonian temporal measure they are not. Rather, they are simply separated by

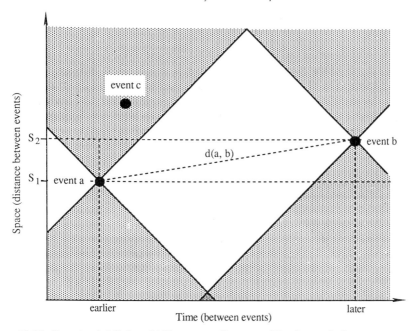

Figure 10.20. *Restricted Minkowski-like event diagrams. The intervals between events in this geometry are restricted. The slopes of the lines define forward (anticipatory) and backward (hereditary) cones within which events may causally interact (light color). The forward causal cone is shown here as defined from the perspective of event a with respect to event b. There are also null cones (dark color) representing regions in which no causal action can take place between events. For instance, since event c lies in the null cone of event a, they cannot causally interact. Rather, they are effectively simultaneous. Worldlines may not cross unless there is a merger of object identity. Objects with mass do not mechanically interact this way since one palpable volume must displace another and cannot occupy the same place at the same time.*

sufficient distance to prohibit causal interaction for the amount of time that separates them. Nothing can transpire between them without violating the limiting speed of light.

Analogously, there is an upward limit on the rate at which one event can be perceived as mechanically influencing another event. No person can perceive a causal interaction between two events faster than the CNS can respond to the information made available by such an interaction (e.g. the motion of an object moving from one place to another). Kolers (1972) has argued that motion perception is related to the CNS formation time for event information. Under this view diagrams for perceptual events, like those for physical events, must also have null cones surrounding any given event to represent the regions in space–time that lie beyond the limits of its ability to causally interact with other events. Figure 10.20 illustrates how such realistic restrictions might be built into an event space–time geometry.

To see how event diagrams might be used for perceptually restricted events, let us consider two examples: the Ternus and the Wertheimer apparent motion effects.

4.2.1   Case 1: Event Diagrams for the Ternus Effects

The Ternus effect is portrayed in Figure 10.21. Despite the fact that dots b and c remain in the same place over time while dots a and d are alternately on and off, the perceived motion is of a coherent three-dot pattern shifting up and down. The puzzle for the event diagramming technique is to explain why the invariant dots b and c do not retain their identity. If they did, then no apparent motion should be seen. Dots a and d lie in each other's null cones and therefore cannot causally interact; thus they should be seen as two successive events. Indeed this effect is reported for some values of on-time and off-time for the dots.

A second and more striking effect is portrayed in Figure 10.22. Here, the identity of invariant dots b and c persists. The timing between dots a and d has been changed so that dot d now lies in the causal cone of dot a. Hence, motion should be perceived between a and d. Indeed it is.

Finally, if the event diagramming technique is to be more than just descriptively adequate, then it should make predictions as well. By altering the timing between the first and second trio of dots so that dots a and d fall into each other's mutual null cones, one would predict that, unlike the second Ternus effect, no motion would be perceived between these end-points because they would be effectively simultaneous. This effect also holds (Figure 10.23).

It is worth noting that the metric for the space–time involved in these diagrams is treated as being essentially flat rather than curved. A variety of additional effects however, can be predicted if one imposes a hyperbolic metric on space–time

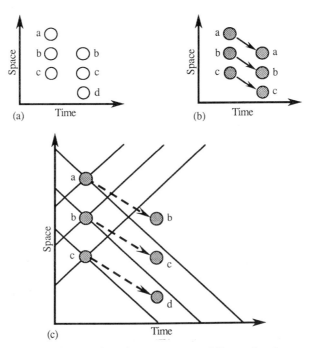

Figure 10.21. *The Ternus effect I. Three dots are seen to shift together from one place to another although the two middle dots are not actually displaced between frames.*

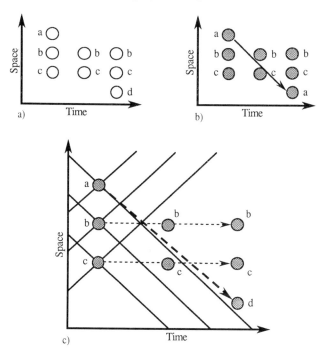

Figure 10.22. *The Ternus effect II. The timing has been changed so that an apparent motion is seen between the dots on the ends even though the two middle dots are not seen to move.*

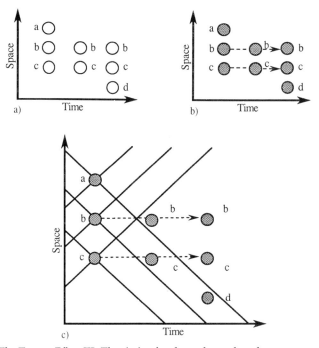

Figure 10.23. *The Ternus Effect III. The timing has been changed so that no apparent motion is seen between the dots on the ends. This effect is achieved by moving these dots into each other's null cones thereby rendering them effectively simultaneous.*

instead (Caelli, 1981). Nevertheless, the diagrams as presented are sufficient for expressing the ordering relationships among apparent and real motion phases (i.e. the order parameter) as the function of a control parameter (e.g. ISI)

4.2.2 Case 2: Diagramming the Phases of Apparent Motion Events

A worldline connects two events that comprise the fore and aft termini of Wertheimer's apparent motion events. The phases of interaction between these events, as expressed by monotonic variation in the ISI, are depicted in Figure 10.24. Compare the parallel between the earlier space and time depictions of Wertheimer's apparent motion effects (Figures 10.13–10.17) and this new event diagram. Phases 1–5 in Figure 10.24 correspond to Figures 10.13–10.17, respectively.

Recall that Korte's 'laws' define the conditions for optimal apparent motion as a linear function of ISI (T), spatial separation (S) and stimulus intensity (I). If we allow the intensity variable to be interpreted as but one example of a more general stimulus salience dimension, then stimulus on-time (e.g. flash duration) may be considered another example as others have argued (Bartley, 1941; Boring, 1942; Neuhaus, 1930). Figure 10.25 provides a graphic interpretation of Korte's laws by event diagrams that have been augmented with tolerance ranges around the velocity angles. A word of caution: the graph of these conditions is presented as being strictly linear. That is, as expressing each phase as exhibiting a *velocity invariance*. This means that the phase in question always lies within the tolerance range around a fixed angle (e.g. optimal motion falls close to the angle whose tangent is approximately 1/2). This is a gross oversimplification for two reasons.

First, in other types of displays, velocity invariance as predicted by Korte's laws has been brought into serious question. Using more complicated (multiple event) lattice displays, Burt and Sperling (1981) have shown that visual angle (i.e. distance between events) seems to have little to do with the apparent motion paths seen in

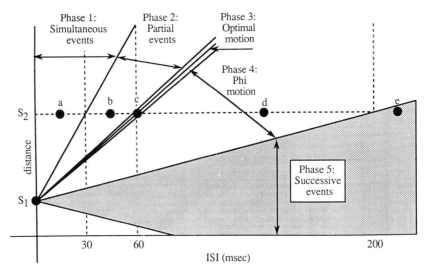

Figure 10.24. *Diagram of the five phases of Wertheimer's (1912) apparent motion event. The phases are defined by the rates at which the transitions take place between stimulus 1 and stimulus 2.*

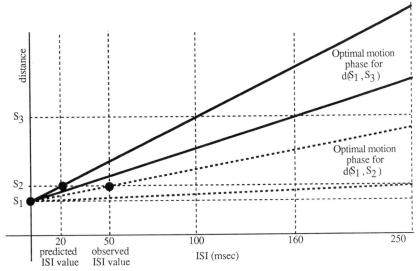

Figure 10.25. *The violation of Korte's (1915) velocity invariance law as a function of change in distance. The predicted upper limit on the optimal motion phase for the distance separating S_1 and S_2 should occur at an ISI of approx. 20 ms. Instead, the observed value of the ISI is approx. 50 ms.*

their displays. Because of this result, they argue that timing parameters are independent of the distance parameter so that *scale invariance* rather than velocity invariance holds. By ignoring the angles in Figure 10.25, we can easily represent the scale invariance hypothesis. Scale invariance would predict that the apparent motion phases should lie between the vertical lines in Figure 10.25 defined at the various values of ISI.

Second, for Wertheimer two-event displays scale invariance does not hold. But, unfortunately, neither does strict velocity invariance. Neuhaus (1930) found the optimal motion phase to lie within ISI values of 50–250 ms for a viewing angle of 0.5°, while at 4° the ISI had to be 100–160 ms. These ranges are plotted in Figure 10.26. (see Section 4.3). To complicate matters even further, we see that not only do the velocity angles vary nonlinearly with a change in distance (visual angle) between the events but so also does the spread of the tolerance regions around these angles. If Korte's laws were velocity invariant over change in distance between events, then one should be able to predict the expected range of ISI values for displays where the events (flashing lights) are moved closer or farther apart. This is clearly not the case for these data. Others have also found optimal motion to hold over a wide range of distances. Zeeman and Roelofs (1953) found the optimal motion phase to hold over 2–18° of visual angle, and Smith (1948) over angles reaching 100°.

What can we conclude from these discrepant results? In general, qualifications must be applied to Korte's 'laws'. These principles are not absolute but require tolerance ranges. Nor do they apply linearly. Still a general trend is predicted by them. Displays with fine patterns and small distances separating them generally require shorter ISIs than displays with coarse patterns and longer distances (Anstis, 1986).

A major difficulty encountered by attempts to diagram apparent motion events is the existence of nonlinear regions where phase transitions occur. The difficulty is compounded by the fact that the boundaries of these phases may themselves be dynamically altered by a change in value of some parameters associated with the displays. These issues are addressed in the next section.

4.3   Graded Determinism, Order Parameters and Distribution Functions

Recall the discussion of slipping-rolling-sliding event phases (Figure 10.12) gone through when an order parameter (R/T) is manipulated via a change in either R or T treated as a free control parameter. Analogously, from our discussion of the two-event apparent motion case, it became clear that the ISI variable can likewise be interpreted as a control parameter for some order parameter yet to be determined. Recall that an order parameter is a measure and a determiner of the phases of orderliness that a dynamical system moves through when a control parameter is manipulated. It provides a quantitative measure of the difference between the phases coalescing at the critical point in the transition from one phase to another (Bruce and Wallace, 1989; Haken, 1977; Landau and Lifschitz, 1985). We would like to generalize the notion of control and order parameters to psychological phenomena in the following way: an independent variable of a dynamical (perceptual) system qualifies as a control parameter if, under extensive variation, the range of values of the dependent variable includes well-demarcated (nonlinear) intensive effects. Such nonlinearly demarcated, intensive effects comprise the *phases* of orderliness. These intensive effects (order parameter), if obtained as nonlinear outcomes from the manipulation of an extensive (control) parameter could be either perceptually or behaviorally demarcated categories (Shaw and Cutting, 1980).

In classic psychophysics the boundaries demarcating perceptual phases were called *thresholds*. Consider the successive phases of object visibility under *change-in-viewing-distance*–the control parameter–as implicating some order parameter. Phase 1: not seeing the object at all because it is too distant; phase 2: the object coming into view but remaining too indistinct to be recognized; and phase 3: the object finally becoming recognizable. Likewise, a change in order parameter can demarcate action phases. For instance, a four-footed animal will go through a well-delineated sequence of successively ordered locomotive phases, called *gaits* (e.g. walk, trot, gallop) as the control parameter of locomotive velocity is monotonically increased. Mathematically speaking: what concepts are needed to express the relationship between control and order parameters?

Control parameters are attached to functionals–order parameters–that govern *distributions* of functions where ordinary parameters attach to single functions that govern data sets. Thus, a control parameter can be construed as a free parameter on an order parameter treated as a generalized function, or what has been called a *distribution function* (Schwartz, 1966). Distributions are continuous linear functionals on a vector space of continuous functions which have continuous derivatives of all orders and vanish appropriately at infinity. They generalize the notion of a radon measure (i.e. a regular Borel measure) and are intimately related to the theory of Lebesgue integrals–the most general integral known. The importance of these two concepts for order parameter theory is: (1) The sets in a distribution may be more complicated than what we typically encounter; they may be functions with many points of discontinuity (e.g. phase transition points). (2) The typical integral usually encountered (the Riemannian integral) is not, in general, defined for distributions. Instead, we must select another integral (the Lebesgue integral that generalizes the Riemannian integral) over discontinuous functions (e.g. distributions).

Laws of nature expressed by distribution functions exhibit a *graded determinism* rather than an absolute determinism (Shaw and Kinsella-Shaw, 1988). This is typical of principles that have the thrust of laws for biological and social sciences. Therefore, we should not expect the same precision that is possible with the laws of physics. Graded deterministic laws are especially sensitive to changes in boundary conditions. For instance, water normally boils at 100°C and freezes at 0°C at one atmosphere of pressure; but under variable atmospheric pressure it will boil and freeze at considerably higher or lower temperatures. Hence, there exists a wide range of values at which the transition from liquid phase to gaseous phase, or from liquid phase to solid phase will be observed.

Just because, in our ignorance, we observe these phase transitions in nature at different altitudes, it does not mean that temperature is disqualified as a legitimate control parameter for the order parameter that determines the observed phase transitions. Rather, we must recognize that when boundary conditions are not or cannot be ideally controlled, then a tolerance range must be placed around the control parameter, thereby making it a distribution function. Our inability to control the boundary conditions of a statistically complex phenomenon does not invalidate the search for order parameters, it merely makes the search more difficult.

Let us apply this concept of control and order parameters to Korte's laws presented earlier. Since the variables S, T and I interact, it is not possible to give definite boundaries to the control parameter ranges that separate one phase of apparent motion from another. These are nonlinear boundaries for which no mathematical expression currently exists. The best we can do is to define the invariant order of phases that a change in one of these variables effects when that variable is used as a control parameter. The order of apparent motion phases has been found to be invariant even if the metric is yet undisclosed (Kolers, 1972; Korte, 1915; Neuhaus, 1930). Nevertheless, for the sake of illustrating how such graded deterministic laws might be expressed, consider the ranges illustrated in Figure 10.25.

Recall that for an appropriate selection of values for stimulus intensity (I) and stimulus separation (S), as illustrated in Figures 10.13–10.17, the interstimulus interval (ISI) acted as a control parameter producing the following order of intensive effects:

Phase 1: above approx. 200 ms → successive events;
Phase 2: approx. 60–200 ms → phi (objectless) motion between the two stimuli;
Phase 3: approx. 60 ms → optimum motion of one object;
Phase 4: approx. 30–60 msec → two partial motions near termini;
Phase 5: less than 30 ms → two simultaneous events with no motion.

The order of phase transitions implicates an order parameter that is quite general, holding equally well for displays with a different selection of distances between events and event salience. The generality of Korte's laws suggests that whatever the order parameter involved, it must be at least as general. This generality extends to apparent motion events that are found to occur for sensory modalities other than vision.

For instance, the cutaneous apparent motion phenomenon is very much like its visual counterpart. It also follows Korte's law. The phase of two vibrators, for example, can be alternated – say, one on the arm and the other on the wrist 15–20 cm apart. If single pulses with an ISI of approximately 100 ms are applied, an apparent tactile motion between sites is experienced (Sherrick, 1968). If we plot the curves of the ISI against the stimulus duration for both tactile and visual optimal motion conditions, the two curves lie nearly on top of each other (Sherrick and Rogers, 1966). 'The conditions that maximize the visual and tactile apparent movement are similar enough to suggest that they are not specific to a modality, but result from the operation of a common set of neurological principles' (Kenshalo, 1972, p. 140).

Related apparent motion phenomena are sensory saltation effects. These involve the impletion of apparent vibratory stimuli between end-point vibrator stimuli. Three identical square wave pulsed tappers are placed approximately 10 cm apart along the forearm. These three tappers are then activated in cyclic successive order for a few milliseconds with a near-zero ISI. The person then experiences a saltation effect: namely, a slow sweeping sequence of taps are felt that successively fill-in between the three actual taps. Analogous saltation effects have been achieved for auditory and visual cases as well (Geldard, 1975).

Thus, we have evidence for various cases of analogous impletion effects across sensory modalities. In all cases the origin of the impletion is assumed to be central and cognitively constructed. But an equally likely hypothesis is that they depend on vibratory information samples that support generative specification.

As pointed out, Korte's laws have been impugned because the values that give rise to the various phases of apparent motion lack specificity (Anstis, 1986; Hochberg, 1986). These criticisms are fair only if you expect the laws of psychology to express an absolute determinism. On the other hand, if you expect laws to express only a graded determinism, then the criticism is unfair. Rather, the ranges of values exist that suggest the need to develop laws governing control variables with tolerance ranges. These laws may be more difficult to formulate but they are no less laws because of this fact. Consider the following example.

Korte's laws entail order parameters that are distribution functions, then, by fixing two of three control parameters, it should be possible to discover the envelope of the distribution function whose tolerance limits the order parameter satisfies. A beautiful example of a distribution function for apparent movement can be found in Kolers (1964; reproduced in Kolers, 1972, p. 29). Kolers conducted an experiment replicating Neuhaus (1930) that indicates an arrangement of event processing curves. Two flashes of light were exposed for different durations and different ISIs. The observer's task was to report whether a smooth continuous motion event was seen. The duration of the flashes varied over the range of 24 to 215 ms. The probability of observers reporting that a motion event had occurred at shorter ISIs was found to increase as the flash durations increased. Notice how the curves are arranged as shown in Figure 10.26. But also notice that the distribution has no clear-cut shape.

Kolers argues that the visual system requires a certain amount of time to process the events (e.g. light flashes) that give rise to apparent motion phases. Consequently, the perception of the imputed velocity of the moving apparent object is

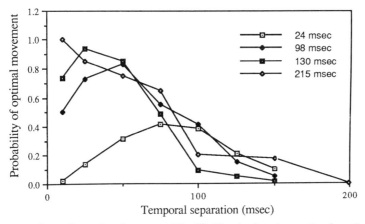

Figure 10.26. *Figure formation functions. The likelihood of seeing optimal motion between two flashes as a function of variation in flash duration and ISI. Note the duration tag on each curve (in 7.ms). The abscissa shows the ISI (offset of first stimulus to onset of second stimulus (in ms). Each curve shows the hypothetical 'figure formation' function for the given stimulus duration and ISI. Assuming that a process is initiated by stimulus onset, then we see that its rise and decay are a direct function of stimulus duration. [From Kolers, 1972, p. 27. © 1972 by the late author.]*

merely a reflection of the perceptual work done during the interval. For example, a 24 ms flash initiates the process (rise of curve) but it fails rapidly (the decay of curve). Compare this with the faster rise and slower decay of the likelihood of detection curve for the process initiated by the 130 ms duration flash. Under these working assumptions the data curves need to be replotted in terms of stimulus onset asychrony (SOA) so that the abscissa includes the onset-to-onset interval.

Upon replotting these same curves a higher-order arrangement clearly emerges. Figure 10.27 shows the shaded envelope around the hypothetical functions that Kolers called 'figure formation' functions – taken collectively they seem to provide a beautiful example of a distribution function determined by an order parameter. This distribution function expresses the tolerance ranges surrounding the phases revealed by variations in a control parameter.

To have a strong case for this envelope actually being a distribution function, certain formal criteria must be met (Schwartz, 1966). One important criterion is to discover the mathematical form of the transformation that maps one curve into the other. Such a transformation would have to apply invariantly to each sampled curve in the distribution. Such a distribution function is a function of functions – a functional.

In other words, a transformational invariant (TI) must exist that expresses explicitly the invariant action that the order parameter has on each of the sampled functions. If so, then the overall shape of the distribution can be geometrically plotted as an envelope over the extreme values of the family of curves. Kolers (1972) came very close to anticipating the generative specification hypothesis for event perception when he called this TI a hypothetical *generator function* for apparent motion.

In principle, the curves can be individuated by experimentally discovering the appropriate weights to be placed on the parameters of the distribution function. Of

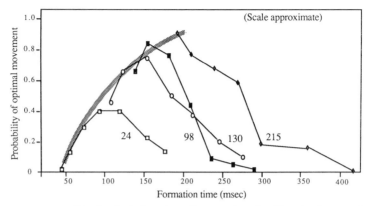

Figure 10.27. *Generator (distribution) function. Curves plotted with stimulus onset asynchrony (SOA) rather than ISI on abscissa. The shaded area shows the envelope of the hypothetical distribution function whose transformational invariant would relate all of the sampled functions in the distribution. The rise and decay of the individual functions seem to be a function of the duration of the stimulus. Presumably the apparent velocity of object motion reflects the processing time of the event information. [From Kolers, 1972, p. 29. © 1972 by the late author.]*

course such work remains to be done before the worth of these conjectures can be ascertained. However, we seem to have little choice but to broaden our tools for formal descriptions if we expect to resolve these long-standing perceptual issues.

5 CONCLUSIONS

In this chapter we have considered the case for a space–time geometry that provides a possible foundation for event information. The hypothesis put forward seeks to expand the dimensions of event perception beyond merely treating events as constructs from static glimpses of local features. Instead, it proposes that events are objects of perception *per se* with their own information transformational and structural invariants. Certain samples of this event information generatively specify a virtual space–time window that the event fills. Under this view, event perception is the filling of this window retrospectively, perspectively and prospectively. This is achieved by detection of a sample that acts as a generator to specify undetected portions bounded retrospectively and prospectively (i.e. filling the virtual window in space–time). How strange an assumption is this? A special emphasis has been given to clarifying the usefulness of the concept of transformational invariant as a fundamentally natural way to define event categories and thereby delimit the subject matter of this new field of scientific endeavor. To express the TIs for different events, the techniques of event diagramming were introduced. In the light of this brief survey, let us summarize the motivation and promise of this graphical technique.

  Classic event space spatializes time by allowing motion over any distance, no matter how far, to take place instantaneously. The arguments offered in our attempts to describe the Ternus effects suggest a need to restrict classic space and time diagrams. Hence, we chose a Minkowski-like event space–time which disallows such impossibly fast events by adding a space–time restriction, namely, the maximum rate of causal action. This limit can be used to express more realistically the rate at which the CNS can handle event information.

In addition, the exercise of attempting to capture Korte's laws indicated that both the precision and the linearity of these laws are suspect. To have explicit principles of this sort will require that they explain the occurrence of the nonlinear phenomena such as phase transitions. By augmenting the Minkowski-like space–time with tolerance ranges, thereby creating a space–time tolerance geometry, the descriptive adequacy of the event diagramming technique is vastly improved. In this way, there is hope that phases may be incorporated into event space–time. The notion was also put forward that tolerance geometries are the natural breeding place not only for phases but for distribution functions as well. Together these two properties provide a means for bringing CNS constraints to bear on event space–time so that the resulting geometry reflects both the environment's and the perceiver's contribution to event perception.

Perhaps the strongest motivation for using event diagrams, however, is to provide researchers who are working on event perception problems with a common means of expressing their findings in some commensurate way. There is little doubt that research and theory in this field would be aided immeasurably if researchers shared a common scientific vocabulary and convenient graphical techniques for portraying event information. Perhaps the suggestions made here may provide a direction for such developments.

ACKNOWLEDGEMENTS

Our thanks to Endre Kadar for his many helpful suggestions on the paper, and to Wolfgang Prinz and Tony Morris whose careful readings of the manuscript helped us to improve it, and to James Todd for his wise comments on many of the topics covered. Any remaining inadequacies, of course, are our sole responsibility.

REFERENCES

Adelson, E. H. Bergen and J. R. (1985). Spatiotemporal energy models for the perception of motion. *Journal of the Optical Society of America*, **2**, 284–299.

Ansbacher, H. L. (1944). Distorting in the perception of real movement. *Journal of Experimental Psychology*, **34**, 1–23.

Anstis, S. (1986). Motion perception in the frontal plane: Sensory aspects. In K. R. Boff, L. Kaufman and J. P. Thomas (Eds), *Handbook of Perception and Human Performance*, vol. 1: *Sensory Processes and Perception* (pp. 16.1–16.27). New York: John Wiley.

Arnold, V. I. (1978). *Mathematical Methods of Classical Mechanics*. New York: Springer.

Bartley, S. H. (1941). *Vision: A Study of its Basics*. New York: Van Nostrand.

Belinfante, J. and Kolman, B. (1972). *A Survey of Lie Groups and Lie Algebras with Applications and Computational Methods*. Phildelphia: Sociey for Industrial and Applied Mathematics.

Bhatia, B. and Verghese, C. A. (1964). Threshold size of a moving object as a function of its speed. *Journal of the Optical Society of America*, **54**, 934–950.

Boring, E. G. (1942). *Sensation and Perception in the History of Experimental Psychology*. New York: Appleton-Century-Crofts.

Braddick, O. J. (1974). A short-range process in apparent motion. *Vision Research*, **14**, 519–527.

Brown, J. F. (1931). The thresholds for visual movement. *Psychologische Forschung*, **14**, 249–268.

Bruce, A. and Wallace, D. (1989). Critical point phenomena: Universal physics at large length scales. In P. Davies (Ed.), *The New Physics* (pp. 236–267). Cambridge: Cambridge University Press.

Bruno, N. and Cutting, J. E. (1988). Minimodularity and the perception of layout. *Journal of Experimental Psychology: General*, **117**, 161–170.

Burke, W. (1987). *Applied Differential Geometry*. Cambridge: Cambridge University Press.

Burt, P. and Sperling, G. (1981). Time, distance, and feature trade-offs in visual apparent motion. *Psychological Review*, **88**, 171–195.

Caelli, T. M. (1981). *Visual Perception: Theory and Practice*. Oxford: Pergamon Press.

Caelli, T. M., Hoffman, W. and Lindman, H. (1978). Subjective Lorentz transformations and the perception of motion. *Journal of the Optical Society of America*, **68**, 402–411.

Capek, M. (1961). *The Philosophical Impact of Contemporary Physics*. Princeton, NJ: Van Nostrand.

Carello, C., Kugler, P. N., Turvey, M. T. and Shaw, R. E. (1984). Inadequacies of the computer metaphor. In M. Gazzaniga (Ed.), *Handbook of Cognitive Neuroscience* (pp. 229–248). New York: Plenum Press.

Cohen, A., Rossignol, S. and Grillner, S. (1988). *Neural Control of Rhythmic Movements in Vertebrates*. New York: John Wiley.

Cutting, J. E. (1983). Four assumptions about invariance in perception. *Journal of Experimental Psychology: Human Perception and Performance*, **9**, 310–317.

Cutting, J. E. (1986). *Perception with an Eye for Motion*. Cambridge, MA: MIT Press.

Cutting, J. E. and Bruno, N. (1988). Additivity, subadditivity, and the use of visual information: A reply to Massaro (1988). *Journal of Experimental Psychology: General*, **117**, 422–424.

Cutting, J. E. and Proffitt, D. R. (1982). The minimum principle and the perception of absolute, common, and relative motions. *Cognitive Psychology*, **14**, 211–246.

Dimmick, R. C. and Karl, J. C. (1930). The effect of exposure time upon the R. L. of visible motion. *Journal of Experimental Psychology*, **13**, 365–369.

Duncker, K. (1929). Über induzierte Bewegung. *Psychologische Forschung*, **12**, 180–259.

Falzett, M. and Lappin, J. S. (1983). Detection of visual forms in space and time. *Vision Research*, **23**, 181–189.

Fodor, J. and Pylyshyn, Z. (1981). How direct is visual perception? *Cognition*, **9**, 139–196.

Fodor, J. and Pylyshyn, Z. (1986). Connectionism and cognitive architecture: A critical analysis. *Cognition*, **28**, 3–71.

Gambaryan, P. (1974). *How Mammals Run: Anatomical Adaptation*. New York: John Wiley.

Geldard, F. A. (1975). *Sensory Saltation: Metastability in the Perceptual World*. Hillsdale, NJ: Erlbaum.

Gerhart, P. M. and Gross, R. J. (1985). *Fundamentals of Fluid Mechanics*. Reading, MA: Addison-Wesley.

Gibson, J. J. (1968). What gives rise to the perception of motion? *Psychological Review*, **75**, 335–346.

Gibson, J. J. (1975). Events are perceived but time is not. In J. T. Fraser and N. Lawrence (Eds), *The Study of Time*, vol. 2. New York: Springer.

Gibson, J. J. (1979). *The Ecological Approach to Visual Perception*. Boston, MA: Houghton Mifflin.

Goldstein, H. (1980). *Classical Mechanics*. Reading, MA: Addison-Wesley.

Gregory, R. L. (1966). *Eye and Brain*. New York: John Wiley.

Haber, R. N. (1983). The impending demise of the icon: A critique of the concept of iconic storage in visual information processing. *Behavioral and Brain Sciences*, **6**, 1–54.

Haken, H. (1977). *Synergetics: An Introduction*. New York: Springer.

Helmholtz, H. von (1866/1925). *A Treatise on Physiological Optics*, vol. 3 3rd edn (J. P. C. Southall, Ed. and Transl.). Menasha, WI: The Optical Society of America, 1925. (Originally published 1866, *Handbuch der physiologischen Optik*. Leipzig: Voss.).

Henderson, D. C. (1973). Visual discriminaton of motion: Stimulus relationships at threshold and the question of luminance–time reciprocity. *Perception and Psychophysics*, **1**, 121–130.

Hildebrand, M. (1965). Symmetrical gaits in horses. *Science*, **150**, 701–708.

Hochberg, J. (1964). *Perception*, 1st edn. Englewood Cliffs, NJ: Prentice-Hall.

Hochberg, J. (1986). Representation of motion and space in video and cinematic displays. In K. R. Boff, L. Kaufman and J. P. Thomas (Eds), *Handbook of Perception and Human Performance*, vol. 1: *Sensory Processes and Perception* (pp. 22.1–22.64). New York: John Wiley.

Hochberg, J. (1987). Perception of motion pictures. In R. L. Gregory (Ed.), *The Oxford Companion to the Mind*. Oxford: Oxford University Press.

Hochberg, J. and Brooks, V. (1978). The perception of motion pictures. In E. C. Carterette and M. P. Friedman (Eds), *Handbook of Perception*, vol. 10 (pp. 259–304). New York: Academic Press.

Johansson, G. (1975). Visual motion perception. *Scientific American*, **232**, 76–88.

Johansson, G. (1985). About visual event perception. In W. H. Warren and R. E. Shaw (Eds), *Persistence and Change: Proceedings of the First International Conference on Event Perception* (pp. 29–54). Hillsdale, NJ: Erlbaum.

Johansson, G., von Hofsten, C. and Jansson, G. (1980). Event perception. *Annual Review of Psychology*, **31**, 27–63.

Kaufmann, A. (1975). *Introduction to the Theory of Fuzzy Sets*, vol. 1. New York: Academic Press.

Kenshalo, D. R. (1972). The cutaneous senses. In J. W. Kling and L. A. Riggs (Eds), *Woodworth and Schlosberg's Experimental Psychology*, vol. 3: Sensation and Perception, 3rd edn. New York: Holt, Rinehart and Winston.

Kinchla, R. A. and Allan, L. G. (1969). A theory of visual movement perception. *Psychological Review*, **76** 537–558.

Koffka, K. (1935). *Principles of Gestalt Psychology*. New York: Harcourt Brace.

Köhler, W. (1917). Die Farbe der Sehdinge beim Schimpansen und beim Haushuhn. *Zeitschrift für Psychologie*, **77**, 248–245.

Kolers, P. A. (1964). The illusion of movement. *Scientific American*, **211**, 98–106.

Kolers, P. A. (1972). *Aspects of Motion Perception*. Oxford: Pergamon Press.

Kolers, P. A. (1974). The illusion of movement. In R. Held and W. Richards (Eds), *Perception: Mechanism and Models* (pp. 316–323). San Francisco, CA: Freeman.

Korte, A. (1915). Kinematoskopische Untersuchungen. *Zeitschrift für Psychologie*, **72**, 194–296.

Kugler, P. N. and Turvey, M. T. (1987). *Information, Natural Law, and the Self-assembly of Rhythmic Movement*. Hillsdale, NJ: Erlbaum.

Kugler, P. N., Turvey, M. T., Carello, C. and Shaw, R. E. (1985). The physics of controlled collisions: A reverie about locomotion. In W. H. Warren and R. E. Shaw (Eds), *Persistence and Change: Proceedings of the First International Conference on Event Perception* (pp. 195–229). Hillsdale, NJ: Erlbaum.

Landau, L. D. and Lifschitz, E. M. (1985). *Statistical Physics*, Part 1, 3rd edn. Oxford: Pergamon Press.

Lappin, J. S., Bell, H. H., Harm, O. J. and Kottas, B. (1975). On the relation between time and space in the visual discrimination of velocity. *Journal of Experimental Psychology: Human Perception and Performance*, **1**, 384–394.

Lee, D. N. (1976). A theory of the visual control of braking based on information about time to collision. *Perception*, **5**, 437–459.

Lee, D. N. (1980). Visuo-motor coordination in space–time. In G. E. Stelmach and J. Requin (Eds), *Tutorials in Motor Behavior*. Amsterdam: North-Holland.

Mark, L. S., Shapiro, B. and Shaw, R. E. (1986). A study of the structural support for the perception of growth. *Journal of Experimental Psychology: Human Perception and Performance* **12**, 149–159.

Mark, L. S., Todd, J. T. and Shaw, R. E. (1981). The perception of growth: A geometric analysis for distinguishing styles of change. *Journal of Experimental Psychology: Human Perception and Performance*, **7**, 355–368.

Marshall, J. A. (1990). Self-organizing neural networks for perception of visual motion. *Neural Networks*, **3**, 45–74.

Mashhour, M. (1964). *Psychophysical Relations in the Perception of Velocity*. Stockholm: Almqvist and Wiksell.

Massaro, D. W. (1988). Ambiguity in perception and experimentation. *Journal of Experimental Psychology: General*, **117**, 417–421.

Moore, D. J. H. (1971). A theory of form. *International Journal for Man–Machine Studies*, **3**, 31–59.

Moore, D. J. H. (1972). An approach to the analysis and extraction of pattern features using integral geometry. *IEEE Transactions on Systems, Man, and Cybernetics*, **SMC-2**, 97–102.

Nakayama, K. (1985). Biological image motion processing: A review. *Vision Research*, **25**, 625–660.

Neuhaus, W. (1930). Experimentelle Untersuchung der Scheinbewegung. *Archiv für die gesamte Psychologie*, **75**, 315–458.

Oatley, K. (1978). *Perceptions and Representations*. New York: The Free Press.

Pittenger, J. B. (1989). Multiple sources of information: Treat or menace? *Newsletter of the International Society for Ecological Psychology (ISEP)*, **4**, 4–6.

Pittenger, J. B. (1990). The demise of the good old days: Consequences of Stoffregen's concept of information. *ISEP Newsletter*, **4**, 8–10.

Pittenger, J. B. and Shaw, R. E. (1975a). Perception of relative and absolute age in facial photographs. *Perception and Psychophysics*, **18**, 137–143.

Pittenger, J. B. and Shaw, R. E. (1975b). Aging faces as viscal-elastic events: Implications for a theory of non-rigid shape perception. *Journal of Experimental Psychology: Human Performance and Perception*, **1**, 374–382.

Proffitt, D. R. and Cutting, J. E. (1980). An invariant for wheel-generated motions and the logic of its determination. *Perception*, **9**, 435–439.

Rock, I. (1975). *Introduction to Perception*. New York: Macmillan.

Rosen, R. (1991). *Life Itself: A Comprehensive Inquiry into the Nature, Origin, and Fabrication of Life*. New York: Columbia Press.

Schmidt, R. C., Carello, C. and Turvey, M. T. (1990). Phase transitions and critical fluctuations in the visual coordination of rhythmic movements between people. *Journal of Experimental Psychology: HP and P*, **16**, 227–247.

Schöner, G., Jiang, W. Y. and Kelso, J. A. S. (1990). Synergetic theory of quadrupedal gaits and gait transitions. *Journal of Theoretical Biology*, **142**, 359–391.

Schwartz, L. (1966). *Theorie des Distributions*, 2 vols. Paris: Herman. (Discussed in V. S. Vladimirov (1984). *Equations of Mathematical Physics*. Moscow: Mir.)

Shaw, R. E. and Cutting, J. (1980). Clues from an ecological theory of event perception. In U. Bellugi and M. Studdert-Kennedy (Eds), *Signed and Spoken Language: Biological Constraints on Linguistic Form* (pp. 57–84). Dahlem Konferenzen, Berlin. Weinheim: Verlag Chemie.

Shaw, R. E. and Kinsella-Shaw, J. (1988). Ecological mechanics: A physical geometry for intentional constraints. *Human Movement Science*, **7**, 155–200.

Shaw, R. E., Kugler, P. N. and Kinsella-Shaw, J. (1990). Reciprocities of intentional systems. In R. Warren and A. H. Wertheim (Eds), *Perception and Control of Self-motion* (pp. 579–619). Hillsdale, NJ: Erlbaum.

Shaw, R. E. and McIntyre, M. (1974). Algoristic foundations to cognitive psychology. In W. B. Weimer and D. S. Palermo (Eds), *Cognition and the Symbolic Processes*, vol. 1 (pp. 305–366). Hillsdale, NJ: Erlbaum.

Shaw, R. E. McIntyre, M. and Mace, W. M. (1974). The role of symmetry in event perception. In R. B. MacLeod and H. L. Pick (Eds), *Perception: Essays in Honor of James J. Gibson*. Ithaca, NY: Cornell University Press.

Shaw, R. E. and Pittenger, J. (1978). Perceiving change. In H. L. Pick and E. Saltzman (Eds), *Modes of Perceiving and Processing Information* (pp. 187–204). Hillsdale, NJ: Erlbaum.

Shaw, R. E. and Turvey, M. T. (1981). Coalitions as models for ecosystems: A realist perspective on perceptual organization. In M. Kubovy and J. Pomerantz (Eds), *Perceptual Organization* (pp. 343–415). Hillsdale, NJ: Erlbaum.

Shaw, R. E., Turvey, M. T. and Mace, W. M. (1982). Ecological psychology: The consequence of a commitment to realism. In W. B. Weimer and D. S. Palermo (Eds), *Cognition and the Symbolic Processes* vol. 2 (pp. 159–226). Hillsdale, NJ: Erlbaum.

Shaw, R. E. and Verbrugge, R. (1975). A symmetry analysis of perceptual information for rolling objects. Meeting of the Midwestern Psychological Association, Chicago, May 1975.

Shaw, R. E. and Wilson, B. E. (1976). Generative conceptual knowledge: How we know what we know. In D. Klar (Ed.), *Carnegie-Mellon Symposium on Information Processing: Cognition and Instruction*. Hillsdale, NJ: Erlbaum.

Sherrick, C. E. (1968). Bilateral apparent haptic movement. *Perception and Psychophysics*, **4**, 159–162.

Sherrick, C. E. and Rogers, R. (1966). Apparent haptic movement. *Perception and Psychophysics*, **1**, 175–180.

Smith, K. R. (1948). Visual apparent motion in the absence of neural interaction. *American Journal of Psychology*, **61**, 73–78.

Stoffregen, T. (1990). Multiple sources of information: For what? *ISEP Newsletter*, **4**, 5–8.

Todd, J. T. (1981). Visual information about moving objects. *Journal of Experimental Psychology: Human Perception and Performance*, **7**, 795–810.

Turvey, M. T. (1990). The challenge of a physical account of action: A personal view. In H. T. A. Whiting, O. G. Meijer and P. C. W. van Wieringen (Eds), *A Natural-Physical Approach to Movement Control* (pp. 57–93). Amsterdam: Free University Press.

Turvey, M. T. and Shaw, R. E. (1979). The primacy of perceiving: An ecological reformulation for understanding memory. In L.-G. Nilsson (Ed.), *Perspectives on Memory Research: Essays in Honor of Uppsala University's 500th anniversary* (pp. 167–222). Hillsdale, NJ: Erlbaum.

Turvey, M. T., Shaw, R. E., Reed, E. and Mace, W. M. (1981). Ecological laws of perceiving and acting: In reply to Fodor and Pylyshyn. *Cognition*, **9**, 237–304.

Ullman, S. (1979). *The Interpretation of Visual Motion*. Cambridge, MA: MIT Press.

Ullman, S. (1980). Against direct perception. *Behavioral and Brain Sciences*, **3**, 373–416.

van Santen, J. P. H. and Sperling, G. (1985). Elaborated Reichardt detectors. *Journal of the Optical Society of America*, **2**, 300–321.

Wallach, H. (1976). On perception. New York: Quadrangle/New York Times Book Co.

Warren, W. H. Jr and Shaw, R. E. (1985). Events as units of analysis for ecological psychology. In W. H. Warren Jr and R. E. Shaw (Eds), *Persistence and Change: Proceedings of the First International Conference on Event Perception* (pp. 1–27). Hillsdale, NJ: Erlbaum.

Wertheimer, M. (1912/1961). Experimentelle Studien über das Sehen von Bewegung. *Zeitschrift für Psychologie*, **61**, 161–265. (Translated in part in T. Snipley (Ed.), *Classics in Psychology*. New York: Philosophical Library, 1961.)

Whitehead, A. N. (1919). *An Enguiry Concerning the Principles of Natural Knowledge*. Cambridge: Cambridge University Press.

Zeeman, W. and Roelofs, C. (1953). Some aspects of apparent motion. *Acta Psychologica*, **9**, 158–181.

Chapter 11

The Perception of Action and Movement

Jürgen Stränger* and Bernhard Hommel†

*Ruhr University, Bochum and †Max Planck Institute for
Psychological Research, Munich

1 INTRODUCTION

The perception of other people's behavior is a particularly important event for coexistence. Although the discussion of the perception of human action has some tradition in practical philosophy (Meggle, 1977), little empirical knowledge is available. Textbooks on perception occasionally mention some aspects under the headings of *biological motion perception, perception of causality* or *person perception* (Bruce and Green, 1990); however, a comprehensive presentation of the various aspects of the perception of human action and body movements is still missing. We hope to close this gap by presenting theoretical and methodical approaches, major findings, and by discussing some problems in this field.

Observers draw a great variety of information from the stream of behavior, for example:

(1) Simple and complex body movements or actions with or without objects such as: WALKING, DANCING, PICKING UP A CUP or TYING A TIE.
(2) Real or pretended internal states, that is, intentions, motives or emotions that are particularly reflected in expressive behavior such as: EFFORT, ANXIETY or HAPPINESS.
(3) Effects of movement or action such as: a fallen vase or a criminal who has been knocked out.
(4) Various verbal and paralinguistic utterances.
(5) Symbolic actions such as: GREETING or SIGNING A CONTRACT.
(6) Social actions such as: HELPING or COOPERATING.

This chapter focuses on the perception of visually presented instrumental behavior. Instrumental behavior can be subdivided – although with fuzzy borders – into *simple body movements (operations), actions* and *activities* (Hacker, 1978; Leont'ev, 1972/1974). Highly automatized *simple body movements* such as WALKING or GRASPING are the basis of simple *intentional actions* such as LIGHTING A CIGARETTE. Perceiving an action requires a linkage of movements, intentions and effects (From, 1971). The perception of *symbolic actions* such as SIGNING A CONTRACT or more complex *activities* that include many actions, such as PREPARING A BIRTHDAY PARTY, requires a semantic integration of visual features of movement and actions, verbal

Handbook of Perception and Action: Volume 1
ISBN 0-12-516161-1

communications and prior knowledge. Without denying the role of semantic integration, this chapter focuses on perceptual aspects. Therefore, complex activities, symbolic actions and verbal communications are excluded.

We will present and compare six approaches addressing the *perception* of visually presented behavior, its intentions and its effects. In view of the multiplicity of these approaches, any prior definition of perception seems rather inappropriate. However, the often implicit concepts of perception will be briefly compared in the discussion.

The first part of this chapter deals with the following six lines of research on different aspects of the perception of behavior:

(1) Johansson's (1973) *biological motion perception* focuses on simple, cyclic body movements such as WALKING. Studies on the perception of personal characteristics such as gender or identity through body motion – mostly through their gait – are also included.

(2) Unlike physical object movements, actions, by definition, have internal determinants that can be drawn from ongoing behavior. Heider and Simmel (1944) first studied the perception of *intention* with moving figural stimuli. More recently, Runeson and Frykholm (1981, 1983) studied this issue with the help of a method taken from biological motion perception. The relationship between feeling, emotional expression and impression is a central problem in research on emotions. Because of the particular importance of this field for the perception of internal determinants of behavior, we will also review some results on the perception of *real* and *pretended emotions*.

(3) Behavior often has intended effects. Therefore, observers must perceive when and whether there is a causal connection between a behavior and its consequences. To our knowledge, the *perception of causality* has not yet been studied with visually presented behavior. Therefore, we include some important results on the perception of causality in object movements that follow the tradition of Michotte (1946/1963).

(4) Any behavioral event extends over time. Therefore, earlier parts of an event have to be linked to later ones. To account for this linkage, Johansson (1973) postulated an integrative short-term memory. Empirical studies on this integration and on the form of memory are part of the *dynamic events models* proposed by Freyd (1983) and Jenkins, Wald and Pittenger (1978). Their major findings will be presented.

(5) Simple concrete actions such as OPENING THE DOOR and more complex ones such as LAYING THE TABLE consist of many body movements. Thus, observers have to perceive not only single body movements, but also have to segment the complex stream of behavior and organize it conceptually. This is a central aspect in Newtson's (1976a) theory of behavior perception, which, in our opinion, is linked to cognitive approaches.

(6) The perception of behavior frequently has action-guiding functions. Thus, behavior is often observed to reproduce it in a similar way, to judge it, or to give behavioral feedback to the performer. Among these functions, *imitation*, that is, observation with immediate reproduction, is an interesting field for research on perception of behavior. Under certain restraints imitation may be regarded as a nonverbal method of reconstructing perceptual experiences, and it is also an interesting link between perception and action.

In Part II we will examine these six fields together. Implicit concepts of perception and methodical approaches are compared and some general issues are discussed with a particular emphasis on the relationship of cognition and perception.

Several related fields are excluded: we do not present research based on mere behavioral *descriptions*. Despite some aspects in common, this particularly concerns studies on *action identification* (see, for example, Miller and Aloise, 1989; Vallacher and Wegner, 1987) and *impression formation*. Although these accomplishments often involve visual perception under natural conditions, this research focuses on semantic rather than perceptual processes. We will also not deal systematically with the *perception of faces* and *facial expression*, as research on facial recognition (Bruce, 1988; Young and Ellis, 1989) and the perception of facial expressions (Buck, 1984; Walbott, 1990) require comprehensive presentations in their own right. Research on *eyewitness accounts* is also excluded, as it deals more with memory than with perceptual issues (Loftus and Ketcham, 1983). Finally, no consideration is given to research on the visual perception of physical motion and events in general (see, for example, Cutting, 1986) or in video and cinematic displays (Hochberg, 1986), as each of these topics would also require a separate chapter.

I   LINES OF RESEARCH

2   PERCEPTION AND IDENTIFICATION OF ACTING PERSONS

2.1   Perception of Biological Motion

We do not perceive human movements as mere changes in the location of parts of the body but, for example, as WALKING, TALKING, PLAYING CARDS or EATING. This classification seems to be effortless, but we have to ask which rules are used to organize such complex and temporally extended sensory information and assign it to specific categories. With regard to body movements, this question was first tackled by the Swedish psychologist Gunnar Johansson (1973). In some demonstrations, he introduced simple patterns of body movement such as WALKING or CYCLING as an object of perception. He coined the term *biological motion* for these patterns.

In his model of perception, which is influenced by Gestalt psychology, Johansson (1973, 1976) differentiates between a mandatory stimulus analysis performed by a basically autonomous perceptual system and central learning-dependent influences. The visual system is assumed to function according to the *principles of vector analysis*. Moving elements of the stimulus field are continuously interrelated, whereby simultaneous movements in the same direction are combined to form a perceptual unit. A hierarchical extraction of the vectors of these simultaneous movements leads to various hierarchically nested perceptual units. For example, when a girl rides a bicycle, the rotation of her feet, the movement of the spokes and the movement of the bicycle can be perceived independently from each other within various reference systems.

Johansson describes human body movements as *hierarchically organized pendulum motions*. If we look at a pedestrian from the side, the upper arm, for example,

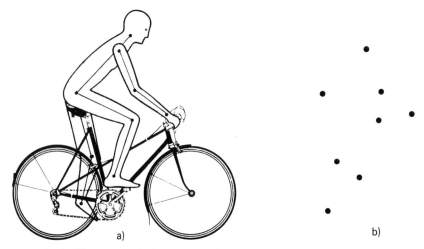

Figure 11.1. *Static illustration of the point-light technique: (a) sketch of the presented scene; (b) point-light presentation.*

describes a pendulum motion relative to the shoulder, the lower arm relative to the upper arm, and the hand relative to the lower arm. Another perceptual unit results from the opposing motions of shoulder and hip. According to Johansson, the vector analysis of such motions is followed by an *integration* of the extracted information in a *short-term memory*. Up to this point, processing is automatic and independent of foreknowledge. In contrast, the vividness of the perceptual impression and the assignment of extracted information to a movement category could be learn-ing-dependent.

In order to exclude influences of knowledge on perception as far as possible and thus study the functioning of the visual system in isolation, Johansson adopted the *point-light technique,* originally introduced by the French physiologist Marey in his early depictions of animal and human movement patterns by photo sequences (Marey, 1894/1994; see also Muybridge, 1897/1979). In this technique, which had already been applied by Taylor (1911) to optimize work sequences, small lamps or light-reflecting patches are attached to the main joints of stimulus persons. By using special lighting and high contrast, the visibility of body movements is reduced until only moving points of light are seen in cinematic or video displays (Figure 11.1).

Johansson particulary varied the type of activity performed by his stimulus persons (1973; Maas *et al.*, 1970, 1971). Subjects either reported generally on what they saw or they judged the identity, gender or activity of the stimulus person. Filmed movement patterns of walking, cycling, climbing and dancing point-light stimulus persons were quickly and easily recognized as human movements – even in movements into spatial depth.

Static figural features of the point-light stimulus provided little help in identifi-cation, completely in contrast to information that is generated by the movement. While walking persons are recognized within 200 ms and discriminated from moving dolls within a maximum of 400 ms, observers did not recognize stationary persons as being human (Johansson, 1976). However, as soon as the stimulus person moved, even 3-month-old infants could discriminate between normal and inverted displays (Bertenthal, Proffitt and Cutting, 1984).

Johansson (1973) found some support for his assumption of a hierarchically ordered representation of complex human movement. For example, he was able to show that the subtraction of a common component from the elements of motions did not impair identification. In this case, the stimulus display was a point-light person who appeared to be walking on the spot. Even the addition of an extra vector by continuously rotating the entire stimulus event had hardly any effect on identifications. Thus, judgments did not depend on the absolute movement relative to the observer but on local aspects of movement, that is, on the internal dynamics of the figure (Cutting and Proffitt, 1981).

2.2   Perception of Gait and Gender Identification

While Johansson analyzed various types of movement, Cutting and his team (Cutting and Proffitt, 1981) focused on the perception of human GAIT, in particular, the identification of biological gender from gait. With their grammar for perceptual events, Cutting and Proffitt (1981) presented a broad theoretical framework for these studies. According to the hierarchically ordered *grammar for event perception*, a visual scene is segmented initially into the event and its ground. The event itself contains the acting figure and the action. Information on the internal dynamics, the component structure and the *center of moment* (see below) is obtained from the figure.

Kozlowski and Cutting (1977) first demonstrated that observers were able to specify beyond chance the biological gender of point-light stimulus persons from their gait, as long as they moved in a natural way. It seems that this identification depends on the detection of an invariant feature in the movement sequence: while the presentation of one-step cycle, for example, was insufficient to permit a valid judgment on gender, two-step cycles were sufficient (Barclay, Cutting and Kozlowski, 1978)

In a search for valid visual movement indicators of gender, Cutting and collaborators studied in vain the contribution of individual features such as arm-swing or walking speed. Barclay, Cutting and Kozlowski (1978) finally measured the width of the shoulders and hips of their male and female stimulus persons and found – as anatomy would lead us to expect – that the quotient of shoulder width/hip width was relatively consistently above 1 in men and below 1 in women. Accordingly, gender identification could be based on the perceptual evaluation of these features. However, this failed to explain why identification was also successful when gait could be viewed only from the side.

Cutting, Proffit and Kozlowski (1978) finally proposed the *center of moment* (C_m) an index that specifies the geometrical point on which the movement of shoulders and hips is drawn. In a frontal perspective, it lies at the intersection of the diagonal lines from shoulder and hip. In a sagittal perspective, the points of maximum extension of shoulder and hip have to be linked diagonally. Thus, the hypothetical point lies within the body, approximately between the navel and the breast bone. This point is lower when shoulders are broader and hips are narrower. An arithmetical description of this relationship is obtained from equation (1):

$$C_m = \text{shoulder width}/(\text{shoulder width} + \text{hip width}) \qquad (1)$$

The index increases numerically as a function of broader shoulders and narrower hips. This relationship can also be drawn from a sagittal perspective and partial information on arm or leg movements if the level of extension of shoulders and hips is taken into account. Therefore, observers may be guided by the relation described with C_m when identifying gender from gait.

2.3   Identifying Oneself and Others Through Movement Perception

The relationship between body movement and biological gender is relatively simple, not least because of gender-specific body proportions. However, point-light movements seem to contain much more specific features that even permit the identification of an individual person.

As Wolff (1932, 1943) has already shown, persons who have not been given information on figural body features recognize themselves much more easily than acquaintances from samples of their filmed gait. This is remarkable, as generally one perceives the movements of other persons much more frequently and more completely than one's own body movements. Cutting and Kozlowski (1977) first compared self- and other identification in the point-light paradigm and found no differences in the precision of judgment. However, this may well have been because they asked for more self- than other identifications and, as a result, different levels of error probability were involved. In any case, Beardsworth and Buckner (1981) confirmed Wolff's findings with controlled error probabilities.

Following Cutting and Kozlowski's study, Frykholm (1983a) found that identification of others was more precise when several activities by each stimulus person were displayed with the point-light technique. On each trial, subjects viewed three film sequences: the first sequence showed the target person performing various actions; the two other sequences showed the same or another person in a random sequence. Subjects had to judge whether the target person appeared in the second or in the third sequence. Using this design, both unknown and known target persons were identified with more than random precision. Even 11-year-olds' identifications of their classmates were better than random. When the children viewed the films again after a 30-month interval, judgments were even more precise.

Frykholm (1983b) also studied the effect of feedback on the identification of point-light stimulus persons. The precision of identifications of friends or strangers decreased over time when subjects received incorrect feedback on their judgments. Nonetheless, the correctness of their judgments remained above random. In addition, some subjects seemed to be immune to incorrect feedback, while others 'gave in' very quickly. Finally, Frykholm showed that the ability to identify strangers correctly not only increased as a function of correct feedback but also generalized to judgments of new actions by the same stimulus persons.

2.4   Discussion

The first studies on the perception of biological motion were designed to test Johansson's (1973) assumption that the visual system functions according to the principle of vector analysis. Experimental procedures were thus based on a clear theoretical ground. Such a comparable base can scarcely be found in more recent studies.

Why, for example, has identifying gender from gait been studied so intensively? Is it really plausible to use kinematic parameters so frequently to determine gender under ecological conditions, although figural, vocal and culturally determined features such as dress and hairstyle should provide valid information more quickly?

Subjects' judgments oppose this: although the average hit rate of 70% compared to an error probability of 50% is certainly significant, this hardly supports the idea that a biologically adapted, direct perceptual process in the sense of Johansson is being studied. Instead, it seems to be a kind of data-induced hypothesis-testing as Cutting and Kozlowski (1977) originally suspected. Perhaps the information made available in the point-light design is, on the one hand, too sparse to permit a direct perception of gender but, on the other hand, sufficient enough to allow a high frequency of correct guesses.

More recent studies on the perception of biological motion are increasingly less concerned with detecting invariant working principles of perceptual systems and more involved in analyzing the assignment of specific perceptual information to specific categories. While both issues are important, they are not identical. Although the categorical decision requires valid perceptual information and, thus, precisely functioning perceptual systems, the decision could still be incorrect despite the availability of valid information because, for example, the analysis of perceptual information has to be learned. Perhaps this issue could be clarified by analyzing the relationships between stimulus information, judgment and feedback on learning trials, as initiated in the work of Frykholm (1983b).

3 PERCEPTION OF THE INTERNAL STATES OF OTHER PERSONS

Everyday interactions do not only require the recognition of specific patterns of movement. Observers frequently also have to identify whether the behavior of other persons was intentional or unintentional if they want to respond to it appropriately. The *perception of intention* was first addressed by Fritz Heider and later by students of Johansson.

3.1 Attribution of Intention

The first studies on the perception of action intentions can be traced back to the Austrian psychologist Fritz Heider who was strongly influenced by Gestalt psychology. According to Heider, the task of the perceptual system is to reconstruct the properties of the distal stimulus from the given sensory information and to form them into a perceptual impression, that is, the *percept*. Thus, a valid perception of events requires that the visual system possesses implicit information on the relationship between sensory information and the object of perception. In the perception of simple objects, Heider (1926/1959, 1930/1959) considered that it was plausible to assume regular relationships between information and object. In contrast, he considered the ability to perceive intentions directly through the perceptions of actions to be less plausible.

Indeed, relationships are very complicated in this case: as a mental cause that cannot be viewed directly, an intention leads to an observable (body) movement that is conveyed by the structure of the information available to the senses. Thus, the perceptual system must reconstruct not only the body movement from the available sensory information but also the intention from the body movement.

According to Heider, especially this second step cannot be performed by an autonomous perceptual system but must be a product of attribution. In his later work, Heider (1944, 1958, 1967) discriminated only rarely and imprecisely between perceptual and cognitive contributions to the percept, because he suspected that perception and cognition both were influenced by the same Gestalt laws. It follows that Gestalt laws of perception can also be used to predict *attributions*, that is, perceptions of intentions.

Heider and Simmel (1944) worked – like many subsequent researchers – with an animated cartoon. In the 150-second film, a large triangle, a small triangle and a circle move around a rectangle at different speeds. The 12 different scenes can be interpreted, for example, as a triangle that moves toward a house, opens a door, enters and closes the door behind it; or as if the two triangles are fighting each other.

One group of subjects should simply report what happens in the film. A second group should interpret the movements of the figures explicitly as human movements and then characterize the figures as persons. In all, only one subject described the contents of the film exclusively in geometrical terms. With the exception of two further subjects (who interpreted the movements as actions by birds), all the remainder interpreted the film as human activity, regardless of whether they were instructed to describe the contents only or to interpret them as human actions. Even a third group, who viewed the film in reverse, exclusively used descriptors of human actions. Comparable findings for displays with no specific prior information are reported by Heider (1967) and Oatley and Yuill (1985).

Heider (1944) attributed this personification to the *law of Prägnanz* from Gestalt psychology. He assumed that persons in contrast to objects are perceived as causes because they organize the stimulus field in the maximally salient ('prägnant' way. According to Heider, an event leads to a situation requiring an explanation that can be 'resolved' by attributing the event to a personal cause. In an ambiguous stimulus situation ('imperfectly structured environment'), this tendency also leads to the personification of objects to which specific intentions are assigned. Thus, each event elicits a need for attribution, and if more plausible causes are not available, material 'agents' are drawn upon to satisfy this need.

The tendency to perceive other persons as absolute causes is revealed not only in animated cartoons but also in more realistic displays such as audiotape (Alexander and Epstein, 1969) or videotape recordings (Storms, 1973) of a conversation between two persons. Depending on the observer's perspective, the contribution of situational factors to the explanation of behavior is underestimated more or less systematically. However, most studies of this *fundamental attribution error* (Ross, 1977) have addressed issues in motivational psychology and used verbal material (Kelley and Michela, 1980; Nisbett and Ross, 1980).

Alongside the law of Prägnanz, Heider and Simmel (1944) found indications of the effectiveness of other Gestalt laws. The *law of similarity* agrees with the finding that subjects tended to perceive the movements of objects that were labeled 'aggressive' as being AGGRESSIVE and the movements of 'passive' objects more as TIMID or COWARDLY. As no prior information was given on the properties of the objects, the 'personality' judgment on the objects must have been conveyed by the judgment on their 'actions'.

The *law of proximity* corresponds to the increased use of interaction-related terms when movements of objects were coordinated in space and time. Simultaneous movements of two objects without contact led, for example, to interpretations such as LEADING or CHASING, depending on whether the 'stronger' or 'more powerful' object was in front or behind. Successive movements of two objects with momentary contact, in contrast, were interpreted as HITTING. Here, Heider and Simmel postulated the additional effect of the *law of good continuation*.

Heider did not trace back the organization of the stimulus field to the activity of a broadly autonomous perceptual apparatus but to a *conceptual, knowledge-controlled,* or – to use a more modern term – *schema-driven integration* of perceptually available data (Heider, 1958, ch. 2). This assumption is supported by findings from studies that varied prior information on the topic of the film or the 'personality' of the 'actors'. For example, Shor (1957) found an increase in the frequency of unfavorable judgments on an object when it had been labeled 'aggressive' before the study. When prior information was given on the 'fair-minded' disposition of the same object, the judgments were markedly more favorable. At the same time, the object's 'interaction partner' received a more negative judgment, and judgments increased in negativity when interaction was more extensive. Naming the topic of the film ('The jealous lover', Oatley and Yuill, 1985) and prior information on the actors' intentions in a realistic film (Zadny and Gerard, 1974) also had a major influence on subjects' judgments.

3.2 Perception of Intention

Runeson and Frykholm (1983) used experiments based on Johansson's research technique to investigate the direct perceptibility of psychological determinants of behavior. These authors interpret psychological determinants of behavior, such as intentions or motives, as dynamic factors in the sense of physical kinetics. In kinetics, dynamic factors determine the kinematic sequence of movements, for example, displacements of mass, speed and acceleration.

If internal states such as intentions unequivocally specify the kinematic properties of actions as dynamic factors, then the opposite inference from kinematic patterns to dynamic determinants is also feasible and testable. Thus, insofar as the psychological determinants of behavior are unequivocally and specifically linked to patterns of body movement, intentions, emotions or motives should be recognizable from the movement pattern on a purely perceptual basis. In addition, a perfect deception of (mental) states would be impossible, as this would violate the principle of the *kinematic specification of dynamics* (KSD) (Runeson, 1977/1983)

Initial empirical findings are very encouraging: Runeson and Frykholm (1981) and Bingham (1987) showed their subjects point-light stimulus persons who were LIFTING and CARRYING a box that was also marked with point-lights. The weight of the box was varied. With such meager stimulus information, observers were able to estimate weights with extreme precision even when the box remained invisible (Runeson and Frykholm, 1983). Estimations on the length of a throw with an invisible sandbag were also very precise. Runeson and Frykholm (1983) instructed their point-light stimulus persons to deceive observers about either the heaviness of the weight they were lifting or their gender. In line with the prediction of the KSD principle, observers gave very precise estimations on both actual and pretended weight. Gender was also determined very precisely as long as subjects were informed about the possibility of deception. However, as soon as this information was not available, there was a clear drop in the hit rate on deception trials.

3.3   Perception of Emotion

Recognizing emotions from facial expressions is a central topic in research on emotion (Buck, 1984; Wallbott, 1990). As a systematic presentation of the perception of facial expressions would go far beyond the bounds of this chapter, we will restrict ourselves to aspects that are related to the KSD principle.

According to this principle, every intensive emotion, such as true happiness, should, as a physiological and emotional state, control different expressive movements. However, as facial expression has a nonverbal communication function as well as an expressive function, the visible sequence will be determined not only by emotion but also by acquired communication rules, that is, *display rules*. According to the KSD principle, it should be impossible to completely hide the expression of an intensive emotion. Rather, a leakage of the hidden emotion is to be anticipated. In research on emotions, this position is represented by Ekman and Friesen (see Ekman, 1982).

In a series of intercultural studies (Ekman, 1972), they first showed that pictures of static prototypes of facial expressions were linked cross-culturally to specific emotions. For example, the state of HAPPINESS was recognized in a face in which both the outer corners of the mouth and the lower eyelids were raised simultaneously. Similar relationships applied to ANGER, DISGUST and SADNESS, while FEAR and SURPRISE were more frequently confused. Thus, the systematic relationship between judged emotional state and facial expression could be confirmed for at least some basic emotions.

Under communication conditions, we always have to expect that expression will be influenced by display rules. The synchronization of expressive movements might be important for the recognition of 'felt' and 'false' emotional states. Thus, the sequence of smiling in the expression of TRUE HAPPINESS differs from other forms of smiling through the face muscles involved (Ekman and Friesen, 1982) and probably also through shifts in time parameters. As spontaneous and intentional facial expressions are based on the same muscular patterns but not on the same neurophysiological foundations (see Buck, 1984, p. 93), happy and polite smiling should differ in their patterns of innervation. Ekman and Friesen (1969) have shown that deception is more difficult to recognize from facial expression alone than from less controlled channels of expression such as foot movements or vocal features (for further findings, see Zuckerman, DePaulo and Rosenthal, 1981). However, the expertness of the observer also plays an important role in the perception of deception, as laypersons are easier to deceive than, for example, CIA experts (Ekman, 1990). Thus, further support for the KSD principle is also to be seen here.

The recognition of emotions is relevant to research on perception from another perspective: early empirical studies were based on ecologically less valid, schematized line drawings (Brunswik and Reiter, 1937) or photographs of faces (Good-enough and Tinker, 1931). It took a long time before the potentials of film and video-recordings for the presentation of expressive movements were used (Isen-hour, 1975; Wallbott, 1990). Indeed, the reduction of sequences of facial expression to static images must be partially responsible for the widespread opinion that the perception of emotions essentially depends on situational context information (Frijda, 1958). However, under natural conditions, static expression is a (pathologi-cal) exception, and it is possible that context information is only particularly necessary for recognizing such exceptions. Although it is claimed that the percep-tion of emotions in nonstatic expression also depends on context cues (Isenhour, 1975; Russel and Fehr, 1987), this seems to be more characteristic for neutral rather than typical emotional facial expression (Ekman and O'Sullivan, 1988). The role of movement information in the perception of emotional expression has been con-firmed by Bassili (1978, 1979), using the point-light technique.

Bassili (1978, 1979) studied whether observers were able to recognize emotions from expressive movements presented by point-light stimulus persons. These models used facial expressions to present various emotions. Their faces were covered with black make-up and up to 100 white spots, and they were presented either under normal lighting conditions, or as displays of moving spots, or as photographs.

Moving point-light displays of the expression of naive (Bassili, 1978) and trained (Bassili, 1979) stimulus persons were identified validly. However, emotions were recognized much more precisely under normal lighting conditions. In this case, even static facial expression was sufficient for identification (Ekman, 1972). How-ever, this did not apply to all expressive movements: while normal lighting facilitated the identification of ANGER, SADNESS, DISGUST and FEAR, SURPRISE and HAPPINESS were just as easily recognized in the point-light display.

3.4 Discussion

Studies on the perception of internal states are based on a wide variety of different theoretical orientations. Studies using Heider's approach have a clear *cognitive orientation*. This is related to their widespread neglect of the concrete properties of the stimulus display and the amount of information that it may contain. Heider and his followers wanted to demonstrate that a specific local event is interpreted as a function of the global event structure and is in no way experienced as a mere relocation of objects. Although available findings are completely in line with this, Heider's (from 1944 onward) assumption that stimulus patterns are necessarily inherently ambiguous, so that perception always requires interpretative elements, remained untested. There are three possible criticisms here:

(1) Possible correspondences between stimulus parameters and judgment were never tested. For example, Heider and Simmel (1944, Scene 10) presented two objects that circled a third object at two successively equal distances. Did the second object FOLLOW the first one, or did it CHASE it? Heider assumed that the spatiotem-poral relationships permitted no clear statement on this. Therefore, the subject had to know, for example, that the first object was 'more powerful' than the second one in order to perceive FOLLOWING. However, it is questionable whether this greater

power is not directly perceivable in the event without any need for inference. Indeed, the decision on CHASING or FOLLOWING could also depend on local stimulus parameters. Michotte (1946/1963), for example, found clear correspondences between specific stimulus parameters and judgments on PROPULSION or LAUNCHING by another object, the TRANSPORT of one object by another one, and the ENTRAINING of a following object by a preceding one. If these cases can be discriminated with available sensory data, why should judgments on CHASING or FOLLOWING not be based on specific local stimulus parameters as well?

(2) It is questionable whether findings obtained with ambiguous stimulus displays can also be generalized to unequivocal scenes. Heider and Simmel's (1944) animated cartoon did not provide the same information as a real hunt or a film of a real hunt. Therefore, it may well have been the experimentally introduced ambiguity of the stimulus materials that forced Heider and Simmel's subjects to make inferences.

(3) Heider and Simmel's stimulus display did not permit any test of the correctness of judgments. In contrast, judgments on the intentions of real persons are frequently controllable. Perhaps Heider and Simmel only really found indications that persons attempt a meaningful understanding of meaningless geometrical displacements.

These criticisms could be tested by manipulating the meaningfulness or the spatial and temporal relationships of the activities of two objects as independent variables. The extent of temporal contingency between the movements of the two 'agents' seems to be decisive for perceiving an interaction. In contrast, the spatial relationship influences the perceived nature of the interaction (Bassili, 1976). The more unequivocal the spatiotemporal relationships between the activities of the objects, the more observers tend to describe only the content of a film. With increasing ambiguity, there is an increase in the percentage of explanations added spontaneously to pure descriptions (Knowles, 1983).

In contrast to the Heider tradition, research by Johansson's followers is based on a *perception-related theory* in which the information content of stimulus events plays an essential role. Of particular theoretical and heuristic interest is the assumption of an unequivocal specification of internal states in the stimulus event (KSD). However, the KSD postulate is only convincing if unequivocal relationships can be confirmed between the causes of dynamic movement and the kinematic sequence of movement as well as correspondences between kinematic information and judgments. It is even more surprising that studies on the perception of internal states have neglected the analysis of stimulus conditions. As long as both relationships are not tested systematically, these studies will raise more questions than answers.

A promising approach – though it requires much further work – seems to be Runeson and Frykholm's attempt to substantiate the KSD principle with findings and hypotheses on action planning and action control. The specific parameters that determine the execution of an action probably also play a central role in its identification. It is therefore possible that parameters that determine the typical female gait or its faking play an equally important role in both production and perception.

Studies on the identification of internal states represent an interesting and stimulating extension of research on the perception of biological motion. This extension should also be encouraged for ecological and theoretical reasons. Studies on the perception of expression are very promising – also for testing the KSD principle. An advantage of this field lies in the fact that muscular foundations of facial expression movements are known and demarcated. This allows facial expressions to be described precisely with, for example, Ekman and Friesen's (1978) facial action coding system (FACS).

4   PERCEPTION OF CAUSALITY

Actions are performed to attain specific goals, that is, to elicit specific effects in the environment. Alongside the action sequence, these effects often provide essential information on the behavioral intentions of the observed person. For example, the aggressive intention underlying a movement frequently only becomes apparent when it leads to specific negative consequences. However, how do we recognize the relationship between an action and its effects? How can we know which effect belongs to which action?

4.1   Theoretical Basis

Up to now, there has been very little direct research on these issues in human behavior. However, Albert Michotte's research program on the perception of causality is closely linked to this field. Michotte investigated the more general issue of whether the causal relationship between two events (e.g. between two ball movements in a game of billiards) is inferred or can be perceived directly. He assumed that the perception of causality, that is, *phenomenal causality*, depends solely on parameters of the stimulus event and on autonomous organizational factors of perception. Accordingly, the causal relationship is directly perceived, that is, it is not added to the percept as a function of experience.

The perception of mechanical causality, as in the example of billiard balls, results from the solution of a *conflict between contradictory organizational tendencies* (Michotte, 1946/1963). On the one hand, the figural features of the billiard balls continue to exist before and after making contact with each other and permit the organization of the stimulus information into two independent objects in the phenomenal world. On the other hand, according to the Gestalt *law of good continuation*, there is a tendency for the movements of the two objects to be integrated into a unified percept of continuous movement.

The conflict between these two organizational tendencies leads to *phenomenal duplication*, that is, object identity and object movement are simultaneously but independently perceived. The movement of an object is accordingly not a constituent element of its identity. The experience of causality results from the integration of the information available from the phenomenal duplication into a unified percept. The integration follows the organizational *principle of ampliation*, a:

> '... process which consists in the dominant movement, that of the active object, appearing to extend itself on to the passive object, while remaining distinct from the change in position which the latter undergoes in its own right.' (Michotte, 1946/1963, p. 217)

This concept serves to predict and explain the experience of mechanical causality.

4.2   Findings on the Perception of Causality

Michotte and collaborators distinguished between two stimulus categories: in LAUNCHING, object *A* moves toward object *B*, stops, and then *B* moves forward in the same direction. In ENTRAINING, both objects move on in the same direction after their contact. After a single presentation of the stimulus pattern, up to 95% spontaneous causal judgments are made in LAUNCHING and up to 65% in ENTRAINING (Crabbé, cited in Michotte, 1966). Until now, size, movement distance, speed, form and color of *A* and *B* have been among the parameters varied. The subjects had to report their perceptual impression that was then tested for causal statements according to some (mostly incompletely specified) criteria. The dependent variable was the percentage of causal judgments, that is, a verbal indicator of the causation experience.

Michotte's approach is based on the assumption of a perceptual conflict in causal events. Accordingly, each manipulation of the prerequisites of this conflict, that is, the phenomenal constancy of the objects that perform the movements and the continuity of movement, should influence the probability of causal judgments. On the other hand, judgments should be resistant to manipulations of stimulus parameters that have no effect on this conflict.

In fact, the frequency of judgments depends not only on the existence of two, discriminable objects (Michotte, 1946/1963, Exp. 3 and 5) but also on the spatiotemporal continuity of the total sequence of movement (Exp. 4, pp. 33–37, ch. 15–16). Thereby the *temporal connection* of the 'effect' to the 'cause' is more important for continuity of movement and causal perception than *spatial proximity* (Yéla, 1952). In general the causal impression is the more compelling, the higher the velocity of *A* compared with *B* (Michotte, 1946/1963; Yéla, 1952). However, as soon as the object that has been launched moves off faster than the object launching it, the observers report an autonomous movement of B that is only contingent on contact with but not caused by *A* (Michotte, 1946/1963, pp. 108–109; Michotte, Knops and Coen-Gelders, 1957).

Michotte also studied stimulus events with more than two objects. Combining two contact events elicits the *tool effect*. In the basic experiment, three objects, *A*, *I* and *B*, are presented. Object *A* moves toward *I* and stops after having made contact. Then *I* moves toward *B* and also stops, while *B* moves on. According to Michotte (1951), subjects agree that, in this case, *I* adopts the role of a passive tool of *A*, with whose help *B* is manipulated. The effect depends above all on the speed of *I* and the distance between *I* and *B*. The effect is no longer found when the interval is large and the speed is low. *I* then goes beyond its (plausible) 'action radius' (Boyle, 1961; Yéla, 1954) and, to some extent, goes 'too far'.

4.3   Discussion

Michotte's (1946/1963) completely inadequate reports on the implementation of his studies, number of subjects, instructions, data collection and evaluation, as well as the forms of sample selection (see Boyle, 1972; Joynson, 1971) do not meet today's methodological requirements. Imprecise reports on the subjects' tasks and how the causal content of their judgments is determined make an assessment of the findings particularly problematic.

According to Michotte (1946/1963, p. 305), the *instructions* are summarized as, 'Say simply what is going on in the apparatus' or some equivalent wording such as 'Say what you see in the apparatus'. Thus, they provide little information on what information should be used to make a judgment (Joynson, 1971). The first version, in particular, is more to be understood as a request for intellectual interpretations of the occurrence than for reports on spontaneous perceptual impressions. Gockeln's findings (1978; cited in Heller and Lohr, 1982, p. 23) have demonstrated the importance of the concrete formulation of the instructions. Gockeln found that unpracticed subjects gave almost exclusively causal answers when they were asked, 'Describe what happens'. Given the instructions, 'Describe what you see', there were very few causal judgments.

For Michotte's theoretical approach, findings that indicate how perceptual impressions depend on the individual are problematic. If the experience of causality actually depends on autonomous organizational processes without any contributions based on knowledge, individual experiences should not be reflected in judgments. This is contradicted by the dependence of judgments on *intelligence level* (Beasley, 1968), *developmental level* (Olum, 1956) and special *strategies* (Gemelli and Cappellini, 1958). Short-term dependencies are also difficult to explain. For example, sometimes the causal impression only occurs after several presentations (Michotte, 1946/1963), and the frequency of causal judgments is influenced by special *training* (Lesser, 1977; Montpellier and Nuttin, 1973) or the type of preceding display (Gruber, Fink and Damm, 1957; Powesland, 1959).

The type of changes determined by practice remains unclear. Major aspects could be the fixation point and the pattern of eye movements. For example, Michotte (1946/1963, Exp. 7) found no causal judgments when the stimulus event was presented peripherally. Hindmarch (1973) reported increased causal judgments when the point of contact was fixated but not the starting point or goal of the total movement. Jansson (1964), nonetheless, also showed that the eye movements of persons who preferred causal judgments did not differ from those of other persons on the first trial. However, on subsequent trials, patterns of eye movement changed. Subjects who did not make causal judgments consistently fixated on object *A*, whereas subjects with causal judgments changed fixations more frequently. Thus, the type of eye movement or the choice of fixation point appears to be the consequence and not the cause of the judgment.

The causal impression does not seem to be completely independent from the skills and perceptual activity of the observer. This questions Michotte's conception, although it in no way excludes the assumption of a direct perception of causality. Perhaps causal experience is perceptually founded but requires experience in the active extraction of relevant stimulus information.

5   DYNAMIC EVENT MODELS

Unlike static images, behavior develops across time and makes different information available to the observer at various points in time. Thus, the perception of a dynamic event requires a medium in which information can be entered from and at different points in time. Simultaneously, a relationship (coherence) has to be constructed between pieces of information from different points in time. Johansson (1973, 1976) has postulated a short-term memory for this function in which information extended over time is integrated. More recent ideas and studies on the short-term representation of events have come from American research teams led by James Jenkins (Jenkins, Wald and Pittenger, 1978) and Jennifer Freyd (1987).

5.1 Theoretical Basis

When we see a walking person again, after he or she had been obscured by a tree trunk for a short while, we are certain that the person had also continued to exist during the interim period. This also applies to a ball whose line of movement is briefly hidden. Thus, we perceive a *phenomenally permanent* environment (Michotte, 1950) or objects with *apparent permanence* (Piaget, 1936/1952), although this perception is not supported continuously by sensory data. What is the basis of the certainty with which we assume the continued existence of objects that are temporally not confirmed by the senses?

On the one hand, this could be due to inference processes. Accordingly, the continued existence of an event that is temporally not represented in the senses is not perceived but is inferred with a certain probability. On the other hand, the way in which, for example, an object disappears from the field of vision and reappears could provide direct information about its continued existence (Gibson *et al.*, 1969; Michotte, 1950). Thus, the sensory effects of a bursting soap bubble are different from those of a soap bubble that is briefly hidden and then reappears. Such information could also be used to construct a mental model of the event.

An *inference approach* assumes a continuous flow of information from the observed event in the environment, across features of the event that are given and represented in the senses, to a percept. According to this approach, missing sensory information has to be replaced by inferences as soon as an object disappears for a short while. According to a *perceptual approach,* event perception does not primarily provide a continuous representation of sensory impressions in a percept but uses perceptual samples to construct an event model that is continuously updated. Although the event model is based on sensory data, it contains only an orientation- or action-relevant excerpt of information about the event in the environment. Thus, the short-term loss of sensory data does not lead to any impairment of perception and requires no inference processes. It is only essential that the model corresponds to the relevant part of reality and provides an orientation for further activity.

The assumption that the environment is *modeled* instead of *represented* requires the model to possess a degree of autonomy from sensory representation. This also applies to the inference approach, as inferences should replace the missing information. In the inference approach, autonomy only arises from a lack of information, and a lack of sensory information may lead to outcomes that deviate from reality. In the perceptual approach, autonomy provides improved orientation, that is, a more precise correspondence between model and modeled event.

If the relationship between the event itself and the event model is closer than the relationship between the sensory representation of the event and its model, the following predictions ensue:

(1) The construction of the model should not depend on the continuity of the flow of sensory information. It should also be possible to construct an event model from visual samples, for example, on the basis of a sequence of static images.

(2) The primacy of the event model over the information represented in the senses should lead to new individual images from the modeled event (e.g. photographs) not being recognized as new but being integrated into the event structure.

(3) The model should exhibit intrinsic dynamic properties, that is, it should reflect the continuity of the event sequence without corresponding to a continuous flow of sensory information. If, for example, a sequence of pictures only represents an event up to a certain point in time, the model should continue this sequence beyond this point.

5.2   Event Models and the Integration of New Information

In studies on the recognition of previously presented and new pictures, Jenkins (1980), Jenkins, Wald and Pittenger (1978) and Pittenger and Jenkins (1979) have found indications of a representation of the total event sequence that extends beyond the individual pictures presented.

In these studies several sequences of behavior were presented as series of slides that had been photographed with a stationary camera. For example, one sequence of 26 pictures showed a woman MAKING A CUP OF TEA. In the subsequent recognition test, eight previously shown pictures, eight new pictures from the same sequence and eight pictures from a similar sequence were presented. The subjects had to indicate which pictures they had already seen. This made it possible to test whether new pictures taken from the event would be recognized as new or would be integrated into the event model because of their similarity of content. Variations of this experimental design presented unrelated sequences of pictures and pictures in which the original spatial relationships were switched (Kraft and Jenkins, 1977) or perspectives were changed (Jenkins, Wald and Pittenger, 1978).

In these studies, the previously shown pictures were identified reliably. In addition, pictures that belonged to the same event but had not been presented before were frequently recognized (incorrectly). This finding is surprising when we recall that Standing (1973) and Standing, Conezio and Haber (1970) found highly accurate recognition of up to 10 000 thematically unorganized pictures. Finally, according to Jenkins' team, new pictures that did not belong to the same event were correctly identified as new. This excluded the possibility that the subjects were generally working imprecisely.

The readiness to recognize pictures that fit the event although they have not been presented before depends on various conditions. In thematically unrelated sequences, it was rarely ever present. Subjects then seemed to recall each picture by itself. In thematically homogeneous sequences, new pictures were recognized as new if they changed the perspective (Jenkins, Wald and Pittenger, 1978) or switched spatial relationships (Kraft and Jenkins, 1977). Finally, as in studies on phenomenal causality (Gemelli and Cappellini, 1958), using an analytical attitude made it possible to counteract the incorrect integration of suitable pictures with mnemonic strategies (Jenkins, 1980).

The studies of Jenkins' team support the idea that new visual samples of an event are integrated into an internal event model. However, an event model that permits the integration of information samples only seems to be created when the visual samples come from the same event in the environment. Subsequently available sensory information is used to update the model if it fills in gaps in the sensory flow of information.

5.3   Dynamic Representation

Freyd (1983) also assumed that presented subsets of an event are not stored discretely but stimulate an internal dynamic representation of the given event. In her experiments, she presented two or more individual pictures of an event in their natural temporal sequence. The last picture in each sequence – the standard – was followed by a comparison picture that was either identical to the standard or showed another stage in the event. If, for example, the standard portrayed a man halfway through JUMPING OFF A WALL, the nonidentical comparison picture showed him either just before landing on the ground or just after he had jumped.

If event models exist and possess a temporal direction, it should be easier to judge the difference of comparison pictures that show an unrealistic temporal continuation of the standard. For example, if an event is presented as a picture stage 1, the internal model should develop autonomously (in anticipation) toward a temporally subsequent stage 2. Therefore, it should be more difficult for a subject to discriminate the representation of the following stage 2 from stage 1 than a prior stage 0 from stage 1.

This assumption is supported by Freyd's studies using pictures of object movements. Subjects required a particularly long time for a 'different' judgment when the comparison picture showed a good temporal and spatial continuation of the previously presented event (Freyd and Finke, 1984, 1985).

The similarity between the standard and the comparison picture was determined, as in Jenkins et al., according to the coherence of the total event. When the standard provided a poor continuation of the prior picture, the effect was not found: 'good' and 'poor' continuations of the standard were then discriminated equally rapidly (Freyd and Finke, 1984). The length of the retention interval was fairly unimportant (Finke and Freyd, 1985). Like the findings of Jenkins, Wald and Pittenger (1978), this raises doubts about whether the effect has a sensory basis. The number of incorrect judgments even increased with longer retention intervals. In contrast, spatial and temporal coherence was decisive: when the three previously presented pictures implied a certain velocity, the judgment effect depended on how well the comparison picture continued the temporal sequence (Finke, Freyd and Shyi, 1986).

In pictures of natural events, also, Freyd (1983) found that nonidentical comparison pictures (stage 0 or 2) were less well discriminated from the standard (stage 1) if they represented a good spatiotemporal continuation of the stage of the event. The good continuation of JUMPING OFF A WALL was discriminated more slowly from the standard than a preceding stage 0. In a similar experiment, Freyd, Pantzer and Cheng (1988) showed a sequence of three slides of flower pots. On the first slide, the flower pot stood on a stand. The second slide was identical to the first except that the stand was missing. The third slide was the same as the second one except that the pot was either above, below or in the same position. Subjects had to memorize the exact position of the pot on the second slide and report whether this was the same as the position on the third slide. An error analysis of 'same' judgments given on trials with objective differences in position showed that flower pots were more often incorrectly linked to the position that they would have occupied if they had fallen off the stand.

The results of studies on the modeling of object movements in which several pictures were shown are compatible with the assumption that the judgment effect has a perceptual basis. The internal modeling of the event had access to larger samples of the prior sequence of events, thus permitting the extrapolation of future development. However, in studies using natural events, a maximum of one or two pictures were presented as the standard from which it was hardly possible to obtain perceptual information about further development. The reported effects are therefore only understandable under the assumption that knowledge about physical laws is used in addition to a temporally oriented event model. Accordingly, the internal model formation does not depend exclusively upon the momentarily available perceptual information but also draws on knowledge about relationships in the environment.

5.4 Discussion

Illusions or distortions of perception are traditionally evaluated as evidence that inferences play a major role in perception. Thus, the demonstration of knowledge-dependent judgment effects in studies on dynamic modeling also initially seems to support an inference approach rather than a perceptual one. Freyd, Pantzer and Cheng (1988) counter this inconsistency by discriminating between knowledge use and inference. They assume that it was not conceptual but perceptual knowledge that was involved in their study. Perceptual knowledge is either innate or is acquired at an early stage of perceptual learning. It determines the way in which the perceptual system works directly without any dependence on intentions or attitudes and thus stipulates a specific structure for event models.

To some extent, this position is the same as Johansson's (1973). In a given situation, both assume a mandatory activity of autonomic perceptual systems. However, in contrast to the influence of Gestalt psychology in Johansson's approach, Freyd *et al.* suspect that the way this system works can be changed by perceptual learning. This makes it very difficult to maintain Johansson's very clear differentiation of the influences of perceptual and conceptual knowledge and increasingly blurs the border between perception and memory. Thus, it is still unclear whether findings on internal modeling can go beyond their significance for memory theory and provide answers to questions on the direct representation of observed behavior.

On the other hand, 'dynamic' approaches force us to reconsider the traditional assumption that perception is a more or less discrete act. This assumption is not implausible for object perception, but the temporal extension of behavior and other events questions the meaningfulness of a strict differentiation between perception and memory, between perceptual and conceptual knowledge (Gibson, 1979; Johansson, 1979; Neisser, 1976). If perception is understood less as a representation of events in the environment and more as an extraction of information about events and their course, then internal modeling approaches can also contribute to an understanding of the perception of behavior.

6   STRUCTURING THE STREAM OF BEHAVIOR

With the exception of Heider and Simmel's (1944) animated cartoon, previous samples of behavior could only be assigned to a single behavior category. However, when perceiving a more complex action, events have to be isolated from the flow of behavior and be related to each other. Roger Barker has discussed the problems of structuring the stream of behavior, while, more recently, Darren Newtson has studied them empirically.

6.1   Theoretical Conceptions

Barker's (1963, 1978) naturalistic observation method refers to Lewin and Heider by assuming that the stream of behavior contains 'gestalt-like' units that 'naive' observers can assess reliably after a short practice. Although Barker admitted that his method presupposed a theory of behavior perception, his research team restricted itself to demonstrating 'natural' units in the stream of behavior. For example, after viewing an 8-minute film, Dickman's (1963) subjects grouped temporally ordered scene descriptions of a movie into an arbitrary number of units. Alongside a large variation in the number of segments, there was a more than random frequency of segmentations at specific locations.

Wright (1967, pp. 68–76) has used numerous observation protocols of behavior in natural situations to work out the following criteria for structuring them into *episodes*, that is, goal-directed actions in concrete situations: (1) change in the sphere of behavior (e.g. verbal, physical); (2) change in the parts of the body predominantly involved; (3) change in the direction of behavior or its tempo; and (4) change in behavior setting and in objects manipulated. The defining criterion of an episode, which Barker viewed as a natural unit of action, is the adherence to the same goal direction. Using an analytical attitude, episodes can be separated into parts (*phases*). By techniques such as time-loop recordings, they can be broken down even further into *actones*. These authors did not speculate about the psychological basis of this unit formation. They also did not test their assumption that the verbally formed units correspond to those found on a visual basis.

An American research team led by Darren Newtson has been analyzing the structuring of the visually presented stream of behavior since 1973 (Newtson, 1976a, 1977; Newtson *et al.*, 1987). According to Newtson (1976b), any action, such as HANGING UP A PICTURE, is defined by a major change in features between at least two points in time. Their empirical work has addressed only postural changes and not object (location) changes, which, however, leads to problems even in HANGING UP A PICTURE. As there are many simultaneous changes in ongoing behavior, observers have to select features whose change they monitor. Behavior perception would accordingly be a *feature monitoring process*.

Drawing on Neisser's (1976) *perceptual cycle model*, Engquist, Newtson and LaCross (1979, unpubl.) introduced *schemata* as the basis of feature selection. Activated schemata are confirmed or rejected by the information available or changed by surprising events (Newtson, 1973; Wilder, 1978a,b). Differences in prior information lead to the perception of different actions if, in each case, other features are specified for monitoring (Cohen and Ebbesen, 1979; Neisser and Becklen, 1975; Newtson, Engquist and Bois, 1977; Newtson and Rindner, 1979).

In agreement with Heider (1958), Newtson (1980) has adopted an interactionist perspective on the relationship between cognitive and perceptual processes. Perceptual organization can be influenced cognitively at any time. Thus, the structuring of ongoing behavior is – unlike in Barker – an outcome of available stimulus features as well as perceptual and cognitive influences.

6.2 Findings on Structuring the Stream of Behavior

6.2.1 General Methods

Newtson's team has mostly used ongoing one-person actions lasting between 30 s and 3 min as stimulus material. These are displayed as film or videotape recordings without any additional structuring aids such as cuts or changes in focus (cf. Hochberg, 1986). Naive observers have to structure the scene 'meaningfully' by pressing a button when they consider that one action has ended and another has begun. Sometimes, the *level of analysis* has been varied through the instructions and demonstrated on the example of OPENING A DOOR. In *natural segmentation*, observers are free to choose the size of units. In *fine* or *large segmentation*, subjects have to mark the finest or largest units. Each button press is temporally precisely assigned to the scene. The individual number of *button presses* is viewed as a measure of the amount of information processed (Newtson, 1973; Newtson, Engquist and Bois, 1977; Newtson and Rindner, 1979). Within an experimental group, all button presses are plotted over constant time intervals of either 0.5, 1.0 or 2.0 s. The resulting irregular *frequency distribution* of the button presses is used to determine the intervals with a particularly large or small frequency. Intervals with a frequency higher than one or two standard deviations above the mean are called *breakpoints* (BP), and intervals one or two standard deviations below the mean are *nonbreakpoints* (NBP).

The method provides stable interindividual differences in the number of segments with a mean retest reliability of 0.72 after 5 weeks, and individual segmentation patterns are also repeated more than randomly (Newtson, Engquist and Bois, 1976).

Alternative methods for determining the segment structure using cluster analysis (Massad, Hubbard, and Newtson, 1979; Newtson *et al.*, 1987, p. 207) or psycholinguistic methods (Carroll, 1980; Corcoran, 1981) have not become popular.

6.2.2 Segments as Coherent Perceptual Units?

Drawing on the click displacement experiments in sentence recognition (Fodor and Bever, 1965), Newtson and Engquist (1976) have studied the organization of units through the detection of deletions of frames from ongoing film at BPs or NBPs. If segments between BPs form a *coherent perceptual unit*, it should be easier to recognize deletions at the borders that define the action rather than within the unit. Newtson and Engquist (1976) have demonstrated for several actions that breaks of 4, 8 and 12 (= 0.5 s) individual frames at three successive BPs are more easily recognized than at matched NBPs. In addition, detection of deletions depended on the length of the deletion for BPs but not for NBPs. Likewise, Carroll (1980) and

Corcoran (1981) confirmed that visual interference was more easily recognized at linguistically defined action borders than within a single unit.

Newtson and Engquist (1976) further suspected that the action-defining BPs are emphasized in ongoing behavior and therefore easier to detect. In the *recognition paradigm*, subjects watch a film display of an action. Ten minutes later, they are presented with slides of BPs and NBPs as well as similar actions by the same stimulus person that were not shown previously. They have to judge whether they have seen them before or not (cf. Jenkins, Wald and Pittenger, 1978). Regardless of whether they segmented the display by button pressing or not, the subjects recognized BPs significantly better than NBPs (Newtson and Engquist, 1976).

Similar to studies on sentence processing in which units are based on the recognition of presented and semantically similar nonpresented words from various parts of sentences, linguistically segmented actions also show that individual pictures from the beginning of the second unit are better recognized than those from the end of the first unit (Carroll, 1980; Corcoran, 1981; Lasher, 1978, 1981). Independently from Newtson, these authors suspect that the perceptual processing of a 'grammatical' action unit proceeds to the subsequent one. The preceding unit is recoded abstractly and holistically, thus impeding precise recognition.

Whether the segmentation procedure provides proof of *coherent perceptual units* remains unclear. On the one hand, feature differences between BPs and NBPs are confirmed (see below). On the other hand, Newtson, Engquist and Bois (1976) report for eight actions a mean unit length of approximately 12 s under natural segmentation, 7 s under fine segmentation, and approximately 26 s under large segmentation. A primarily perceptual organization of units of this length is improbable if a time limit of approximately 3 s is assumed for perceptual organization (Pöppel, 1985).

The psychological foundations of unit formation must therefore be defined more precisely. Is segmentation based – as Newtson suspects – on the comparison of two, temporally separated states, between which a monitored posture feature changed critically, or is it, instead, based on the perception of a holistic 'event Gestalt' (Verlaufsgestalt) (see Johansson, 1973)? It is also necessary to clarify whether action units are perceived directly or are subject to cognitive mediation.

6.2.3   Foundations of Segmentation

According to Newtson's (1976b) *feature monitoring hypothesis*, the perception of an action requires at least one critical posture change between two points in time. To test this hypothesis, posture changes between successive BPs and temporally matched NBPs were coded with the *Eshkol–Wachman movement notation system* (Eshkol, 1973; Rosenfeld, 1982). This goniometric procedure records 15 changes in the angle between the major limbs and their pivot joints. If, for example, the right arm is raised and extended without bending the forearm, a change in the position of the upper arm but not of the forearm is registered. In addition, the frontal orientation and the weight distribution of the body are taken into account. Each comparison of body positions between two points in time thus results in a 17-point vector. Factor and Fourier analyses can be calculated for larger numbers of vectors.

Newtson, Engquist and Bois (1977) tested posture changes between successive BP–BP, NBP–BP, BP–NBP and NBP–NBP pairs in correct and random sequence under all three levels of analysis. As anticipated, the extent of change between correct BP sequences was the highest. For each action, separate factor analyses produced several specific, interpretable factors. For example, in WAITING FOR A PHONE CALL, movements of the right hand and the right forearm formed one factor that, according to Newtson *et al.*, is related to answering the phone. Movements of the head and neck, lower leg and the left upper arm loaded on a second factor. These movements were interpreted as reactions to the ringing of the phone bell.

In an extension of the feature monitoring hypothesis, Newtson *et al.* (1987) looked for periodic changes in ongoing behavior. Posture changes in seven actions were coded with the Eshkol–Wachman system in 1-second intervals. A Fourier analysis of the wave-like course of the posture changes resulted in significant periods for all actions. For CONSTRUCTING STICK FIGURES, for example, these lay at 4 and 16 s. At these intervals there was a repeated increase in posture changes. Other actions showed other significant periods that revealed a nonrandom relationship to the large segments. As the authors did not interpret the content of these periods, we suspect that for CONSTRUCTING STICK FIGURES, one part is added about every 4 s and a whole figure is completed and put aside every 16 s.

In addition to stimulus effects there are also person-dependent effects. For example, instructing subjects to segment finely, naturally or largely leads to the anticipated changes in the number of segments (Hanson and Hirst, 1989; Jensen and Schroeder, 1982; Kogelheide and Strothe, 1980; Koopman and Newtson, 1981; Lassiter, 1988; Newtson, 1973). Thus, the level of analysis is chosen intentionally.

Attitude effects have also been demonstrated. According to Neisser (1976) as well as Engquist, Newtson and LaCross (1979), variations in prior information or observational tasks specify different schemata that should lead to different segmentation patterns (and retention performances). For example, differences in segmentation patterns could be demonstrated following the information that subjects would subsequently have to recall the scene or to judge the person (Atkinson and Allen, 1983; Cohen and Ebbesen, 1979; Engquist, Newtson and LaCross, 1979; Graziano, Moore and Collins, 1988; Markus, Smith, and Moreland, 1985; Massad, Hubbard and Newtson, 1979; with the same tendency, but not significant: Schorneck and Berger, 1980).

Newtson (1973) and Wilder (1978a, b) have also demonstrated that segmentation becomes finer after inserting a *surprising event*. The authors believe that surprised observers try to overcome the uncertainty about the action by a more acute monitoring of the event. Conversely, a known scene should be segmented in larger units, which, as yet, remain unconfirmed. For example, Droste and Holtmann (1980) found no effect of a preceding summary of the scene. Segmentation also did no change significantly during repeated displays (Kogelheide and Strothe, 1980; Nyce and Becklen, 1978). The relationship between segmentation and predictability thus remains open.

6.2.4 Relationships Between Units

Newtson and Engquist (1976) suspected that BPs summarize the action like *comic strips*. Thus, they tested the intelligibility of BP and NBP sequences. Observers saw pairs or triads of BPs or NBPs in natural or randomized sequence. They had to rate the intelligibility of the slides, summarize them into one sentence and judge the correctness of their order. BP sequences scored better than NBP sequences in intelligibility, descriptiveness and in order judgments (Newtson and Engquist,

1976). Variations of the sequence influenced the intelligibility of BPs only and not of NBPs. Scrambled sequences were better recognized in BPs than in NBPs.

Newtson (1977, Exp. 8 and 9) also presented the pictures used in the triads pairwise and found weaker effects. The intelligibility judgments were better for triad displays than those calculated from pairwise presentation of the pictures. Comprehension seems to depend not only on changes from picture to picture: the temporal picture context seems to have an overall effect on comprehension (see Jenkins' concept of coherence).

Further studies investigated whether segmentation varied over a *hierarchical structure*. A 'hierarchical' dependence would be present if a higher than random number of BPs agreed across various segmentation instructions. This has been confirmed repeatedly for fine or large segmentation (see, for example, Hanson and Hirst, 1989; Newtson, 1973; Rindner, 1982, cited in Newtson *et al.*, 1987). Hierarchical dependencies were also found when varying predictability (Wilder, 1978a, b), arousal (Newtson, 1977, Exp. 2), and film projection speed (Newtson and Rindner, 1979).

The type of hierarchical dependence remains undetermined. Hierarchical dependence in the sense of a differentiation of larger segments when performing fine segmentation or summarizing fine units to large ones has not yet been confirmed unequivocally. Although there is a more than random agreement on the number of BPs under large and fine segmentation, the agreement between large breakpoints and fine ones is consistently less than 50% (Hanson and Hirst, 1989: 34%; Kogelheide and Strothe, 1980: 41%; Newtson, 1973: 36%). However, as nearly all previous research has studied mean segmentations in independent groups, a hierarchical organization on the individual level may well remain undetected.

Thus, little is known about the relationships between the units. Findings from Newtson (1977) and Newtson, Gowan and Patterson (1980), like similar findings from Jenkins, Wald and Pittenger (1978), suggest that the relationship between units is determined semantically.

6.3   Discussion: A Cognitive Interpretation of Segmentation

According to Newtson, observers segment when they notice a meaningful change in the postural features monitored. Segmentation assesses a perceptual process that can be influenced cognitively. Although our perspective is compatible with Newtson's findings, we interpret segmentation as a conceptual classification on the basis of activated knowledge structures, and thus as a cognitive process. This elaborates the unpublished schema theory by Engquist, Newtson and LaCross (1979).

Like Barker and Newtson, we assume that ongoing behavior contains anatomical and physical features that are used to identify actions (see the spike structure of posture changes in Newtson *et al.*, 1987; episode criteria in Wright, 1967).

However, which features are attended to and integrated perceptually depends not only on activated knowledge structures and the behavioral intentions of the perceiver but also on the situational context (Cohen, 1981; Engquist, Newtson and LaCross, 1979; Neisser, 1976). As long as the context under natural conditions is not blanked out with the point-light technique or by pantomime (see Becklin, 1983, cited in Newtson *et al.*, 1987; Hilse, 1985; Sakowski, 1985), features of the present situation and experiences with similar action contexts should also activate knowledge structures about probable actions (see *schema* or *script* in Rumelhart, 1980; Rumelhart and Ortony, 1977; Schank and Abelson, 1977). Schank and Abelson (1977) introduced the term *vignette* for the visual properties of actions represented in knowledge structures. We believe that these vignettes, which are embedded in knowledge structure, facilitate the identification of action. In experiments, observers are forced to interpret for themselves the size of a *meaningful action unit*. The example of OPENING A DOOR that is given with the instruction might suggest a finer size of meaningful units than a more complex example like TYPING A LETTER would do (Cohen, 1981; Ebbesen, 1980). Observers might infer further cues from the duration of the event. Thus, A TELEPHONE CALL in a longer office scene might well be segmented into larger units than when it is presented in isolation.

Against this background, our interpretation of segmentation moves away from Newtson's concept: although we do not deny a perceptual basis in the identification of actions, we believe that the button press is cognitively based. Without recourse to knowledge structures, it remains unclear according to which criteria observers discriminate meaningful from meaningless changes. Given the assumption that the visual display activates a domain-specific knowledge structure with visual features, 'meaningful' changes are those that have a correspondence in the knowledge structure. Changes without this correspondence are 'meaningless' and perhaps overlooked. 'Surprising events', which Newtson does not define, do not fit the active script. A hierarchical knowledge structure also permits various, possibly hierarchically nested levels of analysis. The above-mentioned 3-second time limit for the perceptual organization of events and further cues support this cognitive reinterpretation of segmentation as a conceptual classification of visual changes.

Natural conceptual classifications have *fuzzy borders* (Zadeh, 1972). This is also seen in the segmentation of ongoing behavior. According to Stränger, Schorneck and Droste (1983, p. 27), about 30% of BPs conveyed on a 2-second basis are surrounded by intervals of intermediate segmentation frequency (IBP; pattern: IBP–BP–IBP). The BP–BP–IBP and IBP–BP–BP pattern each represent about 13% of the patterns. The pattern NBP–BP–NBP, that should be most prominent if Newtson is right, occurred in less than 4% of the patterns. Accordingly, segmentation seems to be more allotted to time zones than to time points. This is very plausible when we consider that, for example, CLOSING A WINDOW can be segmented somewhere on the way to or from the window. The time of segmentation might depend on what the observer knows about the context of the activity of the actor. If the observer, for example, knows that the actor is irritated by a sudden traffic noise from outside, he may realize the intention of the actor earlier than without that knowledge.

If units are formed on the basis of natural knowledge structures, segments should be *easy to name*. Thus, Schorneck and Berger (1980) showed that observers who had to describe aloud while segmenting mostly gave behavior-synchronous or summarizing descriptions. A detailed analysis of the behavior-synchronous utterances revealed that 63% of the segmentations followed their naming. Accordingly, the conceptual classification seems to be primary; naming or segmenting is secondary.

If conceptual classification is primary, similar segmentation patterns should result on both a verbal and a visual basis. Baggett (1979) has reported a high level of agreement on the segmentation of a 34-minute film using either 367 verbal phrases or 571 single stills. Nonetheless, subjects were presented with a broader, text-linguistic episode concept. If the segmentation pattern of a visually and verbally presented event would also be similar under the instructions given by Newtson, this would be a further confirmation for a cognitive–semantic interpretation of the segmentation.

One of the most notable features of the studies on segmentation is the *high (and reliable) differences in the number of segments*. Stränger, Schorneck and Droste (1983) reported 7 to 80 units for the segmentation of a 10-minute office scene. Similarly high variations can be found in other studies. In free classification tasks, major individual differences in the number of concepts applied are well known (Gardner, 1953/1954; Glixman, 1965). The cognitive style of *category width* was derived from this observation (Pettigrew, 1958). Unfortunately, category width has not yet been correlated with the number of segments in any study on the segmentation of ongoing behavior.

In a theoretical interpretation of observational learning, Stränger has assumed that segments influence memory performance as *chunks* in the sense of Miller (1956). Initial attempts to test this hypothesis on memory for actions with cued recall tests have been unsuccessful (Cohen and Ebbesen, 1979; Droste and Holtmann, 1980; Kogelheide and Strothe, 1980; Schorneck and Berger, 1980; Stränger, 1977), whereas other authors have reported weak relationships (Koopman and Newtson, 1981; Lassiter, Stone and Rogers, 1988). According to Hanson and Hirst (1989), the type of test is a major variable. In free recall, observers recalled more after fine segmentation than after large segmentation. In a cued recall test, these differences could not be found. Thus, segmentation and the representation of an event in memory are probably closely related (Neisser, 1976; Stränger, 1977, 1979). Free recall seems to reflect the memory representation of actions better than tests with prompts. Nonetheless, this discussion is certainly not yet complete (Hanson and Hirst, 1991; Lassiter and Slaw, 1991).

Considering these secondary findings together with some of the findings by Newtson, we assume that visual events in ongoing behavior are primarily classified conceptually. Secondarily, the units are named or marked by the button presses, depending on the instructions (cf. Ebbesen, 1980).

7   BEHAVIOR PERCEPTION AND MOTOR REPRODUCTION

Among the processes that are based on the perception of behavior, direct reproduction, that is, *imitation,* is of particular interest to research on perception. Given certain preconditions, imitation can be regarded as a method of reproducing the perceptual experience. Although each motor imitation requires the perception and storage of observed behavior as well as its transformation into the motor system, these processes are only occasionally addressed in empirical research on imitation. They are mostly neglected in favor of the motivational conditions of imitation (Bandura, 1971, 1986; Scully and Newell, 1985; Stränger, 1977, 1979; Whiting, 1988)

7.1   Imitation Phenomena that are Relevant to
Research on Perception

From a functional perspective, *imitation* is not a unified phenomenon (see Stränger, 1977; for a historical review see Scheerer, 1985).

Sensory Modalities
With reference to the sensory modalities involved, *acoustically, verbally and visually* conveyed forms of *imitation* are often distinguished (see, for example, Guilliaume, 1926/1971; Piaget, 1945/1962). We will only consider the latter.

Relationship Between Perception and the Motor System
Regarding the kind of relationship between perception and the motor system, *automatic, reflex-like* forms of imitation can be discriminated from *conscious, intentional* forms (see, for example, Koffka, 1921/1952; McDougall, 1908; Morgan, 1896; Piaget, 1945/1962). The automatic forms are of particular interest to research on perception as they suggest a connection between perception and the motor system that is originally not mediated by cognition. These automatic forms include:

(1) *Self-imitation*, that is, the repetition of one's own body movement on the basis of its perception (Baldwin, 1895; Guilliaume, 1926/1971; Piaget, 1945/1962).
(2) *Ideomotor*, that is, nonintentional movements or *motor mimicry* that accompany the observation of movements seen in others (James, 1890; McDougall, 1908)
(3) *Movement imitation by infants* (McDougall, 1908) that have received much attention since the studies by Meltzoff and Moore (1977, 1983a,b; see also: Vinter, 1985a, b, 1986; Whiting, 1988)
(4) *Response facilitation*, that is, the elicitation of a behavior in the observer that corresponds roughly to the model (Aronfreed, 1969; Bandura, 1986; Koffka, 1921/1951; McDougall, 1908)

These imitation phenomena particularly occur in early childhood. The similarity between observed and executed behavior is mostly slight.

Type of Agreement
A further important differentiation concerns the type of agreement between model and observer behavior. Process-like *movement imitation* requires the perception and reproduction of spatial and temporal features of a (body) movement. Outcome-oriented *action imitation*, in contrast, emphasizes the reproduction of similar (environmental) effects, while agreement on the course of body movement may be only slight (Aronfreed, 1969; Miller and Dollard, 1941; Morgan, 1896). Different reference systems and forms of representation are linked to this conceptual distinction: if a movement of another person is imitated as a body movement, it should be related to one or more reference points of the actor's body, as for example the center of moment in the imitation of gait (see Johansson and Cutting). These body movements may also be represented dynamically (see Freyd). As a *motor task*, the reproduction of new body movements is not expected to be very successful on the first trials, because the execution also depends on kinesthetic feedback. If a movement of another person is imitated as an object-directed action, it relates, in contrast, to the spatial context outside the actor's body, especially to the displacement and change of the manipulated objects. For an effective representation of these *cognitive tasks*, it is important to discriminate which environmental effects are critical. A rough representation of the changes of objects or their position is sufficient to reproduce similar effects on the first trials with body movements, which may widely diverge from the movements seen in the model.

Observational Learning

In *learning by imitation* or *observational learning,* the observation of a model's behavior plays an important role in the acquisition of a plan for a new body movement or an object-directed action. *Observational learning effects* include the transfer of an available movement or action pattern to a new situation and the recombination of existing movement or action patterns into a new configuration (Bandura, 1971, 1986; Koffka, 1924). In reinforcement theories, these effects are interpreted by generalization (Gewirtz and Stingle, 1968), otherwise by diverse cognitive processes (Aronfreed, 1969; Bandura, 1971, 1986; Stränger, 1977).

7.2 Theoretical Conceptions

Koffka (1924) already emphasized that a central problem in imitation is how perception can issue in a movement similar to the model's behavior. He solved this old *ideomotor problem* by assuming a direct relationship between a perceptual and a movement structure to which Gestalt laws could be applied. In the ontogenetically earlier *compulsory imitation,* the observation of a movement provides an event-Gestalt-like perceptual structure that, according to the *law of configurative supplementation* and the *law of repetition of figures,* directly and necessarily elicits an ideomotor movement. Automatic imitation phenomena could be interpreted in this way (for further theoretical approaches, see Prinz, 1987). In the ontogenetically higher and later *ability to imitate,* that is, *voluntary imitation,* the relationship between perception and movement is mediated by cognitive processes. The central issue here is how the observation leads to a correct perceptual structure. Koffka already pointed to the possibilities of emphasizing the point of attack for the solution, of drawing attention to things not previously connected with the situation, or of pointing out essential features of an action by means of language. The impulse for imitation in these cases mostly comes from sources other than perception. This motivational issue is not a particular problem of imitation but a problem within a general theory of motivated action. However, it has been this motivational aspect that has received the most attention in empirical research on imitation (Bandura, 1986; Halisch, 1990)

   According to Piaget (1945/1962), the development of imitation is based on innate reflexes in which perception and movement are closely linked. Through practice, reflexes are integrated into more flexible sensorimotor schemata, which, like grasping, contain invariant perceptual and motor features. These schemata can be applied with increasing flexibility and purpose to different objects. Through repeated application, the child adjusts his or her sensorimotor schemata to reality (*accomodation*) and simultaneously, but to a lesser extent, adopts new features into his or her schemata (*assimilation*). By repeatedly combining originally isolated sensorimotor schemata, more comprehensive sensorimotor units are formed. This makes the child's behavior increasingly more differentiated and flexible. The perception of another person's or the child's own body movements activates known schemata, which the child first attempts to make persist through similar movements. Originally, this imitation can only be elicited by the perception of own movements (*self-imitation*); later, movements seen in others can also be continued in this way (*imitation of others*). After the sixth stage of sensorimotor development, that is, after approximately 18 months, this procedure is internalized. According to Piaget, the first representations, which also permit *delayed imitation*, are based on this internalization. Because these representations are later linked to language and thought, imitation becomes cognitively mediated, more conscious, and selective.

Koffka and Piaget solved the ideomotor problem by assuming an innate relationship between perception and movement that is later mediated cognitively by language and thought. In this way, they had already provided solutions to a theoretical problem in the early formulation of Bandura' s social learning theory (Stränger, 1977).

Bandura (1962) originally interpreted the mediating representations in observational learning by *stimulus contiguity* (Sheffield, 1961). According to this idea, sensations that are repeatedly elicited by events in close spatiotemporal proximity become associated with each other; this association results in an integrated perception. This conception fails to solve the ideomotor problem unless one assumes a connection between the integrated perception and the motor systems. It also remains unclear why observers are not able to imitate every repeatedly observed behavior at any time. Later, Bandura (1971, 1986) advanced an *information processing interpretation* of observational learning effects. Active observers abstract common features and rules from the model's behavior, transform stimuli into easily remembered schemata, classify and organize actions, and construct ideas about how they should be performed. While originally only visual and verbal representations were taken into account, Bandura (1986) – like Aronfreed (1969) earlier – now also mentions amodal schemata as well as conceptual and propositional representations.

Stränger (1977, 1979) specified Bandura's interpretation in a heuristic model of the processing of visually presented behavior. Taking into account Piaget's *schema concept* and E. J. Gibson's (1969) concept of *perceptual learning*, he proposed a multistorage model with closely interrelated patterns (schemata) of visual and kinesthetic invariances of body movements (and manipulated objects). The schemata have a conceptual character in older children and adults and can frequently be named (e.g. GRASPING, CATCHING A BALL). They permit a conceptual classification and the naming of the observed actions. Fitting in with this conception, Hoenkamp (1978) and Todd (1983) have shown that computer-simulated matchstick-like 'leg or arm movements', whose angle and speed were varied systematically, are also given different names. Accordingly, observers 'know' different visual features of WALKING or RUNNING. Eye movement patterns are considered to be a part of the schema that is constructed through the repeated visual analyses of behavior. These patterns may later control analyses of similar behavior (Neisser, 1976). The selection of analyzing schemata should depend on observational intentions, early stimulus characteristics in the display, and domain-specific perceptual and performance-related experiences. The information available in ongoing behavior either confirms or rejects the schemata underlying the analysis. Visually displayed behavior is thought to be represented in the form of confirmed schemata that are mostly nameable. Up until reproduction, the activated schemata may be maintained through imaging or verbal repetition, and – as long as they are structured hierarchically – may also be organized in higher categories. Kinesthetic components of the active schemata control the motor performance on a strategic level (Miller, Galanter and Pribram, 1960). Depending on the intention of the child or adult observer, behavior is either imitated as an action with similar effects (in the environment) or as a body movement with a similar spatiotemporal structure. In the case of learning, motor reproduction requires kinesthetic and visual feedback as well as adaptations to object properties. This feedback is especially important for movement imitation. Thus, the ideomotor problem is theoretically solved with a schema conception. The differentiation of the schemata may result from mere perceptual learning (see E. J. Gibson, 1969). By emphasizing domain-specific experiences in perception and performance and the need for kinesthetic feedback, the obvious limitations of observational learning are taken into account.

The assumptions of this and similar conceptions can only be tested piecemeal by referring to hypotheses from current research on perception, memory and motor behavior. The available findings are sparse and heterogeneous.

7.3 Findings on Movement and Action Imitation that Relate to Perception

7.3.1 Methods

For a functional analysis of movement and action imitation, known or new behavior is presented with a duration of between 3 s and 4 min. Typically, the sequences last about 20 s in order to avoid intraserial interference (Margolius and Sheffield, 1961).

New body movements with low verbal codability and without objects are appropriate to study the learning of body movements by imitation: for example, the manual language of the deaf (Gerst, 1971), simplified tai chi (Teubner, 1985), or ballet sequences (Gray et al., 1991) and sport exercises (Whiting, 1988) – as well as meaningless hand or arm movements (Prinz and Müsseler, 1988; Vogt, 1988). Action imitation is often studied with namable actions that are related to objects (e.g. tying knots: Roshal, 1961; dismantling and reassembling objects: Margolius and Sheffield, 1961; Jeffery, 1976; Stränger, 1977). As no theoretically based taxonomy of behavior is available, selection depends on practical considerations and individual preferences. For studying visual perception and visual recognition in imitation, patterns with low verbal codability should be preferred.

Older children, adolescents and adults are explicitly told in advance that they must perform the behavior subsequently. Reproduction immediately follows the display, or, when memory is being tested, after a filled time interval of several minutes. In action imitation, the objects are available for the reproduction. Thus, the task is similar to a cued recall test. In contrast, movement imitation is closer to free recall.

If imitation research focuses on differences between acquisition and performance, a *verbal reproduction* may be required as an index of acquisition. In this case, it would be more advantageous to test the *recognition* of presented as compared to similar nonpresented behavior units, as behavior varies in verbal codability and observers have to decide what they consider to be worth reporting. However, this procedure has rarely been applied (see, for example, Hilse, 1985; Weißenfeld, 1984).

In analyses of action imitation, it is mostly tested only how many units or how often previously seen effects roughly agree with the model's demonstration. In contrast, studies on movement imitation also take into account event features such as similarity of posture changes and movement speed (Gray et al., 1991; Teubner, 1985). The dependent variable in observational learning is either the number of trials up to a fixed performance criterion or the quality of reproduction after a set number of demonstrations.

7.3.2 Exemplary Findings

Action Versus Movement Imitation

Infants up to two months of age seem to imitate facial movements more readily than similar object movements (Legerstee, 1991). However, at the end of the first year, infants spontaneously imitate more object-related actions than pure body movements (Abravanel, Levan-Goldschmidt and Stevenson, 1976; Rodgon and Kurdek, 1977). At about the age of four years, children imitate more actions with appropriate objects than equivalent movements without objects (Killen and Uzgiris, 1981; Uzgiris and Silver, 1976, cited in Uzgiris, 1984).

Contrary to Piaget's conception, imitation seems to exist already in the neonate (cf. Field *et al.*, 1982; Meltzoff and Moore, 1977, 1983a; Vinter 1985a,b), and it seems to be based on an inborn intermodal relationship between the perceptual and motor system (cf. Meltzoff and Moore, 1983b). The imitations in neonates may serve communicative functions. In older children, the meaning of an action seems to be essential for imitation.

Extending two experiments from Bandura (Bandura and Jeffery, 1973; Bandura, Jeffery and Bachicha, 1974), Stränger (1977) demonstrated that the reproduction of filmed patterns of 'arm movements' performed in front of a regular background increased as a function of the discriminability of the background. As in Bandura *et al.*, the traceless 'movement' seen had to be reproduced as a trace on paper. With a dotted background, 12-year-olds drew the trace but did not try to reproduce the movement precisely, and some even presented the body movement in the opposite direction. Thus, observers did not copy an arm movement but the linkage between the points. The arm movements could probably have been replaced just as effectively by a moving point-light or a sequence of lamps flashing.

These findings show that older children and adults prefer to reproduce understandable actions rather than meaningless movements (Koffka, 1921/1952). Therefore, studies on movement imitation must explicitly call for the reproduction of the spatial and temporal course of the observed event.

Perceptual aspects

Constant displays of behavior are mostly provided with film or videotape recordings. The *reduction of spatial depth* does not impair reproduction compared to real-life presentation (Martens, Burwitz and Zuckerman, 1976; Stränger, 1977, Exp. 2). However, this might depend on the task and on the developmental level of the observer (Gibson, 1969). Real-life presentations are preferable for the study of movement imitation.

Stränger (1977, Exp. 3) has demonstrated the importance of the *visual display* for action imitation. It was far more difficult to solve a mechanical puzzle on the basis of an effective solution description presented on audiotape than to solve it on the basis of a filmed demonstration.

A prerequisite of any visually conveyed imitation is the *visibility* of the relevant behavior. As kinesthetic sensations are not visible, it is hardly surprising that, for example, in the pursuit-rotor task, observational learning effects on the contact time are not found, although some features of posture are adopted (McGuire, 1961;

Burwitz, 1975, cited in Scully and Newell, 1985). Thus, only the external structure of a behavior is conveyed by observation. Although this structure can clearly be assessed in a more differentiated manner if it is presented repeatedly, successful reproductions of a motor task require own performances.

Body movements and goal-directed actions are imitated better after *dynamic display* than after a sequence of selected stills from the same event (Gray *et al.*, 1991; Roshal, 1961; Stränger, 1977; Thompson, 1940, cited in Miller and Dollard, 1941). If these results can be replicated with selected stills (cf. breakpoints in the sense of Newtson) and controlled presentation times, they suggest that, mediated by perception, the reproduction also profits by dynamic displays.

Williams (1985, cited in Whiting, 1988) displayed target and throwing movements either under normal conditions or with the *point-light technique*. During imitation, he recorded electromyographic and goniometric data. The lack of any significant differences in reproduction suggests that even moving point-lights provide a sufficiently unequivocal specification of the movement.

It thus seems as though dynamic visual presentations facilitate the construction of a coherent and possibly even dynamic representation (Freyd, 1987) that is used to control one's own imitation.

Relationship Between Perception and Motor Performance

When adults learn the manual alphabet for the deaf, they tend to copy the movements already during presentation (Berger, 1966). This particularly applies when other ways of coding are hardly available (Berger *et al.*, 1979). Such accompanying movements also occur covertly: Berger also demonstrated by electromyography that observers show specific innervations in their corresponding muscles during the observaton of different body movements by a model (Berger and Hadley, 1975; Berger, Irwin, and Frommer, 1970; see Jacobson, 1932, on imagined movements). These findings, like imitations of facial movements in human neonates (Field, *et al.*, 1982; Meltzoff and Moore, 1977, 1983a; Vinter, 1985a,b), suggest a direct, not cognitively mediated link between the visual and the motor system even in adults.

Aspects of Motor Reproduction

Initial movement imitations of new skills mostly agree only roughly with the observed behavior (Gray *et al.*, 1991; Teubner, 1985). The construction of new sensorimotor schemata clearly requires *kinesthetic feedback*.

The role of *visual feedback* is documented by studies in which the visual angle between display and reproduction is manipulated. In action imitation, the best results are generally achieved when model and observer stand side by side or the camera follows the corresponding 'subjective' perspective. If, in contrast, the visual angle or the spatial reference system changes between display and reproduction, imitative performance usually deteriorates (Greenwald and Albert, 1968; Poljakova, 1958; Roshal, 1961; Stränger, 1977, Exp. 1). Comparable findings are also available on movement imitation (Jordan, 1977, cited in Whiting, 1988). These designs clearly require *mental transformations* of the visual representation (Shepard and Cooper, 1982) that are time-consuming and subject to interference (Stränger, 1977, Exp. 1)

Such findings also suggest that a primary visual representation of the observed behavior is involved in the control of imitation. It should marginally be noted that action imitation is facilitated by the additional presentation or self-generation of verbal descriptions. The presentation of relevant evidence is beyond the scope of this chapter (see Bandura, 1986; Stränger, 1977).

7.4 Discussion

Systematic functional analysis of imitation performance is impeded by the following deficits. First, there has long been a lack of procedures for systematically describing actions and body movements (see Section 8.2). In addition, there is no theoretically based taxonomy for selecting behaviors. Our differentiation between (body) movement imitation and action imitation is only a first step in this direction. There is also a lack of experimental paradigms for studying theoretically derived issues. From the perspective of research on perception, the following aspects particularly require more attention.

Before far-reaching speculations are made about the cognitive–semantic processing of observed behavior, analyses of eye movements should be used to determine what is actually being observed (Scully and Newell, 1985; Stränger, 1977).

Expert–novice differences in eye movements during the analysis of an event would be particularly interesting here. Everyday experience already suggests such differences: while novices, for example, can scarely differentiate ice-skating figures or types of stroke in tennis, experts easily perceive specific patterns of movement on the basis of visual features. Usually, they can also name these patterns. For the perception and coding of static displays, expert–novice differences have frequently been confirmed empirically (Chase and Simon, 1973; De Groot, 1965; Gibson, 1969); for dynamic displays such studies are at least available on automobile drivers (Shinar, 1978).

Under natural conditions, experts and novices mostly differ in their perceptual experience *and* their motor skills in the domain in question. One becomes expert at a skill through repeated close observation, by extracting invariant patterns, learning labels for these patterns and performing the skill with different forms of feedback. If observational learning is considered to be independent of motor reproduction processes (see Bandura), then *pure perceptual learning* without any motor performance should be sufficient to acquire a behavior. This seems to be true for observational learning of actions. For example, Stränger (1977, Exp. 3) found no group differences in the frequency of solutions of a rather difficult mechanical puzzle after repeated observation of a filmed solution or after a performance trial following each of the five presentations. This might be due to the verbal codability of the task. We were unable to find similar investigations on movement imitation, but would expect obvious differences in the quality of performance in this case.

Another indication of expert–novice differences has been a reported by Scully (1986). Experienced raters differed little in their judgment of a normal gymnastic exercise and the exercise presented with the point-light technique. The ratings of unexperienced subjects were more heterogeneous. Nonetheless, Scully did not test whether the experienced raters themselves had mastered the exercises. Another test of theories that consider observational learning as being independent of motor reproduction, requires a comparison of the visual discrimination of human movement patterns by motorically (but blindly) pretrained 'experts' and by novices without this motor training. As the motor reproduction would handicap the novices, the registration of eye movements during the presentation and/or the recognition of the same and slightly different dynamic displays would provide a more appropriate test of the visual discrimination.

II DISCUSSION: COMPARING THE LINES OF RESEARCH

8 CONCEPTS OF PERCEPTION, METHODS AND THEORETICAL PROBLEMS

8.1 Differences in the Concepts of Perception

The explicit or implicit concepts of perception in the lines of research discussed above can be described and classified in the following manner:

8.1.1 Concepts of Autonomous Perceptual Organization

Groups that approach the perception of behavior from classic perceptual research, such as motion perception, conceive behavior as a complex dynamic event that can be described anatomically and physically in the form of mass displacements with specific acceleration and speed. Behavior is ecologically valid as an object of perception, and its perception may have biological survival value. However, the symbolic meaning of behavior is never mentioned.

Sensory information from the behavioral event is organized by an autonomous perceptual system. Attitudes, inferences, comparisons with stored knowledge and other cognitive influences do not play any major role in the construction of the perceptual experience. Thus, the perceptual system is conceived as being cognitively impenetrable (Fodor and Pylyshyn, 1981). At best, the perception is modifiable through perceptual learning (see Runeson). In the research designs, stimulus parameters of a specific type of behavior are varied systematically and simple perceptual judgments are assessed. Individual influences on perceptual experience are rarely studied at all. A major research goal is to determine invariants of the event, for example, the center of moment in gait.

Variants of this concept of perception are proposed by Johansson, Cutting and Michotte. Their conceptions of autonomous perceptual processes and the focuses of their empirical research programs nonetheless diverge.

In terms of the popular but oversubscribed dichotomy of direct and indirect theories of perception (Bruce and Green, 1990), these concepts seem to be closer to the direct pole.

8.1.2 Concepts of Cognitively Penetrable Perceptual Organization

A second group of authors base their work on a broader concept of perception. Perception does not refer exclusively to autonomous perceptual processes responsible for the detection of visual invariants in stimulus events that can be described completely in anatomical and physical terms. Instead, perceptual processes can be cognitively penetrated. Perceptual experience is based on event features and a species-specific, universal and automatic perceptual processing that is nonetheless influenced by attitudes, prior information, knowledge structures (see our interpretation of Newtson's results) and inferences (see Heider on intention 'perception'). The perception of meaning, which results partially from event features and partially from the knowledge base, is also considered.

The empirical approach is more molar: minute-long scenes are presented that would require an enormous effort to describe systematically. Stimulus displays are rarely varied systematically and related to perceptual judgments. Instead, statements on perception are derived from verbal reports (Heider) or button presses and recognition performance at various points in the stream of events (Newtson). More attention is given to individual influences on perception.

These concepts correspond to indirect theories of perception. If a strict distinction is made between perception and cognition, these concepts would be classified as being closer to cognition. They are also more appropriate for symbolic actions, which are excluded from this chapter. With reference to Fodor and Pylyshyn (1981), who have criticized the unacceptable extension of Gibson's concept of invariance formation with their example of discriminating between a real and a fake picture from Leonardo da Vinci, we suspect that, even for the perception of a relatively simple sequence such as GREETING, the extraction of visual invariants alone is scarcely sufficient to permit a culturally appropriate reaction without referring to symbolic meaning in memory.

8.1.3   Perception in the Service of Other Functions

A third area of research is not particularly concerned with either the perceptual organization of behavior or the cognitive influences on perception. Instead, perception serves the formation of orienting (Freyd, Jenkins) or action-guiding representations (theories on imitation). Ideas on perception are not worked out in detail and precise descriptions of the stimulus event are not given. The inclusion of these approaches in a chapter on behavior perception is above all justified because these fields deal with relationships between perception, memory and the motor system, which require a more detailed empirical analysis.

A premature restriction to a specific concept of perception would hardly be appropriate to the study of perception of action and movement. Nonetheless, the first concept is central to psychophysically oriented research on perception.

8.2   Research Methods

Statements on perception are mostly derived from the relationship between systematically varied properties of the available information and various indicators of perception. Therefore, we will compare some possibilities for describing and varying behavior and discuss the most important indicators of its perception.

8.2.1   Stimulus Description Procedures

In the approaches presented here, the behavioral event is described in different ways. If – as in Heider and in action imitation – no clear borders are drawn between

perception and cognition, researchers mostly dispense with a precise description of
the stimulus event. However, if it is assumed that cognition influences perception,
the available (and used) information should be described in as much detail as
possible. Methods are to be found in other approaches.

The comparably simple structure of events that form the basis of the perception
of causality and the recognition of biological movements permits a detailed
description of the spatial and temporal features of the stimulus event. For example,
Cutting (1978a, b) was able to specify the cyclic movement of gait so precisely in
physical–anatomical terms that differences in the course of point-light movement in
the gait of men and women could be simulated on a computer. This form of
description would require too much effort to be applied to anything other than
simple, cyclic body movements.

The course of more complex, irregular patterns of behavior can be assessed with
systems for the *notation of body movements* (see the Eshkol–Wachman system in
Newtson et al., 1977, 1987). Further movement notation systems have been described by Rosenfeld (1982) and Wallbott (1982). Ekman and Friesen's (1978) facial
action coding system (FACS) is widely used in research on facial expression. Choice
depends on the area of behavior and the research issue in question. However, until
analysis can be performed automatically (see, on the development of automatic
systems, Grieve et al., 1975; Woltring, 1984), these analysis-intensive systems are
only meaningful when research focuses on the perception and reproduction of
spatial and temporal parameters of the course of movement.

For classifying ongoing behavior into categories, which is typical for research on
segmentation and action imitation, an event description with a (hierarchical)
proposition structure is sufficient (Kintsch and van Dijk, 1978). Suggestions on how
to construct a proposition structure can be found in articles on action memory that
use film and text displays (Baggett, 1979; Lichtenstein and Brewer, 1980) as well as
in work on action identification (Vallacher and Wegner, 1987). Such procedures are
appropriate when research focuses on the cognitive organization of observed
behavior.

8.2.2   Experimental Variations in Presented Behavior

Body Movement, Point-light Movement, Removal of Manipulated Objects
As yet, the point-light technique has mostly been used to separate figural body
features and movement. It has been demonstrated repeatedly that recognition is
superior under natural display conditions as compared to the presentation of
point-lights. Therefore, it has to be explained which features are responsible for the
better recognition of natural displays.

The point-light technique, like pantomime, disassociates body movements from
their spatial context. The influence of spatial context and objects on the perception
and reproduction of actions can be tested by systematic comparison between mere
body movements without appropriate objects and real-life actions incorporating the
appropriate objects. For example, Sakowski (1985) confirmed clear retention advantages for real as compared to pantomimic displays of REFUELLING in free recall.
When the title REFUELLING was presented, performances under mimed and real
conditions became more similar. However, there were no differences in recognition
performance (Hilse, 1985). Therefore, context influences have a stronger effect on
verbal retention and less on visual recognition.

The role of body movements in learning object-related actions can be studied by means of animation films. For example, Roshal (1961) showed that learning to tie knots with the help of an animated film demonstration was even superior to a film version with observable hands.

Context Influences
The montage techniques of film directors such as Kuleshov, Eisenstein and Hitchcock assume that individual camera frames are influenced by the surrounding frames. In an analogous manner, the perception of a neutral emotional expression may depend on the contexts that directly surround it (Isenhour, 1975; Russell and Fehr, 1987; Wallbott, 1990). For prototypical sequences of expression, this effect is less probable (Section 3.3). Perhaps the embedding of ambiguous actions in preceding, subsequent and accompanying behavior (in other channels of expression) might influence their identification. As a renewed controversy in the recognition of facial expressions between Russell and Ekman shows (Ekman, O'Sullivan and Matsumoto, 1991; Russell, 1991a, b), it is essential to distinguish multiple kinds of context. An important distinction is made between the context of expression, that is, the time and spatial context of the behavior displayed (in different channels), and the context of judgment, that is, the circumstances of the observer's judgment. Given the intention to find out whether effects in the context of expression are based on judgment (i.e. anchor effects and adaptation level), on memory, or on perception, the use of different test procedures seems to be appropriate.

As in the work of Hilse and Sakowski, different test procedures are needed here to test whether these are judgment and memory effects or perceptual effects.

Static and Dynamic Display with Variations in Speed
Both biological motion perception and imitation research have confirmed repeatedly that dynamic compared with static display facilitates recognition and imitation. However, dynamic and static displays are only two points on a continuum of possible variations in speed. Professional film and video techniques permit displays of single stills with varying sequential speed and dynamic displays ranging from extreme slow-motion to time-lapse recordings.

As Barker already suspected, various aspects of behavior are emphasized at different display speeds. In the analysis of facial expression under natural speed, we see, for example, SMILING. If the constituent muscle movements of this smiling are analyzed with the FACS (Ekman and Friesen, 1978) on successive stills at a speed of 25 pictures per second, changes can be seen that are scarcely detectable at natural speed. On the other hand, in extreme time-lapse recordings of, for example, a therapy session, (synchronized) changes in body posture are much more apparent than when they are displayed at their natural speed (Scheflen, 1964). Barker's team has proposed that the 'normal behavior perspective' specifies natural behavior units with basic evolutionary significance (see Wright, 1967, p. 78).

Variable display speeds open up interesting possibilities for studying the perception of behavior. For example, subjects can be asked to scan behavioral events at self-selected, variable speeds, and the observation times for single sections can be related to performance variables. Stränger (1977, Exp. 2), for example, has shown that children who learn a difficult mechanical puzzle look at slides of the single solution stages for different lengths of time given a free choice of display times. If they are permitted to attempt a solution after each observational trial, the peak of display times shifts successively toward later solution stages. This was observed less frequently during multiple observations without performances. The children seemed to scan the event as a function of their reproduction progress. Further, children performed slightly better under self-controlled display times compared with constant display. Under self-controlled display times, subjects with higher variability in times also attained the learning criterion more rapidly. Advanced film and video techniques also permit such studies on dynamic events.

Further Variations

Masking (Cutting, Moore and Morrison, 1988; Johansson, 1976) or *selective point-light marking* of specific parts of the body (Johansson, 1975), can be used to determine the stimulus features on which behavior identification depends. Identifying breaks at specific points in ongoing behavior (Newtson and Engquist, 1976) permits statements on differences in the information content of an event. Superimposing two behaviors can provide information on the selective perception and processing of simultaneously presented behavior (Neisser and Becklen, 1975).

8.2.3   Registering Indicators of Perception

Eye-movement Analyses

Studies of eye movements, like those used to study the perception of causality, are also desirable in other fields. Modern systems of eye-movement analysis make it possible to present a video scene to observers and to play back their fixation point in the observed scene on a second video screen. This permits a precise identification of which features observers monitor in a complex scene. This method is useful for studies on perceptual learning and to determine differences between experts and novices in the perception of behavior.

Phenomenal Report, Describing and Naming

Michotte based the causality statements on his subjects' reports on what they had experienced. The criteria for reporting, however, remain unclear. Heider derived perceptions of intention from intentional descriptions. In biological motion perception, display patterns are either named freely (Johansson) or assigned to one of several verbal categories (Cutting)

However, linking verbal utterances to properties of the percept is problematic for two reasons: unlike visual perception, statements on perception are always categorical. For example, when subjects state after perceiving gait that the stimulus person is a woman, we do not know whether they had also recognized features of the individual gait that they did not report. A second problem is that although, in natural speech, subjects prefer to describe specific stimulus configurations causally or intentionally, perception is described differently, depending on the instructions (see Section 4.3).

Perceptual experience and description are thus at best correlated but not identical. Reports on spatial and temporal relationships of observed behavior, in particular, are mostly poor when given verbally.

Recognition

Spatial and temporal properties of perceptual experience are easier to derive from the recognition of identical or similar visual displays (see Jenkins, Freyd, Newtson).

A major advantage of these methods is that both stimulus material and testing procedures are presented in the visual modality and are therefore directly comparable. However, previous studies have almost exclusively used static recognition material, despite the fact that film and video techniques also permit the construction of dynamic comparisons (Hilse, 1985; Sakowski, 1985). By using dynamic comparison stimuli with slightly changed spatial and temporal features, it should be possible to derive specific characteristics of the visual representation of the event. Although the criticism that this would involve memory effects is appropriate, it is secondary for two reasons: (1) when testing the perception of a behavior that extends over time, memory effects always have to be assumed (Johansson, 1973); and (2) other criteria, such as phenomenal report or motor reproduction, are also subject to these memory effects.

One main problem in recognition methods is the selection of the comparison stimuli. The more they are made similar to the display materials, the higher the error rate; the more the differences are emphasized, the higher the hit rate and the lower the error rate. One solution is to consider the procedures used in signal detection theory.

Segmentation

The cognitive organization of ongoing behavior could possibly be studied with a combination of Newtson's segmentation procedure and accompanying description. It would be particularly interesting to develop methods for the assessment of cognitive organizations on hierarchically nested levels of abstraction.

Imitation as Motor Reproduction

Imitation permits statements on perception as long as the behavior is easy to perform motorically, as is the case for simple arm movements (Prinz and Müsseler, 1988; Vogt, 1988). In difficult motor tasks, imitation does not merely include perceptual features but also features of the motor tranformation.

At least as far as older children and adults are concerned, the type of imitation is probably very dependent on the instructions: unless explicitly instructed, subjects have to find out whether the imitation requires a reproduction of a movement outcome, for example, an imaged movement trace or the reproduction of the spatial and temporal features.

8.2.4 Comparisons Between Stimulus Dislay and Indicators of Perception

It is easier to draw conclusions on perceptual processes if the stimulus display and the indicators of perception can be described in the same medium. If, for example, it is intended to study the perception of temporal and spatial features of an easily performed movement pattern, it is advantageous if the movement pattern and the reproduction are described with a differentiated movement notation system. By this procedure, it should be possible to clarify which features of the event are imitated. An elegant variant has been developed by Prinz and Müsseler (1988) and by Hösl (1988) to study movement imitation. They demonstrated a simple arm movement with a computer mouse. The subjects had to perform an exact movement imitation.

A computer program was developed that permitted a precise determination of spatial and temporal deviation in the imitation. However, this procedure is restricted to movements in two-dimensional space and, in addition, they could equally well be displayed as a moving point-light. Systems for notating body movements are not subject to this restriction. Nonetheless, they do not provide such a detailed assessment of the temporal course of movement.

If a study is only concerned with categorical recognition and not the representation of spatial and temporal features, then a proposition structure of the behavioral event is an appropriate standard with which the verbal indicators of perception can be compared. Properties of the primary visual representation can, as mentioned above, best be assessed with the recognition of dynamic displays.

8.3   Theoretical Problems

Most previous studies on the perception of behavior have been designed as demonstration experiments. Systematic research programs are rare or restricted to narrow aspects such as the perception of gait. Contacts between the various research traditions are still slight; related research is barely taken into account. This may be because behavior is a very complex object of perception, thus permitting the study of different aspects. In addition, the approaches have their origins in different theoretical traditions – above all, Gestalt theory – more recent information processing approaches and neo-Gibsonian concepts.

However, the perception of behavior could gain a greater theoretical importance as a particular type of event: behavior is an ecologically valid event, whose recognition probably has biological survival value. In contrast to traditional movement perception, multiple simultaneous reference systems and the possibility of mental determination should be taken into account. The perception of temporally extended behavior requires a reconceptualization of the rigid separation between perception and memory. Perhaps even the primary visual representation of behavior takes a dynamic form. Finally, certain kinds of imitation suggest a noncognitively mediated relationship between perception and the motor system. This is not the place to discuss all these points in detail. We consider the issue of the relationship between perceptual and cognitive determinants in the occurrence of perceptual events to be of basic and primary importance for this and other areas of perceptual psychology. As this aspect reappears continuously in the research traditions, we shall pay particular attention to it.

8.3.1   The Relationship Between Cognitive and Perceptual Processes

Behavior provides information that is perceptually organized, selected, interpreted and finally forms the basis for conscious perception. This perceptual experience, the percept, is the foundation for various actions that may serve as indicators of perception, as they permit inferences on the properties of the percept and the perceptual process. These perceptual indicators include description, recognition, segmentation or imitative reproduction.

Cognitive determinants such as expectations, attitudes or conceptual knowledge could enter into the perceptual process at four points. (1) It is conceivable, though hardly confirmed empirically, that they influence the organization and integration of sensory data (see Section 8.3.2). (2) They might interfere in the selection of stimulus features (see Section 8.3.3). (3) They could also influence the interpretation of organized information (see Section 8.3.4). (4) Finally, cognitions could also influence the indicators of perception, that is, they could influence the use of the percept for solving a specific task (see Section 8.3.5).

8.3.2   The Autonomy of Perceptual Organization and Integration

Unlike other processes, the organization and integration of the data available to the senses is probably largely independent of cognitive influences. Various types of autonomy have to be differentiated here:

(1) According to *genetic autonomy*, the perceptual system is practically unchangeable in ontogenesis. This autonomy could, for example, be responsible for the perceptual organization of an event into figure and ground or for the perception of causality. This autonomous perceptual organization prepares the information available to and registered by the senses and thus determines the percept. In the perception of behavior, this assumption of autonomy is most closely found in the modeling of the functions of the perceptual system (Cutting, 1981; Hochberg and Fallon, 1976; Hoffman and Flinchbaugh, 1982; Johansson, 1973; Vaina and Bennour, 1985).

(2) A weaker form of autonomy permits modifications of the autonomous perceptual system through perceptual experiences while simultaneously maintaining its independence from cognitive influences. This *functional autonomy* would be reconcilable with age- or practice-dependent differences and with experiences of highly 'compelling' perceptual impressions, as frequently reported in, for example, Michotte's paradigm. Changes in the perceptual system could be based on *perceptual learning* in the sense of Gibson (1969) and Wolff (1984), that is, on an adaptation of the functions of the perceptual system to relevant structures in the environment.

An empirical discrimination between genetic and functional autonomy calls for systematic developmental studies or perception training programs. If effects of development or training cannot be demonstrated in either eye-movement patterns or recognition performance, this would support genetic autonomy. Strong developmental or training effects in eye-movement patterns and/or recognition performance would, in contrast, support functional autonomy. Cognitive effects on the autonomously conceived organization of perception would be present if findings analogous to developmental and training effects could be demonstrated as a pure function of instructions.

Functional autonomy could also be tested with *induced perceptual conflicts*. For example, Michotte (e.g. 1946/1963, p. 71) systematically varied the relationships between stimulus parameters and cognitive information in order to determine which information was more dominant in the perceptual judgment. Systematic analyses of the effect of contradictions between perceptual and cognitive information still have to be performed in other areas. Particular attention should also be paid to the selection of the indicators of perception. Results based on judgments alone have little power, as they render it difficult to decide which features have guided the subjects. Perceptual conflicts can also be constructed with correct versus false feedback, as applied by Frykholm (1983a, b) in the identification of point-light stimulus persons. This would make it possible to test whether feedback that was either consistent with or contradicted the perceptual impression would lead to experienced and reported disassociations between subjects' spontaneous perceptual impressions and their beliefs.

8.3.3 Cognitive Influences on Selective Attention to Behavior

Possibly, conceptual knowledge, expectations and attitudes influence the selection of specific aspects of events. The situational context and other prior information could activate schemata that, in turn, specify features that are monitored for changes in ongoing behavior (Engquist, Newtson and LaCross, 1979; Neisser, 1976; Neisser and Becklen, 1975; Stränger, Schorneck and Droste 1983). The perceptual organization of features selected in this way could, in turn, be mandatory and autonomous.

Empirical confirmation could be provided by analyses of eye movements. If, given constant stimulus display, the eye movements vary systematically with the prior information or the observation tasks, this would support cognitive influences on feature selection.

8.3.4 Cognitive Influences on the Interpretation of Organized and Selected Information

The probable autonomy of the organization of perception does not exclude cognitive contributions to its outcomes. Nonetheless, it would be necessary to clarify: (1) under which conditions cognitive influences might occur; (2) what is their purpose; and (3) how far they are dependent on the task requirements.

(1) Regarding the *conditions*, some studies on the perception of causality (Knowles, 1983; Levelt, 1962) suggest that cognitive influences are more probable in ambiguous stimulus displays. Similar ideas are discussed for the perception of emotions (Ekman and O'Sullivan, 1988; Russell and Fehr, 1987). Experimental variations of the *ambiguity of the stimulus event* can be used to test across paradigms whether cognitive influences occur more frequently in ambiguous displays. Michotte (1946/1963) already differentiated in this sense between stimulus-dependent and experience-dependent causal judgments. A comparative study of the contributions of stimulus information and explicit knowledge requires a more detailed description of the stimulus display than that found in previous studies on the perception of intention, on segmentation and on imitation.

(2) As well as demonstrating conditions under which perceptual organization can be influenced cognitively, the function of such influences should also be analyzed. Perhaps, *concepts of causality* or *intention* do not serve just to supplement or replace incomplete perceptual information. Conceptual and situational knowledge could also ensure a more effective and directed extraction of environmental information. Thus, Jansson (1964), for example, demonstrated in a study of the perception of causality that the pattern of eye movements changes as a function of the preceding judgment. The acquisition of situation-specific knowledge about the causal relationship of two events is thus not only a consequence of preceding activity but also a basis for subsequent action. If this acquisition of knowledge is

equated with the formation of internal event models, this would simultaneously be an indication of the action-guiding function of such models. Thus, the dynamic properties of internal models postulated by Freyd (1987) perhaps permit not only a reliable prediction of the temporal development of an event but also probably the planning of one's own perceptual activity.

(3) The control of a precise movement imitation also requires the use of information on behavior, while the quality of reproduction simultaneously increases as a function of practice. Schema theoretical approaches trace this back to the development of a behavior-specific schema that possibly also permits a more effective use of the information given by the model. This relationship is similar to that between situational knowledge and eye movements according to Jansson (1964). This similarity may well not be arbitrary, as the schemata underlying imitation could also be event models in which the behavior-controlling function comes to the fore.

8.3.5   Cognitive Influences on the Use of Information

The dependent variables on the perception of behavior are always founded on the results of *intentional actions* that are based on a percept without representing it directly. If, for example, the same film of a woman playing billiards serves as stimulus material in studies on the perception of causality, intention, emotion, biological motion, segmentation and imitation, the perceptual indicators would clearly seem to depend on the specific task.

In Heider's paradigm, the subjects might report that a woman was playing billiards; their judgments would thus be gender- and action-related. Perhaps the observers would not fail to notice, however, that the woman intentionally aims the balls toward the pockets and is pleased when she is successful, or that the ball movements have a causal effect on each other. However, the observer would hardly report on this spontaneously. Following a nonspecific imitation instruction, the observer would probably play billiards without precisely reproducing the observed movements. After corresponding instructions and some practice, they could nonetheless achieve this. Thus, each individual indicator of perception gives only an incomplete report on what the observer *saw*.

Each action and thereby each indicator of perception requires *comprehending the instructions*, the *ability to extract appropriate stimulus information*, and the *adequate use of this information*. For example, subjects in studies on the perception of emotions must comprehend what is asked of them and report the emotions they perceive in a comprehensible way. This requires the inclusion of explicit *conceptual knowledge*. In contrast, lay persons should hardly be able to report which stimulus information was precisely taken into account in the judgment, as this *perceptual knowledge* is often implicit.

Perhaps it also applies to other areas of the perception of behavior that comprehending the instructions and appropriately using the percept require conceptual knowledge. Organizing and integrating the complex stimulus event into a percept, in contrast, requires a perceptual system that is probably autonomous. The working rules of this system need to be detected through studies in perceptual psychology.

If we follow this differentiation between conceptual knowledge in the use of the percept and implicit rules in its formation, observers should, for example, visibly perceive the emotions of others even when they possess no concept of emotions and are therefore unable to communicate their experience verbally.

The concept that only an indicator of perception and not the formation of the percept can be influenced cognitively would be supported by the following data pattern:

(1) Eye and head movements while observing an identical event are independent of instructions to perform different perceptual actions, that is, they are relatively constant. Thus, the perceptual actions do not influence the selection of information.

(2) Different indicators of perception vary in the strength with which they are influenced by systematically varied expectations and attitudes. Indicators of perception that are broadly independent of instruction and attitude effects best reflect the perceptual properties of the perceptual experience. In the discussion of methods, this is suspected for recognition.

Cognitive influences on indicators of perception and thus on the use of the percept are highly plausible but previously not proven unequivocally, as demonstrated cognitive effects could already be due to the selection of features.

8.3.6 Outlook: Perception and Action

Many of the aspects discussed lead up to the issue of the relationship between perception- and action-related event models, or – in Neisser's (1985) terminology – perception and action schemata. Perhaps perception does not lead just to action; the action competencies may also influence perception and thus the relationship between the two functional areas might be cyclic (Neisser, 1976; von Weizsäcker, 1940).

Reproductions of observed point-light movements (Scully and Newell, 1985; Williams, 1985, cited in Whiting, 1988) are an appropriate way to study the relationship between perception and own performance. To test the possible influence of domain-specific action competence on perceptual differentiation, the expert–novice dichotomy could be used to study, in particular, how far the identification of (point-light) movement patterns depends on the observer's level of mastering the actions (see Section 7.4).

Available studies on the perception of movement and action are not sufficient to provide satisfactory answers to the questions formulated here. At first glance, the approaches and methods seem to be too heterogeneous. On the other hand, this multiplicity provides the opportunity to analyze perceptual processes on different levels without losing sight of their complexity. In everyday perception and action, the criteria of perception also change continuously; intention, causality and sequences of movement are inseparably entangled in actions. At the same time, perception, cognition, memory and action are closely related. To analyze such relationships, we consider it to be meaningful and promising to engage in further experimental studies of the perception of behavior.

REFERENCES

Abravanel, E., Levan-Goldschmidt, E. and Stevenson, M. B. (1976). Action imitation: The early phase of infancy. *Child Development*, **47**, 1032–1044.

Alexander, C. N. and Epstein, J. (1969). Problems of dispositional inference in person perception research. *Sociometry*, **32**, 381–395.

Aronfreed, J. (1969). The problem of imitation. In L. P. Lipsit and H. W. Reese (Eds), *Advances in Child Development and Behavior*, vol. 4 (pp. 209–319). New York: Academic Press.

Atkinson, M. L. and Allen, V. L. (1983). Perceived structure of nonverbal behavior. *Journal of Personality and Social Psychology*, **45**, 458–463.

Baggett, P. (1979). Structurally equivalent stories in movie and text and the effect of the medium on recall. *Journal of Verbal Learning and Verbal Behavior*, **18**, 333–356.

Baldwin, J. M. (1895). *Mental Development in the Child and in the Race*. New York: Macmillan.

Bandura, A. (1962). Social learning through imitation. In M. R. Jones (Ed.), *Nebraska Symposium on Motivation*, vol. 10 (pp. 211–269). Lincoln, NE: University of Nebraska Press.

Bandura, A. (1971). Analysis of modeling processes. In A. Bandura (Ed.), *Psychological Modeling* (pp. 1–62). Chicago, IL: Aldine.

Bandura, A. (1986). *Social Foundations of Thought and Action. A Social Cognitive Theory*, ch. 2: Observational learning (pp. 47–105). Englewood Cliffs, NJ: Prentice-Hall.

Bandura, A., and Jeffery, R. W. (1973). Role of symbolic coding and rehearsal processes in observational learning. *Journal of Personality and Social Psychology*, **26**, 122–130.

Bandura, A., Jeffery, R. W. and Bachicha, D. L. (1974). Analysis of memory codes and cumulative rehearsal in observational learning. *Journal of Research in Personality*, **7**, 295–305.

Barclay, C. D., Cutting, J. E. and Kozlowski, L. T. (1978). Temporal and spatial factors in gait perception that influence gender recognition. *Perception and Psychophysics*, **23**, 145–152.

Barker, R. G. (1963). The stream of behavior as an empirical problem. In R. G. Barker (Ed.), *The Stream of Behavior* (pp. 1–22). New York: Appleton.

Barker, R. G. (1978). Stream of individual behavior. In R. G. Barker and associates (Eds), *Habitats, Environments and Human Behavior* (pp. 3–16). San Francisco, CA: Jossey-Bass.

Bassili, J. N. (1976). Temporal and spatial contingencies in the perception of social events. *Journal of Personality and Social Psychology*, **33**, 680–685.

Bassili, J. N. (1978). Facial motion in the perception of faces and of emotional expression. *Journal of Experimental Psychology: Human Perception and Performance*, **4**, 373–379.

Bassili, J. N. (1979). Emotion recognition: The role of facial movement and the relative importance of upper and lower areas of the face. *Journal of Personality and Social Psychology*, **37**, 2049–2058.

Beardsworth, T. and Buckner, T. (1981). The ability to recognize oneself from a video recording of one's movements without seeing one's body. *Bulletin of the Psychonomic Society*, **18**, 19–22.

Beasley, N. A. (1968). The extent of individual differences in the perception of causality. *Canadian Journal of Psychology*, **22**, 399–407.

Berger, S. M. (1966). Observer practices and learning during exposure to a model. *Journal of Personality and Social Psychology*, **3**, 696–701.

Berger, S. M., Carli, L. L., Hammersla, K. S., Karshmer, J. F. and Sanchez, M. E. (1979). Motoric and symbolic mediation in observational learning. *Journal of Personality and Social Psychology*, **37**, 735–746.

Berger, S. M. and Hadley, S. W. (1975). Some effects of a model's performance on an observer's electromyographic activity. *American Journal of Psychology*, **88**, 263–276.

Berger, S. M., Irwin, D. S. and Frommer, G. P. (1970). Electromyographic activity during observational learning. *American Journal of Psychology*, **83**, 86–94.

Bertenthal, B. I., Proffitt, D. R. and Cutting, J. E. (1984). Infant sensitivity to figural coherence in biomechanical motions. *Journal of Experimental Child Psychology*, **37**, 213–230.

Bingham, G. P. (1987). Kinematic form and scaling: Further investigations on the visual perception of lifted weight. *Journal of Experimental Psychology: Human Perception and Performance*, **13**, 155–177.

Boyle, D. G. (1961). The concept of the 'radius of action' in the causal impression. *British Journal of Psychology*, **52**, 219–226.

Boyle, D. G. (1972). Michotte's ideas. *Bulletin of the British Psychological Society*, **25**, 89–91.

Bruce, V. (1988). *Recognising Faces*. Hillsdale, NJ: Erlbaum.

Bruce, V. and Green, P. R. (1990). *Visual Perception. Physiology, Psychology and Ecology*, 2nd edn. Hillsdale, NJ: Erlbaum.

Brunswik, E. and Reiter, L. (1937). Eindruckscharaktere schematisierter Gesichter. [Impression formation by schematized faces.] *Zeitschrift für Psychologie*, **142**, 67–134.

Buck, R. (1984). *The Communication of Emotion*. New York: Guilford Press.

Carroll, J. M. (1980). *Toward a Structural Psychology of Cinema*. The Hague, Netherlands: Mouton.

Chase, W. G. and Simon, H. A. (1973). Perception in chess. *Cognitive Psychology*, **4**, 55–81.

Cohen, C. E. (1981). Goals and schemata in person perception: Making sense from the stream of behavior. In N. Cantor and J. F. Kihlstrom (Eds), *Personality, Cognition and Social Interaction* (pp. 45–68). Hillsdale, NJ: Erlbaum.

Cohen, C. E. and Ebbesen, E. B. (1979). Observational goals and schema activation: A theoretical framework for behavior perception. *Journal of Experimental Social Psychology*, **15**, 305–329.

Corcoran, F. (1981). Processing information from screen media: A psycholinguistic approach. *Educational Communication and Technology Journal*, **29**, 117–128.

Cutting, J. E. (1978a). Generation of synthetic male and female walkers through manipulation of a biomechanical invariant. *Perception*, **7**, 393–405.

Cutting, J. E. (1978b). A program to generate synthetic walkers as dynamic point-light displays. *Behavior Research Methods and Instrumentation*, **10**, 91–94.

Cutting, J. E. (1981). Coding theory adapted to gait perception. *Journal of Experimental Psychology: Human Perception and Performance*, **7**, 71–87.

Cutting, J. E. (1986). *Perception with an Eye for Motion*. Cambridge, MA: MIT Press.

Cutting, J. E. and Kozlowski, L. T. (1977). Recognizing friends by their walk: Gait perception without familiarity cues. *Bulletin of the Psychonomic Society*, **9**, 353–356.

Cutting, J. E., Moore, C. and Morrison, R. (1988). Masking the motions of human gait. *Perception and Psychophysics*, **44**, 339–347.

Cutting, J. E. and Proffitt, D. R. (1981). Gait perception as an example of how we may perceive events. In R. D. Walk and H. L. Pick (Eds), *Intersensory Perception and Sensory Integration* (pp. 249–273). New York: Plenum Press.

Cutting, J. E., Proffitt, D. R. and Kozlowski, L. T. (1978). A biomechanical invariant for gait perception. *Journal of Experimental Psychology: Human Perception and Performance*, **4**, 357–372.

De Groot, A. D. (1965). *Thought and Choice in Chess*. The Hague, Netherlands: Mouton.

Dickman, H. R. (1963). The perception of behavioral units. In R. G. Barker (Ed.), *The Stream of Behavior* (pp. 23–41). New York: Appleton.

Droste, I. and Holtmann, R. (1980). Kognitive Mechanismen in der Handlungswahrnehmung: Der Einfluß von Struktur und Modalität einer Vorinformation auf die Wahrnehmungsorganisation und die Erinnerungsleistung von Handlungen. [Cognitive processes in perception of action: The infuence of the structure and modality of preinformation on the perceptual organization and memory for actions.] Unpublished master's thesis, Dept. of Psychology, Ruhr-University Bochum, Germany.

Ebbesen, E. B. (1980). Cognitive processes in understanding ongoing behavior. In R. Hastie, T. M. Ostrom, E. B. Ebbesen, R. S. Wyer, D. L. Hamilton and D. E. Carlston (Eds), *Person Memory. The Cognitive Basis of Social Perception* (pp. 179–225). Hillsdale, NJ: Erlbaum.

Ekman, P. (1972). Universals and cultural differences in facial expressions of emotion. In J. Cole (Ed.), *Nebraska Symposium on Motivation, 1971*, vol. 19 (pp. 207–283). Lincoln, NA: University of Nebraska Press.

Ekman, P. (Ed.) (1982). *Emotion in the Human Face*, 2nd edn. Cambridge: Cambridge University Press.

Ekman, P. (1990). New findings and work in progress using FACS. Paper presented at the 4th European Conference on Facial Expression – Measurement and Meaning. Berlin, Germany.

Ekman, P. and Friesen, W. V. (1969). Nonverbal leakage and clues to deception. *Psychiatry*, **32,** 88–106.

Ekman, P. and Friesen, W. V. (1978). *Facial Action Coding System*. Palo Alto, CA: Consulting Psychologists Press.

Ekman, P. and Friesen, W. V. (1982). Felt, false, and miserable smiles. *Journal of Nonverbal Behavior*, **6,** 238–252.

Ekman, P. and O'Sullivan, M. (1988). The role of context in interpreting facial expression: Comment on Russell and Fehr (1987). *Journal of Experimental Psychology: General*, **117,** 86–88.

Ekman, P., O'Sullivan, M. and Matsumoto, D. (1991). Confusions about context in the judgment of facial expression: A reply to 'The contempt expression and the relativity thesis'. *Motivation and Emotion*, **15,** 169–176.

Engquist, G., Newtson, D. and LaCross, K. (1979). Prior expectations and the perceptual segmentation of ongoing behavior. Unpublished manuscript, Univerity of Virginia, Charlottesville, VA.

Eshkol, N. (1973). *Moving, Writing, Reading*. Tel Aviv, Israel: Movement Notation Society.

Field, T. M., Woodson, R., Greenberg, R. and Cohen, D. (1982). Discrimination and imitation of facial expressions by neonates. *Science*, **218,** 179–181.

Finke, R. A. and Freyd, J. J. (1985). Transformations of visual memory induced by implied motions of pattern elements. *Journal of Experimental Psychology: Learning, Memory, and Cognition*, **11,** 780–794.

Finke, R. A., Freyd, J. J. and Shyi, G. C.-W. (1986). Implied velocity and acceleration induce transformations of visual memory. *Journal of Experimental Psychology: General*, **115,** 175–188.

Fodor, J. A. and Bever, T. G. (1965). The psychological reality of linguistic segments. *Journal of Verbal Learning and Verbal Behavior*, **4,** 414–420.

Fodor, J. A. and Pylyshyn, Z. W. (1981). How direct is visual perception? Some reflections on Gibson's 'ecological approach'. *Cognition*, **9,** 139–196.

Freyd, J. J. (1983). The mental representation of movement when static stimuli are viewed. *Perception and Psychophysics*, **33,** 575–581.

Freyd, J. J. (1987). Dynamic mental representation. *Psychological Review*, **94,** 427–438.

Freyd, J. J. and Finke, R. A. (1984). Representational momentum. *Journal of Experimental Psychology: Learning, Memory, and Cognition*, **10,** 126–132.

Freyd, J. J. and Finke, R. A. (1985). A velocity effect for representational momentum. *Bulletin of the Psychonomic Society*, **23,** 443–446.

Freyd, J. J., Pantzer, T. M. and Cheng, J. L. (1988). Representing statics as forces in equilibrium. *Journal of Experimental Psychology: General*, **117,** 395–407.

Frijda, N. H. (1958). Facial expression and situational cues. *Journal of Abnormal and Social Psychology*, **57,** 149–154.

From, F. (1971). *The Perception of Other People*. New York: Columbia University Press. (Original work published in Danish, without year.)

Frykholm, G. (1983a). *Perceived Identity I: Recognition of Others by their Kinematic Patterns*. Uppsala, Sweden: Uppsala Psychological Reports, No. 351.

Frykholm, G. (1983b). *Perceived Identity II: Learning to Recognize Others by their Kinematic Patterns*. Uppsala, Sweden: Uppsala Psychological Reports, No. 352.

Gardner, R. W. (1953/1954). Cognitive styles in categorizing behavior. *Journal of Personality*, **22**, 214–233.

Gemelli, A. and Cappellini, A. (1958). The influence of the subjects attitude in perception. *Acta Psychologica*, **14**, 12–23.

Gerst, M. S. (1971). Symbolic coding processes in observational learning. *Journal of Personality and Social Psychology*, **19**, 7–17.

Gewirtz, J. L. and Stingle, K. G. (1968). Learning of generalized imitation as the basis for identification. *Psychological Review*, **75**, 374–397.

Gibson, E. J. (1969). *Principles of Perceptual Learning and Development*. New York: Appleton-Century-Crofts.

Gibson, J. J. (1979). *The Ecological Approach to Visual Perception*. Boston, MA: Houghton Mifflin.

Gibson, J. J., Kaplan, G. A., Reynolds, H. N. and Wheeler, K. (1969). The change from visible to invisible: A study of optical transitions. *Perception and Psychophysics*, **5**, 113–116.

Glixman, A. T. (1965). Categorization behavior as a function of the meaning domain. *Journal of Personality and Social Psychology*, **2**, 370–377.

Goodenough, F. L. and Tinker, M. A. (1931). The relative potency of facial expression and verbal description of stimulus in the judgment of emotion. *Comparative Psychology*, **12**, 365–370.

Gray, J. T., Neisser, U., Shapiro, B. A. and Kouns, S. (1991). Observational learning of ballet sequences: The role of kinematic information. *Ecological Psychology*, **3**, 121–134.

Graziano, W. G., Moore, J. S. and Collins, J. E. Jr (1988). Social cognition as segmentation of the stream of behavior. *Developmental Psychology*, **24**, 568–573.

Greenwald, A. G. and Albert, S. M. (1968). Observational learning: A technique for elucidating S–R mediation processes. *Journal of Experimental Psychology*, **76**, 267–272.

Grieve, D. W., Miller, D. I., Mitchelson, D., Paul, J. P. and Smith, A. J. (Eds) (1975). *Techniques for the Analysis of Human Movement*. London: Lepus Books.

Gruber, H. E., Fink, C. D. and Damm, V. (1957). Effects of experience on perception of causality. *Journal of Experimental Psychology*, **53**, 89–93.

Guilliaume, P. (1926/1971). *Imitation in Children*. Chicago, IL: University of Chicago Press, 1971. (Original work published 1926.)

Hacker, W. (1978). *Allgemeine Arbeits- und Ingenieurspsychologie*. [General work and engineering psychology, 2nd edn.] Bern, Switzerland: Huber.

Halisch, F. (1990). Beobachtungslernen und die Wirkung von Vorbildern. [Observational learning and the impact of models.] In H. Spada (Ed.), *Allgemeine Psychologie* (pp. 373–402). Bern, Switzerland: Huber.

Hanson, C. and Hirst, W. (1989). On the representation of events: A study of orientation, recall and recognition. *Journal of Experimental Psychology: General*, **118**, 136–147.

Hanson, C. and Hirst, W. (1991). Recognizing differences in recognition tasks: A reply to Lassister and Slaw. *Journal of Experimental Psychology: General*, **120**, 211–212.

Heider, F. (1926/1959). Thing and medium. *Psychological Issues*, 1959 Monograph 3 (pp. 1–34). (Original work published 1926.)

Heider, F. (1930/1959). The function of the perceptual system. *Psychological Issues*, 1959, Monograph 3 (pp. 35–52). (Original work published 1930.)

Heider, F. (1944). Social perception and phenomenal causality. *Psychological Review*, **51**, 358–374.

Heider, F. (1958). *The Psychology of Interpersonal Relations*. New York: John Wiley.

Heider, F. (1967). On social cognition. *American Psychologist*, **22**, 25–31.

Heider, F. and Simmel, M. (1944). An experimental study of apparent behavior. *American Journal of Psychology*, **57**, 243–259.

Heller, O. and Lohr, W. (1982). Das Werk Michottes und seiner Mitarbeiter: Eine Einführung in den Gegenstand. [The work of Michotte and his colleagues: An introuction to the topic.] In O. Heller and W. Lohr (Eds), *Albert Michotte, Gesammelte Werke*, vol. 1 (pp. 15–41). [Albert Michotte, Collected works]. Bern, Switzerland: Huber.

Heller, O. and Lohr, W. (Eds) (1982). *Albert Michotte, Gesammelte Werke*, Bd. 4. [Albert Michotte, Collected Works, vol. 4]. Bern, Switzerland: Huber.

Hilse, B. (1985). Beobachtungslernen: Wiedererkennen von Routinehandlungen nach Wissens-aktualisierung durch den Kontext. [Observational learning: Recognition of scripted actions after knowledge instigation by the context.] Unpublished master's thesis. Dept. of Psychology, Ruhr-University Bochum, Germany.

Hindmarch, I. (1973). Eye movements and the perception of phenomenal causality. *Psychologica Belgica*, **13**, 17–23.

Hochberg, J. (1986). Representation of motion and space in video and cinematic displays. In K. R. Boff, L. Kaufman, and J. P. Thomas (Eds), *Handbook of Perception and Human Performance)* vol. I: *Sensory Processes and Perception*, ch. 22 (pp. 1–64). New York: John Wiley.

Hochberg, J. and Fallon, P. (1976). Perceptual analysis of moving patterns. *Science*, **194**, 1081–1083.

Hoenkamp, E. (1978). Perceptual cues that determine the labeling of human gait. *Journal of Human Movement Studies*, **4**, 59–69.

Hoffman, D. D. and Flinchbaugh, B. E. (1982). The interpretation of biological motion. *Biological Cybernetics*, **42**, 195–204.

Hösl, K. (1988). Frequenzanalytische Untersuchungen zur Bewegungsnachahmung. [Frequency analyses of movement imitation.] Unpublished master's thesis. Dept. of Psychology and Physical Education, University of Bielefeld, Germany.

Isenhour, J. P. (1975). The effects of context and order in film editing. *AV Communication Review*, **23**, 69–80.

Jacobson, E. (1932). Electrophysiology of mental activities. *American Journal of Psychology*, **44**, 677–694.

James, W. (1890). *The Principles of Psychology*. New York: Holt.

Jansson, G. (1964). Measurement of eye movements during a Michotte launching event. *Scandinavian Journal of Psychology*, **5**, 153–160.

Jeffery, R. W. (1976). The influence of symbolic and motor rehearsal in observational learning. *Journal of Research in Personality*, **10**, 116–127.

Jenkins, J. J. (1980). Can we have a fruitful cognitive psychology? In H. E. Howe (Ed.), *Nebraska Symposium on Motivation, 1979*, vol. 27 (pp. 211–238). Lincoln, NE: University of Nebraska Press.

Jenkins, J. J., Wald, J. and Pittenger, J. B. (1978). Apprehending pictorial events: An instance of psychological cohesion. In C. W. Savage (Ed.), *Minnesota Studies in the Philosophy of Science*, vol. 9 (pp. 129–163). Minneapolis, MN: University of Minnesota Press.

Jensen, T. D. and Schroeder, D. A. (1982). Behavior segmentation in a dyadic situation. *Personality and Social Psychology Bulletin*, **8**, 264–272.

Johansson, G. (1973). Visual perception of biological motion and a model for its analysis. *Perception and Psychophysics*, **14**, 201–211.

Johansson, G. (1975). Visual motion perception. *Scientific American*, **232**, 76–88.

Johansson, G. (1976). Spatiotemporal differentiation and integration in visual motion perception. *Psychological Research*, **38**, 379–393.

Johansson, G. (1979). Memory functions in visual perception. In L.-G. Nilsson (Ed.), *Perspectives on Memory Research* (pp. 93-103). Hillsdale, NJ: Erlbaum.

Joynson, R. B. (1971). Michotte's experimental methods. *British Journal of Psychology*, **62**, 293–302.

Kelley, H. H. and Michela, J. L. (1980). Attribution theory and research. *Annual Review of Psychology*, **31**, 457–501.

Killen, M. and Uzgiris, I. C. (1981). Imitation of actions with objects: The role of social meaning. *Journal of Genetic Psychology*, **138**, 219–229.

Kintsch, W. and Van Dijk, T. (1978). Toward a model of text comprehension and production. *Psychological Review*, **85**, 363–394.

Knowles, P. L. (1983). Measuring human social perception directly. *Human Movement Studies*, **2**, 161–170.

Koffka, K. (1921/1924, 1928/1952). *The Growth of Mind*. 'The problem of imitation'. London: Routledge and Kegan Paul. (Original work published 1921; 2nd edn 1928.)

Kogelheide, P. and Strothe, Ch. (1980). Kognitive Mechanismen in der Handlungswahrnehmung: Der Einfluß von wiederholter Darbietung und Strukturierungsauftrag auf die Wahrnehmungsorganisation und Erinnerungsleistung von Handlungen. [Cognitive processes in action perception: The influence of repeated presentation and segmentation instructions on the perceptual organization and memory for actions.] Unpublished master's thesis. Dept. of Psychology, Ruhr-University, Bochum, Germany.

Koopman, C. and Newtson, D. (1981). Level of analysis in the perception of ongoing instruction: An exploratory study. *Journal of Educational Psychology*, **73**, 212–223.

Kozlowski, L. T. and Cutting, J. E. (1977). Recognizing the sex of a walker from a dynamic point-light display. *Perception and Psychophysics*, **21**, 575–580.

Kraft, R. N. and Jenkins, J. J. (1977). Memory for lateral orientation of slides in picture stories. *Memory and Cognition*, **5**, 379–403.

Lasher, M. D. (1978). The pause in the moving structure of dance. *Semiotica*, **22**, 107–126.

Lasher, M. D. (1981). The cognitive representation of an event involving human action. *Cognitive Psychology*, **13**, 391–406.

Lassiter, G. D. (1988). Behavior perception, affect, and memory. *Social Cognition*, **6**, 150–176.

Lassiter, G. D. and Slaw, R. D. (1991). The unitization and memory of events. *Journal of Experimental Psychology: General*, **120**, 80–82.

Lassiter, G. D., Stone, J. I. and Rogers, S. L. (1988). Memorial consequences of variation in behavior perception. *Journal of Experimental Social Psychology*, **24**, 222–239.

Legerstee, M. (1991). The role of person and object in eliciting early imitation. *Journal of Experimental Child Psychology*, **51**, 423–433.

Leont'ev, A. N. (1972/1974). The problem of activity in psychology. *Soviet Psychology*, 1974/75, **13**, 4–33. (Original work published 1972.)

Lesser, H. (1977). The growth of perceived causality in children. *Journal of Genetic Psychology*, **130**, 145–152.

Levelt, W. J. M. (1962). Motion braking and the perception of causality. In A. Michotte *et al.* (Eds), *Causalité, Permanence et Réalité Phénoménale* (pp. 244–258). Louvain, Belgium: Publications Universitaires.

Lichtenstein, E. H. and Brewer, W. F. (1980). Memory for goal-directed events. *Cognitive Psychology*, **12**, 412–445.

Loftus, E. F. and Ketcham, K. E. (1983). The malleability of eye witness accounts. In S. M. A. Lloyd-Bostock and B. R. Clifford (Eds), *Evaluating Witness Evidence* (pp. 159–171). New York: John Wiley.

Maas, J. B., Johansson, G. Jansson, G. and Runeson, S. (1970). *Motion Perception I*. [Film]. Boston, MA: Houghton Mifflin.

Maas, J. B., Johansson, G., Jansson, G. and Runeson, S. (1971). *Motion Perception II*. [Film]. Boston, MA: Houghton Mifflin.

Marey, E.-J. (1894/1994). Le mouvement. Nimes, France: J. Chambon. (Original work published 1894.)

Margolius, G. J. and Sheffield, F. D. (1961). Optimum methods of combining practice with filmed demonstration in teaching complex response sequences: Serial learning of a mechanical-assembly task. In A. A. Lumsdaine (Ed.), *Student Response in Programmed Instruction* (pp. 33–53). Washington, DC: National Academy of Sciences – National Research Council, Publ. No. 943.

Markus, H., Smith, J. and Moreland, R. L. (1985). Role of the self-concept in the perception of others. *Journal of Personality and Social Psychology*, **49**, 1494–1512.

Martens R., Burwitz, L. and Zuckerman, J. (1976). Modeling effects on motor performance. *Research Quarterly*, **47**, 277–291.

Massad, Ch. M., Hubbard, M. and Newtson, D. (1979). Selective perception of events. *Journal of Experimental Social Psychology*, **15**, 513–532.

McDougall, W. (1908). *An Introduction to Social Psychology*. London: Methuen.

McGuire, W. (1961). Some factors influencing the effectiveness of demonstrational films: Repetition of instructions, slow motion, distribution of showings, and explanatory narration. In A. A. Lumsdaine (Ed.), *Student Response in Programmed Instruction* (pp. 187–207). Washington, DC: National Academy of Sciences – National Research Council, Publ. No. 943.

Meggle, G. (Ed.) (1977). *Analytische Handlungstheorie*. [Analytic theory of action.] Frankfurt, Germany: Suhrkamp.

Meltzoff, A. N. and Moore, M. K. (1977). Imitation of facial and manual gestures by human neonates. *Science*, **198**, 75–78.

Meltzoff, A. N. and Moore, M. K. (1983a). Newborn infants imitate adult facial gestures. *Child Development*, **54**, 702–709.

Meltzoff, A. N. and Moore, M. K. (1983b). The origins of imitation in infancy: Paradigm, phenomena, and theories. In L. P. Lipsitt and C. Rovée-Collier (Eds), *Advances in Infancy Research* vol. 2 (pp. 265–301). Norwood, NJ: Ablex.

Michotte, A. (1946/1963). *The Perception of Causality*. London: Methuen. (Original work published 1946.)

Michotte, A. (1950). A propos de la permanence phénoménale, faits et théories. [On phenomenal permanence, facts and theories.] *Acta Psychologica*, **7**, 298–322.

Michotte, A. (1951). La perception de la fonction 'outil'. [The perception of the 'tool function'.] In G. Ekman *et al.* (Eds), *Essays in Psychology, Dedicated to David Katz* (pp. 193–213). Uppsala, Sweden: Almquist and Wicksells.

Michotte, A. (1966). Die Kausalitätswahrnehmung. [Perception of causality.] In W. Metzger and H. Erke (Eds), *Handbuch der Psychologie*, vol. 1/1 (pp. 954–977). Göttingen, Germany: Hogrefe.

Michotte, A., Knops, L. and Coen-Gelders, A. (1957). Etude comparative de divers situations expérimentales donnant lieu à des impressions d'entrainement. [A comparative study of various experimental conditions giving rise to the impressions of 'entraining'.] In *Rencontre – Encounter – Begegnung. Contributions à une Psychologie Humaine, Dédiées au Professeur F. J. J. Buytendijk* (pp. 284–294). Utrecht, Netherlands: Het Spectrum.

Miller, G. A. (1956). The magical number seven, plus minus two: Some limits on our capacity for processing information. *Psychological Review*, **63**, 81–97.

Miller, G. A., Galanter, E. and Pribram, K. H. (1960). *Plans and the Structure of Behavior*. New York: Holt.

Miller, N. E. and Dollard, J. (1941). *Social Learning and Imitation*. New Haven, CT: Yale University Press.

Miller, P. H. and Aloise, P. A. (1989). Young children's understanding of the psychological causes of behavior: A review. *Child Development*, **60**, 257–285.

Montpellier, G. de and Nuttin, J. R. (1973). A note on 'Michotte's experimental methods' and 'Michotte's ideas'. *British Journal of Psychology*, **64**, 287–289.

Morgan, C. L. (1896). *Habit and Instinct*. London: Arnold.

Muybridge, E. (1897/1979). *Muybridge's Complete Human and Animal Locomotion*. New York: Dover Publications.

Neisser, U. (1976). *Cognition and Reality*. San Francisco, CA: Freeman.

Neisser, U. (1985). The role of invariant structures in the control of movement. In M. Frese and J. Sabini (Eds), *Goal-directed Behavior: The Concept of Action in Psychology* (pp. 97–108). Hillsdale, NJ: Erlbaum.

Neisser, U. and Becklen, R. (1975). Selective looking: Attending to visually specified events. *Cognitive Psychology*, **7**, 480–494.

Newtson, D. (1973). Attribution and the unit of perception of ongoing behavior. *Journal of Personality and Social Psychology*, **28**, 28–38.

Newtson, D. (1976a). Foundations of attribution: The perception of ongoing behavior. In J. H. Harvey, W. J. Ickes, and R. F. Kidd (Eds), *New Directions in Attribution Research,* vol. 1 (pp. 223–247). Hillsdale, NJ: Erlbaum.

Newtson, D. (1976b). The process of behavior observation. *Journal of Human Movement Studies,* **2,** 114–122.

Newtson, D. (1977). *Task and Observer Skill Factors in Accuracy of Assessment of Performance,* Technical Report TR-77-A7. US Army Research Institute for the Behavioral and Social Sciences.

Newtson, D. (1980). An interactionist perspective on social knowing. *Personality and Social Psychology Bulletin,* **6,** 520–531.

Newtson, D. and Engquist, G. (1976). The perceptual organization of ongoing behavior. *Journal of Experimental Social Psychology,* **12,** 436–450.

Newtson, D., Engquist, G. and Bois, J. (1976). The reliability of a measure of behavior perception. *JSAS Catalog of Selected Documents in Psychology,* **6,** MS 1173, 1–30.

Newtson, D., Engquist, G. and Bois, J. (1977). The objective basis of behavior units. *Journal of Personality and Social Psychology,* **35,** 847–862.

Newtson, D., Gowan, D. and Patterson, C. (1980). The development of action discrimination (abstract). *Personality and Social Psychology Bulletin,* **6,** 192–193.

Newtson, D., Hairfield, J., Bloomingdale, J. and Cutino, S. (1987). The structure of action and interaction. *Social Cognition,* **5,** 191–237.

Newtson, D. and Rindner, R. J. (1979). Variation of behavior perception and ability attribution. *Journal of Personality and Social Psychology,* **37,** 1847–1858.

Nisbett, R. and Ross, L. (1980). *Human Inference: Strategies and Shortcomings of Social Judgment.* Englewood Cliffs, NJ: Prentice-Hall.

Nyce, D. and Becklen, R. (1978). Effects of familiarity on behavior segmentation. Unpublished manuscript, Dept. of Psychology, Cornell University, Ithaca.

Oatley, K. and Yuill, N. (1985). Perception of personal and interpersonal action in a cartoon film. *British Journal of Social Psychology,* **24,** 115–124.

Olum, V. (1956). Developmental differences in the perception of causality. *American Journal of Psychology,* **69,** 417–425.

Pettigrew, T. F. (1958). The measurement and correlates of category width as a cognitive variable. *Journal of Personality,* **26,** 532–544.

Piaget, J. (1936/1952). *The Origins of Intelligence in Children.* New York: International Universities Press, 1952. (Original work published 1936.)

Piaget, J. (1945/1962). *Play, Dreams, and Imitation in Childhood.* London: Heinemann, 1951; New York: Norton, 1962. (Original work published 1945.)

Pittenger, J. B. and Jenkins, J. J. (1979). Apprehension of pictorial events: The case of a moving observer in a static environment. *Bulletin of the Psychonomic Society,* **13,** 117–120.

Poljakova, A. G. (1958). Analiz processa usvoenija navyjov putem podrazanija u detej doskol'nogo vozrasta. [The analysis of skill acquisition by imitation in preschoolers.] *Voprosy Psichologii,* **5,** 88–97.

Pöppel, E. (1985). *Grenzen des Bewußtseins.* [The borders of consciousness.] Stuttgart, Germany: dva.

Powesland, P. F. (1959). The effect of practice upon the perception of causality. *Canadian Journal of Psychology,* **13,** 155–168.

Prinz, W. (1987). Ideo-motor action. In H. Heuer and A. F. Sanders (Eds), *Perspectives on Perception and Action* (pp. 47–76). Hillsdale NJ: Erlbaum.

Prinz, W. and Müsseler, J. (1988). Nachahmungen einfacher Köprerbewegungen [Imitations of simple body movement.] Unpublished DFG-Research report, Dept. of Psychology and Physical Education, University of Bielefeld, Germany.

Rodgon, M. M. and Kurdek, L. A. (1977). Vocal and gestural imitation in 8-, 14-, and 20-month-old children. *Journal of Genetic Psychology,* **131,** 115–123.

Rosenfeld, H. M. (1982). Measurement of body motion and orientation. In K. R. Scherer and P. Ekman (Eds), *Handbook of Methods in Nonverbal Behavior Research* (pp. 199–286). London: Cambridge University Press.

Roshal, S. M. (1961). Film-mediated learning with varying representation of the task: Viewing angle, portrayal of demonstration, motion, and student participation. In A. A. Lumsdaine (Ed.), *Student Response in Programmed Instruction* (pp. 155–175). Washington, DC: National Academy of Sciences – National Research Council, Publ. No. 943.

Ross, L. (1977). The intuitive psychologist and his shortcomings: Distortions in the attribution process. In L. Berkowitz (Ed.), *Advances in Experimental Social Psychology*, vol. 10 (pp. 173–220). New York: Academic Press.

Rumelhart, D. E. (1980). Schemata: The building blocks of cognition. In R. J. Spiro, B. C. Bruce, and W. F. Brewer (Eds), *Theoretical Issues in Reading Comprehension* (pp. 33–58). Hillsdale, NJ: Erlbaum.

Rumelhart, D. E. and Ortony, A. (1977). The representation of knowledge in memory. In R. C. Anderson, R. J. Spiro and W. E. Montague (Eds), *Schooling and the Acquisition of Knowledge* (pp. 99–136). Hillsdale, NJ: Erlbaum.

Runeson, S. (1977/1983). *On Visual Perception of Dynamic Events*. Acta Universitatis Upsaliensis, Sweden: Studia Psychologica Upsaliensia, Serial No. 9. (Original work published 1977.)

Runeson, S. and Frykholm, G. (1981). Visual perception of lifted weight. *Journal of Experimental Psychology: Human Perception and Performance*, **7**, 733–740.

Runeson, S. and Frykholm, G. (1983). Kinematic specification of dynamics as an informational basis for person-and-action perception: Expectation, gender recognition, and deceptive intention. *Journal of Experimental Psychology: General*, **112**, 585–615.

Russell, J. A. (1991a). The contempt expression and the relativity thesis. *Motivation and Emotion*, **15**, 149–168.

Russell, J. A. (1991b). Rejoinder to Ekman, O'Sullivan, and Matsumoto. *Motivation and Emotion*, **15**, 177–184.

Russell, J. A. and Fehr, B. (1987). Relativity in the perception of emotion in facial expressions. *Journal of Experimental Psychology: General*, **116**, 233–237

Sakowski, H. (1985). Beobachtungslernen: Freie Wiedergabe von Routinehandlungen nach Wissensaktualisierung durch den Kontext. [Observational learning: Free recall of scripted actions after knowledge instigation by the context.] Unpublished master's thesis, Dept. of Psychology, Ruhr-University Bochum, Germany.

Schank, R. C. and Abelson, R. P. (1977). *Scripts, Plans, Goals and Understanding. An Inquiry into Human Knowledge*. Hillsdale, NJ: Erlbaum.

Scheerer, E. (1985). Pre-evolutionary conceptions of imitation. In G. Eckhardt, W. G. Bringmann and L. Sprung (Eds), *Contributions to a History of Developmental Psychology: International William T. Preyer Symposium* (pp. 27–53). The Hague, Netherlands: Mouton.

Scheflen, A. E. (1964). The significance of posture in communication systems. *Psychiatry*, **27**, 316–331.

Schorneck, D. and Berger, G. (1980). Kognitive Mechanismen in der Handlungswahrnehmung: Der Einfluß von Lern- un Beschreibungsauftrag auf die Wahrnehmungsorganisation und die Erinnerung von Handlungen. [Cognitive processes in action perception: The influence of learning and description instructions on the perceptual organization and memory for actions.] Unpublished master's thesis, Dept. of Psychology, Ruhr-University Bochum, Germany.

Scully, D. M. (1986). Visual perception of technical execution and aesthetic quality in biological motion. *Human Movement Science*, **5**, 185–206.

Scully, D. M. and Newell, K. M. (1985). Observational learning and the acquisition of motor skills: Toward a visual perception perspective. *Journal of Human Movement Studies*, **11**, 169–186.

Sheffield, F. D. (1961). Theoretical considerations in the learning of complex sequential tasks from demonstration and practice. In A. A. Lumsdaine (Ed.), *Student Response in Programmed Instruction* (pp. 13–32). Washington, DC: National Academy of Sciences – National Resarch Council, Publ. No. 943.

Shepard, R. N. and Cooper, L. A. (1982). *Mental Images and their Transformations*. Cambridge, MA: MIT Press.

Shinar, D. (1978). *Psychology on the Road*. New York: John Wiley.

Shor, R. E. (1957). Effect of preinformation upon human characteristics attributed to animated geometrical figures. *Journal of Abnormal and Social Psychology*, **54**, 124–126.

Standing, L. (1973). Learning 10 000 pictures. *Quarterly Journal of Experimental Psychology*, **25**, 207–222.

Standing, L., Conezio, J. and Haber, R. N. (1970). Perception and memory for pictures: Single-trial learning of 2500 visual stimuli. *Psychonomic Science*, **19**, 73–74.

Storms, M. D. (1973). Videotape and the attribution process: Reversing actors' and observers' points of view. *Journal of Personality and Social Psychology*, **27**, 165–175.

Stränger, J. (1977). Beobachtungslernen: Kognitive Analyse des Erwerbs von Handlungsplänen durch intentionale: Modellbeobachtung bei elf- bis dreizehnjährigen Schülern. [Observational learning: Cognitive analysis of the acquisition of actions plans by intentional model observation in 11- to 13-year-old students.] Unpublished doctoral dissertation, Dept. of Psychology, Ruhr-University Bochum, Germany.

Stränger, J. (1979). Intentionales Beobachtungslernen bei Schülern: Die Entstehung von Handlungsplänen durch Modellbeobachtung. [Intentional observational learning: The acquisition of action plans by observation of a model.] In K. J. Klauer and H. J. Kornadt (Eds), *Jahrbuch für Empirische Erziehungswissenschaft* (pp. 143–182). Düsseldorf, Germany: Schwann.

Stränger, J., Schorneck, D. and Droste, I. (1983). Wahrnehmungsstrukturierung und Erinnerung konkreter Handlungen. [Perceptual organization and memory for concrete actions.] *Zeitschrift für Sozialpsychologie*, **14**, 2–33.

Taylor, F. W. (1911). *The Principles of Scientific Management*. New York: Harper.

Teubner, C. (1985). Beobachtungslernen: Kodierungshilfen in der Anfangsphase des Erwerbs von Tai-Chi-Komponenten. [Observational learning: Coding aids in the initial phase of the acquisition of tai-chi-components.] Unpublished master's thesis, Dept. of Psychology, Ruhr-University Bochum, Germany.

Todd, J. T. (1983). Perception of gait. *Journal of Experimental Psychology: Human Perception and Performance*, **9**, 31–42.

Uzgiris, I. C. (1984). Imitation in infancy: Its interpersonal aspects. In M. Perlmutter (Ed.), *Parent–Child Interaction and Parent–Child Relations in Child Development* (pp. 1–32). Hillsdale, NJ: Erlbaum.

Vaina, L. and Bennour, Y. (1985). A computational approach to visual recognition of arm movements. *Perceptual and Motor Skills*, **60**, 203–228.

Vallacher, R. R. and Wegner, D. M. (1987). What do people think they're doing? Action identification and human behavior. *Psychological Review*, **94**, 3–15.

Vinter, A. (1985a). *L'imitation chez le nouveau-né*. [Imitation in the neonate.] Paris: Delachaux et Niestlé.

Vinter, A. (1985b). La capacité d'imitation à la naissance: Elle existe, mais que signifie-t-elle? [The capacity of imitation at birth: It exists but what does it mean?] *Revue Canadienne de Psychologie*, **39**, 16–33.

Vinter, A. (1986). The role of movement in eliciting early imitations. *Child Development*, **57**, 66–71.

Vogt, S. (1988). *Einige gestaltpsychologische Aspekte der zeitlichen Organisation zyklischer Bewegungsabläufe*. [Some Gestalt-psychological aspects of the temporal organization of cyclic movements.] Bremen, Germany: Bremer Beiträge zur Psychologie, No. 77.

von Weizsäcker, V. (1940). *Der Gestaltkreis. Theorie der Einheit von Wahrnehmen und Bewegen*. [The Gestalt circle. Theory of the unit of perception and action.] Stuttgart, Germany: Thieme.

Wallbott, H. G. (1982). *Bewegungsstil und Bewegungsqualität. Untersuchungen zum Ausdruck und Eindruck gestischen Verhaltens*. [Movement style and movement quality. Research on the expression and impression of gesture.] Weinheim, Germany: Beltz Forschungsberichte.

Wallbott, H. G. (1990). *Mimik im Kontext.* [Facial expression in context.] Göttingen, Germany: Hogrefe.

Weißenfeld, G. (1984). Beobachtungsauftrag, Schemaaktivierung und die Wiedergabe beobachteter Handlungen mit Abrufhilfen. [Observational task, script instigation and the recognition of observed actions.] Unpublished master's thesis, Dept. of Psychology, Ruhr-University Bochum, Germany.

Whiting, H. T. A. (1988). Imitation and the learning of complex cyclical actions. In O. G. Meijer and K. Roth (Eds), *Complex Movement Behaviour: The Motor-action Controversy* (pp. 381–401). Amsterdam: North Holland.

Wilder, D. (1978a). Effect of predictability on the units of perception and attribution. *Personality and Social Psychology Bulletin, 4,* 281–284.

Wilder, D. (1978b). Predictability of behaviors, goals, and unit of perception. *Personality and Social Psychology Bulletin, 4,* 604–607.

Wolff, P. (1984). Saccadic eye movements and visual stability: Preliminary considerations towards a cognitive approach. In W. Prinz and A. F. Sanders (Eds), *Cognition and Motor Processes* (pp. 121–137). Berlin: Springer.

Wolff, W. (1932). Selbstbeurteilung und Fremdbeurteilung im wissentlichen und unwissentlichen Versuch. Physiognomische Untersuchungen an der Stimme, dem Profil, den Händen und der freien Nacherzählung. [Judgments about self and others in a witting and unwitting investigation. Physiognomic inquiries of voice, profile, hands, and free recall.] *Psychologische Forschung, 16,* 251–328.

Wolff, W. (1943). *The Expression of Personality.* New York: Harper.

Woltring, H. J. (1984). On methodology in the study of human movement. In H. T. A. Whiting (Ed.), *Human Motor Actions – Bernstein Reassessed* (pp. 35–73). Amsterdam, Netherlands: Elsevier.

Wright, H. F. (1967). *Recording and Analyzing Child Behavior,* ch. 4 (pp. 56–98). New York: Harper.

Yéla, M. (1952). Phenomenal causation at a distance. *Quarterly Journal of Experimental Psychology, 4,* 139–154.

Yéla, M. (1954). La nature du 'rayon d'action' dans l'impression de causalité mécanique. [The nature of the 'radius of action' in the impression of mechanical causality.] *Journal de Psychologie Normale et Pathologique, 47,* 330–348.

Young, A. W. and Ellis, H. D. (Eds) (1989). *Handbook of Research on Face Processing.* Amsterdam: Elsevier.

Zadeh, L. A. (1972). A fuzzy-set-theoretic interpretation of linguistic hedges. *Journal of Cybernetics, 2,* 4–34.

Zadny, J. and Gerard, H. B. (1974). Attributed intentions and informational selectivity. *Journal of Experimental Social Psychology, 10,* 34–52.

Zuckerman, M., DePaulo, B. M. and Rosenthal, R. (1981). Verbal and nonverbal communication of deception. In L. Berkowitz (Ed.), *Advances in Experimental Social Psychology,* vol. 14 (pp. 1–59). New York: Academic Press.

Index

For core concepts and keywords, please refer to the Table of Contents as well.